EMR Complete
A Worktext

EMR Complete
A Worktext

DANIEL LIMMER

Medical Editor
Edward T. Dickinson, MD, FACEP

Brady
is an imprint of

Pearson

Boston Columbus Indianapolis New York San Francisco Upper Saddle River
Amsterdam Cape Town Dubai London Madrid Milan Munich Paris
Montreal Toronto Delhi Mexico City Sao Paulo Sydney Hong Kong
Seoul Singapore Taipei Tokyo

Library of Congress Cataloging-in-Publication Data

Limmer, Daniel.
   EMR complete : a worktext/Daniel Limmer; medical editor, Edward T.
Dickinson.
       p. ; cm.
   Includes bibliographical references and index.
   ISBN-13: 978-0-13-503771-3
   ISBN-10: 0-13-503771-9
   1. Emergency medicine. 2. Emergency medical technician. I.
Dickinson, Edward T. II. Title.
   [DNLM: 1. Emergency Treatment—methods—Problems and Exercises. 2.
Emergency Medical Services—methods—Problems and Exercises. 3.
Emergency Medical Technicians—Problems and Exercises. WB 18.2 L734e
2011]
   RC86.7.L5595 2011
   616.02'5—dc22   2009039847

Publisher: Julie Levin Alexander
Publisher's Assistant: Regina Bruno
Editor-in-Chief: Marlene McHugh Pratt
Acquisitions Editor: Sladjana Repic
Senior Managing Editor for Development: Lois Berlowitz
Project Manager: Triple SSS Press Media Development, Inc.
Editorial Assistant: Jonathan Cheung
Director of Marketing: David Gesell
Executive Marketing Manager: Katrin Beacom
Marketing Manager: Stephen G. Smith
Marketing Specialist: Michael Sirinides
Marketing Assistant: Judy Noh
Managing Editor for Production: Patrick Walsh
Production Liaison: Faye Gemmellaro
Production Editor: Heather Willison, S4Carlisle Publishing Services
Manufacturing Manager: Ilene Sanford
Manufacturing Buyer: Pat Brown
Editorial Media Manager: Amy Peltier

Media Project Manager: Lorena Cerisano
Art Director: Christopher Weigand
Cover Design: Blair Brown
Cover Images: iStockPhoto
Interior Design: Nesbitt Graphics
Managing Photography Editor: Michal Heron
Photographers: Nathan Eldridge, Michael Gallitelli, Michal Heron, Ray Kemp
Opener Images: Daniel Limmer (scene photos); Getty Images (ambulance photos)
Manager, Image Rights and Permissions: Zina Arabia
Manager, Visual Research: Beth Brenzel
Image Permission Coordinator: Jan Marc Quisumbing
Composition: S4Carlisle Publishing Services
Printer/Binder: Courier/Kendallville
Cover Printer: Lehigh-Phoenix Color/Hagerstown

Many of the designations by manufacturers and sellers to distinguish their products are claimed as trademarks. Where those designations appear in this book, and the publisher was aware of a trademark claim, the designations have been printed in initial caps or all caps.

Notice: The author and the publisher of this book have taken care to make certain that the information given is correct and compatible with the standards generally accepted at the time of publication. Nevertheless, as new information becomes available, changes in treatment and in the use of equipment and procedures become necessary. The reader is advised to carefully consult the instruction and information material included with each piece of equipment or device before administration. Students are warned that the use of any techniques must be authorized by their medical adviser, where appropriate, in accord with local laws and regulations. The publisher disclaims any liability, loss, injury, or damage incurred as a consequence, directly or indirectly, of the use and application of any of the contents of this book.

Brady
is an imprint of

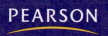

www.bradybooks.com

10 9 8
ISBN 13: 978-0-13-503771-3
ISBN 10: 0-13-503771-9

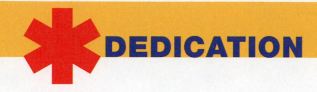

DEDICATION

To those who arrive first. To those who see the scene and patients at their worst while consistently striving to do their best. To you, the Emergency Medical Responder.

BRIEF CONTENTS

DETAILED CONTENTS

Section 2   Airway and Cardiac Resuscitation   136

CHAPTER 7   AIRWAY   138

CHAPTER 8   CARDIAC RESUSCITATION AND DEFIBRILLATION   181

Section 3   Patient Assessment   218

CHAPTER 9   PATIENT ASSESSMENT: SCENE SIZE-UP   220

Section 5 Trauma 414

Section 6   Special Patient Populations   588

CHAPTER 24   OBSTETRICS AND NEONATAL CARE   590

CHAPTER 27   SPECIAL POPULATIONS AND SITUATIONS   677

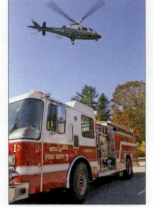

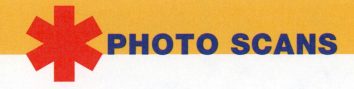

PHOTO SCANS

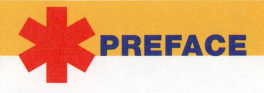

PREFACE

The Vision for EMR Complete

EMR Complete is designed to be a worktext—a book and workbook combined with a feature called *Stop, Review, Remember*. We believe that the ability to read a book in short segments followed by immediate review in which you can write and then check your answers helps you learn.

This book includes several other components designed to help you further:

- The book is written in a friendly instructional tone. You will note that the book presents material in the way an instructor or mentor might teach you. Relating EMS concepts and skills to everyday life is one of the ways we present material in this understandable fashion.

- The *Big Picture* feature has never been done in a textbook. Scans help define a step-by-step process and are very valuable. But we wanted to take the next step in visual learning. The *Big Picture* starts you off with an example of a scene or patient and then shows some of the steps or decisions you must make superimposed around the photo. We wanted to start the learning right away by showing you both the steps *and* the context you will be performing them in.

- The *Ask Yourself* feature in the margins ties back in all cases to one of the chapter objectives. At the end of that reading, "ask yourself" if you can now answer that question or questions. If not, you'll know to review the information again.

- Because you will make important decisions in the field, two features will help you practice this decision making: *Emergency Medical Responder Practice* and *Critical Thinking*.

You will notice that this book is written with acute awareness of the importance of the first few minutes of the call—and for those who perform care in that challenging time. The author and each contributor have worked diligently to ensure the knowledge and skills presented in this text maintain the perspective of perhaps the most important person in the EMS system—the one who arrives *first*.

ACKNOWLEDGMENTS

Books are a huge undertaking. A new book created to accompany new education standards raised the bar even further. Fortunately a tremendous team of people were assembled to put the book you see before you together.

I would like to thank the contributors to this book. Some have been with me for a while on projects; some stepped up to the plate for the first time. I would like to offer my sincere thanks to Dan Batsie, Tony Crystal, Andy Stern, Richard Belle, Daren Potter, Melissa Alexander, Marc Minkler, and Eric Mayhew.

Ed Dickinson, MD, FACEP, is a personal friend and medical editor for this and many other books. I consider myself so incredibly fortunate to know Ed and be able to work with him on projects such as this. Ed brings the true nexus of medical brilliance and street practicality into his work which results in the streetwise, medically accurate text you have before you now.

Brady has a wonderful group of people I have had the good fortune to work with over the years. The team assembled for this edition maintains the tradition. Editor Sladjana Repic took the acquisitions editor role when Marlene Pratt was promoted to editor-in-chief. Congratulations, Marlene, and welcome, Sladjana. It is great to work with you. Lois Berlowitz is one of the few people at Brady who has been there longer than I have been writing. She is the backbone of the editorial process. I am grateful for everything Lois does. Long ago she said, "Dan, that is an interesting idea . . . but it doesn't make good book sense." I *always* listen to Lois's book sense.

Julie Alexander is the publisher at Brady. Even though she has responsibilities throughout a large company, Julie is always there, involved, and passionate about projects such as this one. Thank you to Jonathan Cheung, Monica Moosang, and Regina Bruno.

The production department puts the book together and does a wonderful job. Faye Gemmellaro and Pat Walsh are truly dedicated and professional. Faye is so patient and organized. Pat holds everything together and now smiles. He didn't smile for the first 10 years we worked together.

Michal Heron is responsible for the photo program you see in the book. When you notice a photo that really draws you in, this is because of Michal's tireless efforts and attention to even the most minute detail—as any EMS provider/model who has spent a day on the set can attest to! Michal's influence is on every page of this book. Michal's mentoring an aspiring photographer is also greatly appreciated.

Susan Simpfenderfer is the developmental editor for the text. Susan takes my work and that of the contributors and massages it into the form you see before you. The role of the developmental editor is huge in a project such as this. It involves extreme organization, knowledge of grammar, and without a license or certification, an immersion into the terms and concepts of EMS. I have always joked that our developmental editors should get some sort of EMS certification when they are done with a project. Susan has looked at the material so much I am sure she could pass the exam! Thank you, Susan.

Our sales force does more than sell books. They are the way your instructor is most likely to hear from Brady. Our reps are talented and dedicated but most importantly they are passionate about their products and the people they serve. Tom Kennally, their fearless leader, is always at the helm. To this wonderful group of people, my thanks.

Finally, I would like to offer my most sincere thanks to you, the future Emergency Medical Responder, for the adventure you are embarking on and to your instructor for choosing my book for your education. Creating this book is a responsibility I take with the utmost seriousness. Be safe. Care for people. And have fun while you're doing it. It is an amazing journey.

Dan Limmer
danlimmer@mac.com

Thank You
CONTENT CONTRIBUTORS

Thanks to the following people for their contributions to *EMR Complete: A Worktext*.

Medical Editor
Edward T. Dickinson, MD, FACEP

Chapters 4–6, 15, 16, 23
Tony Crystal, ScD, EMT-P
St. Mary's Hospital
Decatur, IL

Chapters 9, 11, 18–22
Dan Batsie, NREMT-P
Education Coordinator
North East Maine EMS
Bangor, ME

Chapters 24–26
Andrew W. Stern, MPA, MA, NREMT-P
Senior Paramedic
Town of Colonie Emergency Medical Services
Colonie, NY

Chapters 27–31
Eric T. Mayhew, AAS, NREMT-P, CICP
Training Coordinator
Pender EMS and Rescue
Rocky Point, NC

Select Chapter Questions and Key Term Definitions
Daren C. Potter, EMT-P, CLI
West Glens Falls EMS
Queensbury, NY

Learning Objectives and Section Review Tests
Melissa Alexander, NREMT-P
University of New Mexico
Department of Emergency Medicine

REVIEWERS

Thanks to the following reviewers for providing invaluable feedback, insight, and suggestions in the preparation of *EMR Complete: A Worktext*.

Evelyn D. Barnum, EMT-P
Lansing Community College
Lansing, MI

John L. Beckman, FF/EMT-P, AA, BS
Affiliated with Addison Fire Protection
    District
Fire Science Instructor, Technology Center
    of DuPage
Addison, IL

Cheryl Blazek, EMT-P, EMS Training
    Program Coordinator
Southwestern Community College
Creston, IA

Leo M. Brown
Administrative Deputy Chief (retired)
Longboat Key Fire Rescue
Sarasota, FL

David J. Casella, NREMT-B
Opportunities in Emergency Health Care
    Program
Osseo, MN

Tony Crystal, ScD, EMT-P
St. Mary's Hospital
Decatur, IL

Lyndal M. Curry, M.A., NREMT-P
EMS Degree Program Director
College of Allied Health Professions
University of South Alabama
Mobile, AL

Doyle Dennis, AAS, NREMT-P
Medical Program Coordinator
Safety Management Systems Training
    Academy
Lafayette, LA

Mike Grill
EMS Program Coordinator
Cochise Community College
Sierra Vista, AZ

Gregory LaMay
TEEX-ESTI
College Station, TX

Lawrence Linder PhD (c), NREMT-P
Educator
Hillsborough Community College
Tampa, Florida

Eric T. Mayhew, AAS, NREMT-P, CICP
Training Coordinator
Pender EMS Advanced Education
    Institution
Rocky Point, NC

Joseph McConomy Jr., MICP, EMT-B (I)
Senior EMT Instructor
Burlington County Emergency Services
    Training Center
Westampton, NJ

Jack H. Meersman, NREMT-P
Director of Training
Gold Cross Ambulance
Salt Lake City, UT

Edward Mello Jr., MSN., RN APN
Director of Basic EMT Program
Westfield State College

Jeff Och, NREMT-B, RN
Carver, MN

Guy Peifer
Paramedic Program Coordinator
Borough of Manhattan Community College
City University of New York
New York, NY

Cheryl Pittman, EMT1, PhD
Assistant Professor, EMT and First
    Responder Program Director
East Los Angeles College
Monterey Park, CA 91754

Capt. Robert W. Rosier, NREMT-P
Martinez-Columbia Fire Rescue
EMS Director
Level II EMS Instructor
Martinez, GA

Kristie Skala
AIMS Community College
Greeley, CO

Wade Skinner, EMT-B
West Jordan, UT

Andrew W. Stern, MPA, MA, NREMT-P
Senior Paramedic
Town of Colonie Emergency Medical
    Services
Colonie, NY

David L. Sullivan, PhD(c), NREMT-P
EMS/CME Program Director
Pinellas County EMS
St. Petersburg College
Pinellas Park, FL

Robert G. West, Med., EMT-I, I/C
Educator
North Shore Community College
Danvers, MA

PHOTO ACKNOWLEDGMENTS

All photographs not credited adjacent to the photograph or in the following photo credit section were photographed on assignment for Brady/Pearson Education.

PHOTO CREDITS

Figures 9-3, 15-14a–b, 20-16, 22-6a–i, 30-5, and 30-10 photographed for Pearson by Ray Kemp/911 Imaging.

ORGANIZATIONS

We wish to thank the following organizations for their assistance in creating the photo program for this first edition:

Delta Ambulance, Waterville, ME. Paul Thompson, EMT-P, Fleet Coordinator

Fairfield Fire Rescue, Fairfield, ME. Chief Duane Bickford

Falmouth Fire-EMS, Falmouth, ME. Asst. Chief Doug Patey, EMT-P, I/C

Kennebec Valley Emergency Medical Services Council, Winslow, ME. Rick Petrie, EMT-P

Kennebunk Fire and Rescue, Kennebunk, ME. Deputy Chief David Cluff

NorthStar Ambulance, Farmington, ME. Michael Senecal, EMT-P, Director

Oakland Fire Rescue, Oakland, ME. Chief David Coughlin

Sanford Fire Department, Sanford, ME. Chief Raymond Parent, Regional Coordinator

Waterville Fire Department, Waterville, ME. Chief David Lafountain

Winslow Fire Department, Winslow, ME. Chief David Lafountain

TECHNICAL ADVISORS

Thanks to the following people for providing technical support during the photo shoots for this first edition:

Brian Chamberlin, EMT-P, KVEMSC/Augusta Rescue
Steven Diaz, MD, Maine General Medical Center & Maine EMS Medical Director
Carl French, CCEMTP/FF EMT-T, Sanford Fire Department, Sanford, ME
Judy French, EMT-I, Alfred Rescue, Alfred, ME
Lt. Paul Goldstein, FF/EMT, Falmouth, ME
Mark King, EMT-P, KVEMSC/Winthrop Ambulance, Winthrop, ME
Marc Minkler, EMT-P, Portland Fire Department, Portland, ME
Asst. Chief Doug Patey, EMT-P, I/C, Falmouth Fire-EMS, Falmouth, ME
Rick Petrie, EMT-P, KVEMSC/United Ambulance, Winslow, ME
Carol Pillsbury, EMT-P, NorthStar Ambulance
Tiffany Stebbins, EMT-P, KVEMSC

LOCATIONS

Thanks to the following people who provided locations for our photographs:

Barry Acker, The Landing School, Arundel, ME
David Cluff, Duffy's Tavern & Grill, Kennebunk, ME
Colby College, Waterville, ME
Paul Goldstein, Falmouth, ME
David Groder, EMT-P, Oakland, ME
Jay Hallett, Handy Boat Yard, Falmouth, ME
Maineline Technology Group, Falmouth, ME
Allie Moore, EMT-B, Oakland, ME
OceanView at Falmouth, ME
Francis Pooler, Fairfield, ME
Sappi Fine Paper, Skowhegan, ME
Erick and Kim Van Sickle, Leyland British Auto, Arundel, ME

MODELS

Thanks to the following people who portrayed patients and EMS providers in our photographs:

Richard Battle
Jessica Blomerth
Erica Bohlman
Jeremy R. Buzzell
Emily L. Carter
Brian Chamberlin
Eric Cheney
Vivian Chicoine
Amanda Chretien
Cody Chretien
Shanelle Coolidge
Stephanie Cordwell
Drew Corey
Gary H. Cushing
Jack Davis
Jonathan Denham
Diane Deyoe
Erin Deyoe
Shannon Deyoe
Steven Diaz
Thomas H. Doak
George Donovan
Paul J. Dubois
Casey Dugas
Chip Eames

Jane Fenn
Regina M. Fife
Gary Foss
Robert G. Fox
Carl French
Judy French
Maurice Froppier
Sherry Given
Nancy Goldstein
Paul Goldstein
Jennifer L. Grey
Kristen Hagan
Ann E. Harrison-Billiat
Kevin L'Heureux
Helena Hollauer
Adolph Holmes
Alex Johnson
Mark King
Susan King
Rod Koehn
John Lacombe
Matthew Leach
Sarah Kaylee Leary
Travis Leary
Sarah K. Limmer

Kenneth Lovell
Kalem Malcolm
Allyson P. Moore
Gary Paradis
Thaddeus J. Pawlick
Jason C. Pfingst
Fran Pooler
Kathryn Pow
Nicole Prescott
Zachary Pushee
David Rackliffe
Gerald Roderick
Jim Scully
Stephen L. Smith
Kenneth Solorzano
McKenzie Stebbins
Andrew Stevenson
Edward Strapp
Todd Tracy
Erick Van Sickle
Kim Van Sickle
John G. Vatulas
Michelle Vrbanek
Llewellyn Wilson

PHOTO COORDINATORS

Thanks to the following for valuable assistance coordinating models, props, and locations for our photo shoots: Judy French, Alfred Rescue, and Kelly Roderick, KVEMSC.

PHOTO ASSISTANT/COMPUTER POST-PRODUCTION

Isaac Turner and Frank Menair

Daniel Limmer

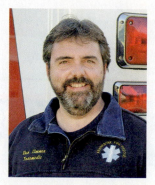

Daniel Limmer, EMT-P, has been involved in EMS for 31 years. He is active as a paramedic with Kennebunk Fire-Rescue in Kennebunk, Maine. A passionate educator, Dan teaches basic, advanced, and continuing education EMS courses throughout Maine. He previously taught at the George Washington University in Washington, DC, where he coordinated international EMS education programs, and at the Hudson Valley Community College in Troy, New York. He is a charter member of the National Association of EMS Educators.

Dan has also been involved in law enforcement, serving both as a dispatcher and police officer in Colonie, New York. Dan received several awards and honors in law enforcement including the distinguished service award (officer of the year), life saving award, and three command recognition awards. He served in the communications, patrol, juvenile, narcotics, and training units in the police department. Dan retired from police work in New York but remains active as a police officer on a part-time basis in Maine.

In addition to authoring numerous EMS journal articles, Dan has co-authored numerous EMS texts including *Emergency Care, First Responder—A Skills Approach, EMT Complete: A Basic Worktext, Advanced Medical Life Support,* and *Active Learning Manual for EMTs.*

Edward T. Dickinson, Medical Editor

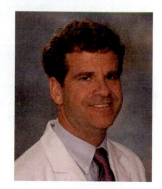

Edward T. Dickinson, MD, NREMT-P, FACEP, is currently associate professor and director of EMS field operations in the Department of Emergency Medicine of the University of Pennsylvania School of Medicine in Philadelphia. He is medical director of the Malvern Fire Company, the Berwyn Fire Company, and the Township of Haverford paramedics in Pennsylvania. He is a residency-trained, board-certified emergency medicine physician who is a fellow of the American College of Emergency Physicians.

Dr. Dickinson began his career in emergency services in 1979 as a firefighter-EMT in upstate New York. He has remained active in fire service and EMS for the past 30 years. He frequently rides with EMS units and has maintained his certification as a National Registry EMT-Paramedic.

He has served as medical editor for numerous Brady EMT-B and First Responder texts and is the author of *Fire Service Emergency Care* and co-author of *Emergency Care, Fire Service Edition,* and *Emergency Incident Rehabilitation.* He is co-editor of *ALS Case Studies in Emergency Care.*

CHAPTER 10

Patient Assessment: The Primary Assessment

NAVIGATION GUIDE

The following items provide an overview to the purpose and content of this chapter. The Education Standard and Competency are from the National EMS Education Standards.

Education Standard Assessment (Primary Assessment)

Competency Uses scene information and simple patient assessment findings to identify and manage immediate life threats and injuries within the scope of practice of the EMR.

Knowledge Area Primary Assessment
- Level of consciousness
- ABCs
- Identifying life threats
- Assessment of vital functions
- Begin interventions needed to preserve life

Objectives After reading this chapter, you should be able to:

1. Define key terms introduced in this chapter.
2. Describe the purpose of the primary patient assessment.
3. Explain the importance of scene safety and using personal protective equipment.
4. Identify patients for whom you should take spinal precautions.
5. Explain each of the eight basic components of a primary patient assessment.
6. Determine patients' chief complaints.
7. Perform each of the following components of the primary patient assessment:
   a. Form a general impression of the patient.
   b. Determine level of consciousness.
   c. Assess the airway status.
   d. Assess adequacy of breathing.
   e. Assess adequacy of circulation.
   f. Assess for disability.
   g. Expose the patient to assess for pertinent findings.
   h. Update the incoming EMS units with pertinent information from your assessment.
8. Use primary assessment findings to identify patients who are in serious, or potentially serious, condition.
9. Intervene as necessary in the primary assessment to maintain airway, breathing, and circulation.

Navigation Guide

This toolbox helps students navigate through the chapter materials. Placed at the beginning of each chapter, the Navigation Guide refers readers to the Education Standards, Competencies, Knowledge Areas, Objectives, Key Terms, and Media Resources. These elements provide a foundation for learning chapter content.

NAVIGATION GUIDE *(continued)*

Key Terms Page references indicate first major use in this chapter. The Margin Glossary in this chapter provides definitions as you read.

general impression p. 246   *level of consciousness* p. 247   *agonal* p. 254
chief complaint p. 246   *patent* p. 248

Media Resources Please go to **www.bradybooks.com** to access mykit for this text. You will find quizzes, critical thinking scenarios, weblinks, animations, and videos related to this chapter—and much more. Look for online information on patient assessment techniques. You will also find video clips on assessment of pain and conducting a detailed physical exam.

INTRODUCTION

Once you have completed the scene size-up, you will perform a primary assessment. The primary assessment is the most important part of patient care because it must identify and correct life threats the patient may be experiencing. It is worth repeating: the primary assessment is about identifying and correcting conditions that can kill your patient. You must perform it before you do anything else.

Not every patient will have life-threatening conditions. Some will have a minor illness or injury, others will be in serious condition, and others will fall somewhere in between. Your assessment will help you identify how to treat each patient. (See The Big Picture: Primary Assessment of the Medical Patient and The Big Picture: Primary Assessment of the Trauma Patient.)

ASK YOURSELF
- What is the purpose of the primary patient assessment?
- How would you explain the importance of scene safety and using personal protective equipment?
- How would you explain each of the eight basic components of a primary patient assessment?

CASE STUDY

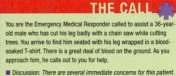

THE CALL

You are the Emergency Medical Responder called to assist a 36-year-old male who has cut his leg badly with a chain saw while cutting trees. You arrive to find him seated with his leg wrapped in a blood-soaked T-shirt. There is a great deal of blood on the ground. As you approach him, he calls out to you for help.

- Discussion: *There are several immediate concerns for this patient. How should you begin your assessment?*

Eight Components of the Primary Assessment

The primary assessment has eight basic components:

- General impression
- Level of consciousness
- Airway
- Breathing
- Circulation
- Disability
- Expose
- Update incoming EMS units

Objectives

Objectives form the basis of each chapter and were developed around the Education Standards and Instructional Guidelines.

Objectives After reading this chapter, you should be able to:

1. Define key terms introduced in this chapter.
2. Describe the purpose of the primary patient assessment.
3. Explain the importance of scene safety and using personal protective equipment.
4. Identify patients for whom you should take spinal precautions.
5. Explain each of the eight basic components of a primary patient assessment.
6. Determine patients' chief complaints.
7. Perform each of the following components of the primary patient assessment:
   a. Form a general impression of the patient.
   b. Determine level of consciousness.
   c. Assess the airway status.
   d. Assess adequacy of breathing.
   e. Assess adequacy of circulation.
   f. Assess for disability.
   g. Expose the patient to assess for pertinent findings.
   h. Update the incoming EMS units with pertinent information from your assessment.
8. Use primary assessment findings to identify patients who are in serious, or potentially serious, condition.
9. Intervene as necessary in the primary assessment to maintain airway, breathing, and circulation.

Key Terms Page references indicate first major use in this chapter. The Margin Glossary in this chapter provides definitions as you read.

general impression p. 246	*level of consciousness p. 247*	*agonal p. 254*
chief complaint p. 246	*patent p. 248*	

Key Terms

Page numbers are included to identify the term's first major use in the chapter.

Media Resources

Media Resources can be found under **mybradykit** at **www.bradybooks.com**. Students and instructors can access weblinks, animations, and videos related to chapter content.

Media Resources Please go to **www.bradybooks.com** to access mykit for this text. You will find quizzes, critical thinking scenarios, weblinks, animations, and videos related to this chapter—and much more. Look for online information on patient assessment techniques. You will also find video clips on assessment of pain and conducting a detailed physical exam.

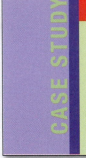

Case Study

Case material opens with The Call, followed by The Response, and concluding with Transition. Each case segment ends with a question that promotes critical thinking.

CASE STUDY

THE CALL

You are the Emergency Medical Responder called to assist a 36-year-old male who has cut his leg badly with a chain saw while cutting trees. You arrive to find him seated with his leg wrapped in a blood-soaked T-shirt. There is a great deal of blood on the ground. As you approach him, he calls out to you for help.

■ Discussion: *There are several immediate concerns for this patient. How should you begin your assessment?*

CASE STUDY

THE RESPONSE

Once bleeding is controlled, you continue your assessment of vital signs and symptoms. You note that the patient is anxious and pale and has a heart rate of 128.

■ Discussion: *What does this patient presentation tell you? Is there a significance to the patient's anxiety? To his heart rate?*

CASE STUDY

TRANSITION

The ambulance arrives on scene. You have only been able to complete the primary assessment and didn't get to do a history, blood pressure, or any further examinations. You update the EMS units.

■ Discussion: *Do you think the incoming EMS units will be upset because you only did a primary assessment? Would you tell the incoming EMS units that the patient was stable or unstable?*

Ask Yourself

This appears in the margin after a chapter objective has been first covered. These questions are used to reinforce chapter objectives.

ASK YOURSELF

- What are some ways you will intervene as necessary in the primary assessment to maintain airway, breathing, and circulation?

general impression how the patient looks to you as you approach.

chief complaint the patient's response to your question about how he is feeling or what is wrong.

Running Glossary

Definitions for key terms are provided in the margins, next to the text in which they're introduced.

EMR Note

This feature highlights important need-to-know information.

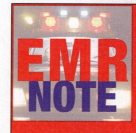

EMR NOTE

You will learn the patient assessment skills in a step-by-step manner. This will help ensure a structured and thorough approach to your patient assessment. When you encounter a serious patient in a stressful situation, your knowledge of these steps will help you provide lifesaving care. You will also find unusual situations and patients with varied problems. The same steps will apply, but you will have to adapt them to each situation you encounter.

Stop, Review, Remember

The "work" part of the Worktext, these are integrated throughout chapters at several key places, enabling readers to instantly assess their learning before going on. Multiple-choice, fill-in-the-blank, matching, and critical-thinking questions provide readers with immediate feedback.

Stop, Review, Remember

Multiple Choice

Place a check next to the correct answer.

1. The mnemonic for remembering the levels of consciousness is:
   - _____ a. SAMPLE.
   - _____ b. ABC.
   - _____ c. 4-CONS.
   - _____ d. AVPU.

2. The patient who responds only to a pinch of the muscles near the neck is responsive to:
   - _____ a. voice.
   - _____ b. pain.
   - _____ c. carotid stimulation.
   - _____ d. pressure.

3. Which of the following steps is NOT part of the "A" or airway portion of the primary assessment?
   - _____ a. Inserting an oral airway
   - _____ b. Suctioning
   - _____ c. Checking a pulse
   - _____ d. Jaw-thrust maneuver

4. The general impression is best described as:
   - _____ a. how the patient looks as you approach.
   - _____ b. the patient's status after the primary assessment.
   - _____ c. key information you will call or radio to the incoming EMS units.
   - _____ d. a check of the patient's mental status.

5. Which of the following would indicate a potentially serious patient? Each of these patients is alert and oriented.
   - _____ a. A patient who is complaining of a broken arm
   - _____ b. A patient who was punched in the nose with moderate bleeding
   - _____ c. A patient who was involved in a minor car crash and complains of neck pain
   - _____ d. A patient who complains of abdominal pain and has cool, moist skin

SCAN 7-3   Suctioning

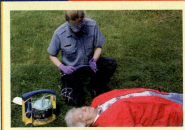

7-3a Prepare suction unit.

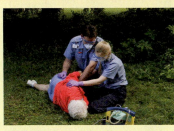

7-3b Roll the patient to his/her side.

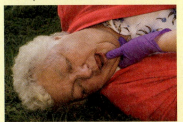

7-3c Open mouth.

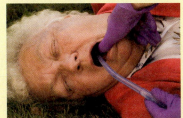

7-3d Place tip in the mouth only as far as you can see.

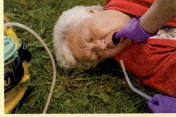

7-3e Suction while moving the tip out.

Scans

Procedures are performed step by step with explanations and photographs.

The Big Picture

This feature is an innovative way to present the "big picture" of an EMS scene superimposed with the critical steps Emergency Medical Responders will perform at that scene. It is a visual element designed to practically present what instructors have been telling students for decades: You will respond to a call and be faced with a challenging situation in which you must perform what you have been taught in class. The Big Picture helps convey that message.

The Last Word

This is a summary of important points learned in each chapter.

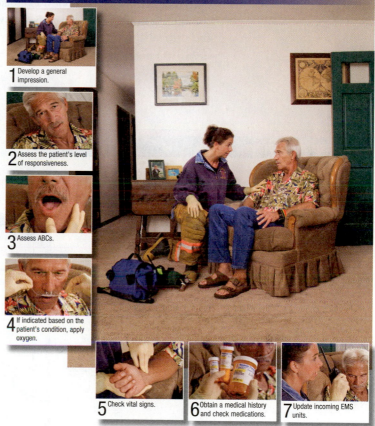

The Big Picture
Primary Assessment of the Medical Patient

1 Develop a general impression.

2 Assess the patient's level of responsiveness.

3 Assess ABCs.

4 If indicated based on the patient's condition, apply oxygen.

5 Check vital signs.

6 Obtain a medical history and check medications.

7 Update incoming EMS units.

THE LAST WORD

You should now have enough information to determine if your patient is potentially seriously ill or injured or if he seems more stable. Seriously ill or injured patients will require additional assessment and care, usually at a rapid pace. More stable patients require further care that can be done at a more relaxed pace.

Chapter Review
Each chapter ends with review exercises containing multiple-choice, short answer, and critical-thinking questions.

✳ Chapter Review

Multiple Choice

Place a check next to the correct answer.

1. How do your findings in the general impression affect the rest of the patient assessment?
   _____ a. The general impression tells you whether further assessment is necessary.
   _____ b. The general impression helps determine the priority of the patient and a general direction for assessment techniques and speed.
   _____ c. The general impression determines if the scene is safe and if any additional resources are necessary.
   _____ d. The general impression helps you determine whether Standard Precautions are necessary.

2. Suction would first be performed in the _____ part of the primary assessment.
   _____ a. general impression
   _____ b. airway
   _____ c. breathing
   _____ d. circulation

3. The radial pulse is located at the:
   _____ a. neck.
   _____ b. groin.
   _____ c. upper arm.
   _____ d. wrist.

4. When exposing the patient, you will expose:
   _____ a. the upper torso.
   _____ b. the lower extremities.
   _____ c. all relevant areas.
   _____ d. only the chest.

5. You are caring for a patient who fell a considerable distance. You suspect a neck and/or spine injury is likely. You are unable to open the airway enough with a jaw thrust to assist breathing. You should:
   _____ a. continue trying the jaw thrust.
   _____ b. place a towel under the patient's head and try the jaw thrust again.
   _____ c. use the head-tilt, chin-lift maneuver instead.
   _____ d. wait for the paramedics to use advanced airway techniques.

Short Answer

1. What are the differences between the scene size-up and the primary assessment?

2. Can a patient who is breathing not have a pulse?

3. Why do you expose a patient as part of the primary assessment?

Critical Thinking

1. It has been said that the primary assessment is the most important part of the patient assessment process. Do you agree? Why or why not?

2. You are alone caring for a patient until EMS responds. Your patient is breathing inadequately. You are assisting ventilations when you notice a leg that is badly angulated (bent) and looks broken. What should you do?

3. What can pulse rate, skin color, skin temperature, and skin condition tell you about a patient?

Case Study

You are an Emergency Medical Responder at a high school where a student is believed to have consumed alcohol. You arrive at the health office and find the patient will only respond to loud verbal stimulus by moaning. You observe stains on the front of his shirt where he appears to have vomited before you arrived.

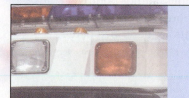

SECTION 2
Review and Practice Examination

Assess what you have learned in this section by checking the best answer for each multiple-choice question. When you are done, check your answers against the key provided in Appendix B.

1. When the intercostal muscles of the chest contract and the diaphragm drops, which of the following occurs?
   _____ a. Inhalation
   _____ b. Air is forced out of the lungs
   _____ c. Decreased size of the chest cavity
   _____ d. Increased pressure of the chest cavity

2. The vocal cords are contained within the:
   _____ a. pharynx.
   _____ b. trachea.
   _____ c. bronchi.
   _____ d. larynx.

3. Oxygen is moved from the lungs to the bloodstream when air reaches the:
   _____ a. bronchi.
   _____ b. bronchioles.
   _____ c. alveoli.
   _____ d. pharynx.

4. Which of the following is an expected body response to hypoxia?
   _____ a. Increased respiratory rate, decreased heart rate
   _____ b. Decreased respiratory rate, decreased heart rate
   _____ c. Decreased respiratory rate, increased heart rate
   _____ d. Increased respiratory rate, increased heart rate

5. Upon arriving at the scene of a medical emergency, you see a patient who is unresponsive and snoring. Which of the following should you do first?
   _____ a. Check the carotid pulse.
   _____ b. Begin bag-valve-mask ventilations.
   _____ c. Use a head-tilt, chin-lift to open the airway.
   _____ d. Apply oxygen using a nonrebreather mask.

6. You have arrived at the home of a 72-year-old patient whose wife called 911 because she couldn't wake him up. The patient is slumped to the side in his recliner and does not respond to your voice or a pinch to his shoulder. Which of the following should you do next?
   _____ a. Apply oxygen by nonrebreather mask.
   _____ b. Tilt the recliner all the way back and open the patient's airway.
   _____ c. Move the patient to the floor and open the patient's airway.
   _____ d. Advise incoming EMS units that the patient is in cardiac arrest.

7. A 14-year-old male patient with a history of asthma is wheezing, but he is agitated with you. He does not want you to place an oxygen mask on his face. Which of the following should you assume?

   _____ a. The patient may be hypoxic and needs your help, even though he appears to be refusing oxygen.
   _____ b. The patient does not need oxygen by mask and you should respect his wishes.
   _____ c. Whoever called 911 was mistaken about the cause of the emergency.
   _____ d. You could be sued if you try to get the patient to accept oxygen when he does not want it.

8. A patient who was struck several times in the face during a barroom fight is lying on his back and you can hear gurgling noises when he breathes. Which should you do first?
   _____ a. Perform the head-tilt, chin-lift maneuver.
   _____ b. Begin ventilations with a bag-valve-mask device.
   _____ c. Stabilize the spine and suction the airway.
   _____ d. Insert an oral airway.

9. Your patient is a 17-year-old female who has consumed an excessive amount of alcohol at a party. She is unresponsive and vomiting. Which of the following is the best course of action?
   _____ a. Turn the patient on her side and suction until the airway is clear.
   _____ b. Preoxygenate the patient using a bag-valve-mask device and then suction until the airway is clear.
   _____ c. Preoxygenate the patient using a bag-valve-mask device and then suction for 15 seconds.
   _____ d. Place the patient supine and suction for 15 seconds before applying oxygen with a nonrebreather mask.

10. A patient with a history of depression was found lying in bed and his wife was unable to wake him. When you enter the room you hear loud snoring. Which of the following are the most likely explanation and course of action?
    _____ a. The patient is choking on a foreign body; you should perform abdominal thrusts (the Heimlich maneuver).
    _____ b. The patient has adequate breathing since you can hear him snore with every breath; you should apply oxygen.

    _____ c. The patient's tongue is obstructing his airway; you should perform a head-tilt, chin-lift maneuver.
    _____ d. The patient has vomited; begin suctioning immediately.

11. Your patient is a 30-year-old man who fell from his second-story roof as he was cleaning out his gutters. On your arrival, the patient was unresponsive and had inadequate breathing. You have attempted to perform a jaw-thrust maneuver, but are unable to ventilate the patient. What should you do next?
    _____ a. Suction the mouth to remove secretions.
    _____ b. Place the patient on his side and await the incoming EMS crew for further instructions.
    _____ c. Apply an oxygen mask with a flow rate of at least 10 liters per minute.
    _____ d. Perform a head-tilt, chin-lift.

12. As you are ventilating a patient, she vomits a large amount of undigested food. Which of the following is the best course of action?
    _____ a. Turn the patient on her side, manually remove as much material as you can from the airway, and then suction the rest with a rigid suction catheter before resuming ventilations.
    _____ b. Use a flexible suction catheter to remove the material as you continue to ventilate.
    _____ c. Suction using a rigid suction catheter for no more than 15 seconds before resuming ventilations. Reoxygenate the patient before suctioning again.
    _____ d. Suction using a rigid suction catheter for as long as it takes to remove the material, applying suction both while inserting and withdrawing the catheter.

13. Which of the following best describes the depth of insertion of a rigid suction catheter to remove fluids from the airway?
    _____ a. It is used only between the cheek and gums.
    _____ b. It is inserted until you feel resistance.
    _____ c. It is inserted only as far as you can see.
    _____ d. It is inserted to the level of the epiglottis.

Section Review
After each section, a test is provided to ensure that learning is cumulative throughout the text.

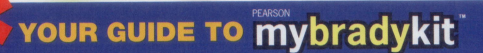

YOUR GUIDE TO PEARSON mybradykit™

Mybradykit provides online chapter support materials and resources in one location. Students can prepare for class and exams with skills and objectives checklists, multiple-choice questions, case study activities, web links, animations, author podcasts, study aids, trauma gallery, chapter summary in Spanish, and more! To access **mybradykit**, please visit **www.bradybooks.com**. A few key components are described here …

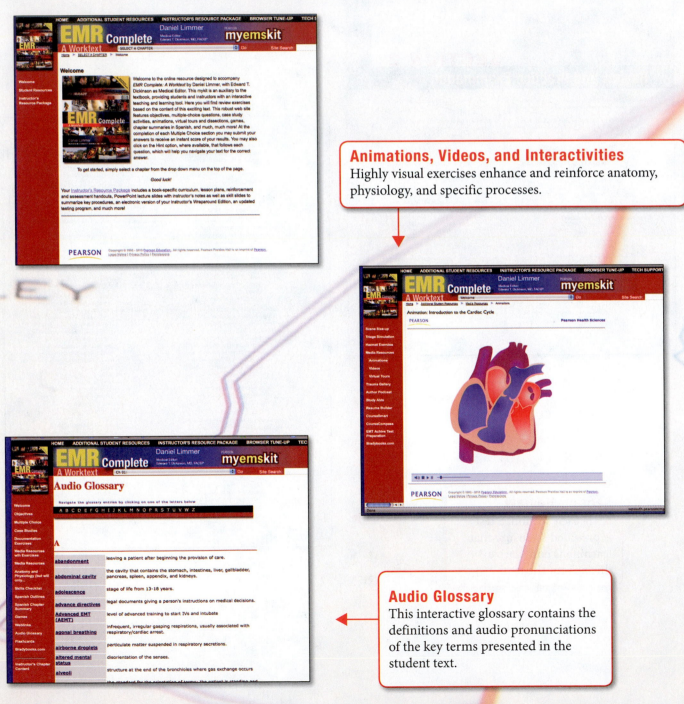

Animations, Videos, and Interactivities
Highly visual exercises enhance and reinforce anatomy, physiology, and specific processes.

Audio Glossary
This interactive glossary contains the definitions and audio pronunciations of the key terms presented in the student text.

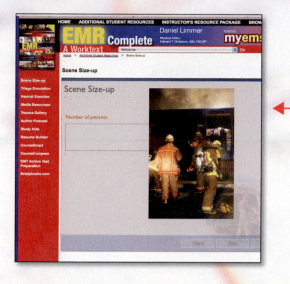

Scene Size-Up

This component tests the student's ability by flashing scenes on screen and asking questions regarding number of patients, resource determination, Standard Precautions, scene safety, and mechanism of injury.

Virtual Tours

3D animations, including a Heart and Airway virtual tour, offer a deeper understanding and graphical view of difficult concepts.

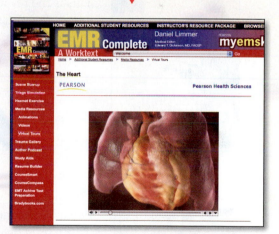

Chapter Quizzes

Chapter-specific multiple-choice quizzes test and reinforce knowledge.

✳ Other features

Anatomy Labeling Exercises

Drag-and-drop activities test knowledge of human anatomy.

Case Study with Documentation Exercise

Designed to develop critical thinking, each case study offers questions that help to hone the student's assessment skills.

Podcasts

Listen as Brady authors discuss key EMR topics.

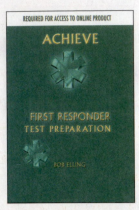

Achieve: First Responder Test Preparation ISBN 0-13-198894-8

This dynamic online test preparation program allows you to practice taking national- and state-type tests and quizzes. Rationale and remediation is included. Check it out at **www.bradybooks.com**.

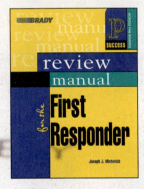

Review Manual for First Responder ISBN 0-13-118439-3

This is the resource to help you pass your national or state certification exam. All items are written and tested by educators and offer proven authoritative information with rationales.

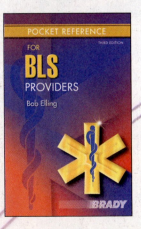

Pocket Reference for BLS Providers, 3rd edition ISBN 0-13-173730-9

This handy field reference is on water-resistant paper and includes skills checklist, common medications, abbreviations and acronyms, and anatomy charts.

All student resources are available for purchase at www.bradybooks.com

EMR Complete
A Worktext

SECTION 1
Preparatory

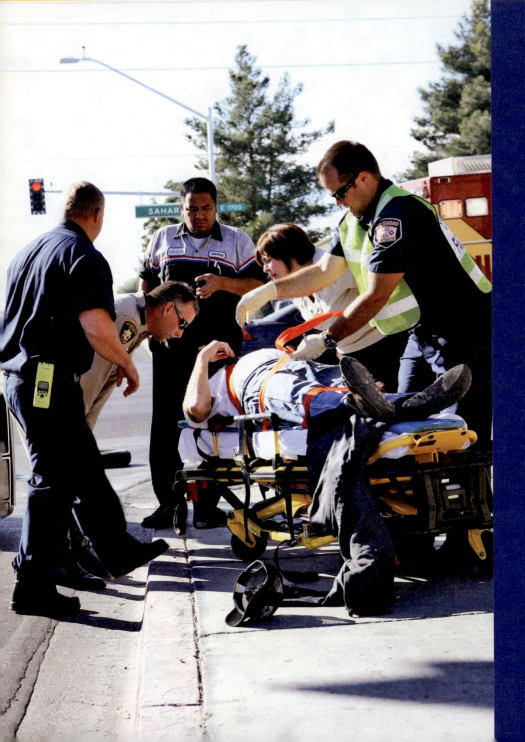

SECTION OUTLINE

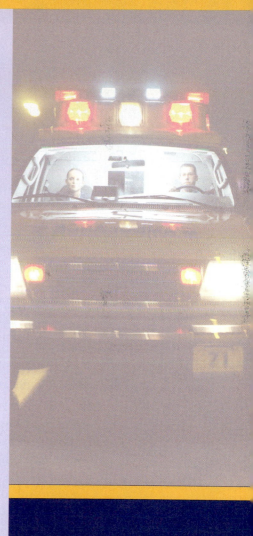

In this section, you will cover the following EMS Education Standards:

- **Preparatory**
- **Anatomy and Physiology**
- **Medical Terminology**
- **Pathophysiology**
- **Lifespan Development**
- **Public Health**

Introduction to EMS Systems

NAVIGATION GUIDE

The following items provide an overview to the purpose and content of this chapter. The Education Standards and Competencies are from the National EMS Education Standards.

Education Standards Preparatory (EMS Systems, Research); Public Health

Competencies Uses simple knowledge of the EMS system, safety/well-being of the Emergency Medical Responder (EMR), medical/legal issues at the scene of an emergency while awaiting a higher level of care.

Has an awareness of local public health resources and the role EMS personnel play in public health emergencies.

Knowledge Area EMS Systems
- Roles/responsibilities/professionalism of EMS personnel
- Quality improvement
Research
- Impact of research on EMR care
- Data collection

Objectives After reading this chapter, you should be able to:

1. Define key terms introduced in this chapter.
2. Describe the importance of public safety answering points (PSAPs) and specially trained emergency medical dispatchers (EMDs) in EMS systems.
3. Compare and contrast the training and responsibilities of EMRs, EMTs, AEMTs, and Paramedics.
4. Provide examples of different EMS systems.
5. Give examples of how the resources of specialty hospitals, such as trauma centers, can benefit patients.
6. Explain the importance of each of the ten classic EMS system components listed in the text.
7. Relate each of the following factors to the practice of EMRs:
   a. Your state's legislation
   b. Your state's EMS organization or agency
   c. Regional/local EMS oversight agencies
   d. Medical oversight
   e. The agency with which you will volunteer or be employed
8. Explain the roles and responsibilities of Emergency Medical Responders (EMRs).

NAVIGATION GUIDE *(continued)*

9. Give examples of professionalism in EMR practice.
10. Discuss the purpose of quality improvement in EMS.
11. Give examples of ways you can reduce the likelihood of errors in your practice as an EMR.
12. List ways in which research may influence EMR practice.

Key Terms Page references indicate first major use in this chapter. The Margin Glossary in this chapter provides definitions as you read.

Media Resources Please go to **www.bradybooks.com** to access mykit for this text. You will find quizzes, critical thinking scenarios, weblinks, animations, and videos related to this chapter—and much more. Look for online information on the EMS Agenda for the Future. You will also find a video clip on the Healthy People 2010 initiative.

INTRODUCTION

The **Emergency Medical Responder (EMR)** is a vital part of the **emergency medical services (EMS) system**. The EMR is trained to get there first—the point when a difference can be made between life and death (Figures 1-1a and 1-1b ■). (See The Big Picture: The EMS System).

The training you are about to undergo is focused on just that—the knowledge and skills to save a life, to comfort a patient at the height of crisis, and to provide care that flows seamlessly into the care given by emergency personnel on the ambulance.

Emergency Medical Responder (EMR)
training level to be a first responder to most calls.

emergency medical services (EMS) system
grouping of medical providers from 911 to the emergency department.

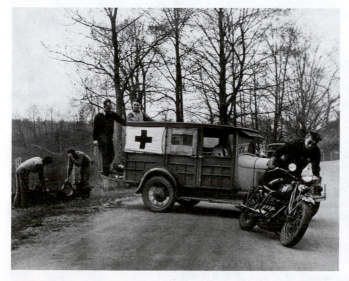

■ **Figure 1-1a** Early 1900s ambulance at the scene of an accident. (© Underwood & Underwood/Corbis)

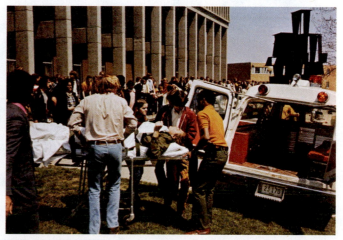

■ **Figure 1-1b** Ambulance at the scene of the Kent State University shooting in 1970. (© Bettman/Corbis)

The Big Picture
The EMS System

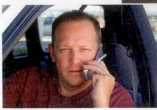

1 A citizen calls 9-1-1.

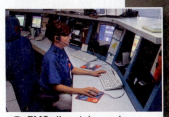

2 EMS dispatch sends an Emergency Medical Responder to the scene.

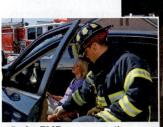

3 An EMR assesses the patients.

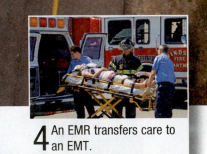

4 An EMR transfers care to an EMT.

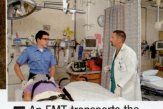

5 An EMT transports the patient to the emergency department.

As an EMR, you are the first part of the EMS system who will respond to the patient's side. Your training will prepare you to respond first and provide lifesaving care. Your training will focus on knowledge and skills that will have the most impact on the patient in those first minutes, including preventing further injury; ensuring airway, breathing, and circulation; controlling bleeding; assessing the patient; monitoring vital signs; and providing other elements of patient care.

Emergency Medical Responders come from many backgrounds. Some are firefighters or police officers who respond on emergency vehicles with medical equipment. Others work as part of industrial response teams, in correctional facilities, or as community members wanting to make a difference (Figures 1-2a to 1-2d ■).

Regardless of the reason you are reading this book, you will be given the training to truly make a difference.

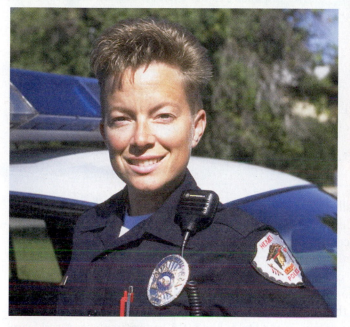

■ **Figure 1-2a** EMR police officer.

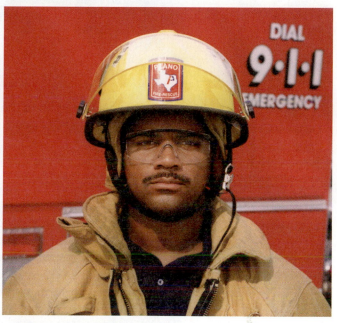

■ **Figure 1-2b** EMR firefighter.

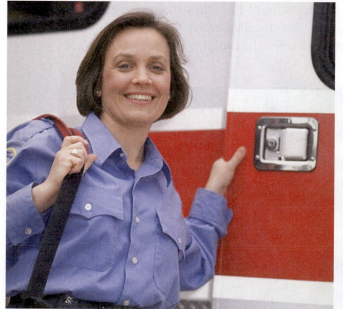

■ **Figure 1-2c** EMR community volunteer.

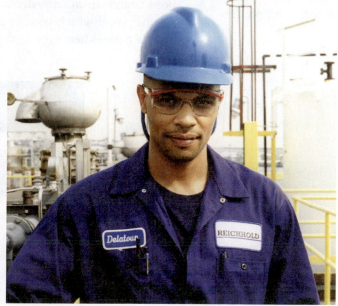

■ **Figure 1-2d** EMR industrial worker.

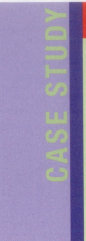
THE CALL

You are volunteering as an Emergency Medical Responder at the county fair. You are an EMR at work, so you help the community for these 10 days a year.

Your radio crackles for a "man down" near the grandstand. No further information is available and you don't know whether he fell from the stands, got into a fight, or maybe simply got sick. Since you are only a few hundred yards away, you pick up the pace.

■ Discussion: *What do you think you need to do if you are the first responder to the scene?*

ASK YOURSELF

■ How would you describe the importance of public safety answering points (PSAPs) and specially trained emergency medical dispatchers (EMDs) in EMS systems?

public safety answering point location where emergency calls are answered.

emergency medical dispatcher person who is trained to answer and prioritize emergency calls.

The EMS System

Since you will be a part of the EMS system, it is important to know all of its components and how it works. The depth of the system and the varied personnel involved may surprise you.

911

The system begins with the call for EMS. The patient may call EMS. Other times a family member, friend, or bystander calls 911. These calls are answered at a **public safety answering point** (PSAP). These centers receive calls for police, fire, and EMS.

Many of the dispatchers at these centers are trained as **emergency medical dispatchers** (EMDs). When an emergency call comes into a PSAP, these specially trained dispatchers obtain valuable information to give to responding EMS units; they also provide lifesaving medical instructions over the phone until help arrives (Figure 1-3 ■).

An overwhelming majority of the United States has a 911 system in place. A call from any phone using this number will put you in contact with professionals at a communications center. In most systems, calling 911 will also allow the dispatcher to identify the number from which you are calling. This is called enhanced-911 and is valuable in the event a patient becomes unresponsive before he can give his location.

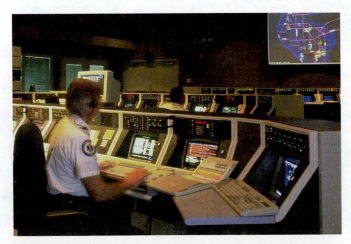

■ **Figure 1-3** Communication center.

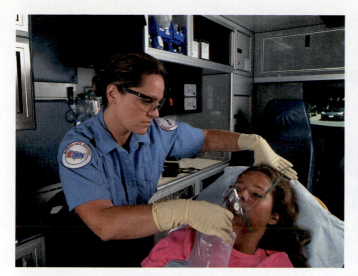

Figure 1-4 Emergency Medical Technician (EMT).

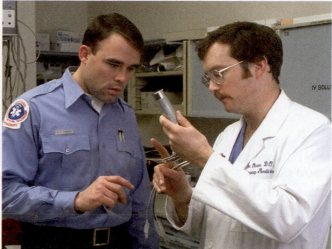

Figure 1-5 Advanced EMT (AEMT).

EMS Systems

When the ambulance arrives, it contains an array of sophisticated medical equipment—much of which you will be trained to use—and EMS providers at one of three levels:

- The **Emergency Medical Technician (EMT)** receives approximately 150 hours of training (Figure 1-4 ■). EMTs learn all of the material you learn in this class plus they receive more in-depth training in medical and trauma care, pharmacology, and other topics.
- The **Advanced EMT (AEMT)** is an EMS provider who is trained in some advanced skills such as administering intravenous (IV) fluid and some medications as well as advanced airway and assessment techniques (Figure 1-5 ■).
- The **Paramedic** is the highest level of EMS provider. The Paramedic performs the skills that the AEMT provides but also administers a greater number of medications, monitors and interprets electrocardiograms (ECGs), and does all of these things with minimal radio or phone contact with a physician (Figure 1-6 ■).

The levels of training listed here were developed as part of the National EMS Scope of Practice project. The Federal Department of Transportation, National Highway Traffic Safety Administration—who is responsible for the development of EMS training curricula and

ASK YOURSELF

- Compare and contrast the training and responsibilities of EMRs, EMTs, AEMTs, and Paramedics.

Emergency Medical Technician (EMT)
minimum training level to staff an ambulance.

Advanced EMT (AEMT)
level of advanced training to start IVs and intubate.

Paramedic highest level of nationally recognized training.

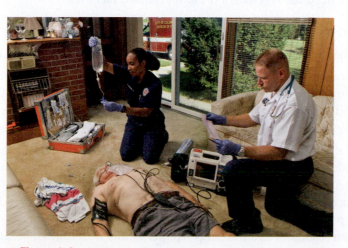

Figure 1-6 Paramedic.

standards—had education standards for each level developed. Those standards are upon what this textbook is based.

Classic Components of an EMS System

There are many different types of EMS systems. The system itself may be based in the fire department, it may be a third service (a municipal or private ambulance), or it may be a hospital-based system.

Many EMS systems provide a **tiered response** that has more than one level. An example is the system where a police officer or the fire service provides first response (at the EMR or EMT level), an ambulance responds with EMTs, and a Paramedic responds in a separate vehicle if needed. There are no set rules and many variations within EMS systems around the country.

As an EMR, you may be volunteer or paid, work in a fire department or industry, and respond in anything from an emergency vehicle to your personal vehicle or even on foot.

The EMS system continues into the hospital emergency department—and beyond. The nurses, physicians, and health-related professionals in the emergency department are responsible for taking care of the patient when he arrives at the hospital.

The hospital provides additional diagnostic services such as X-rays, computed tomography (CT) scans, ultrasounds, blood testing, and more to help determine what is wrong with the patient. The patient can be admitted to the hospital or discharged home to follow up with his personal physician.

While hospitals may look similar from the outside, the abilities within are sometimes quite different. The following are types of specialty hospitals available in some EMS systems:

- A **trauma center** has around-the-clock availability of a range of physician specialists (such as orthopedists, neurologists, and so on) and an operating room that is available and staffed 24 hours a day. Many serious trauma patients are saved only when a surgeon is able to operate and address internal injuries causing severe bleeding—and ultimately death—if not corrected. Trauma centers are available for this reason and more.
- A **pediatric center** offers highly specialized care for children who are ill or injured.
- A **burn center** provides specialized care for patients who have been severely burned.
- A **cardiovascular care center** provides emergent care for heart attack patients.
- A **stroke center** provides specialized care for those suspected of having a stroke.

As you study each of the chapters in this text, you will learn to care for a variety of patients who may need the services of these specialized facilities.

Ten Classic EMS System Components

The National Highway Traffic Safety Administration (NHTSA), through the U.S. Department of Transportation (DOT), developed ten classic components of any EMS system. These components were developed during a period when EMS was rapidly developing and provided a framework for the growth of EMS systems in the United States. The following components are still valid today:

1. Regulation and policy—Each state must have laws, regulations, policies, and procedures that govern its EMS system. It also is required to provide leadership to local jurisdictions.
2. Resource management—Each state must have central control of EMS resources so all patients have equal access to acceptable emergency care.
3. Human resources and training—All personnel who staff ambulances and transport patients must be trained to at least the EMT level.

tiered response system where EMTs and Paramedics respond separately.

trauma center hospital specializing in trauma care.

pediatric center hospital specializing in pediatric care.

burn center hospital specializing in burn care.

cardiovascular care center hospital specializing in advanced cardiac care.

stroke center hospital specializing in advanced stroke care.

ASK YOURSELF

- What are some examples of different types of EMS systems.
- How can the resources of specialty hospitals, such as trauma centers, benefit patients?
- What is the importance of each of the ten classic EMS system components listed in the text?

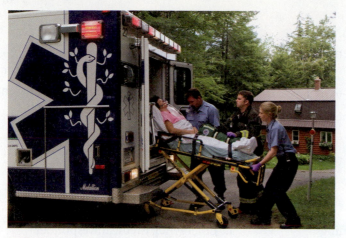

■ **Figure 1-7** Transport of a patient.

4. Transportation—patients must be safely and reliably transported by ground or air ambulance (Figure 1-7 ■).
5. Facilities—Every seriously ill or injured patient must be delivered in a timely manner to an appropriate medical facility.
6. Communications—A system for public access to the EMS system must be in place. Communication among dispatcher, ambulance crew, and hospital also must be possible.
7. Public information and education—EMS personnel should participate in programs designed to educate the public. The programs must focus on injury prevention and how to properly access the EMS system.
8. Medical oversight—Each EMS system must have a physician as a medical director.
9. Trauma systems—Each state must develop a system of specialized care for trauma patients, including one or more trauma centers and rehabilitation programs. It must also develop systems for assigning and transporting patients to those facilities.
10. Evaluation—Each state must have a quality improvement system in place for continuing evaluation and upgrading of its EMS system.

✳ Stop, Review, Remember

Multiple Choice

Place a check next to the correct answer.

1. There are _____ commonly recognized levels of EMS training.

    _____ a. 3

    _____ b. 4

    _____ c. 5

    _____ d. 8

2. 911 calls are answered:

    _____ a. at a public safety answering point.

    _____ b. at the closest police or fire station.

    _____ c. by phone company employees who route the call to the appropriate agency.

    _____ d. by an automated system that routes your call based on your location or the closest cell tower.

3. A third service EMS agency is one that:

_____ a. is based in a fire department.

_____ b. responds from a hospital.

_____ c. is a separate municipal service.

_____ d. provides care at the Paramedic level.

4. The minimum EMS level required for staffing an ambulance is the:

_____ a. Emergency Medical Responder.

_____ b. Emergency Medical Technician.

_____ c. Advanced Emergency Medical Technician.

_____ d. Paramedic.

Matching

Match the following descriptions with the appropriate level of training.

1. _____ Has the minimum level of training required to staff an ambulance

2. _____ Is most likely to get to a scene first

3. _____ Has the greatest number of hours of training

4. _____ Performs the most skills with minimal contact with a physician

5. _____ Has more training hours than an EMT but less than a Paramedic

a. Emergency Medical Responder

b. Emergency Medical Technician

c. Advanced Emergency Medical Technician

d. Paramedic

Critical Thinking

1. An EMS system describes itself as having a "tiered response." What does that mean?

_____

_____

_____

_____

2. Describe the components of the EMS system that your patient and his family would meet from the beginning of their journey to the end.

_____

_____

_____

_____

3. How does the Emergency Medical Responder level of certification differ from other levels of EMS training?

_____

_____

_____

_____

Emergency Medical Responder Practice

You are taking a course that will, upon successful completion, allow you to practice as an Emergency Medical Responder. This means that you will be given the entry-level training to become certified as an EMR. A number of other factors will guide your practice as an EMR. These include the following:

- State legislation—In many states your authorization and/or scope of practice is written and adopted into law. (Scope of Practice will be discussed in Chapter 3.)

- State EMS agencies—All states have some sort of organization that oversees EMS within that state. These agencies are often responsible for oversight of training and issuance of certificates or licenses.

- Regional or local medical agencies—Some areas also have EMS oversight and administration at the local level, whether it be region, county, or city.

- Medical oversight—The role of the physician medical director is vital to an EMS system. The medical director is involved in quality improvement and the development of protocols.

- Agency rules and regulations—Emergency Medical Responders come from a wide range of agencies where some EMRs are paid and some provide volunteer services. Many EMRs work as part of a volunteer medical response team at their place of employment. Regardless of how or where you provide care, there will be rules set by your agency or employer.

ASK YOURSELF

- How would you relate each of the following factors to the practice of EMRs?
  - Your state's legislation
  - Your state's EMS organization or agency
  - Any regional or local EMS oversight agencies
  - Medical oversight
  - The agency with which you will volunteer or be employed
- What are the roles and responsibilities of EMRs?

Roles and Responsibilities of the Emergency Medical Responder

The fact that becoming an Emergency Medical Responder as part of the EMS system is a big responsibility has already been mentioned. But what are these responsibilities? They will see that they involve everything from your appearance and attitude to your commitment to quality and the way you are trained to care for our patients. They include the following:

- Ensure personal safety as well as concern for the safety of your patient and others. As an EMR you will arrive first. The initial survey of the scene for safety is your responsibility. You must take appropriate actions to protect yourself, patients, and bystanders from danger.

- Maintain equipment readiness—As an EMR you provide lifesaving care. In order to properly provide this care, you must ensure your equipment is kept clean and in good working condition. Equipment (such as suction and a defibrillator) is worthless without the proper accessories and charged batteries.

- Evaluate and size up the scene—Emergency scenes are also sized up for other hazards such as hazardous materials and fire. You will determine how many patients are present and look for clues to the cause of their illness or injury.

- Gain access to patients—As the first to arrive you will make determinations about how to reach patients. Patients are generally easy to access whether at home, at work, or in a car. You will occasionally find patients entrapped or in a situation that would be dangerous to access (for example, a patient in a steep ravine or pinned by machinery). In these cases, you would call the appropriate teams to handle the situation.

- Perform patient assessment—Prompt and accurate assessment of your patient is crucial. You will begin by looking for and treating life-threatening conditions and then assess for less serious conditions. Assessment and reassessment continue until the ambulance arrives.

- Administer care—Your care is based on your assessment findings. Some patients will require lifesaving care such as oxygen, defibrillation, or control of serious bleeding whereas others will largely require only reassurance until the ambulance arrives.

- Provide emotional support—People remember how much you care more than they remember the medical care you provide.

- Maintain continuity of care—Once you provide care, you must continue care until you turn it over to another qualified provider. Keep records of the care you provide and be sure all relevant information is turned over to the EMTs when they arrive so the patient receives uninterrupted and efficient care.

- Maintain medical legal standards in patient care—Care must be provided in accordance with all applicable rules and laws. You may provide only the care you are allowed to perform, and you must maintain strict patient confidentiality.

- Community relations—Whether providing care or simply wearing the uniform of your agency, you are visible to the public. Everyone in your system will be judged on your actions and behaviors. You may also have the opportunity to present community education programs or classes at local schools, business organizations, and senior citizen centers.

professionalism treating others as you would want to be treated.

ASK YOURSELF

- What are some examples of professionalism in EMR practice?

Professionalism is another important term when discussing the roles and responsibilities of the EMR. Professionalism is a wide-ranging term, which means that the EMR is perceived as a caring and competent member of the EMS system.

This perception is based on many factors, including:

- Integrity
- Empathy
- Motivation
- Appearance and hygiene
- Patient advocacy
- Communication and teamwork
- A demeanor that is confident, tactful, and respectful
- Knowledge of your individual limitations

Successful EMS providers at any level treat people the way they would expect to be treated themselves—in both medical care and compassion. By using this rule, you will seldom go wrong.

Your professionalism extends into the medical areas of care including many of the topics which follow including quality improvement, honesty, and avoiding medical errors.

As an Emergency Medical Responder you will likely be required to obtain ongoing or continuing education (CE). This may be done through conferences, self-study or refresher classes. The science of medicine changes frequently. Professionals keep up with these changes.

THE RESPONSE ✳

You get to the patient's side at about the same time as the sheriff's deputy. Although you are not sure what happened, the man looks really sick. He appears to be about 75 years old and is very pale and sweaty. Sometimes you know when people are sick. He was obviously sick.

The patient tells you that he isn't sure what happened. He woke up on the ground. His wife, who looks worried, says he passed out when getting up from a picnic table. You can see he is breathing deeply. After checking his pulse at the wrist, you determine that it is a bit fast and weak.

The deputy is also an EMR. She administers oxygen while you get more of the history. The patient says he's had heart problems and high blood pressure. He doesn't have any pain—he just feels weak. You continue getting vital signs when the ambulance pulls up.

■ Discussion: *What do you think a pulse that is fast and weak means? What if the deputy had been a Paramedic? What would your role have been?*

Quality Improvement

One of the most important traits of an EMS system is that it strives to provide quality care. This is done with a process called quality improvement (QI). Formally defined as a dynamic system for continually evaluating and improving care, a QI plan looks at all aspects of an agency including patient assessment and care, documentation, patient satisfaction, and other areas to make sure the highest quality care is being delivered daily.

Quality improvement is done in many ways. Agencies often convene a QI committee. The committee is usually composed of members of an organization, both administrative and field staff, the medical director, and others.

The committee reviews run reports and other indicators of quality. An example might be reviewing documentation for proper procedures in a particular type of call (such as cardiac arrest) or ensuring that incoming EMS units are promptly and accurately notified about the patient's condition. If the committee finds any potential issues, they will recommend policy or procedural changes or additional training to get the agency to the level of quality expected.

QI committees are not to be feared and should never be operated in a punitive manner. In fact, all EMRs should participate in quality improvement. This is done by staying current on the knowledge and skills you learn as an EMR, completing accurate documentation, and providing care that would make you proud. You may also choose to serve on your QI committee.

Errors in EMS

Those who practice EMS are human . . . and humans make mistakes. It is estimated that the cost of medical errors may reach into the billions of dollars annually. Medical errors cause anguish to both the patients involved and to those who provided care.

ASK YOURSELF
■ What is the purpose of quality improvement in EMS?
■ What are some ways you can reduce the likelihood of errors in your practice as an EMR?

In an overwhelming majority of calls, patient care is provided without error.

Errors do occur, of course. They may be small and seem relatively insignificant, or they can be life threatening. Errors may be in skill performance, knowledge, or decision making. One thing is certain—it is up to you to prevent errors. This may be done in the following ways:

- Double-check important facts or decisions.
- Use pocket reference guides, protocol books, or "cheat sheets."
- Question assumptions—especially in serious situations.
- Ask for help or for assistance.
- Debrief calls afterward and look for ways to improve processes and decisions.

Research in EMS

ASK YOURSELF
- How may research impact EMR practice?

Much of what you learn in EMS is based on research. As EMS grows and matures as a profession the amount of research performed will increase—and the care you provide will be based more and more on research.

You will see examples of research as you practice as an EMR. Every few years the American Heart Association issues changes in guidelines for cardiopulmonary resuscitation (CPR) and emergency cardiac care. If you have held a CPR card in the past, you may have noticed changes in the number and timing of chest compressions and ventilations.

Another example of research-influenced care is covered in the portion of this textbook that has to do with bleeding and shock. You will be trained to use a tourniquet (a device that is wrapped around an extremity and tightened to control bleeding). If you had taken a similar course only a few years ago, you would have been instructed that tourniquets are extremely dangerous and should rarely be used. Today we believe tourniquets are not as dangerous as previously thought and have a place in patient care when used properly.

When you practice as an EMR, the protocols you use and the decisions and advice given by medical oversight physicians are also based on research and experience.

Research and You

As an EMR, you may be involved in research. Perhaps an EMS provider in your area or a physician at a local emergency department would like to study some part of your EMS system response or the assessment and care you provide. To do this, you may be asked to complete a form after a certain type of call or you may be asked to demonstrate a skill. Researchers may also look at the documentation and data collection from certain types of calls. There are many ways researchers study EMS.

Similar to QI, this research is not something where you will personally be graded or examined. You will likely be one person or one response in a large number of calls that will be evaluated to help determine how best to provide emergency care in the future.

You can help research efforts every day by providing thorough, accurate documentation on each call (Figure 1-8 ■). Some research (called retrospective research) uses a review of past calls as a means to gather data.

TRANSITION

The ambulance staff asks about the situation. You tell them it appears that the patient passed out immediately after getting up from the picnic table. He is complaining of weakness and denies any pain. He has a history of heart problems and high blood pressure. He didn't hurt himself when he fell to the ground.

You tell the EMTs to check with the deputy to make sure you didn't miss anything. The man starts to look a little better and is talking about not going to the hospital. His wife doesn't let him get away with that.

■ Discussion: *While it will be discussed in detail in another chapter, what would you think you would need to do if the patient refused to be transported?*

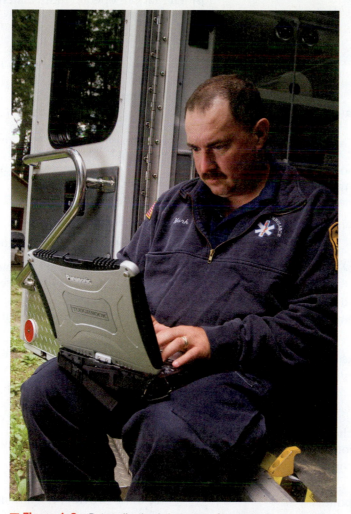

■ **Figure 1-8**   Data collection is important. Completing a prehospital care report (PCR) is a critical part of your responsibilities.

Remember, your training will prepare you to respond first and provide lifesaving care using the knowledge and skills you will gain in this course and from this text. Within those first minutes, you will have the most impact, focusing on preventing further injury; ensuring airway, breathing, and circulation; controlling bleeding; assessing the patient; checking vital signs; and providing other elements of patient care.

✳ Chapter Review

Multiple Choice

Place a check next to the correct answer.

1. Which of the following statements is false?

   _____ a. The EMS system includes the hospital emergency department.

   _____ b. EMRs are part of the EMS system.

   _____ c. EMRs are trained to respond to an emergency scene first.

   _____ d. Emergency medical dispatchers are also EMRs.

2. As an Emergency Medical Responder, you will respond to the scene of various types of emergencies. Your primary goal during your patient interaction should be to:

   _____ a. obtain an ECG and give appropriate medications.

   _____ b. obtain an in-depth history of the patient's medication history.

   _____ c. prevent further injury and make lifesaving interventions consistent with your training.

   _____ d. perform the interventions you think the emergency department would do if the patient were there.

3. The patient is in need of an intervention to open her airway that will allow her to breathe with ease. At what minimum level would a responder be trained to provide this type of lifesaving intervention?

   _____ a. Emergency Medical Responder

   _____ b. Emergency Medical Technician

   _____ c. Paramedic

   _____ d. Emergency physician

4. You are at the scene of a motor vehicle collision at 2:00 a.m. The patient requires rapid transport to a hospital that can operate immediately on his traumatic injuries. Which hospital is best suited to receive this patient?

   _____ a. Burn center

   _____ b. Stroke center

   _____ c. Trauma center

   _____ d. Cardiovascular center

5. Laws that are written and adopted governing scope of practice and/or authorization are created by:

   _____ a. state EMS agencies.

   _____ b. state legislation.

   _____ c. local agency directors.

   _____ d. regional medical directors.

6. You are working as an EMR at a private industrial recycling facility. The company has created a guidebook telling you and the company's other EMRs what you are allowed to do. This is an example of:

   _____ a. agency rules and regulations.

   _____ b. state scope of practice.

   _____ c. regional care protocols.

   _____ d. national training curriculum.

7. A quality improvement plan continually evaluates all of the following areas except:

   _____ a. patient satisfaction.

   _____ b. EMS provider documentation.

   _____ c. completion of duty requirements.

   _____ d. patient assessment.

8. The quality improvement committee makes the determination of proper or improper care primarily by:

_____ a. calling members that were on a call to testify before the committee.

_____ b. reviewing the shift logs relevant to call volume.

_____ c. asking the provider's partner his personal opinion of the person's character.

_____ d. reviewing the patient care run reports for an individual call.

9. It is not acceptable to use a pocket reference guide to help prevent errors in patient assessment and care.

_____ a. True

_____ b. False

10. What level of provider will typically administer intravenous medications to a medical patient with little or no physician contact?

_____ a. Paramedic

_____ b. Advanced EMT

_____ c. EMT

_____ d. EMR

Matching

Match the following descriptions with the appropriate term.

1. _____ Responder that is trained to more than an EMT level but less than a Paramedic level
2. _____ Hospital with around-the-clock staff available to treat a variety of heart problems
3. _____ Hospital capable of receiving patients who have sustained injuries such as stab wounds, gunshot wounds, and long falls
4. _____ Physician that oversees the development of protocols to guide care
5. _____ Center that receives emergency call requesting assistance for police, fire, or EMS
6. _____ Hospital whose specialty is patients below the age of 18
7. _____ Hospital whose specialty is patients that have come in contact with flame or another burning process
8. _____ Minimum level of care necessary to staff an ambulance
9. _____ Hospital whose primary concern is those having suffered a stroke
10. _____ Person who receives and dispatches a call for emergency assistance
11. _____ Responder who is primarily trained to be the first responder on a call
12. _____ The highest level of nationally recognized EMS training

a. Trauma center
b. Pediatric center
c. Burn center
d. Cardiovascular center
e. Stroke center
f. Emergency Medical Responder
g. Emergency Medical Technician
h. Advanced Emergency Medical Technician
i. Paramedic
j. Public service answering point
k. Emergency medical dispatcher
l. Medical director

Critical Thinking

You arrive on the scene of a patient who has been stabbed by an assailant. You find a male lying on the ground with blood coming from his stomach area. There is another emergency responder arriving in a Paramedic Fly-Car and an ambulance is visible coming down the road.

1. What should be your primary concern?

   _____

   _____

   _____

2. What is the name for this type of response with people arriving at different times in different vehicles?

   _____

   _____

   _____

3. This patient will most likely require transport to what type of hospital?

   _____

   _____

   _____

EMR Safety and Wellness

✳ NAVIGATION GUIDE

The following items provide an overview to the purpose and content of this chapter. The Education Standards and Competencies are from the National EMS Education Standards.

Education Standards Preparatory (Workforce Safety and Wellness); Public Health

Competencies Uses simple knowledge of the EMS system, safety/well-being of the EMR, medical/legal issues at the scene of an emergency while awaiting a higher level of care.

Has an awareness of local public health resources and the role EMS personnel play in public health emergencies.

Knowledge Area Workforce Safety and Wellness
- Standard safety precautions
- Personal protective equipment
- Stress management
- Dealing with death and dying
- Prevention of response-related injuries
- Lifting and moving patients

Objectives After reading this chapter, you should be able to:

1. Define key terms introduced in this chapter.
2. List indications of the potential for danger to yourself or others at the scene of an EMS call.
3. Given a scenario of an emergency call, describe how you could use each of the following principles to protect yourself:
   a. Cover
   b. Concealment
   c. Distraction
   d. Retreat
4. Explain the importance of assessing an emergency scene from a distance.

5. Describe the role of each of the following measures in protecting yourself from disease and injury in your work as an EMR:
   a. Regular physical examination
   b. Vaccinations
   c. Personal protective equipment (gloves, eye and face protection, respiratory protection, gown)
   d. Hand washing
   e. Reporting exposure to communicable disease

6. Give examples of common stressors for EMS personnel.
7. Recognize behaviors in yourself or others that are signs of stress.
8. Describe actions that you can take, and things you should avoid, to prevent and reduce stress.
9. Describe signs that a patient is dead and cannot be resuscitated.
10. Explain each of the following reactions to grief:
    a. Denial
    b. Anger
    c. Bargaining
    d. Depression
    e. Acceptance

11. Give examples of instances when you may need to use an emergent or urgent move to relocate or reposition a patient before additional help arrives.
12. Demonstrate the use of good body mechanics when lifting.
13. Given a scenario in which a patient must be moved or repositioned, explain the principles you will follow to move the patient with regard to both your safety and well-being and the patient's.
14. Explain the basic principles of patient restraint.

Key Terms Page references indicate first major use in this chapter. The Margin Glossary in this chapter provides definitions as you read.

cover, p. 24
concealment, p. 24
distraction, p. 24
retreat, p. 24
hazardous materials, p. 25
placards, p. 25
carbon monoxide, p. 26
Standard Precautions, p. 26
body fluids, p. 26
airborne droplets, p. 26
infection, p. 26
vaccination, p. 28

pathogens, p. 28
personal protective equipment, p. 28
high-efficiency particulate air (HEPA), p. 32
bacteria, p. 32
exposure, p. 32
needlestick, p. 32
decay, p. 37
rigor mortis, p. 37
decapitation, p. 37
body mechanics, p. 38

bariatric patient, p. 39
emergency moves, p. 41
urgent moves, p. 41
long axis, p. 42
inadequate breathing, p. 43
altered mental status, p. 43
shock, p. 43
hypothermia, p. 43
frostbite, p. 43
recovery position, p. 44
supine, p. 44

Media Resources Please go to **www.bradybooks.com** to access mykit for this text. You will find quizzes, critical thinking scenarios, weblinks, animations, and videos related to this chapter—and much more. Look for online information on stress management. You will also find a video clip on transmission and treatment for AIDS.

INTRODUCTION

Scene safety is arguably the most important thing you will consider at an emergency call.

Although most calls go by uneventfully, you will one day be on a call where there is a potential for danger. Sometimes the dangers are obvious such as violence or an overturned tanker carrying hazardous materials.

Other sources of harm could easily be overlooked. Injuring your back could cause lifelong disability. The effects of stress are often downplayed or ignored.

The time you spend as an EMR has the potential to be incredibly rewarding and interesting—especially when you take good care of yourself. In this chapter, you will learn how to maintain your safety and wellness.

THE CALL ✴

Your unit is dispatched to respond to a "man down" at 4226 Adams Street. The dispatcher advises that they are still on the phone with the scene. A female caller is telling the dispatcher that her husband is on the floor in the bathroom. She can't wake him up.

■ Discussion: *What are the first questions that you will need to ask?*

Scene Safety

You can't help but watch television news and wonder if you will encounter any of the hazards you see there as you practice as an EMR. Generally, EMS is a safe profession that responds to patients' calls for help and does tremendous good for people. However, you do have the potential to encounter danger or hazards at the scene of an emergency.

Chapter 9, "Patient Assessment: Scene Size-Up," will provide additional information on how—and when—to protect yourself from dangers during your response to a call.

This chapter discusses threats such as violence, hazardous materials, and other scene hazards (Figures 2-1a to 2-1c ■).

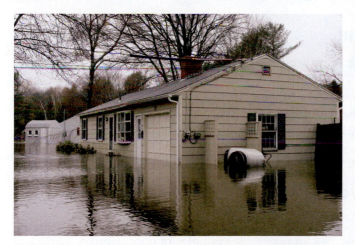

■ **Figure 2-1a** Hazardous materials pose a threat to emergency medical responders. *(© Daniel Limmer)*

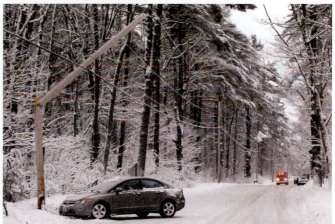

■ **Figure 2-1b** You may encounter dangers from motor vehicle collisions. *(© Daniel Limmer)*

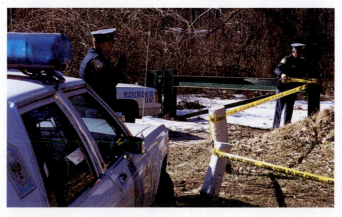

■ **Figure 2-1c** A crime scene.

Protecting Yourself from Violence

Although this section will teach responses to violence, the best way to protect yourself is to avoid it altogether. Observation is the best method to do this.

Your observations will begin as you approach the scene and begin to size it up. Begin your observations from a distance as you approach the scene in your vehicle or on foot. As you approach the scene, look for:

- Obvious signs of violence such as fighting or shouting
- The use or threatened use of weapons
- Large or unruly crowds; people fleeing from the scene
- Signs of drug or alcohol use by the patient, family, or bystanders

If these signs seem obvious to you, they are. You likely have a sense of other items that may be added to the list. Each scene is different, and violence can present differently.

Experienced EMRs also get a sense of danger from other things. Emergencies are generally active scenes. When someone greets you at the door and shows you to the patient, it may seem normal—and potentially safe. If you get to a scene and the house is quiet and dark, it may also be a sign of danger.

Approach slowly and carefully, using all of your senses. At the first indication of danger, stop. You will need to take actions to protect yourself and your crew from danger. Four basic procedures are used in response to danger: **cover**, **concealment**, **distraction**, and **retreat**. You will also need to use a portable radio or cell phone to call for assistance and warn others who may be responding to the scene.

Cover and Concealment

One of the steps you will take to protect yourself is to "take cover." You have probably heard this said in the movies. The definition of cover is to take a position that hides your body and is thick or dense enough to offer protection. While it is a rare occurrence that someone would shoot you, the true measure of good cover is that it will stop a bullet. Concealment hides your body but offers no protection.

Examples of adequate cover include:

- a brick wall
- the engine block of your vehicle
- a sturdy tree (Figure 2-2a ■).

A large shrub or the interior walls of a house are examples of concealment. These will hide you but offer minimal protection (Figure 2-2b ■).

Distraction and Retreat

It only makes sense to get away from the danger. You must do so in a safe and strategic manner integrating principles of cover and concealment.

Distraction is using a piece of equipment or another item at the scene to block an aggressor and buy you more time. You may be carrying a piece of equipment that you can throw at a dangerous person to slow him up and help your retreat. If the ambulance is at the scene, the stretcher may be wedged in a doorway or pushed toward a person. Closing doors behind you can help to gain more time. If you are truly in danger, every second counts.

If you spot danger in advance or are suddenly confronted by it, immediately move away from the danger to a position of cover. You must not stop there. Immediately look for your next position of cover (preferred) or concealment. When it is safe to do so, move to it. Do this until you are totally safe from the danger (Figure 2-2c ■).

ASK YOURSELF

- Can you define all key terms introduced in this chapter?
- Ask a fellow student if he can list indications of the potential for danger to himself or others at the scene of an EMS call.
- Given a scenario of an emergency call, how would you use each of the following principles to protect yourself?
  - Cover
  - Concealment
  - Distraction
  - Retreat
- How would you explain the importance of assessing an emergency scene from a distance?

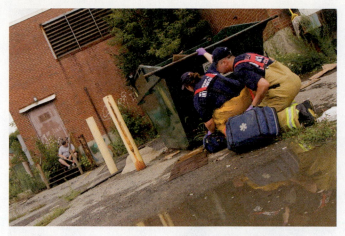

Figure 2-2a The EMR takes cover.

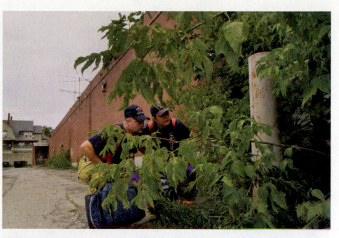

Figure 2-2b The EMR must look for a place of concealment.

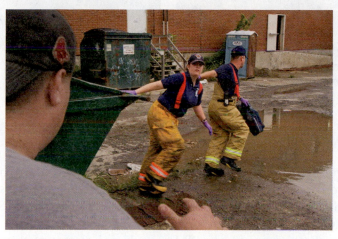

Figure 2-2c The EMR retreats from a visibly dangerous area.

Don't forget to call for help and to warn others of the danger so incoming police, fire, and EMS personnel are not in harm's way.

Other Scene Hazards

Violence isn't the only—or the most frequent—hazard. You can come across anything from fire to **hazardous materials** to collisions that involve unstable vehicles or downed power lines.

The most important principle of scene safety—don't enter a scene until it is safe to do so. The dangers from hazardous materials and downed power lines can extend a considerable distance from the scene. You must assess the scene from a distance. Use binoculars to increase your ability to scan the scene from a distance. When observing the scene for hazards, look for:

- Signs of hazardous materials, including the types of vehicles involved in a crash or warning devices (for example, **placards**) on buildings or vehicles (Figure 2-3 ■)
- Signs of wires down in an area, including darkness (indicating the power is out), asymmetry of (unequal distance between) telephone poles, damaged utility poles, and wires hanging low or on the ground (Figure 2-4 ■)
- Unstable vehicles, including those that are on anything other than all four wheels (Vehicles that are on the roof or side are at risk of further movement which could cause serious injury. Also be alert for vehicles that are on nonlevel surfaces or leaking fuel or fluids of any kind.)

hazardous materials substances that are harmful to health.

placards signs indicating a type of material in a container.

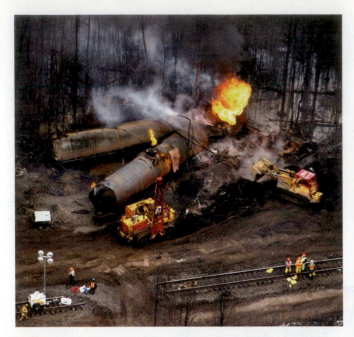

■ **Figure 2-3** A scene containing hazardous materials. *(© Syracuse Newspapers/Mike Greenlar/The Image Works)*

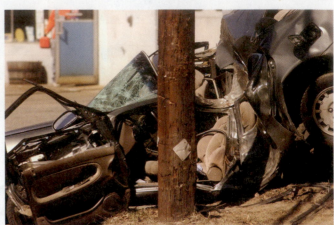

■ **Figure 2-4** Collisions involving utility poles may cause downed power lines. *(© Mark C. Ide)*

carbon monoxide
odorless gas that is harmful to one's health.

■ Patients that are in dangerous places, including fires, unsafe atmospheres (such as confined spaces or **carbon monoxide**), and heights

Personal protection from these dangers involves observation and avoiding the danger. If you enter the scene and become involved when a vehicle is unstable, hazardous materials are present, or wires are down, the risks to you are grave. It may be too late. Observation and prevention are key.

Your observations will be conducted as part of the scene size-up, which will be discussed in greater detail in Chapter 9, "Patient Assessment: Scene Size-Up". Additional information on hazardous materials will be covered in Chapter 30, "Special Operations."

Protection from Disease

You likely will have questions and concerns about protecting yourself from disease. After all, you will be encountering patients who have diseases or are bleeding—or both.

Rest assured that you can both safely provide patient care and protect yourself from disease. Medical professionals—in and out of the hospital—have been doing just that for years.

Standard Precautions
contact precautions to prevent spread of disease.

Standard Precautions, in the past also referred to as body substance isolation, are practices to prevent exposure to disease during patient contact. They are called Standard Precautions because they apply to all patients.

You can't tell by looking at a patient whether he has a disease. Diseases infect people regardless of race, sex, and socioeconomic status. We treat all patients with compassion and care and while doing so we protect ourselves from disease.

body fluids
blood, saliva, urine, and other substances produced by the body.

airborne droplets
particulate matter suspended in respiratory secretions.

infection
organisms invading the immune system, causing illness.

Diseases may be transmitted to EMS providers through **body fluids** or **airborne droplets** from the patient that are allowed to enter the body and cause **infection**. Table 2-1 lists some of the diseases you may be concerned about and the mode of transmission.

The entry into your body may be through an open wound (it may be a small cut or crack in the skin) or through mucous membranes, including the eyes, nose, and mouth. You can also be exposed to disease through an accidental needlestick (Figures 2-5a to 2-5c ■).

TABLE 2-1 Communicable Diseases

DISEASE	MODE OF TRANSMISSION	INCUBATION
AIDS (acquired immune deficiency syndrome)	HIV-infected blood via intravenous drug use, unprotected sexual contact, blood transfusions, or, rarely, accidental needlesticks. Mothers may also pass HIV to their unborn children.	Several months or years
Chicken pox (varicella)	Airborne droplets. Can also be spread by contact with open sores	11 to 21 days
German measles (rubella)	Airborne droplets. Mothers may pass the disease to unborn children.	10 to 12 days
Hepatitis	Blood, stool, or other body fluids, or contaminated objects	Weeks to months, depending on type
Meningitis, bacterial	Oral or nasal secretions	2 to 10 days
Mumps	Droplets of saliva or objects contaminated by saliva	14 to 24 days
Pneumonia, bacterial and viral	Oral or nasal droplets and secretions	Several days
Staphylococcal skin infections	Direct contact with infected wounds or sores or with contaminated objects	Several days
Tuberculosis (TB)	Respiratory secretions, airborne or on contaminated objects	2 to 6 weeks
Whooping cough (pertussis)	Respiratory secretions or airborne droplets	6 to 20 days

Other methods that diseases are transmitted outside of a patient care setting include contaminated food and sexual contact.

It is the goal of this section to properly instruct you on these Standard Precautions and keep you safe on every call. This section will cover all the material you need to protect yourself from disease.

Before the Response

As an EMR, you may be required to have a regular physical examination. This examination will check for common medical conditions and identify any potential problems before they become serious. Different organizations will require different examinations. An EMR who is part of a hazardous materials team will likely have a more rigorous examination (because of use of a respirator and protective clothing) than someone who responds to community medical and traumatic emergencies.

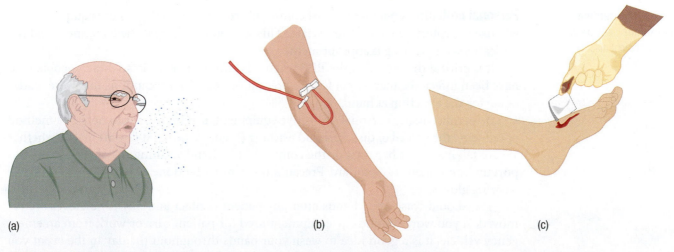

(a)   (b)   (c)

■ **Figure 2-5** (a) Droplet infection. (b) Blood-to-blood contact. (c) Open wounds and exposed tissue.

- How would you describe the role of each of the following measures in protecting yourself from disease and injury in your work as an EMR?
  - Regular physical examination
  - Vaccinations
  - Personal protective equipment (gloves, eye and face protection, respiratory protection, gown)
  - Hand washing
  - Reporting exposure to communicable disease

vaccination injection to help prevent disease and illness.

pathogens disease-causing agents.

personal protective equipment equipment used to prevent disease.

In general, it is good to get an examination on a regular basis as part of your personal health care.

You will also receive **vaccinations** to help prevent disease. These vaccinations are required or highly recommended for those providing health care in any setting. Recommended vaccinations include:

- Tetanus
- Hepatitis A
- Hepatitis B
- Measles, mumps, and rubella (MMR)
- Chickenpox
- Influenza

You will also be screened yearly for tuberculosis through a skin test.

Your agency will have policies and procedures in place to help prevent exposure to bloodborne and airborne **pathogens**. These are required by federal agencies such as the Occupational Safety and Health Administration (OSHA) as well as agencies at the state level. These requirements are based on the most recent health recommendations of experts such as those at the Centers for Disease Control and Prevention (CDC). You will be trained on these procedures and on the proper operation and use of all equipment on an annual basis.

Your employer or agency is required to have strategic controls in place to help prevent exposure to disease long before the potential contact occurs. Training is one of these requirements. Another is making equipment available whenever and wherever it is needed. For example, protective gloves, eyewear, masks, and gowns must be placed where they can be retrieved when needed. If you arrive alone, for example, as part of an industrial team or even in your own vehicle, you will be issued protective equipment for use at the scene since EMS will not be present.

If you respond as part of the EMS system on an emergency vehicle, the vehicle and the medical kits must have protective equipment readily available. This equipment will be discussed in detail in the next section.

The rules for protection from disease also apply to cleaning up spills and equipment after a call. Follow your agency's guidelines during postcall cleanup. This will be discussed further in Chapter 28, "Operations."

During the Response—Personal Protective Equipment

Personal protective equipment, most commonly referred to as PPE, is the equipment you will use to protect yourself from disease. This section will discuss the equipment and the indications for wearing it appropriately.

It is critical that you don the PPE when it is appropriate to do so. Many people who have been infected either forgot to take precautions or took precautions that were inadequate for the situation at hand.

Before discussing personal protective equipment, it is important to note one method of reducing the spread of disease: hand washing (Figure 2-6a ■). It doesn't matter whether we are talking about hepatitis or the common cold, hand washing may be the most important component of Standard Precautions. It must be done whether or not you are wearing gloves.

You should wash your hands after any patient contact and any time gloves are removed. If you work around the equipment used for patient care or work from an emergency vehicle, it is a good idea to wash your hands throughout the day in the event you come in contact with a substance inadvertently left behind by another crew.

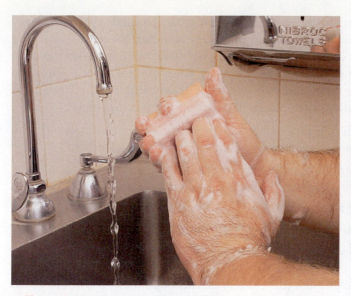

Figure 2-6a Wash your hands thoroughly.

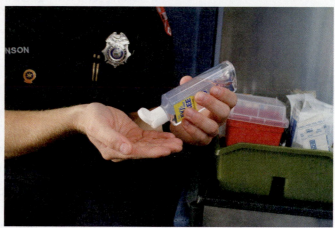

Figure 2-6b Use foam, liquid, or an alcohol-based washing agent.

While you may feel that you have been adequately washing your hands for some time, hand washing for health care personnel must be performed in a specific order to prevent recontamination:

1. Use warm water.
2. Thoroughly lather and scrub your hands—and any other skin that could have become exposed.
3. Use a brush to clean under your nails if necessary.
4. Rinse your hands thoroughly.
5. Dry your hands.
6. Turn off the water using the towel to avoid touching the faucet you touched earlier with soiled hands.

If you are in the field and soap and water isn't available, use an alcohol-based hand cleaner until soap and water is available (Figure 2-6b ■).

Gloves

Protective gloves are the most commonly used means of personal protection at emergency scenes. They are required when there is a chance that your hands may come in contact with the blood or body fluids of another. This may happen when assessing or caring for a patient or when moving a patient (Figure 2-7 ■).

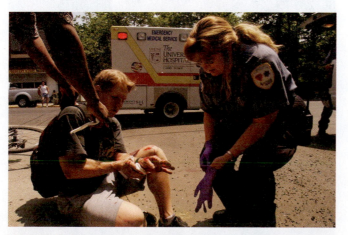

Figure 2-7 Always demonstrate Standard Precautions. (© Mark C. Ide)

Many EMS personnel don gloves when getting out of their vehicle even before approaching the scene. In that case it isn't technically taking Standard Precautions because you haven't seen the patient to know if precautions are needed. Donning gloves too early also poses the risk of damaging the gloves as you carry your kits and other equipment. Even a small tear in your gloves will render them useless as protection.

Consider the following patient encounters. In which would you don gloves?

- You are called to an industrial accident. A man is bleeding from his lower leg where it had been caught in a machine.
- You are called to a motor vehicle collision. You don't see blood on the patient but there is quite a bit of broken glass in the passenger compartment.
- You are called to a home for a woman who feels weak. She has no other complaints except feeling tired. You do not observe any blood or body fluids.

The industrial accident would clearly require gloves. The broken glass at the motor vehicle collision would lead you to think there could be blood somewhere you don't see. In both of these cases it would be prudent to wear gloves. Although many providers would wear gloves in the third example, the patient with weakness, it wouldn't be required by the principles of Standard Precautions unless a specific exposure risk was present.

In essence, the Standard Precautions you choose to take are based on your observations and experience. It is an important decision you will make on every call initially and consider throughout the call.

If the woman who felt weak began to vomit or suddenly became unresponsive, you would have your personal protective equipment available and don it immediately and discard appropriately. (Figure 2-8 ■). In the case of vomiting or airway care and suction, you would wear glasses and possibly face protection as well. These will be discussed next.

When responding to an emergency, you should carry two pairs of gloves in the event one tears or becomes soiled and requires changing.

Contaminated gloves must be removed carefully to avoid contamination (Scan 2-1). With a gloved hand, grip the cuff of the glove on the other hand and begin to roll it inside out. Avoid snapping the glove or similar quick motions that could spray blood or fluids. Once that glove has been partially removed, do the same on the other hand. You can now remove the gloves because the noncontaminated inside is facing out and may be safely gripped. Roll the gloves inside out into each other and dispose of them appropriately.

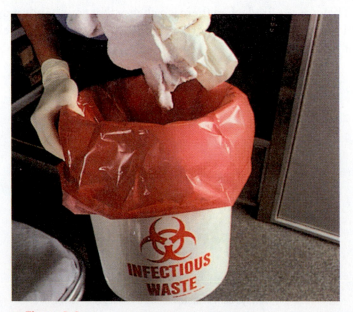

■ **Figure 2-8** Discard all contaminated items safely.

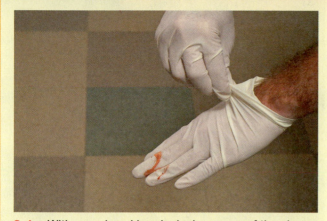

2-1a With one gloved hand, pinch an area of the glove on your other hand near the cuff. Do not touch your skin.

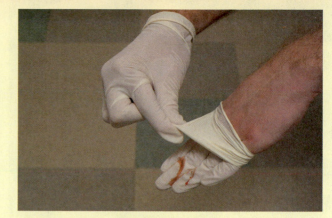

2-1b Pull the glove off inside out.

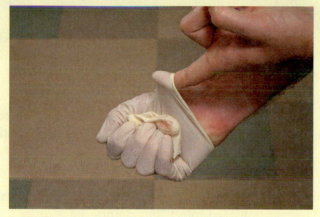

2-1c Find a noncontaminated area of the remaining glove and pull it off inside out. The first glove should end up inside the second glove.

Eye and Face Protection

As mentioned earlier, you can be exposed to a disease by a splash or spray of body fluids into mucous membranes of the face. This can occur when bleeding is severe or spurting, when patients vomit, during suctioning, and during childbirth, to name a few possibilities. Remember, it is up to you to recognize the potential for exposure in these situations and take the appropriate precautions.

There are two basic types of devices for eye and face protection used in EMS. The first, protective eyewear, entails special protective glasses or an EMR's eyeglasses with clip-on side protection. Since your eyes are always open, this protection is vital. Eye protection is always worn when suctioning or dealing with any splashing body fluids.

The face shield combines eye protection via a plastic shield with a surgical-type mask (Figure 2-9 ■). This device protects the entire face and is used in situations where there is a high likelihood of fluids splashing onto the face.

Respiratory Protection

Some diseases are airborne. This means they are in the air, often in tiny droplets sprayed from another person during a cough or sneeze.

Because the pathogens in these droplets are so small, a simple surgical mask or face shield will not filter out these disease-causing organisms. This is why you may be fitted

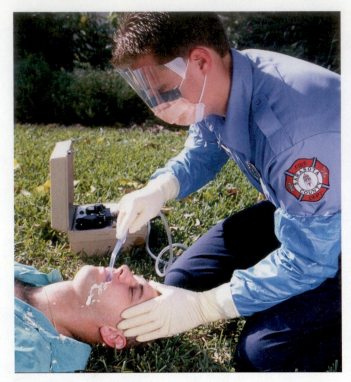

■ **Figure 2-9** Wear a face shield as necessary.

■ **Figure 2-10** N95 respirator.

high-efficiency particulate air (HEPA) respirator or mask that filters ultrafine particles in the air.

bacteria organisms causing infection.

for a **high-efficiency particulate air (HEPA)** respirator or an N95 mask (Figure 2-10 ■). These masks are specially designed for filtering out very small items such as the **bacteria** that causes tuberculosis.

Gown

Gowns protect your clothing from contamination. On calls where there is a considerable amount of blood or fluid, you will wear a gown to protect your clothes and yourself.

Major trauma calls and childbirth are examples of when a gown might be necessary.

The clothing you wear does provide a barrier between you and blood and body fluids—but it isn't designed to do so. Should your clothing become contaminated, remove it as soon as possible. Shower or wash any areas of skin that were contaminated. Wash the contaminated clothes by themselves in a separate load—preferably at the station rather than at home.

Exposure to an Infectious Substance

In the unlikely event you are exposed to the blood or body fluids of another, there are procedures that must be followed. Your agency should have a policy in place for events such as this. Figure 2-11 ■ describes a general procedure to take when you believe you have been exposed to disease. Always follow your agency's guidelines.

exposure contact with a substance.

The policy will define **exposure**. Not every time you come in contact with a substance will be considered an exposure. For example, if you get blood on your clothes over intact skin it would not be considered an exposure. However, you will be considered to have had an exposure if you suffer an accidental **needlestick** with a contaminated needle, have substances splash into your face (eyes, nose, or mouth), or have substances come in contact with an open wound on your skin.

needlestick accidental penetration of a needle.

Becoming exposed does not mean you will catch a disease. This depends on many factors, including whether your patient has any conditions such as HIV or hepatitis, the location of the exposure on your body, and the amount of infectious material involved.

INFECTIOUS DISEASE EXPOSURE PROCEDURE

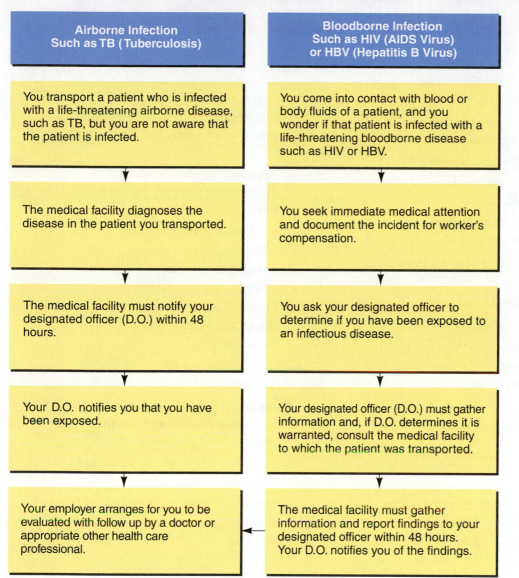

Airborne Infection Such as TB (Tuberculosis)	Bloodborne Infection Such as HIV (AIDS Virus) or HBV (Hepatitis B Virus)
You transport a patient who is infected with a life-threatening airborne disease, such as TB, but you are not aware that the patient is infected.	You come into contact with blood or body fluids of a patient, and you wonder if that patient is infected with a life-threatening bloodborne disease such as HIV or HBV.
The medical facility diagnoses the disease in the patient you transported.	You seek immediate medical attention and document the incident for worker's compensation.
The medical facility must notify your designated officer (D.O.) within 48 hours.	You ask your designated officer to determine if you have been exposed to an infectious disease.
Your D.O. notifies you that you have been exposed.	Your designated officer (D.O.) must gather information and, if D.O. determines it is warranted, consult the medical facility to which the patient was transported.
Your employer arranges for you to be evaluated with follow up by a doctor or appropriate other health care professional.	The medical facility must gather information and report findings to your designated officer within 48 hours. Your D.O. notifies you of the findings.

■ **Figure 2-11** Sample procedure for infectious disease exposure.

When you first realize you have been contaminated, you should immediately clean the area thoroughly. If skin is involved, wash with soap and water or shower. If your eyes are involved, irrigate them for at least 20 minutes.

You will also need to seek the care of a physician or other health care practitioner trained to evaluate and treat occupational exposures immediately following the exposure. If you have been exposed to a disease, obtaining care promptly is crucial. Follow your agency's exposure control plan which may include going to the same emergency department as the patient for care. You should also notify the appropriate personnel in your agency.

After you receive care, you will need to document the events around the exposure including the time and date, a description of the event, actions taken after the exposure, and other information as required by your department.

Multiple Choice

Place a check next to the correct answer.

1. Well-being is best defined as:

    _____ a. protection from violence and hazardous materials.

    _____ b. staying psychologically stress free.

    _____ c. a general concept of safety and health in EMS.

    _____ d. preventing disease through the proper use of equipment.

2. The best method to protect yourself from danger is to:

    _____ a. know defensive tactics.

    _____ b. practice concealment.

    _____ c. know exactly how far you can go before encountering danger.

    _____ d. be observant and avoid danger altogether.

3. The difference between cover and concealment is that:

    _____ a. concealment hides your body; cover protects it.

    _____ b. concealment protects your body; cover hides it.

    _____ c. concealment would stop a bullet; cover won't.

    _____ d. cover is rarely found at emergency scenes; concealment is common.

4. Which of the following is NOT an acceptable method of determining a hazard during the size-up of a vehicle crash on the highway?

    _____ a. Approaching the vehicle to examine the shipping papers for hazardous materials

    _____ b. Looking at placards from a distance

    _____ c. Looking for asymmetry of phone poles

    _____ d. Observing power outages in the area as you approach the scene

5. Standard Precautions are best defined as:

    _____ a. taking all possible precautions against disease whether or not there is a risk of transmission.

    _____ b. a practice to prevent exposure to disease.

    _____ c. wearing gloves on any call.

    _____ d. wearing gloves and eyewear on any call.

Emergency Medical Responder Practice

For each of the following, write whether the incident as described would constitute a reportable exposure.

1. An EMR gets blood and saliva sprayed across a face shield he is wearing.

    _____

    _____

    _____

2. An EMR has a small cut on his arm. Blood is splashed on his shirt over the cut and soaks through.

    _____

    _____

    _____

3. An EMR is working with advanced life support personnel and moves a pile of medical equipment. A contaminated needle is in the pile and punctures the skin of the EMR.

_____

_____

_____

4. An EMR notices that there is a tear in his protective gloves and a small amount of blood has seeped through over intact skin.

_____

_____

_____

Short Answer

For each of the following diseases, choose whether it is spread by bloodborne or airborne transmission.

a. Tuberculosis

_____

b. HIV

_____

c. Hepatitis B

_____

d. Hepatitis C

_____

e. Influenza

_____

f. Chickenpox

_____

Stress

EMS can be stressful. Having just finished reading the previous section, you may even be a bit stressed now thinking about catching a disease on a call. Fortunately, that is very rare—and preventable—much like the stress of EMS.

Every EMR is different. What causes stress for one will have a minimal effect on another. Some common stressors for emergency services personnel at all levels include:

- Dangerous situations or having your life threatened
- Seriously ill or injured patients
- The death of a patient or coworker
- Multiple patients
- Pediatric patients
- Seeing the stress and anguish of a patient, family member, or bystander

The EMR will be required to deal with the medical and personal needs of the patient and family during an emergency in a calm and controlled manner. Patients rarely remember

ASK YOURSELF

- What are some examples of common stressors for EMS personnel?

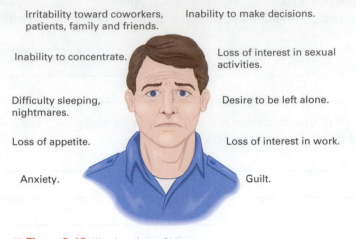

Irritability toward coworkers, patients, family and friends.

Inability to make decisions.

Inability to concentrate.

Loss of interest in sexual activities.

Difficulty sleeping, nightmares.

Desire to be left alone.

Loss of appetite.

Loss of interest in work.

Anxiety.

Guilt.

■ **Figure 2-12** Warning signs of stress.

the care you provided them for their illness or injury but almost always remember the compassion you showed them.

During a call be calm and nonjudgmental—even if the behavior of a patient or family member seems unreasonable. Allow patients and family members to express feelings unless this causes a behavior that is harmful to you, the patient, or others.

After the call, sometimes immediately—and even days to weeks later—you could begin to experience signs of stress (Figure 2-12 ■). It may start slowly or suddenly; many times providers experiencing stress know something is wrong but don't attribute it to stress. Some of the signs of stress include:

- Difficulty sleeping and/or nightmares
- Irritability
- Feelings of sadness, anxiety, and guilt
- Indecisiveness
- Loss of appetite
- Loss of interest in sexual activity
- Isolation
- Loss of interest in work
- Inability to concentrate
- Feelings of hopelessness
- Misuse of alcohol or drugs
- Signs of physical illness

Dealing with Stress

Every EMR experiences stress at some point. When it occurs, it is important to deal with it appropriately.

There are many lifestyle changes you can make—some of which can actually help prevent stress before it happens. If you take care of yourself, you will respond better to stress. Limit caffeine and alcohol intake. Participating in regular exercise (Figure 2-13 ■) and relaxation techniques are among the ways you may reduce or prevent stress.

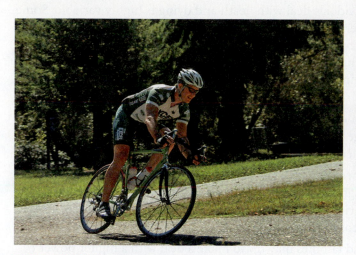

■ **Figure 2-13** Regular exercise helps manage stress.

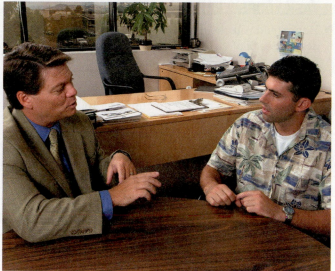

■ **Figure 2-14** It's important to seek help when feeling the effects of stress.

There may come a time when you feel you need to talk with someone about your feelings (Figure 2-14 ■). Other times your agency or employer may ask you to speak with a counselor. This happens to many EMRs and is not a sign of weakness.

Speaking with a professional counselor can help you recognize that the feelings and symptoms you experience are a normal reaction to stress. The counselor can help provide you additional ways of dealing with stress.

For many years EMS providers participated in critical incident stress debriefings. A debriefing is a meeting held after a particularly traumatic call that brings providers together with peer counselors to talk about the event in an attempt to reduce stress.

Many organizations have stopped the debriefing process and instead now use the services of professional counselors. This was done because of the lack of research proving a benefit to the debriefing process.

Death and Dying

At some point in your time as an EMR, you will be called to a person who is near death or has died. It is a stark fact that patients die despite our best efforts.

Although we attempt to resuscitate patients who are not breathing and are without a pulse, there are some patients who simply cannot be saved. They may have injuries that are too serious, or they may have been without a pulse for too long to recover.

It is a difficult decision determining whether to resuscitate a patient or not. Some general signs a person is deceased and can't be resuscitated include:

- Tissue **decay** (peeling, decaying skin).
- **Rigor mortis** (stiffening of the joints which occurs after death). Note: Check more than one joint.
- Injuries that are obviously incompatible with recovery (for example, **decapitation**).

Follow established local protocols when making a decision whether to initiate care in patients with potential signs of obvious prolonged death.

ASK YOURSELF

■ What are the signs that a patient is dead and cannot be resuscitated?

decay degrading of the skin and organ systems.

rigor mortis stiffening of the muscles and joints after death.

decapitation injury causing separation of the head and neck.

ASK YOURSELF

- How would you describe each of the following stages of grief?
  - Denial
  - Anger
  - Bargaining
  - Depression
  - Acceptance

Dealing with Grief

Much like stress, the way individuals deal with death and dying is highly variable. Some may react with rage while others quietly withdraw. There are certain stages that both patients and families go through upon receiving news of a terminal condition—or that a relative goes through after learning of the death of a loved one. People do not necessarily go through the following stages in order, nor do all people necessarily go through all the stages. These stages include:

- Denial—The person denies the existence or seriousness of the condition or situation. This may range from denying the diagnosis of a disease to denying a loved one has actually died.

- Anger—The patient lashes out against the disease, or family members experience an outburst after the diagnosis or death of a loved one. In most cases the anger is not directed at EMS providers but you should always be alert and prepared in the event the anger does become physical toward you or others.

- Bargaining—Patients and families may try to make a deal with a higher power or even an EMS provider to extend life. Assure patients and family members that you and the entire system will do everything in your power to help them. Maintain a nonjudgmental attitude.

- Depression—Patients and family members at some point will react with sadness and grief. This may be seen as crying, sadness, or withdrawal from others. Understand that these too are normal reactions. Listen to the patient and assure him the feelings are normal.

- Acceptance—Although one might never truly accept impending death, the patient and family get to a point when they realize death is imminent. Many times the patient and family members will not arrive at this final stage at the same time. Listen to the patient and family members and maintain a nonjudgmental attitude in reference to anything that is said as people begin to cope with a pending tragedy.

Lifting and Moving Patients

Properly lifting and moving patients is part of maintaining your well-being. EMRs can become injured while lifting and moving patients. Back injuries caused by improperly lifting and moving patients can cause lifelong disability.

With proper decision making and techniques, you can safely lift and move patients. There are many situations in which you may be called upon to lift. Consider the following situations as you read this section. These events may all occur at the same call:

- You arrive at the scene and family members are yelling at you to hurry because the patient isn't responding to them. You need to carry your first-in kit, suction equipment, and automated defibrillator while hurrying to the patient's side.

- You arrive at the patient's side. He is slumped over in the chair and unresponsive. He is making gurgling noises as he breathes. You must move him to the floor to provide airway care and assessment.

- You are asked to stay and assist the ambulance crew by moving the stretcher and equipment to the ambulance.

Body Mechanics

body mechanics proper use of the body to lift.

Body mechanics is a term that describes the proper use of your body to lift. Lifting is a mechanical process and your body is the device that does the hard work. Something as

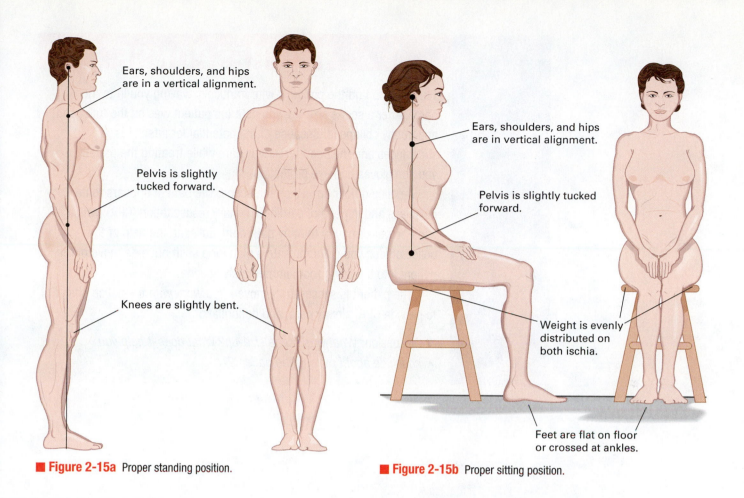

Figure 2-15a Proper standing position.

Ears, shoulders, and hips are in a vertical alignment.

Pelvis is slightly tucked forward.

Knees are slightly bent.

Figure 2-15b Proper sitting position.

Ears, shoulders, and hips are in vertical alignment.

Pelvis is slightly tucked forward.

Weight is evenly distributed on both ischia.

Feet are flat on floor or crossed at ankles.

simple as posture has a profound effect on your body and how it works (Figures 2-15a and 2-15b ■).

The following concepts comprise body mechanics:

- You should keep your back straight and in line. Maintain good posture (Figure 2-16 ■).
- Grip the person or object you are lifting firmly and securely (Figure 2-17 ■).
- Make sure you have good and solid footing. Keep your feet shoulder-width apart.
- Don't twist while you move.
- Communicate and coordinate with others who are assisting you in lifting.

Each situation you encounter will be unique. The amount of space you have available to you, the weight and size of the patient, and how much help you have will be a little different in each situation. Each time you must lift or move, you will look at all of these factors and make a decision on the best way to move the patient. As you size up the situation, you will consider the following:

- The approximate weight of the patient or item to be lifted
- The help you have available (if any)
- Your physical abilities and limitations in lifting and moving
- The physical space you will be lifting in (This may be a large living room, a tiny bedroom, or even a vehicle.)

ASK YOURSELF

- With a fellow student, can you demonstrate the use of good body mechanics when lifting?
- Given a scenario in which a patient must be moved or repositioned, can you explain the principles you will follow to move the patient with regard to both your safety and well-being and the patient's?

bariatric patient a patient who is extremely overweight or obese.

THE RESPONSE ✴

You arrive to find the patient's wife frantically waving you in to the home. After a scene size-up, you note the patient was on the toilet and apparently collapsed. Because of the potential for infectious substances and the need for airway care while treating the patient, you don gloves and eye protection.

A police officer arrives on the scene. The patient appears to be pulseless and in need of cardiopulmonary resuscitation (CPR), which can't be performed in the tiny bathroom. Enlisting the help of the police officer, you communicate a plan for a swift but safe move of the patient into the living room immediately outside.

The patient is successfully moved. You work with the police officer to provide CPR, airway care, and defibrillation.

■ Discussion: *What was scene size-up? What does it help you conclude about moving the patient?*

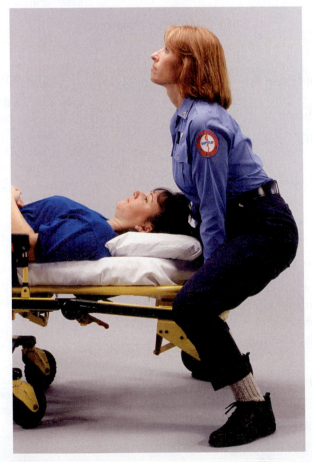

■ **Figure 2-16** Power lift.

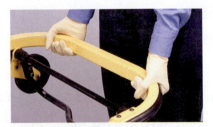

■ **Figure 2-17** Power grip.

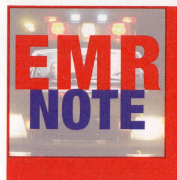
The Lift

Once you have sized up the scene and are about to make the move, you will place your feet approximately shoulder-width apart, grip the person or item to be lifted firmly, keep the weight in close to your body, and lift with your legs, not your back. Avoid lifting and twisting at the same time.

Just as there are ways of staying safe and uninjured during the lifting process, there are ways injury is more likely. These include:

- Twisting while lifting or moving
- Lifting without firm footing or a solid grip
- Lifting while reaching or stretching
- Lifting while the object or person is too far from your body
- Using your back to lift

Positioning Patients for Safety and Comfort

Now that you have learned to safely move patients, it is important to know *when* to use these procedures. There are times when you will need to move patients quickly, like when they are at risk of being burned in a fire. Other times the patient is safe where he is and can wait for the arrival of the ambulance before any movement occurs.

The decision on whether to physically move a patient is based on benefit versus risk. Your thinking for a patient with traumatic injuries may be, "If I move this patient it could further injure his spine . . . but if I don't the vehicle he is near could roll over on top of him." In this case, moving the patient would make sense since he is truly in danger. Most of the time the patient will be safe where he is and movement is not necessary.

There are two types of moves you will be called upon to make. These are referred to as emergent or **emergency moves** and **urgent moves**. The emergency move is for extreme conditions. The urgent move is done quickly, but it allows for some protection of the patient's spine to be taken.

Examples of situations that require emergency moves include:

- Fire or risk of fire or explosion
- Unstable vehicles or surfaces
- Cardiac arrest
- The need to access other patients (for example, in a motor vehicle crash you may need to move a patient to access a critically injured patient)

This is not an all-inclusive list. You will have to make decisions based on the situations you are presented with on any given call.

emergency moves
moves done in extreme, life-threatening conditions.

urgent moves moves done quickly but providing protection.

ASK YOURSELF

- What are some instances when you may need to use an emergency or urgent move to relocate or reposition a patient before additional help arrives?

long axis moving the patient while preserving the spine in-line position.

Since emergency moves must be done immediately, there usually is minimal equipment—and sometimes minimal help—available. Although these moves must be done quickly, there are ways to help protect the spine during the move. The most common—and practical—is moving the patient along what is known as the **long axis**. This means you move the patient so that the spine stays in a straight line, minimizing potential for injury. This is generally done by pulling or dragging from the shoulders, supporting the head when possible, so that the spine stays in line.

The firefighter's carry is shown in Scan 2-2. Figures 2-18a to 2-18h ■ show examples of other emergency moves including:

1. Shirt (clothing) drag
2. Sheet (or blanket) drag
3. Firefighter's drag
4. Cradle carry

At times, you will move patients because of their medical or traumatic condition. Earlier in this section, we discussed moving an unresponsive patient from a chair to the floor for airway care. This is an example of an urgent move.

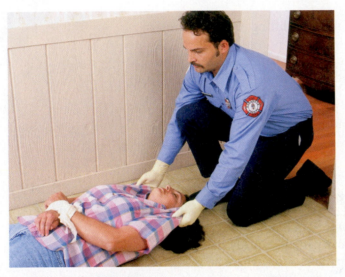

■ **Figure 2-18a** Shirt drag.

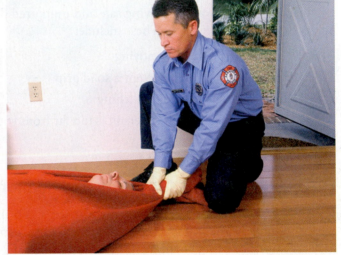

■ **Figure 2-18b** Blanket drag.

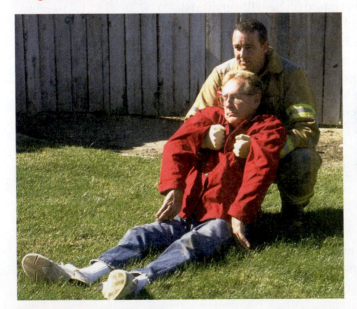

■ **Figure 2-18c** Shoulder drag.

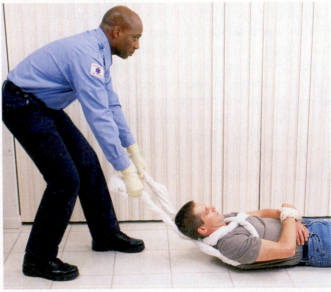

■ **Figure 2-18d** Sheet drag.

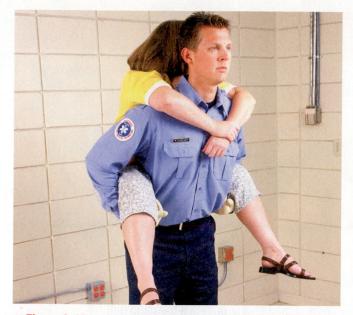

■ **Figure 2-18e** Piggyback carry.

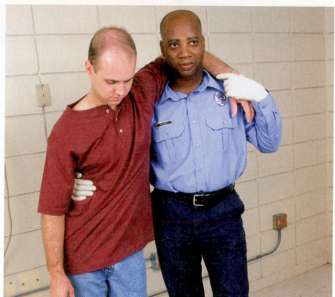

■ **Figure 2-18f** One-rescuer crutch.

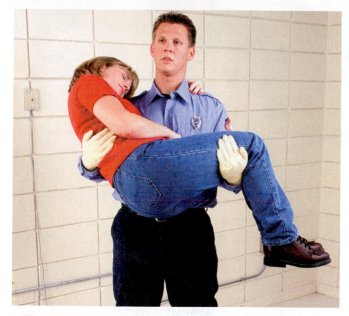

■ **Figure 2-18g** Cradle carry.

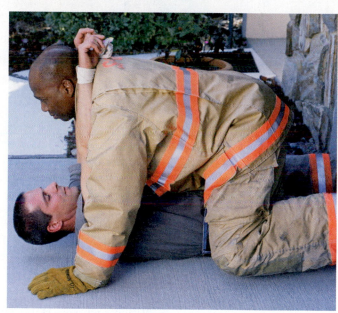

■ **Figure 2-18h** Firefighter's drag.

You will still provide spinal protection when possible. The urgent move allows a little more time for this than the emergency move. As the name implies it must be done promptly, but not with the haste of an emergency move.

The following are examples of when an urgent move would be performed:

- Positioning a patient for airway care or **inadequate breathing**
- Positioning a patient with an **altered mental status**
- Positioning a patient for treatment of **shock**
- Removing a patient from a situation that may worsen his condition (for example, moving a patient from snow or ice to avoid **hypothermia** and **frostbite**)

There are other general rules for positioning patients.

inadequate breathing
respiration pattern not consistent with life.

altered mental status disorientation of the senses.

shock inadequate perfusion of the body.

hypothermia decreased body temperature.

frostbite injury caused by extreme cold exposure.

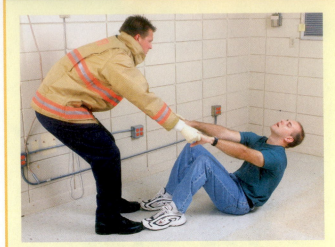

2-2a Grasp the patient's wrists.

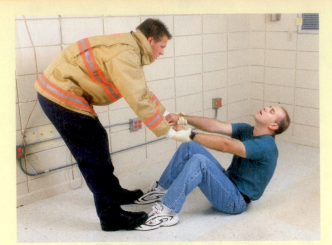

2-2b Stand on the patient's toes and pull.

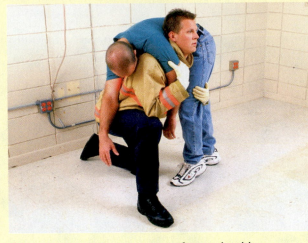

2-2c Put the patient over one of your shoulders.

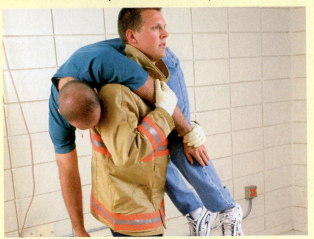

2-2d Pass an arm between the patient's legs and grasp the arm nearest to you.

Patients who are stable and alert can usually choose what is referred to as their "position of comfort." Patients who have breathing problems usually prefer to sit up—and this is best for them.

When patients are breathing adequately but are unresponsive, they are placed in the **recovery position**. This position is when the patient is placed on his side to prevent secretions from going down into the throat and lungs.

Patients who have traumatic injuries often are suspected of having damage to the spine. When possible these patients are placed in a **supine** position (flat on the back). You will help protect the spine by holding the patient's head in place and preventing movement. This is called cervical spine (c-spine) stabilization (Figure 2-19 ■).

Perform this stabilization by placing a gloved hand on each side of the patient's head. If the patient is conscious, advise him of what you will be doing and instruct him not to move his head.

Further information on caring for spine injuries will be discussed throughout this book.

recovery position   lying on left side to prevent inhalation of secretions.

supine   flat on back.

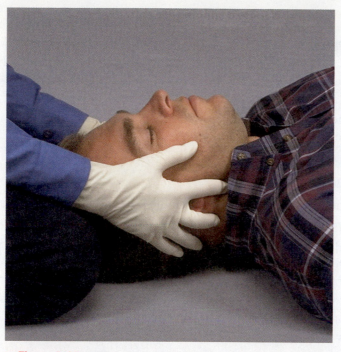

■ **Figure 2-19** Cervical spine stabilization.

✳ Stop, Review, Remember

Multiple Choice

Place a check next to the correct answer.

1. Which of the following statements about stress is true?

   ____ a. Calls involving multiple patients cause significant stress for all providers.

   ____ b. Two EMRs may respond to a serious call involving a pediatric patient differently.

   ____ c. EMRs are trained and expected not to experience stress on emergency calls.

   ____ d. Extreme stress helps all providers to function efficiently in an emergency.

2. Lifestyle changes to deal with stress include all of the following EXCEPT:

   ____ a. increasing caffeine intake.

   ____ b. reducing alcohol intake.

   ____ c. exercise.

   ____ d. relaxation techniques.

3. Which of the following is a sign of obvious death?

   ____ a. Two broken legs and a broken arm

   ____ b. A knife sticking out of a patient's chest

   ____ c. A patient who is unresponsive

   ____ d. A patient who sustained a severe head injury and whose brain can be seen

4. In the recovery position the patient is placed:

   ____ a. with the head lower than the legs.

   ____ b. with the legs raised.

   ____ c. on his side.

   ____ d. on his front (prone).

5. Which of the following is the main difference between an emergency move and an urgent move?

_____ a. Emergency moves are always done with spinal precautions.

_____ b. Urgent moves are performed when the patient is in immediate physical danger.

_____ c. Urgent moves allow a little more time for spinal precautions.

_____ d. Emergency moves are done when a patient has a compromised airway.

Emergency Medical Responder Practice

To move or not to move? For each patient in the following list, determine if he should be moved or left in place until the ambulance arrives.

1. Your patient was skateboarding and is on the sidewalk complaining of a broken leg.

_____

2. You arrive to find a car wrapped around a telephone pole. You only have access to the driver's side of the car. The driver is complaining of neck pain. The passenger is unresponsive and bleeding severely. Do you move the driver?

_____

3. Your patient is sitting in a chair and is not breathing.

_____

4. Your patient was ejected from a truck and is found lying in a dark roadway at night.

_____

5. Your patient is outside in the snow. EMS is more than 20 minutes away.

_____

Matching

You are providing care for family members and patients who are dealing with death and dying. Based on the following statements, match each with one of the stages of death and dying.

1. _____ Please, please. I'll give you anything to save him.

2. _____ If I can just see my granddaughter's wedding, I'll die peacefully.

3. _____ I don't think the diagnosis is correct. No one in my family gets cancer.

4. _____ Get out! Get out! Get out! I don't want any help.

5. _____ Excuse my wife. She is very upset. I'm tired and I've been fighting this for a long, long time.

6. _____ It can't be true. He's not dead. The doctor said he had 6 more months.

a. Denial
b. Anger
c. Bargaining
d. Depression
e. Acceptance

Patient Restraint

There are times when you may be called upon to participate in the restraint of a patient. Patients may require restraint for a variety of reasons ranging from psychiatric conditions to violence to medical conditions that cause dangerous behavior. No matter the exact reason, restraint is done for the protection of the patient and those around him.

ASK YOURSELF
- What are the basic principles of patient restraint?

It is most important to realize that your safety comes first. Restraint is a physical process and injury may occur. The legal right to restrain patients is granted by laws or regulations in your state. Your protocols may also provide guidance on when—or when not—to restrain a patient.

In most areas the right to restrain a patient and to have a patient taken against his will to a hospital for care lies with the police. Contacting medical direction for advice may also be beneficial—or even required in your area. Always follow your local protocols.

The process of restraint should be done in a careful, coordinated manner. Generally it is best to have four to five rescuers present to restrain a patient. Fewer may result in injuries to the patient or rescuers as more force may be required with fewer people. Too many rescuers can cause confusion and should be avoided.

The EMS provider in charge of the scene or the police officer will coordinate the restraint including providing assignments (for example, restraining lower extremities, calming the patient). Stay out of the patient's reach until all rescuers are ready to go.

When the order is given to move toward the patient, do so swiftly and decisively. Remember that restraint is designed only to control a person so he may get the treatment he needs. Restraint should never be violent or punitive. Calmly explain what you are doing each step of the way—even if the patient doesn't appear to understand what you say.

The patient should be brought carefully down to the ground or preferably onto a stretcher. The patient will then be secured using restraints. These may be commercially made devices or straps. You may also use items you have available, including cravats to restrain a patient's limbs.

Regardless of the restraints you choose, be sure they are soft and thick to prevent injury. Do not use rope, wire, or other thin items as they will cause injury if the patient continues to struggle against the restraints.

Always restrain patients face up. Patients who are placed face down are difficult to monitor. There have been situations where patients who have been placed face down or restrained forcefully have died during the restraint process. Monitor your restrained patient's airway, breathing, and circulation (ABCs) throughout your time with him. Be sure the patient is breathing adequately at all times. A sudden change in a patient's condition (for example, suddenly quiet after fighting against the restraints) may be an indication the patient's condition has deteriorated. If there is a sudden change in the patient's condition, immediately reassess the ABCs and initiate care as indicated (such as bag-valve-mask ventilation for the patient who has suddenly stopped breathing after being restrained).

Remember that the patient has a medical or psychiatric condition that requires your assessment and care. Provide that care as you would for any patient. Deliver oxygen if necessary and obtain vital signs. If you are normally required to provide written documentation of your patient care, be careful to document both the reasons for the restraint and that you carefully monitored the patient at all times after the patient was restrained.

TRANSITION ✳

EMS arrives and observes you performing CPR. You advise them of how the patient was found and moved. You estimate, based on the wife's account, the patient has been down for about 4–5 minutes. You advise them of the care you have provided and offer to continue to help at the scene, for which the EMS crew is grateful.

■ **Discussion:** *This case study doesn't discuss the outcome for the patient. What do you think happened after you gave a verbal report? What else must you do to document the case?*

THE LAST WORD

There is nothing more important than keeping safe and healthy while you are providing EMS care. You can't help if you are sick or injured, and the consequences of injuries that occur while providing EMS are lifelong.

The topics in this chapter were wide-ranging but important. Remember to adequately protect yourself from disease, remain safe when dealing with scene hazards, and recognize the stresses that you, your patients, and family members feel.

Finally, remember that lifting and moving patients and helping with patient restraint are big responsibilities. There are clinical implications as well as a direct impact on the safety of both you and your patient.

✳ Chapter Review

Multiple Choice

Place a check next to the correct answer.

1. Which of the following is usually not a sign of stress in the EMR?

   _____ a. Irritability

   _____ b. Loss of appetite

   _____ c. Making decisions rapidly

   _____ d. Difficulty sleeping

2. Which of the following is not recommended as a method of dealing with stress in EMS?

   _____ a. Exercise

   _____ b. Relaxation techniques

   _____ c. Speaking with a counselor

   _____ d. Going out drinking with colleagues

3. A pathogen is a:

   _____ a. scientific test for a disease.

   _____ b. method of protection against a disease.

   _____ c. disease-causing organism.

   _____ d. sign or symptom of a disease.

4. One method to prevent disease that can be taken before the call is:

   _____ a. assuming all patients in "bad" sections of town are likely to carry infectious diseases.

   _____ b. getting vaccinations.

   _____ c. wearing gloves whenever you are in the station or rescue vehicle.

   _____ d. getting a tuberculosis test.

5. The appropriate personal protective device you should wear when you suspect a patient has tuberculosis is:

_____ a. a HEPA or N95 mask.

_____ b. a surgical mask.

_____ c. a face shield/surgical mask combination.

_____ d. none of the above. You do not need to wear protection; put a surgical mask on the patient.

6. A gown would most likely be worn in which of the following calls?

_____ a. A conscious man experiencing a heart attack

_____ b. A child who fell and has a wound on her leg with steady flowing blood

_____ c. A patient who requires suction

_____ d. A woman about to give birth

7. Which of the following is not a sign of obvious death where resuscitation should not be initiated?

_____ a. Absent pulse

_____ b. Decapitation

_____ c. Tissue decay

_____ d. Rigor mortis

8. The stages of death and dying include all of the following except:

_____ a. denial.

_____ b. acceptance.

_____ c. depression.

_____ d. mortality.

9. Body mechanics refers to:

_____ a. how your body is used to lift.

_____ b. using mechanical devices to lift patients' bodies.

_____ c. knowledge of the working of muscles and bones in the body.

_____ d. lifting with your legs, not your back.

10. Which of the following is a procedure you should follow while lifting?

_____ a. Keep the weight as far from your body as possible.

_____ b. Lift with the strong muscles of your back.

_____ c. Consider the weight you are lifting before you lift.

_____ d. Spread your legs as far apart as they will comfortably go to lower your center of gravity.

Emergency Medical Responder Practice

For each of the following situations, determine whether the patient would require no move, an urgent move, or an emergency move.

1. You encounter a patient in a car that is on fire.

_____

2. You find a patient without a pulse and not breathing in bed.

_____

3. You find a patient who hurt his leg skateboarding. He is in the traffic lane of a busy highway.

_____

4. You find a patient who has difficulty breathing sitting on a park bench.

_____

5. You observe a patient in a vehicle that was involved in a crash. He is unresponsive and has blood in his mouth that appears to be flowing back to his throat.

_____

6. You are treating a patient you encounter on a camping trip. He appears to have a heat emergency and is out in the hot sun.

_____

Short Answer

1. List three things you should consider before lifting a patient.

_____

_____

_____

2. Explain the term "Standard Precautions."

_____

_____

_____

3. List the five stages of death and dying.

_____

_____

_____

4. Explain what is meant by long axis drag.

_____

_____

_____

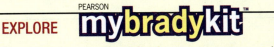

EXPLORE PEARSON **mybradykit**™

Please go to **www.bradybooks.com** to access mykit for this text. You will find quizzes, critical thinking scenarios, weblinks, animations, and videos related to this chapter— and much more. Look for online information on stress management as well as a video clip on transmission and treatment for AIDs.

Register your access code from the front of your book by going to **www.bradybooks.com** and selecting the mykit links.

Medical, Legal, and Ethical Issues

NAVIGATION GUIDE

The following items provide an overview to the purpose and content of this chapter. The Education Standards and Competencies are from the National EMS Education Standards.

Education Standards Preparatory (Medical/Legal and Ethics); Public Health

Competencies Uses simple knowledge of the EMS system, safety/well-being of the EMR, medical/legal issues at the scene of an emergency while awaiting a higher level of care.

Has an awareness of local public health resources and the role EMS personnel play in public health emergencies.

Knowledge Area Medical/Legal and Ethics
- Consent/refusal of care
- Confidentiality
- Advance directives
- Tort and criminal actions
- Evidence preservation
- Statutory responsibilities
- Mandatory reporting
- Ethical principles/moral obligations
- End-of-life issues

Objectives After reading this chapter, you should be able to:

1. Define key terms introduced in this chapter.
2. Explain the importance to EMRs of understanding the legal and ethical aspects of emergency medical care.
3. Differentiate between actions that are within the EMR's scope of practice and those that are not.
4. Explain the importance of only providing emergency medical care that is within your scope of practice.
5. Explain the importance of medical oversight in EMS systems.
6. Give examples of off-line and on-line medical oversight.
7. Explain the components required in order to obtain expressed consent.
8. Predict potential consequences of failing to obtain the proper type of consent to provide emergency medical care.

NAVIGATION GUIDE *(continued)*

9. Given a patient care scenario, identify the type of consent that applies to the situation.
10. Describe the actions that you should and should not take when a patient refuses your care.
11. Differentiate between situations in which you can and cannot share a patient's protected health information with someone else.
12. Explain the EMR's obligations with respect to advance directives.
13. Given a scenario involving a health care provider's interactions with a patient, identify potential ethical issues in the situation.
14. Give examples of actions or inactions that can lead to specific types of tort claims.
15. Describe how EMRs can provide patient care while minimizing disruption of crime scenes and destruction of evidence.
16. Give examples of situations in which EMRs may be required to make a mandatory report to law enforcement or other authorities.

Key Terms Page references indicate first major use in this chapter. The Margin Glossary in this chapter provides definitions as you read.

scope of practice p. 53
protocols p. 53
off-line medical direction p. 53
on-line medical direction p. 53
expressed consent p. 54
implied consent p. 54
emancipated minor p.54
refusal of care p. 54
patient refusal p. 54

Health Insurance Portability and Accountability Act (HIPAA) p. 57
advance directives p. 59
do not resuscitate order p. 59
living will p. 60
durable power of attorney p. 60
health care proxy p. 61
ethics p. 61

tort p. 62
assault p. 62
battery p. 62
abandonment p. 62
negligence p. 62
duty to act p. 62
breach of duty p. 62
proximate causation p. 62

Media Resources Please go to **www.bradybooks.com** to access mykit for this text. You will find quizzes, critical thinking scenarios, weblinks, animations, and videos related to this chapter—and much more. Look for online information on HIPAA and organ donation.

INTRODUCTION

As you practice as an EMR, most everything you do has a foundation in legal or ethical guidelines. This chapter will explain these important concepts and how to apply them while protecting you and helping your patient.

CASE STUDY

THE CALL ✳

Your emergency medical response unit is called to 1426 Abercrombie Circle for a man who "doesn't feel well." The dispatcher advises that the man has been feeling weak and nauseous for about 2 hours.

■ Discussion: *What else would you like to know about this patient from the dispatcher?*

Providing Legal and Ethical Care

From the moment you approach a patient to begin care prior to the handoff to the EMTs, legal and ethical considerations weave their way into your care and decision making. Consider the following scenarios and questions as you read this section:

- You are called to a sick man. You approach him and identify yourself as an Emergency Medical Responder. Do you need his permission to help him?

- You are called to a scene where a child is having an allergic reaction. A babysitter asks if you can give the child a shot to make him better. What do you say?

- You arrive at the scene of a call. There is a man on the couch who appears lifeless. A family member says, "Please don't do anything. He has cancer. Let him die in peace." What do you do?

- You are out with friends after work. They saw you on the highway at a car crash earlier. "What happened?" they ask. Can you tell them?

Each of the preceding points involves a legal or ethical issue that the EMR must deal with successfully. This section will describe in detail how to handle these issues in the field.

Scope of Practice

A **scope of practice** is the set of rules, regulations, and laws that designate how you legally function as an EMR.

In some states there is one state law that defines how you practice (the assessments, skills, and interventions you are allowed to perform). Other areas may have regulations at the state level, but agencies at the regional, county, or local level also contribute to the scope of practice.

As the name of this chapter implies, the EMR has duties in medical, legal, and ethical areas. Medically you have a responsibility to provide care to your patient not only to the best of your abilities, but to standards and expectations of your EMS system and current medical practice.

When you respond to a call you are likely governed by **protocols**. Protocols are written guidelines or instructions that describe appropriate assessment and care in specific situations. You may have a protocol that tells you which patients should receive oxygen or that provides care guidelines when treating patients who are having an allergic reaction.

Medical Oversight

Your system's medical director plays a vital role in ensuring the delivery of high-quality patient care. Your medical director may be responsible for developing the protocols that guide your practice. These protocols are also referred to as **off-line medical direction** because they are written. You do not need to personally contact a physician for these instructions.

There are times, however, when you will call a physician for instructions or advice on a call. When you receive orders over the radio or phone this is called **on-line medical direction**. You may contact on-line medical direction for specific advice on treating a patient or assistance with patient refusal or other on-scene issues.

Consent

Simply stated, you need permission to assess and care for a patient. Of course nothing is as simple as it seems. There are actually several different types of consent.

ASK YOURSELF

- Can you define key terms introduced in this chapter?

- Why is it important to understand the legal and ethical aspects of emergency medical care?

- How do you differentiate between actions that are within the EMR's scope of practice and those that are not?

- What is the importance of only providing emergency medical care that is within your scope of practice?

- What is the importance of medical oversight in EMS systems?

- What are some examples of off-line and on-line medical oversight?

- What are the components required in order to obtain expressed consent?

scope of practice rules, regulations, and laws that designate how you legally function.

protocols written guidelines or instructions describing assessment and care.

off-line medical direction written physician orders directing care and assessment based on a general set of signs and symptoms.

on-line medical direction physician orders received specific to an active patient's signs and symptoms.

expressed consent when a patient gives permission for care.

implied consent assuming permission of an unresponsive patient requiring care.

emancipated minor a minor who may receive the rights of an adult.

refusal of care patient not permitting care.

patient refusal see *refusal of care.*

ASK YOURSELF

■ What are the potential consequences of failing to obtain the proper type of consent to provide emergency medical care?

■ Given a patient care scenario, how can you determine the type of consent that applies to the situation?

■ What are the actions that you should and should not take when a patient refuses your care?

Expressed consent is when a patient gives permission for care. In order to do this the patient must be old enough (usually 18 years of age), have the mental capacity necessary to make the decision, and not be impaired by alcohol, drugs, or the effects of injury or illness. If the patient does have any of these conditions, he may not legally be able to give consent.

Determining if a patient is capable of making a decision is challenging. The EMTs or Paramedics on the ambulance will be able to help with this decision as will medical direction if necessary. Generally a person who is competent understands the nature of his condition and the consequences of not seeking help. This is also known as understanding the risks versus benefits of care.

If a patient is unresponsive due to a medical or traumatic condition, you may begin care based on the principle of **implied consent**. The law allows us to assume the patient would consent if he were able.

During your time as an EMR, you will also be called to treat pediatric patients. As mentioned earlier, pediatric patients are not able to consent to care on their own. The law gives this right to the parent of the child until the child turns 18. This is sometimes referred to as parental control. If a parent is present on an emergency scene, you will ask the parent if it is OK to assess and treat the child.

Other situations may arise such as a child at a day care center where a form is on file that grants consent for emergencies. If a child becomes ill or injured in a location where a parent is not present, seek to immediately contact the parents through the dispatcher or cell phone. Do not delay lifesaving care if a parent isn't immediately available.

Some pediatric patients may be **emancipated minors**. This means that a court has ruled they are legally considered to have the rights of an adult. This may be a formal court order or may be allowed in some areas if minors are married, are pregnant, have children themselves, or are in military service. Emancipated minors would be allowed to give consent for their own care.

Refusal of Care

You must receive a patient's consent to provide any assessment and care. In most cases patients will consent and allow you to help. There will be times when a patient will not. This is called **refusal of care** or **patient refusal** (Figure 3-1 ■).

Patients have the right to refuse assessment and/or care as long as they meet specific criteria—criteria that are essentially the same as for consent: the patient must be

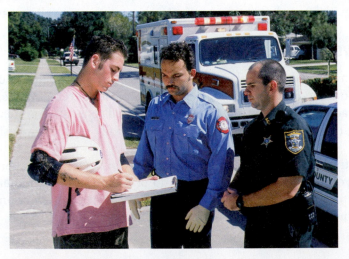

■ **Figure 3-1** There must be a witness when a patient signs a refusal of care form.

an adult, able to understand the consequences of refusal, and able to make an informed decision.

Patients may accept your assessment but then later refuse transportation to the hospital when the EMTs arrive. In this case the EMTs would document the refusal of transport. You would not document a refusal since the patient accepted your care on scene.

If a patient decides to refuse your assessment or care, you must advise him of the risks of doing so. In most cases this includes worsening of the condition or injury, and in some cases unconsciousness and death. Complete your documentation by noting any observations and assessments you have performed, efforts you have taken to attempt to convince the patient to accept care, and that the patient was told he could call back at any time if he feels the need.

Some agencies have a specific form to be used in the event of patient refusal (Figure 3-2 ■).

This often includes a checklist of steps to perform and a place for the patient to sign indicating that he has refused care and/or transport. This signature must usually be witnessed by a party other than the patient (Figure 3-3 ■). Many systems recommend the use of a police officer, firefighter, or other official at the scene when possible.

Many systems require you to contact medical direction or to wait for the ambulance before leaving the scene.

Patient refusals are a significant cause of liability against EMS providers. Patients who refuse care may sue the personnel who were at the scene if their condition worsens. There are certain situations where the patient should not be allowed to refuse care. These include:

- Patients who have an altered mental status. This might be anything from the patient appearing confused or lethargic to unresponsive.
- Patients who have ingested alcohol or drugs.
- Patients who may have judgment impaired by their condition (such as pain or lack of oxygen).

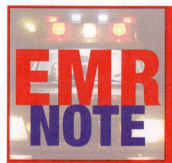

Patients may refuse care even though it would be in their best interest to accept care and transportation to the hospital. This is done for a number of reasons including fear, denial, and concern over the cost of care and transportation.

You should attempt to convince your patient to accept care and transportation. Determining why the patient may be refusing will help you overcome the resistance to care.

- If the patient appears to be afraid or in denial, you may be able to have a friend or family member convince him to accept your care.
- When the patient is concerned about cost, explain to him it may actually be more expensive later when the condition gets worse.
- In all cases, explain the consequences of not accepting care. If the patient appears to have a serious illness or injury, be frank with the patient; the condition could be fatal.

EMS PATIENT REFUSAL CHECKLIST

PATIENT'S NAME: _____ AGE: _____

LOCATION OF CALL: _____ DATE: _____

AGENCY INCIDENT #: _____ AGENCY CODE: _____

NAME OF PERSON FILLING OUT FORM: _____

I.   ASSESSMENT OF PATIENT (Check appropriate response for each item)

    1.   Oriented to: Person? ☐ Yes ☐ No
                                  Place? ☐ Yes ☐ No
                                  Time? ☐ Yes ☐ No
                                  Situation? ☐ Yes ☐ No

    2.   Altered level of consciousness? ☐ Yes ☐ No

    3.   Head injury? ☐ Yes ☐ No

    4.   Alcohol or drug ingestion by exam or history? ☐ Yes ☐ No

II.   PATIENT INFORMED (Check appropriate response for each item)

☐ Yes ☐ No   Medical treatment/evaluation needed

☐ Yes ☐ No   Ambulance transport needed

☐ Yes ☐ No   Further harm could result without medical treatment/evaluation

☐ Yes ☐ No   Transport by means other than ambulance could be hazardous in light of patient's illness/injury

☐ Yes ☐ No   Patient provided with Refusal Information Sheet

☐ Yes ☐ No   Patient accepted Refusal Information Sheet

III. DISPOSITION

☐ Refused all EMS assistance

☐ Refused field treatment, but accepted transport

☐ Refused transport, but accepted field treatment

☐ Refused transport to recommended facility

☐ Patient transported by private vehicle to _____

☐ Released in care or custody of self

☐ Released in care or custody of relative or friend

    Name: _____ Relationship: _____

☐ Released in custody of law enforcement agency

    Agency: _____ Officer: _____

☐ Released in custody of other agency

    Agency: _____ Officer: _____

IV.   COMMENTS: _____

_____

_____

_____

■ **Figure 3-2** A patient refusal form.

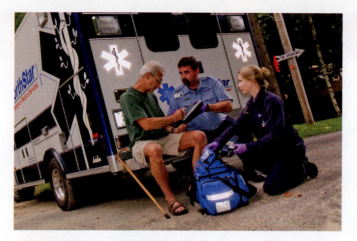

■ **Figure 3-3** EMRs and EMTs may work a refusal scenario together.

While these conditions do not legally give you a right to force a patient to accept your care, if you are later sued, the patient will not be considered capable of refusing care. This is a dilemma faced frequently by EMS providers in the field.

In this situation make sure the ambulance responds to the scene. Do not cancel them. You may also seek the assistance of the police as well as that of medical direction via cell phone or radio.

Confidentiality

When you respond to a home, an office, or even the highway for a call you will find patients who need your care. They will tell you what is wrong and divulge their medical history. You will get a glimpse into their life. These patients depend on you for their medical care—and to maintain the strictest confidence of what you see, hear, and do.

There are laws regarding confidentiality, the most significant of which is the **Health Insurance Portability and Accountability Act** (more commonly known as **HIPAA**). This law identifies protected health information (PHI) which cannot be disclosed to others except in certain situations. The PHI includes anything that identifies the patient and anything that relates to the assessment and care of the patient. This confidentiality includes anything you see (including written medical histories and medications) and hear.

The penalties for violation of the act are severe.

There are times when it is acceptable to disclose protected health information. These include:

- Transferring relevant and pertinent information to others directly involved in the patient's care
- Upon patient approval to insurers and those responsible for payment
- Operational reasons within EMS agencies including quality improvement and research
- Mandatory reporting situations such as crimes of violence, abuse, or public health situations (for example, a contagious disease outbreak)
- When required to do so by legal subpoena

ASK YOURSELF

■ How do you differentiate situations in which you can and cannot share a patient's protected health information with someone else?

Health Insurance Portability and Accountability Act (HIPAA) law regarding confidentiality of protected health information.

Multiple Choice

Place a check next to the correct answer.

1. Rules and regulations that are set to designate how an emergency responder can legally function are called:

   ____ a. on-line medical control.

   ____ b. off-line medical control.

   ____ c. protocols.

   ____ d. scope of practice.

2. Written orders that are established by a physician for the purpose of guiding your practice are referred to as:

   ____ a. on-line medical control.

   ____ b. off-line medical control.

   ____ c. protocols.

   ____ d. scope of practice.

3. An unconscious patient involved in a motor vehicle collision is able to be treated under:

   ____ a. expressed consent.

   ____ b. implied consent.

   ____ c. emancipated consent.

   ____ d. written consent.

4. Protected health information (PHI) may be disclosed to all of the following except:

   ____ a. the transporting ambulance.

   ____ b. quality improvement (QI) research forms.

   ____ c. the finance department for billing.

   ____ d. various agency members.

5. A lawyer visits your ambulance station. He states that the court has issued a subpoena for one of your patient care run reports but he doesn't have a copy of the subpoena for you to see. In this case, you should:

   ____ a. give him the report.

   ____ b. shut the door without saying a word.

   ____ c. call the police to report him for trespassing.

   ____ d. request he return later with the actual document.

Matching

Match the following descriptions with the appropriate term.

1. _____ Permission for care given directly by the patient

2. _____ Patient who the court has ruled may legally have the rights of an adult regardless of the patient's age

3. _____ Physician orders or advice received via cell phone or radio while on a call

4. _____ Information that relates to a particular patient or the patient's assessment and care

5. _____ Written guidelines that describe appropriate assessment and care in specific situations

6. _____ Permission for care that is given on the assumption the injured person would want lifesaving care to be provided

a. Scope of practice

b. Protocols

c. On-line medical control

d. Expressed consent

e. Implied consent

f. Emancipated minor

g. Patient refusal

h. Protected health information

7. _____ Term describing a patient's wishes to receive no assessment or treatment

8. _____ Rules and regulations that govern how you will legally function as an EMR

Case Study

You arrive at a standby for an apartment fire. The ambulance is en route but still a distance away. The fire chief brings you a 17-year-old female and her 1-year-old son. They both are displaying symptoms of smoke inhalation and are conscious, alert, and crying. The female states she doesn't want to be evaluated because they are waiting for her husband to get home and she doesn't want to miss him arriving.

1. Is she in a position to legally consent for her own care and why?

_____

_____

_____

_____

2. Is she in a position to legally consent for the care of her child and why?

_____

_____

_____

_____

3. If she were allowed to refuse care, who would be best suited to witness the refusal signatures?

_____ a. Fire chief

_____ b. Patient's husband

_____ c. Patient's son

_____ d. You

Advance Directives

Advance directives are legal documents that either provide instruction on a patient's medical decisions (for example, whether CPR should be performed) or appoint a person to make that decision in the event the patient is unable to do so.

The directive most commonly applicable in the field is the **do not resuscitate order**, also called a DNR or DNAR (Do not attempt to resuscitate order) (Figure 3-4 ■). This order is requested by a patient and is signed by a physician when the resuscitation is unlikely to succeed or if it would only temporarily extend life and while doing so cause unnecessary suffering and disability.

DNR orders are most commonly seen in chronic conditions such as cancer. Patients and families are instructed to keep the order available to show EMS providers who respond to the scene. You should quickly check the order to be sure it applies to the patient in question, is valid and unexpired, and is signed by a physician. Note that DNR orders may have specific instructions for resuscitation (for example, no advanced airways or feeding tubes). Make sure it applies to the care you would provide the patient.

advance directives legal documents giving a person's instructions on medical decisions.

do not resuscitate order written document of a patient requesting cardiac resuscitation not be performed.

ASK YOURSELF

- What are the EMR's obligations with respect to advance directives?

PREHOSPITAL DO NOT RESUSCITATE ORDERS

ATTENDING PHYSICIAN

In completing this prehospital DNR form, please check part A if no intervention by prehospital personnel is indicated. Please check Part A and options from Part B if specific interventions by prehospital personnel are indicated. To give a valid prehospital DNR order, this form must be completed by the patient's attending physician and must be provided to prehospital personnel.

A) _____ **Do Not Resuscitate (DNR):**
No Cardiopulmonary Resuscitation or Advanced Cardiac Life Support be performed by prehospital personnel

B) _____ **Modified Support:**
Prehospital personnel administer the following checked options:
_____Oxygen administration
_____Full airway support: intubation, airways, bag/valve/mask
_____Venipuncture: IV crystalloids and/or blood draw
_____External cardiac pacing
_____Cardiopulmonary resuscitation
_____Cardiac defibrillator
_____Pneumatic anti-shock garment
_____Ventilator
_____ACLS meds
_____Other interventions/medications (physician specify)
_____

Prehospital personnel are informed that (print patient name)_____
should receive no resuscitation (DNR) or should receive Modified Support as indicated. This directive is medically appropriate and is further documented by a physician's order and a progress note on the patient's permanent medical record. Informed consent from the capacitated patient or the incapacitated patient's legitimate surrogate is documented on the patient's permanent medical record. The DNR order is in full force and effect as of the date indicated below.

_____   _____

Attending Physician's Signature   _____

_____   _____

Print Attending Physician's Name   Print Patient's Name and Location
                                          (Home Address or Health Care Facility)

_____

Attending Physician's Telephone

_____   _____

Date   Expiration Date (6 Mos from Signature)

■ **Figure 3-4** An example of an advance directive.

living will legal document created in advance in the event a person in unable to communicate their health care wishes at a time of injury or illness.

durable power of attorney document designating a legal decision maker.

You may ask why someone would call for EMS if the patient isn't supposed to be resuscitated. It is actually a common occurrence because families are nervous and not prepared for the death of their loved one. Because of this, your compassion when examining the DNR and dealing with these family members is very important.

If the DNR order is expired or does not seem to apply, you should begin appropriate care or resuscitation.

There are other types of legal documents you may see. These include **living wills** and **durable power of attorney**.

A living will is a document that provides directives as to the patient's wishes in regard to medical care in the event the patient isn't able to state them. The difference between a

DNR and a living will is that the living will can be created by anyone in any medical condition. The DNR is only created when a medical condition creates a futile situation where resuscitation will not work.

A durable power of attorney designates a surrogate decision maker if a person suddenly becomes incapacitated. The power of attorney is a legal document that can designate a person to act in a variety of settings from financial to health care. The **health care proxy** is another document, similar to a power of attorney, that assigns decision-making capabilities for health care decisions only.

Many areas do not allow EMS personnel to act based on living wills, power of attorney, or health care proxies when at the scene of a patient who is unable to speak for himself and requires care and/or resuscitation. Follow your local protocols.

health care proxy
document designating a legal decision maker for medical decisions.

CASE STUDY

THE RESPONSE

You arrive to find the scene safe. The patient appears to have vomited, so you don gloves and eye protection and introduce yourself. The man says, "My *wife* called for you. I didn't. I don't want to go to the hospital." He seems to be in some distress and may have some difficulty breathing.

You tell the patient that you are an Emergency Medical Responder and are here to help before the ambulance arrives. He agrees to your assessment while you wait for the ambulance. You notice that the patient's skin is pale, moist, and cool. You know these are not good signs.

You place him on some oxygen. He protests a bit but eventually agrees. Then you begin to take a history and get vital signs while you wait for the ambulance.

■ Discussion: *Why is pale, moist, and cool skin not a good sign?*

Ethics

The practice of EMS must be based on science and law. These are relatively easy to define. But EMS must also be practiced ethically. Ethical principles are a bit trickier to define.

Some define **ethics** with examples of things that an EMR shouldn't do: Don't steal from patients or treat them unkindly. Others use examples of things an EMR should do: Treat patients as you would want to be treated.

Ethics are based on morals. Morals are attitudes based on the concept of right and wrong. This compass should be foremost in your mind when making decisions and dealing with patients, family, and other medical personnel. The following traits are also important in an ethical approach to EMS:

Honesty—being truthful with patients and hospital staff and in documentation/reporting

Kindness and compassion—treating patients as you would want to be treated

Advocacy—helping patients solve problems or be heard when they cannot do it themselves

Patients who feel they have been well taken care of (treated respectfully and listened to) usually rate their medical care higher and are less likely to bring a lawsuit against someone who provided emergency care to them.

ethics   moral judgments.

ASK YOURSELF

■ Given a scenario involving a health care provider's interactions with a patient, how do you identify potential ethical issues in the situation?

Liability and Negligence

While it is rare, you could be sued as a result of your actions as an Emergency Medical Responder. This section details the legal processes involved in a lawsuit and how to reduce the risk of being sued.

A **tort** is a wrongdoing for which a legal action can be brought to court for damages. A tort is a civil (as opposed to criminal) wrongdoing. Criminal charges are even more rare against EMS providers. The most common are for **assault** or **battery**. These would most commonly be charged for treating or transporting a patient against his will.

There are two main areas that EMS providers are exposed to liability: abandonment and negligence.

Abandonment is when you leave a patient after providing care without turning that patient over to another provider or medical professional of equal or greater certification or licensure. Never leave a patient without ensuring quality and continuing care.

Negligence is defined as failing to follow a standard of care, which causes or worsens the patient's injuries or conditions. The injuries may be physical or emotional. There are four elements required to prove negligence:

1. The provider had a **duty to act**. This means that the provider was required to perform care by law or because of job duties or expectations. An EMR who is paid for his time (such as a firefighter or police officer) or is in an on-duty status as a volunteer would have a duty to act.
2. There was a **breach of duty**, which could be a failure to perform a required assessment or treatment or performing an action incorrectly.
3. Harm was caused to the patient. This harm may be physical or psychological.
4. **Proximate causation** means that the harm was caused by action or inaction of the EMR.

As mentioned earlier, lawsuits are rare—and most can be prevented. Acting in good faith and in the patient's best interest are crucial. To prevent lawsuits:

- Treat people with kindness and respect.
- Follow your local protocols.
- Document activities and events thoroughly on your run report form.

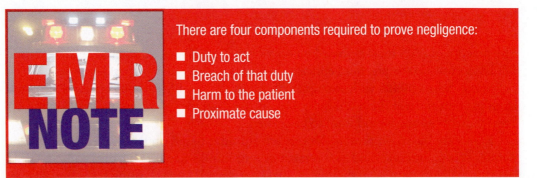

EMR NOTE

There are four components required to prove negligence:
- Duty to act
- Breach of that duty
- Harm to the patient
- Proximate cause

Consider the following situations. Do you think the four components of negligence are met?

1. You are carrying a patient from a bedroom to the living room. You accidentally drop the patient and he breaks his wrist.
2. You are called for an unresponsive man. You arrive to find him in cardiac arrest. You do CPR prior to the arrival of the ambulance but the man dies.
3. You are called to a patient who doesn't feel well. You examine the patient while you wait for the EMTs. He decides he doesn't want to go to the hospital. He doesn't go and dies a short time later from a heart attack.

---

tort a legal wrongdoing.

assault the threat or act of physical harm.

battery unlawful touching of a person.

abandonment leaving a patient after beginning the provision of care.

negligence failure to follow a standard of care.

duty to act legal requirement to perform care.

breach of duty failure to perform or incorrectly performing an action.

proximate causation harm caused by the action or inaction of a provider.

ASK YOURSELF

- What are some examples of actions or inactions that can lead to specific types of tort claims?
- How can EMRs provide patient care while minimizing disruption of crime scenes and destruction of evidence?
- What are examples of situations in which EMRs may be required to make a mandatory report to law enforcement or other authorities?

In the first case, depending on the circumstances, an argument could be made that the EMR was negligent. You learned how to safely move patients in the previous chapter. In the second case, there is no basis for negligence because the patient's death was caused by a medical condition and not an action or inaction by the EMR.

The third case could go either way depending on the actions and documentation of the EMR. The EMR would have to explain the risks of refusal and ensure the patient was competent to refuse care. Documentation of these facts is crucial—and predictive of the potential outcome of a lawsuit.

The conclusion of this section is a good place to mention the Latin phrase *primum non nocere,* which means "first do no harm." It refers to a fundamental tenet of medicine: that we should care for our patients and while doing so should never do harm. In more modern terms, it is always best to turn your patients over to the EMTs or the hospital in better shape than you found them.

✳ Stop, Review, Remember

Multiple Choice

Place a check next to the correct answer.

1. Patients can possess multiple legal documents outlining their wishes should they be unable to speak for themselves. Which document provides the medical decision-making responsibilities to another person?

   _____ a. Living will

   _____ b. Do not resuscitate order

   _____ c. Health care proxy

   _____ d. Power of attorney

2. Do not resuscitate orders are considered valid if they are unexpired and:

   _____ a. signed by a physician.

   _____ b. signed by the patient.

   _____ c. signed by an attorney.

   _____ d. signed by a nurse.

3. Treating patients as you would want to be treated is an example of:

   _____ a. negligence.

   _____ b. proximate causation.

   _____ c. ethics.

   _____ d. tort.

4. Treating a patient against his will and then transporting him is considered to be:

   _____ a. abandonment.

   _____ b. assault or battery.

   _____ c. negligence.

   _____ d. breach of duty.

5. A patient that is injured further because an EMR was unable to properly and safely operate a stretcher can be considered to have _____ against the EMR.

   _____ a. breach of duty

   _____ b. proximate causation

   _____ c. abandonment

   _____ d. ethics violation

True/False

Mark whether each of the following statements is true (T) or false (F).

1. _____ Not completing a portion of your required care because you don't feel like taking time to fully complete it is a breach of duty.

2. _____ A responder who is working in a given area is able to decide which calls for assistance he will answer and which he will ignore.

3. _____ A wrongdoing that can bring legal action upon someone is considered a causation.

4. _____ Good ethics are based upon the person possessing good morals.

5. _____ Do not resuscitate orders are widely accepted in the prehospital environment.

Case Study

Fred, an EMR, responds to the scene of a call for assistance. The police have secured a male who assaulted his wife. The man is requesting evaluation for injuries that he received. Fred doesn't feel that he is injured and wishes to refuse to provide him care.

1. What type of violation resulting in liability has Fred committed? Explain why.

   _____

   _____

   _____

   Fred thinks the situation through further and decides to treat the man. In retaliation for the things he has done, Fred decides to improperly care for his wounds and cause him further injury and discomfort.

2. What type of violation resulting in liability is this, and why?

   _____

   _____

   _____

   Fred again has a change of heart and decides he doesn't want to treat his patient anymore. He walks away to his vehicle and leaves the scene without completing his care or any documentation.

3. What type of violation resulting in liability is this, and why?

   _____

   _____

   _____

EMS at the Crime Scene

At some point you will provide care at the scene of a crime. This crime may be an assault with minor injuries or a patient seriously injured by a knife or pistol) .

A taser is a device that uses electrical current to disrupt muscle control and incapacitate a violent individual. This device is now in widespread use by police. You may be called to care for a patient with whom a taser was used.

In a majority of the patients, recovery is quick and without serious injury. If you are called to care for someone who has been hit with the taser probes or electrodes (Figure 3-5a ■):

1. Assure your own safety. The patient will have been restrained by the police but was once violent and can become violent again.
2. Assure the ABCs. In the event of a co-existing medical problem or an incustody death situation you should always initially perform the ABCs and carefully monitor them throughout the call.
3. Assess injuries and complaint as you normally would.
4. Do not remove taser electrodes unless you have been trained to do so.

In addition to providing care to your patient, you will also be expected to preserve evidence that may be present at the scene.

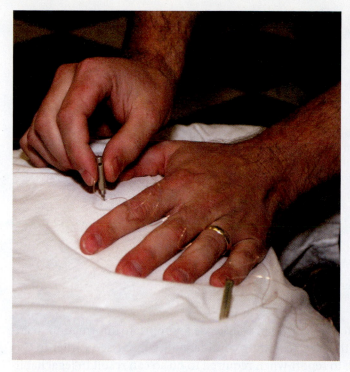

■ **Figure 3-5a** Police may use a taser; the perpetrator may have an injury resulting from that use. (© Daniel Limmer)

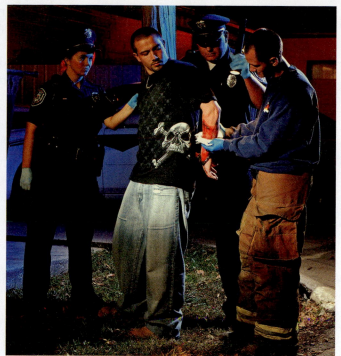

■ **Figure 3-5b** As an EMR, you may provide treatment to an injured perpetrator.

When you enter a crime scene, you have two main goals: providing care to your patient and minimizing your impact on the crime scene as you do so.

Good general rules are not to touch anything you don't have to and to be observant as you provide care.

Evidence Identification and Preservation

To preserve evidence, you must be familiar with types of evidence and where it may be located. It is difficult to watch the news or prime-time television without seeing something about evidence. There are many types of evidence, including:

Fingerprints—A fingerprint is moisture and oils left behind on a surface. It carries the distinct patterns of the person who left the "print," which can be used to identify a suspect. Since fingerprints are only moisture, it is quite easy to smear the prints by touching them. This ruins any potential evidence value. Fingerprints can be obtained off a variety of surfaces such as rough surfaces, paper, and even skin. To preserve prints, avoid touching anything you don't absolutely have to.

Blood and body fluids—These fluids can be examined for blood type, DNA, pattern of spatter, and more. Prevent contamination of blood and fluids (Figure 3-5b ■). Avoid stepping in blood or fluids. When cutting off clothes, place different clothing items in different places to avoid contamination between different samples.

Wounds—When exposing the patient, avoid cutting directly through bullet or knife holes in clothing. Try to cut at least 6 inches away from these holes.

Conditions at the scene—As an Emergency Medical Responder you will arrive at the scene early and observe the scene as those who arrive later won't. Make mental notes about the scene and what you see. Report these observations to the police when your patient care activities are through.

Statements of the patient and those at the scene—As you care for your patient, you may hear the patient or those around him make statements. These statements may amount to a confession, a threat, or other information that could be vital to the investigation. Document statements by the patients and others in quotes when including them in your report.

Be sure to follow the guidelines of your local EMS and law enforcement authorities in regard to your actions at crime scenes.

Mandatory Reporting

You will have situations where you are required by law to make a report to authorities. Although the laws vary by state, many providers are mandated to report suspected crimes of the following types:

- Child abuse or neglect
- Domestic violence
- Elder abuse
- Sexual assault
- Gunshot wounds or other violence
- Infectious diseases

When you are mandated to report, you may disclose appropriate information to authorities and aren't subject to the laws regarding confidentiality discussed earlier in this chapter (Figure 3-6 ■). Failure to report when required to do so can result in legal liability or penalty. Check with your instructor about specifics for your state.

Your documentation will be vital in cases such as this. It will also be challenging because of the potential for emotions you may feel in cases of abuse and neglect. Always document objectively (factually) in these cases. Avoid emotion or statements based on opinion. If you note statements of others, put them in quotes and identify them as such by writing "patient states" or "the patient's mother stated."

CASE STUDY

TRANSITION

The ambulance arrives, which causes the patient to again say how much he doesn't want to go to the hospital. The patient's wife shoots you nervous glances. She has told you she thinks it is serious because this was how he looked before his last heart attack.

You introduce the patient to the EMTs. You spent some time talking with the patient while waiting for the ambulance trying to convince him to accept the care and transportation of the EMTs. The patient still says he doesn't want to go, but you can see the EMTs share your concern for the patient.

You provide your vitals and history information to the EMTs and stick around to help the patient and his wife where you can. He eventually does accept care and transportation from the EMTs—after coaxing from his wife—which is a good thing because he is having a heart attack.

- Discussion: *For how long should you try to convince the patient to accept care before you accept his decision to refuse care? What are the steps you must follow if he were to refuse care?*

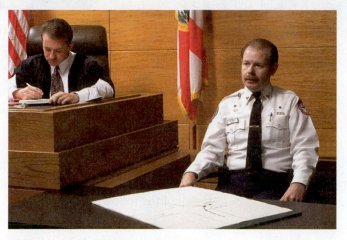

Figure 3-6 An EMR testifying in court.

THE LAST WORD

No one wants to get sued. Fortunately it is rare and preventable. This chapter discussed ways to practice EMS that would prevent lawsuits and always help you keep professionalism and patient care in mind. It also touched upon important issues such as the legal system, ethics, how to provide EMS at a crime scene, and more.

The general rule is to provide quality care and treat people well. And remember, *primum non nocere*: first, do no harm.

✦ *Chapter Review*

Multiple Choice

Place a check next to the correct answer.

1. Rules, regulations, and laws, though they may vary from state to state or region to region, that govern the practice of emergency responders are considered to be:

   _____ a. scope of practice.

   _____ b. proximate causation.

   _____ c. negligence.

   _____ d. protocols.

2. Communication obtained from a physician while on a call that provides assistance with your assessment or care of a patient is said to be:

   _____ a. protocols.

   _____ b. on-line medical control.

   _____ c. off-line medical control.

   _____ d. scope of practice.

3. Written guidelines created by a medical director to provide an EMR with a plan of care for specific medical situations are called:

   _____ a. on-line medical control.

   _____ b. scope of practice.

   _____ c. written consent.

   _____ d. protocols.

4. Permission for treatment obtained directly from a patient who is in need of care is:

   _____ a. written consent.

   _____ b. expressed consent.

   _____ c. implied consent.

   _____ d. emancipated consent.

5. Patients who are able to legally consent for their treatment are also able to decline treatment. This is more commonly referred to as:

_____ a. refusal of care.

_____ b. health care proxy.

_____ c. expressed consent.

_____ d. advance directives.

6. Health care providers often come in contact with their patients' personal information. This information is commonly referred to as:

_____ a. a health care proxy.

_____ b. a do not resuscitate order.

_____ c. ethics.

_____ d. protected health information.

7. An on-duty provider of medical assistance is said to have a(n) _____ when there is an emergency call for assistance.

_____ a. proximate causation

_____ b. duty to act

_____ c. tort

_____ d. abandonment

8. When responding to the scene of crime, in addition to caring for the patient, the emergency responders should also be aware to:

_____ a. preserve evidence and note changes they made to the scene.

_____ b. solve the mystery of the crime.

_____ c. put themselves in harm's way to protect bystanders.

_____ d. act recklessly when it is in the patient's interest.

9. In many states, there are laws that require emergency responders to be mandated reporters for all of the following except:

_____ a. suspected child abuse.

_____ b. suspected elder abuse.

_____ c. suspected acts of domestic violence.

_____ d. incidents of illness in the pediatric population.

10. When an emergency responder begins the care of a patient and does not complete the care provided, he has put himself at risk of charges for:

_____ a. negligence.

_____ b. proximate causation.

_____ c. abandonment.

_____ d. breach of duty.

Case Study

Your EMR unit responds to the scene of a shooting. The police have requested you to the scene, stating there is a male with traumatic injuries. You arrive to find him lying near a knife and some cartridges from a rifle. You begin to treat him, and the ambulance arrives to transport him.

1. What should your paramount concern be given this description of the scene?

_____

_____

_____

_____

2. If this patient is unconscious, what type of consent can you consider to be in place?

_____

_____

_____

_____

3. In an effort to create a "better working environment" is it permissible for you to move the objects surrounding your patient?

_____

_____

_____

_____

4. What steps should you have taken prior to approaching the patient?

_____

_____

_____

_____

5. While you are treating this patient, what steps can you take to preserve any evidence found on the patient's clothing or body?

_____

_____

_____

_____

 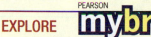

Medical Terminology

NAVIGATION GUIDE

The following items provide an overview to the purpose and content of this chapter. The Education Standard and Competency are from the National EMS Education Standards.

Education Standard Medical Terminology

Competency Uses simple medical and anatomical terms.

Objectives After reading this chapter, you should be able to:

1. Define key terms introduced in this chapter.
2. Explain the importance of understanding medical terminology to communicate with other health care team members.
3. Apply knowledge of common prefixes, suffixes, and root or stem words to interpret medical terms.
4. Recognize common anatomical terms, including:
   a. Right and left
   b. Prone and supine
   c. Lateral recumbent
   d. Medial and lateral
   e. Superior and inferior
   f. Distal and proximal
   g. Anterior (ventral) and posterior (dorsal)
   h. Superficial and deep
   i. Internal and external
5. Identify each of the main body cavities:
   a. Cranial cavity
   b. Thoracic (chest) cavity
   c. Abdominal cavity
   d. Pelvic cavity
6. List the major organs contained within each of the main body cavities.

Key Terms Page references indicate first major use in this chapter. The Margin Glossary in this chapter provides definitions as you read.

anatomical position, p. 72

right, p. 72

left, p. 72

supine, p. 72

prone, p. 72

right lateral recumbent, p. 72

left lateral recumbent, p. 72

medial, p. 73

lateral, p. 74

superior, p. 74

inferior, p. 74

distal, p. 74

proximal, p. 74

anterior/ventral, p. 74

posterior/dorsal, p. 74

superficial, p. 74

deep, p. 74

internal, p. 74

external, p. 74

cranial cavity, p. 75

thoracic (chest) cavity, p. 75

abdominal cavity, p. 75

pelvic cavity, p. 78

NAVIGATION GUIDE *(continued)*

Media Resources Please go to **www.bradybooks.com** to access mykit for this text. You will find quizzes, critical thinking scenarios, weblinks, animations, and videos related to this chapter—and much more. Look for online information on medical terminology and body systems.

INTRODUCTION

Like automobile mechanics who talk about torque wrenches and catalytic converters, and computer specialists who talk about gigabytes and RAM, health care providers have a language of their own. As an EMR, you will need to have a basic understanding of medical terminology to communicate with other health care providers.

CASE STUDY

THE CALL

While hiking in a state park, you come upon a man lying face down in the vegetation along the trail. As you approach the patient, you look for any hazards that may be present. You also call to the man to see if he will respond . . . he does not.

You gently shake the man's shoulder and try to elicit a response. You carefully roll him into a face-up (supine) position and notice his color is grayish blue. You call 911 from your cell phone and advise the dispatcher of your location and that you have found an unresponsive male along the trail.

■ Discussion: *Should you begin an assessment? If so, what will you do?*

ASK YOURSELF

■ Can you define the key terms introduced in this chapter?

■ How would you explain the importance of understanding medical terminology to communicate with other health care team members?

■ How can you apply knowledge of common prefixes, suffixes, and root or stem words to interpret medical terms?

Medical Terminology

Medical terms often include a root word and a prefix (connected in front of the root word) or a suffix (connected behind the root word). Prefixes or suffixes are connected to the root by a connecting vowel (usually an "o" or "i"). Like the toy blocks you once played with, these root, prefix, and suffix "blocks" can be combined in a variety of ways to form many different terms.

As your experience in emergency medical services grows, so will your medical vocabulary. Table 4-1 shows some basic roots, prefixes, and suffixes used to build common medical terms.

Try not to become overwhelmed with medical terminology. Let's take a look at an example of how medical terms can be broken down.

TABLE 4-1 Common Root Words, Prefixes, and Suffixes

WORD PART	WORD PART TYPE	MEANING
Cardio	Root	Heart
Neuro	Root	Nerve
Naso	Root	Nose/nasal
Oro	Root	Mouth/oral
Hyper-	Prefix	Above normal, high
Hypo-	Prefix	Below normal, low
Tachy-	Prefix	Above normal, rapid
Brady-	Prefix	Below normal, slow
-ac	Suffix	Pertaining to
-ology	Suffix	Study of
-al	Suffix	Pertaining to
-ist	Suffix	One who specializes in

ASK YOURSELF

- How do you define the following common anatomical terms?
  - Right and left
  - Prone and supine
  - Lateral recumbent
  - Medial and lateral
  - Superior and inferior
  - Distal and proximal
  - Anterior (ventral) and posterior (dorsal)
  - Superficial and deep
  - Internal and external

anatomical position the standard for the orientation of terms; the patient is standing and facing forward, with legs shoulder-width apart, arms at the sides, and palms turned forward.

right the patient's right.

left the patient's left.

supine lying on back, facing up.

prone lying on stomach.

right lateral recumbent lying on right side.

left lateral recumbent lying on left side.

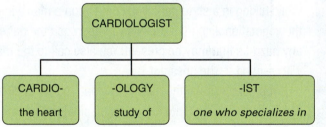

Given the root and suffix definitions, a cardiologist is *one who specializes in the study of the heart.*

Anatomical Terms

To appropriately communicate your patient assessment and management to the EMTs or other health care providers, you need to have a basic understanding of commonly used anatomical terms. This is also important in your documentation, as you will learn in Chapter 13.

Anatomical position is the standard used when referring to a location on your patient. In anatomical position the patient is standing and facing forward, with legs shoulder-width apart, arms at the sides, and palms turned forward. When you refer to **right** and **left**, keep in mind this is the patient's right and left.

Terms that relate to body position include the following:

- **Supine**. The patient is lying on her back, facing up (Figure 4-1a ■). This is also the position you place the patient to perform cardiopulmonary resuscitation (CPR).
- **Prone**. The patient is lying on her stomach (Figure 4-1b ■).
- **Right lateral recumbent**. The patient is lying on her right side (Figure 4-1c ■). This is also known as the recovery position.
- **Left lateral recumbent**. The patient is lying on her left side (Figure 4-1d ■). This is also known as the recovery position.

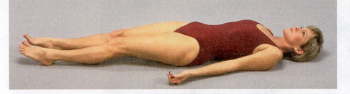

Figure 4-1a Patient in supine position.

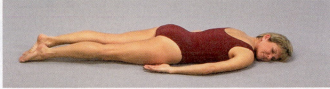

Figure 4-1b Patient in prone position.

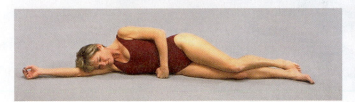

Figure 4-1c Patient in right lateral recumbent position.

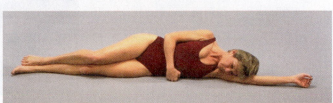

Figure 4-1d Patient in left lateral recumbent position.

Directional Terms

Terms that relate to direction or location include (Figure 4-2 ■):

■ **Medial**. Toward the midline. The midline is an imaginary vertical line drawn through the center of the body, dividing it into equal left and right parts. In anatomical position, the little finger is on the medial side of the hand (Figure 4-3 ■).

medial   toward the midline.

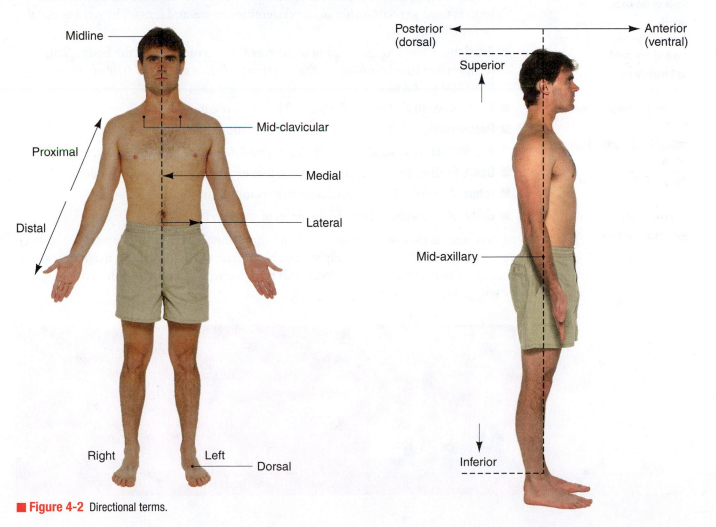

Figure 4-2 Directional terms.

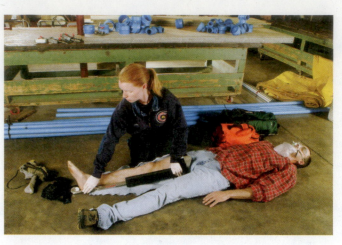

Figure 4-3 Placing a splint medially.

lateral away from the midline.

superior toward the head.

inferior toward the feet.

distal farther from the point of attachment (torso or trunk of the body).

proximal closer to the point of attachment (torso or trunk of the body).

anterior/ventral toward the front.

posterior/dorsal toward the back.

superficial toward the surface.

deep farther from the surface.

internal inside.

external outside.

- **Lateral**. Away from the midline. In anatomical position, the thumb is on the lateral side of the hand.
- **Superior**. Toward the head. The chest is superior to the abdomen.
- **Inferior**. Toward the feet. The xiphoid process (pointed end of the sternum) is inferior to the manubrium (top part of the sternum).
- **Distal**. Farther from the point of attachment (torso or trunk of the body). This term is used in relationship to the extremities (arms and legs). The wrist is distal to the elbow.
- **Proximal**. Closer to the point of attachment (torso or trunk of the body). This term is used in relationship to the extremities (arms and legs). The elbow is proximal to the wrist.
- **Anterior/ventral**. Toward the front. The chest is anterior.
- **Posterior/dorsal**. Toward the back. The shoulder blades are posterior.
- **Superficial**. Toward the surface. A scraped knee would be superficial.
- **Deep**. Farther from the surface. A cut that exposes muscle would be deep.
- **Internal**. Inside. Smoke inhalation may result in internal burns.
- **External**. Outside. A burn to the palm of the hand.

You may notice that these anatomical and directional terms are in pairs. If you keep this in mind, it will be easier to learn the basic terms. The more you use medical terminology, the more comfortable you will become with it and the more your vocabulary will grow.

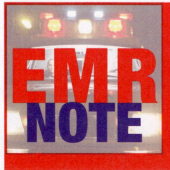

EMR NOTE

Patient care is more important than knowing a specific term. If you are unsure of the proper medical term, using common terms to describe the location or position is better than using an inappropriate term.

�֍ Stop, Review, Remember

True/False

Mark whether each of the following statements is true (T) or false (F).

1. _____ A patient lying on his back, facing up, is in the prone position.

2. _____ Medial means toward the midline.

3. _____ Anything inside the body would be internal.

4. _____ A patient lying on his left side is in the left lateral recumbent position.

5. _____ Inferior is toward the head.

6. _____ A cut that exposes the bone would be considered superficial.

7. _____ The wrist is proximal to the elbow.

8. _____ Anterior refers to the front.

CASE STUDY

THE RESPONSE ✳

You open the patient's airway and notice he is not breathing. Using the rescue mask you have in your backpack, you provide two ventilations and observe the patient's chest rise with each. You check for a carotid pulse, and find it absent. Finding the appropriate landmark, you begin chest compressions.

■ Discussion: *Compare these steps to what you think you should do initially. Are they the same? Chapter 10 discusses primary assessment in detail.*

Body Regions and Cavities

In addition to an understanding of body positions and locations, you need to have an understanding of body regions (external sections of the body illustrated in Figure 4-4 ■), topography (external landmarks illustrated in Figure 4-5 ■), and body cavities (internal body sections illustrated in Figure 4-6 ■).

The internal organs are contained in the main body cavities:

■ **Cranial cavity**. This cavity contains the brain.

■ **Thoracic (chest) cavity**. This cavity contains the heart, lungs, great vessels trachea, and esophagus (Figure 4-7 ■).

■ **Abdominal cavity**. This cavity contains the stomach, intestines, liver, gallbladder, pancreas, spleen, appendix, and kidneys. The plane formed by the lower spine, hip bones, and pubis divides the abdominal and pelvic cavities. The abdominal cavity is also divided into quadrants. If you draw an imaginary line horizontally that intersects the midline at the umbilicus (navel), you divide the cavity into four

ASK YOURSELF

■ How do you describe the main body cavities?
  ■ Cranial cavity
  ■ Thoracic (chest) cavity
  ■ Abdominal cavity

cranial cavity   the cavity that contains the brain.

thoracic (chest) cavity   the cavity that contains the heart, lungs, great vessels, and esophagus.

abdominal cavity   the cavity that contains the stomach, intestines, liver, gallbladder, pancreas, spleen, appendix, and kidneys.

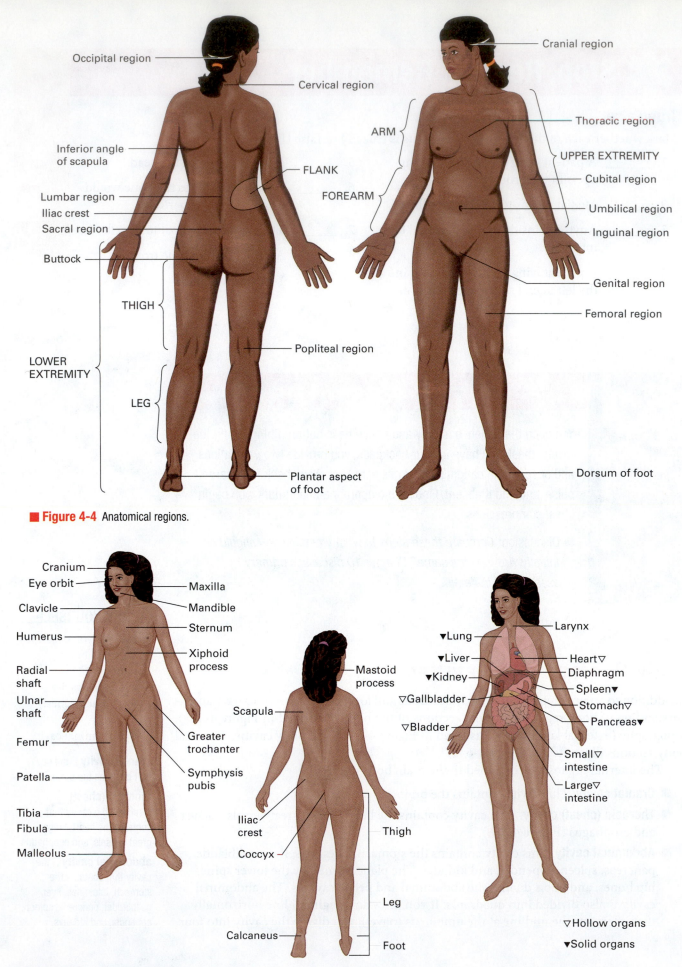

Figure 4-4 Anatomical regions.

Occipital region
Cervical region
Inferior angle of scapula
FLANK
Lumbar region
Iliac crest
Sacral region
Buttock
THIGH
LOWER EXTREMITY
LEG
Popliteal region
Plantar aspect of foot

Cranial region
ARM
Thoracic region
UPPER EXTREMITY
FOREARM
Cubital region
Umbilical region
Inguinal region
Genital region
Femoral region
Dorsum of foot

Figure 4-5 Topographic anatomy.

Cranium
Eye orbit
Maxilla
Clavicle
Mandible
Humerus
Sternum
Radial shaft
Xiphoid process
Ulnar shaft
Femur
Greater trochanter
Patella
Symphysis pubis
Tibia
Fibula
Malleolus

Mastoid process
Scapula
Iliac crest
Coccyx
Calcaneus
Thigh
Leg
Foot

▼Lung
Larynx
▼Liver
Heart▽
▼Kidney
Diaphragm
▽Gallbladder
Spleen▼
▽Bladder
Stomach▽
Pancreas▼
Small▽ intestine
Large▽ intestine

▽Hollow organs
▼Solid organs

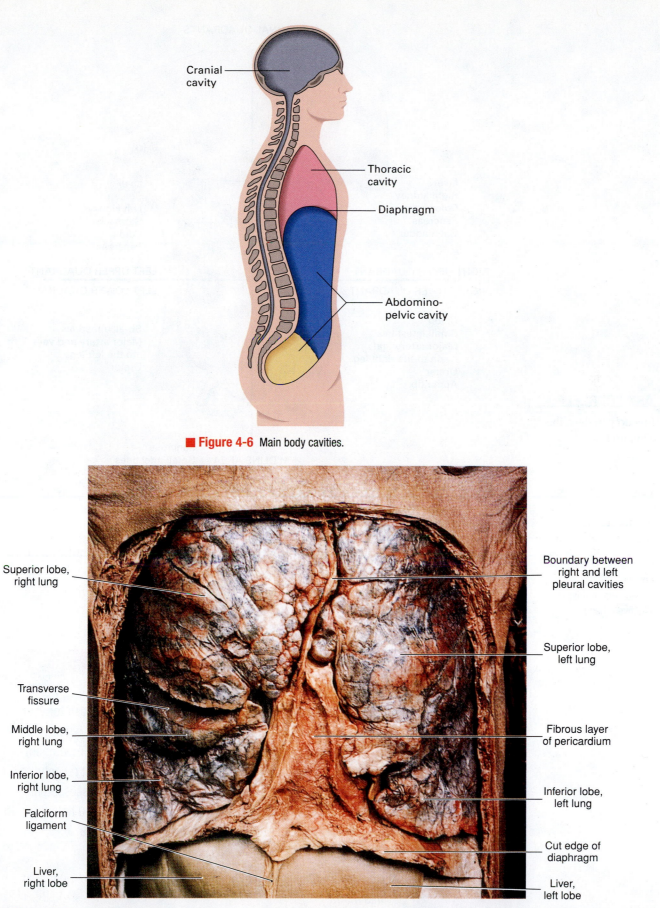

Cranial
cavity

Thoracic
cavity

Diaphragm

Abdomino-
pelvic cavity

■ **Figure 4-6** Main body cavities.

Superior lobe,
right lung

Boundary between
right and left
pleural cavities

Superior lobe,
left lung

Transverse
fissure

Middle lobe,
right lung

Fibrous layer
of pericardium

Inferior lobe,
right lung

Falciform
ligament

Inferior lobe,
left lung

Cut edge of
diaphragm

Liver,
right lobe

Liver,
left lobe

■ **Figure 4-7** The thoracic cavity.

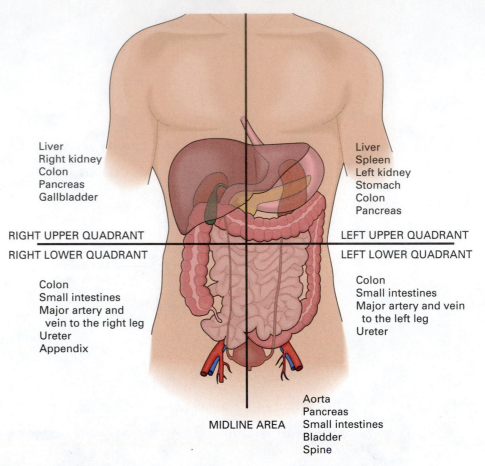

ABDOMINAL QUADRANTS

Liver
Right kidney
Colon
Pancreas
Gallbladder

Liver
Spleen
Left kidney
Stomach
Colon
Pancreas

RIGHT UPPER QUADRANT

LEFT UPPER QUADRANT

RIGHT LOWER QUADRANT

LEFT LOWER QUADRANT

Colon
Small intestines
Major artery and
  vein to the right leg
Ureter
Appendix

Colon
Small intestines
Major artery and vein
  to the left leg
Ureter

MIDLINE AREA

Aorta
Pancreas
Small intestines
Bladder
Spine

■ **Figure 4-8** The abdominal quadrants.

ASK YOURSELF

■ How do you describe the main body cavities?
  ■ Pelvic cavity

■ What are the major organs contained within each of the main body cavities?

pelvic cavity the cavity that contains the bladder, rectum, and internal female reproductive organs.

quadrants: right upper quadrant, right lower quadrant, left upper quadrant, and left lower quadrant (Figure 4-8 ■).

■ **Pelvic cavity**. This cavity contains the bladder, rectum, and internal female reproductive organs.

CASE STUDY

TRANSITION ✴

When the EMTs arrive, they take over the CPR efforts and ask for your verbal report. You advise them you were hiking on the trail when you noticed the patient lying in the vegetation in a right lateral recumbent position facing away from the trail. You tell them he did not respond to you so you rolled him into a supine position; called 911; assessed his airway, breathing, and circulation; and then began CPR. You help the EMTs prepare the patient for transport down the trail to the ambulance.

■ Discussion: *Should you or the EMTs try to determine the identity of this man?*

Stop, Review, Remember

Matching

Match the following organs with the body cavity in which they are contained.

1. _____ Bladder
2. _____ Kidneys
3. _____ Brain
4. _____ Heart
5. _____ Esophagus
6. _____ Rectum
7. _____ Liver
8. _____ Appendix

a. Cranial cavity
b. Thoracic cavity
c. Abdominal cavity
d. Pelvic cavity

THE LAST WORD

Medical terminology is the language of health care providers. As a vital link in overall patient care, the Emergency Medical Responder needs a basic understanding of medical terminology, body positions, body regions, and body cavities.

This knowledge will improve your understanding of patient assessment and patient care, as well as provide for a smooth transition to the EMTs who continue the patient care you started.

It will take you time to develop your vocabulary; however, the more you use medical terminology, the easier this new language will become.

Chapter Review

Multiple Choice

Place a check next to the correct answer.

1. The medical prefix that means "above normal" is:
   _____ a. tachy-.
   _____ b. hypo-.
   _____ c. hyper-.
   _____ d. brady-.

2. In anatomical position, the patient is:
   _____ a. standing and facing forward, with legs shoulder-width apart, arms crossed in front, and palms turned forward.
   _____ b. standing and facing forward, with legs shoulder-width apart, arms crossed in back, and palms turned backward.
   _____ c. standing and facing forward, with legs shoulder-width apart, arms at the sides, and palms turned forward.
   _____ d. standing and facing forward, with legs shoulder-width apart, arms at the sides, and palms turned backward.

3. The heart, lungs, great vessels, and esophagus are contained in the:

_____ a. cranial cavity.

_____ b. pelvic cavity.

_____ c. thoracic cavity.

_____ d. abdominal cavity.

4. Your patient has a minor cut on his right forearm. When describing the location of this injury you would say it is:

_____ a. distal to the elbow.

_____ b. distal to the wrist.

_____ c. lateral to the elbow.

_____ d. medial to the wrist.

5. In the prone position, the patient is:

_____ a. lying on the back.

_____ b. lying on the stomach.

_____ c. sitting with the back partially upright.

_____ d. sitting with the back upright.

6. When compared to the bladder, the heart is:

_____ a. superior.

_____ b. inferior.

_____ c. medial.

_____ d. lateral.

7. You are treating a 6-year-old who fell off her bicycle and scraped the front of her knee. This injury would be considered:

_____ a. anterior.

_____ b. posterior.

_____ c. deep.

_____ d. superficial.

8. The stomach, intestines, liver, gallbladder, pancreas, spleen, appendix, and kidneys are contained in the:

_____ a. cranial cavity.

_____ b. pelvic cavity.

_____ c. thoracic cavity.

_____ d. abdominal cavity.

9. The patient found in the left lateral recumbent position is:

_____ a. sitting down with the left leg and left arm extended.

_____ b. in a semisitting position and leaning to the left.

_____ c. lying on the left side with the head on the left arm.

_____ d. lying flat on the back with arms at the sides.

10. The bladder, rectum, and internal female reproductive organs are contained in the:

_____ a. cranial cavity.

_____ b. pelvic cavity.

_____ c. thoracic cavity.

_____ d. abdominal cavity.

Matching

Match the following descriptions with the appropriate term.

1. _____ The patient's right
2. _____ Toward the back
3. _____ The patient's left
4. _____ Lying on stomach
5. _____ Lying on right side
6. _____ The standard for the orientation of terms
7. _____ Lying on left side
8. _____ Toward the midline
9. _____ Away from the midline
10. _____ Outside
11. _____ Toward the head

a. Anatomical position
b. Right
c. Left
d. Supine
e. Prone
f. Right lateral recumbent
g. Left lateral recumbent
h. Medial
i. Lateral
j. Superior
k. Inferior

12. _____ Lying on back, facing up   l. Distal
13. _____ Toward the feet   m. Proximal
14. _____ Farther from the point of attachment   n. Anterior/ventral
15. _____ Toward the front   o. Posterior/dorsal
16. _____ Toward the surface   p. Superficial
17. _____ Closer to the point of attachment   q. Deep
18. _____ Farther from the surface   r. Internal
19. _____ Inside   s. External

Emergency Medical Responder Practice

You and your partner respond to an emergency call at the local elementary school playground for a child who fell from the jungle gym. When you arrive, you are led to the patient who is lying on her right side crying in pain. You notice discoloration and deformity to her right leg below her knee.

1. What is the appropriate term for the position in which you found the patient?

   _____

   _____

   _____

   _____

2. How would you relate the injury location to the knee?

   _____

   _____

   _____

   _____

3. How would you relate the injury location to the foot?

   _____

   _____

   _____

   _____

Anatomy and Physiology

NAVIGATION GUIDE

The following items provide an overview to the purpose and content of this chapter. The Education Standard and Competency are from the National EMS Education Standards.

Education Standard Anatomy and Physiology

Competency Uses simple knowledge of the anatomy and function of the upper airway, heart, vessels, blood, lungs, skin, muscles, and bones as the foundation of emergency care.

Objectives After reading this chapter, you should be able to:

1. Define key terms introduced in this chapter.
2. Give examples of structures that are studied in topographic, gross, and microscopic anatomy.
3. Give an example of the relationship between anatomy and physiology.
4. Define homeostasis.
5. Describe the basic structure and functions of the major systems of the human body:
   a. Skeletal
   b. Muscular
   c. Respiratory
   d. Cardiovascular
   e. Nervous
   f. Integumentary
   g. Digestive
   h. Urinary
   i. Lymphatic/immune
   j. Endocrine
   k. Reproductive (male and female)
6. Describe the life support chain.
7. List factors that can interfere with the life support chain.

Key Terms Page references indicate first major use in this chapter. The Margin Glossary in this chapter provides definitions as you read.

NAVIGATION GUIDE *(continued)*

Media Resources Please go to **www.bradybooks.com** to access mykit for this text. You will find quizzes, critical thinking scenarios, weblinks, animations, and videos related to this chapter—and much more. Look for online information on identifying body systems. You will also find animations on the heart and endocrine system.

INTRODUCTION

As an EMR, you need a basic understanding of anatomy and physiology to better understand the effects of illness or injury, to provide appropriate emergency care, and to communicate with other health care providers. In Chapter 4, you learned about key medical terminology. This chapter will give you the information you need to know about the human body in order to provide care and to communicate effectively with other EMS personnel.

CASE STUDY

THE CALL

You are working with your local volunteer fire department that is providing standby medical care during a bicycle motocross (BMX) race. The day is partly cloudy with mild temperatures. The fans have been cheering their local favorites and the races have progressed without incident.

As the riders are racing around a tight berm, one of the riders rides high on the track and leaves the raceway. The rider collides with a track official who is knocked down onto the ground. You are called to the track to provide care.

■ Discussion: *How many patients do you anticipate helping? Which patient will take priority?*

anatomy *the study of structure.*

topographic anatomy *anatomy that looks at the external surfaces and the shapes given by underlying structures.*

gross anatomy *anatomy that looks at the structures visible to the naked eye.*

microscopic anatomy *anatomy that looks at the structures only visible through a microscope.*

physiology *the study of function.*

homeostasis *the body's state of balance between all the body processes.*

ligaments *structures that attach bone to bone.*

cranium *part of the skull containing the brain.*

ASK YOURSELF

- Can you define the key terms introduced in this chapter?

- What are some examples of structures that are studied in topographic, gross, and microscopic anatomy?

- What is an example of the relationship between anatomy and physiology?

- How would you explain homeostasis to

- How would you explain the basic structure and functions of the major systems of the human body to a fellow

- What are the structure and functions of the skeletal system?

The Human Body

The study of anatomy and physiology fills textbooks and college classrooms alike. In this chapter you will learn some basic principles that will help you provide better patient care. As your emergency medical services career develops, you may wish to enhance your knowledge through additional reading or courses. An excellent text to further your journey is Brady's *Anatomy & Physiology for Emergency Care*, second edition.

Anatomy is the study of structure, or more simply, how the body part looks. Anatomy can be divided into three general types: topographic, gross, and microscopic. **Topographic anatomy** looks at the external surfaces and the shapes given by underlying structures, such as the bumps and indentations over the joints in your fingers. **Gross anatomy** looks at the structures visible to the naked eye, such as the muscles, bones, and body organs. **Microscopic anatomy** looks at the structures only visible through a microscope, such as blood and tissue cells.

Physiology is the study of function, or how the body part works. A major concept of physiology is **homeostasis**, the body's state of balance between all the body processes. Whether your patient has lost a large amount of blood from an injury or has an underlying medical condition, the body systems are always attempting to maintain balance, or homeostasis.

Anatomy and physiology are interrelated. What a body part looks like relates to what it does, and what it does relates to what it looks like. One of the more obvious examples is the pelvic girdle (pelvis). The female pelvic girdle is designed to support the developing fetus and related structures during pregnancy and allow for delivery of the baby, whereas the male pelvic girdle is designed for lifting and carrying, and not changes related to pregnancy. This is a major method used by investigators to determine whether a skeleton was a female or male.

There are 11 systems in the body that all must work together. Think about a football team. There are 11 players on the field that must all work together so the team can score a touchdown. If one or more players do not work in coordination with the rest of the team, the play will be unsuccessful. When body systems do not work in coordination the body may become ill, may have to work to repair an injury, or may even die.

The Skeletal System

Like the building studs and trusses supporting the walls and roof of your residence, the skeleton provides the basic framework for support of the body. The skeleton also protects many of your vital organs, such as the cranium protecting the brain and the rib cage protecting the heart and lungs. The bones of the skeleton consist of both living tissue and nonliving materials. The living tissue has a blood and nerve supply similar to all other body tissues. The nonliving materials include storage of calcium, a mineral that helps strengthen the bone. The bone marrow, the inside part of the bone, produces the red blood cells.

There are 206 bones in the adult skeleton (Figure 5-1 ■). The pediatric skeleton has slightly fewer bones as some bones are not formed. Bones have to be strong enough to support the body and protect vital organs, flexible enough to respond to stress and pressure, and jointed to allow for movement. Bones are attached to each other by **ligaments**. Muscles are connected to bones by tendons.

The major components of the skeleton include the following:

- *Skull.* The skull consists of several bones that form the cranium and the face. The **cranium** is composed of several bones that are fused together to form a vault that protects the brain. At birth, several of these cranial bones are not fused together, thus allowing the skull to flex as it passes through the birth canal. The face

Skeletal System

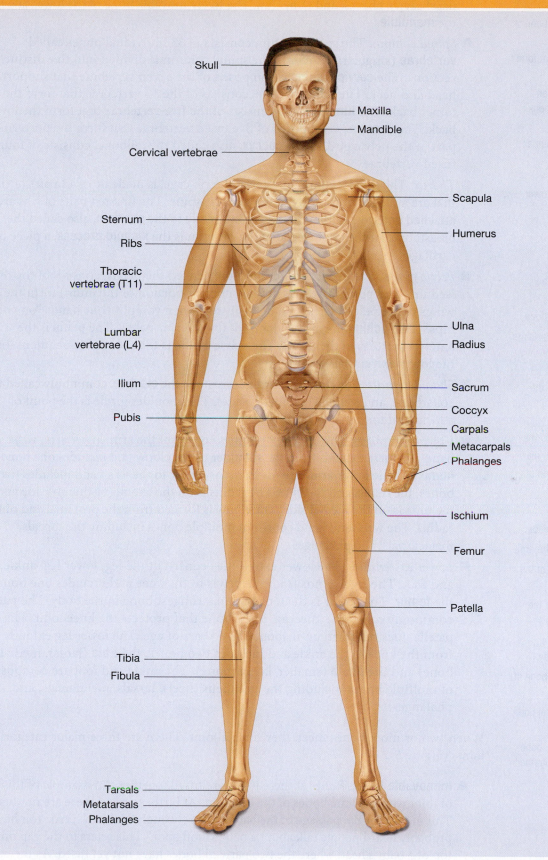

Skull

Maxilla

Mandible

Cervical vertebrae

Scapula

Sternum

Humerus

Ribs

Thoracic
vertebrae (T11)

Lumbar
vertebrae (L4)

Ulna

Radius

Ilium

Sacrum

Pubis

Coccyx

Carpals

Metacarpals

Phalanges

Ischium

Femur

Patella

Tibia

Fibula

Tarsals

Metatarsals

Phalanges

Figure 5-1 The skeletal system.

mandible movable bone of the lower jaw.

vertebrae bones that form the spinal column.

cervical spine seven vertebrae forming the neck.

thoracic spine 12 vertebrae forming the upper back.

lumbar spine five vertebrae forming the lower back.

sacrum five fused vertebrae forming the posterior pelvic girdle.

coccyx four vertebrae forming the tailbone.

sternum the breastbone.

xiphoid process cartilage at the inferior end of the sternum.

ilium major bone of the pelvic girdle; contains the iliac crests.

ischium bone that forms the loops on the inferior pelvis.

pubis anterior portion of the pelvis.

clavicle collarbone.

scapula shoulder blade.

humerus bone of the arm.

radius lateral bone of the lower arm.

ulna medial bone of the lower arm.

femur bone of the leg; largest bone in the body.

tibia larger, medial bone of the lower leg.

fibula smaller, lateral bone of the lower leg.

immovable joints bone joints that are fused together.

consists of several bones that are fused together to form the lower eye sockets, nasal cavity, cheeks, and upper jaw. The freely movable bone of the lower jaw is the **mandible**.

■ *Spinal column.* The spinal column consists of 33 individual bones called **vertebrae** (singular: *vertebra*). The spinal column is divided into five distinct sections. The **cervical spine** is composed of the seven vertebrae that support the head and neck. The **thoracic spine** consists of the 12 vertebrae that form the upper back. The **lumbar spine** consists of the five vertebrae that form the lower back. The **sacrum** is composed of five fused vertebrae that form the posterior part of the pelvic girdle. The **coccyx**, also called the tailbone, consists of four fused vertebrae.

■ *Thorax.* The thorax, commonly called the rib cage, is made up of 12 pairs of ribs that are attached posteriorly to the thoracic spine. The first ten pairs of ribs are attached anteriorly either directly or indirectly to the **sternum,** also called the breastbone. At the inferior end of the sternum is the **xiphoid process**, a piece of cartilage.

■ *Pelvic girdle.* The pelvic girdle, commonly called the pelvis, consists of the **ilium**, ischium, and pubis. The iliac crests (superior portion of the ilium) form the wings of the pelvis. These can be easily felt when you put your hands "on your hips." The **ischium** forms two loops of the inferior pelvis. The **pubis** is the anterior portion of the pelvis. The pelvic girdle is the point of attachment for the lower extremities.

■ *Shoulder girdle.* The shoulder girdle consists of the **clavicle**, commonly called the collarbone, and **scapula** (shoulder blade). The shoulder girdle is the point of attachment for the upper extremities.

■ *Upper extremities.* The upper extremities consist of the arm, lower arm, wrist, and hand. The arm extends from the shoulder to the elbow and includes one bone, the **humerus**. The lower arm extends from the elbow to the wrist and includes two bones, the **radius** and the **ulna**. The radius is on the lateral (or thumb) side and the ulna is on the medial side. The elbow is formed from the proximal end of the radius. The wrist and hand consist of multiple bones including the carpals, metacarpals, and phalanges.

■ *Lower extremities.* The lower extremities consist of the leg, lower leg, ankle, and foot. The leg extends from the pelvis to the knee and includes one bone, the **femur**. The femur is the longest and strongest bone in the body. The patella, commonly called the kneecap, is the bone that protects the knee joint. The patella does not form until about 2 to 6 years of age. The lower leg extends from the knee to the ankle and includes two bones, the **tibia** (larger, medial bone) and the **fibula** (smaller, lateral bone). The ankle and foot are composed of multiple bones including the calcaneus (heel), tarsals, metatarsals, and phalanges.

When two or more bones meet, they form a joint. There are three major categories of joints (Figure 5-2 ■):

■ **Immovable joints**. Bones at these joints are fused together. An example of this type of joint would be the bones of the cranium. At birth, some of these are not fused. This allows for the passage of the baby's head through the birth canal. You have probably heard people talk about a baby's "soft spot." This refers to the gap on the top of a baby's head where the two parietal bones have not yet fused. As the baby develops, this gap closes and the parietal bones fuse together.

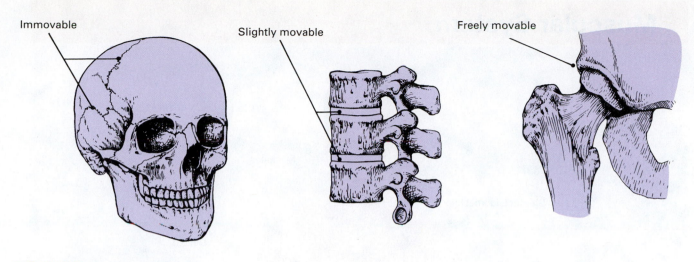

Immovable

Slightly movable

Freely movable

■ **Figure 5-2** The three types of joints.

■ **Slightly movable joints**. Bones at these joints have a limited range of motion. An example of this type of joint would be the vertebrae that make up the spinal column. Although the entire spinal column has great range of motion (for example, you can touch your toes and bend side to side), the amount of movement between each vertebra is very limited.

■ **Freely movable joints**. Bones at these joints have a great range of motion. Types of freely movable joints include hinge joints (fingers, toes, elbow, and knee), ball-and-socket joints (hip and shoulder), gliding (wrist and ankle), and saddle (thumb).

The Muscular System

The muscular system works in conjunction with the skeletal system to provide support for the body and movement. Because these two systems have such an interdependent relationship, they are often referred to as the musculoskeletal system. When muscles contract, they generate heat. This can be noticed when you increase muscle activity during a workout and start sweating or when you step outside on a chilly day and your muscles shiver to increase warmth.

There are 600 muscles in the body (Figure 5-3 ■). Most of these work in pairs. As one muscle contracts, the opposing muscle relaxes. Muscles are made up of a bundle of muscle fibers. Think about a telephone cable that contains numerous individual wires all bundled in the insulating cover. There is a nerve attached to each muscle, and when stimulated causes the muscle to contract. The strength of this impulse will dictate how many muscle fibers in the bundle are stimulated to contract. Muscle contraction is an "all or nothing" process. If you need to lift a cervical collar from your response bag, some of the muscle fibers are stimulated to contract. If you need to lift a patient into the ambulance, more muscle fibers are stimulated to contract. Muscles are attached to bones by **tendons**.

There are three types of muscles (Figure 5-4 ■):

■ **Voluntary muscle** is also called skeletal or striated muscle. As the name indicates, these muscles are under voluntary control. They are attached to the bones of the skeleton and permit movement. When you respond to a call, your brain sends impulses to the muscles, allowing you to get up from your current position and move to the response vehicle. These muscles may be somewhat flat, like the muscles of the chest and abdomen, or round, like the muscles of the arms or legs. A voluntary muscle has stripes, called striations, thus the name striated muscle.

■ **Involuntary muscle** is also called smooth muscle. Unlike voluntary muscle, we have no or very little control over involuntary muscle. These muscles are smooth in

slightly movable joints
bone joints that have a limited range of motion.

freely movable joints
bone joints that have a great range of motion.

ASK YOURSELF
■ What are the structure and functions of the muscular system?

tendons   cords of tissue that connect muscles to bones.

voluntary muscle   muscle type under conscious control.

involuntary muscle   muscle type not under conscious control.

Muscular System

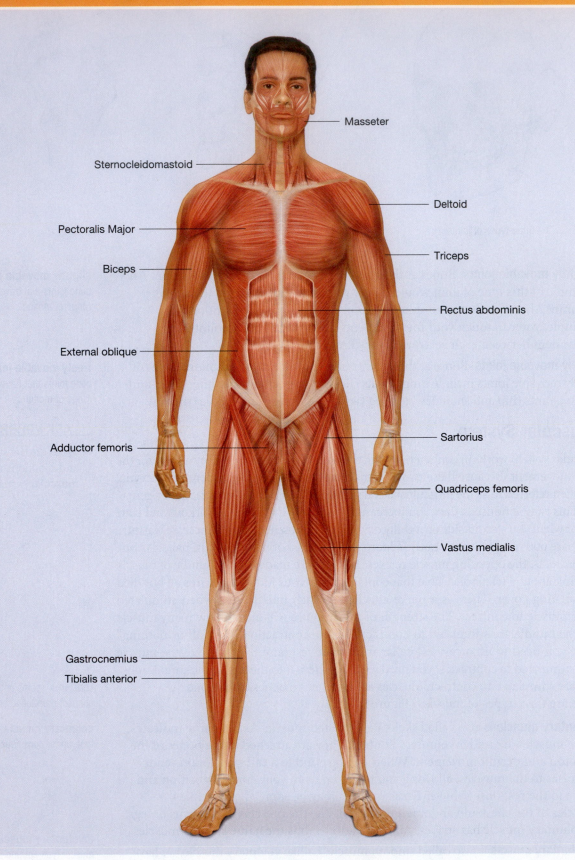

Masseter

Sternocleidomastoid

Deltoid

Pectoralis Major

Triceps

Biceps

Rectus abdominis

External oblique

Sartorius

Adductor femoris

Quadriceps femoris

Vastus medialis

Gastrocnemius

Tibialis anterior

■ **Figure 5-3** The muscular system.

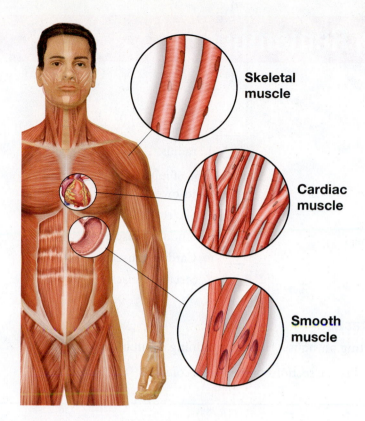

Figure 5-4 The three types of muscles.

appearance and do not have striations. Involuntary muscles may be found in the airways of the respiratory system, the digestive tract, and the blood vessels. These muscles are stimulated to contract without our conscious thought. Just imagine if you had to consciously think and contract the appropriate muscles for each breath.

- **Cardiac muscle** is only found in the heart. Cardiac muscle looks similar to voluntary muscle and acts more like involuntary muscle. Cardiac muscle has special features that allow it to generate its own stimulus to contract and to rapidly respond to the demands upon the circulatory system.

cardiac muscle muscle type found only in the heart.

CASE STUDY

THE RESPONSE

The races have been stopped while you tend to a patient. When you arrive at the patient's side, he is lying on the ground complaining of severe pain in the left arm. You notice some discoloration and swelling distal to the elbow. The patient is alert and able to answer questions appropriately, but thinks he may have briefly been unconscious after hitting the hard ground. There are no other obvious injuries.

You appropriately stabilize the arm and move the patient to the medical tent for further assessment and treatment.

- Discussion: *What is missing from this description? Was there a proper assessment of whether there was one patient or two?*

Stop, Review, Remember

Multiple Choice

Place a check next to the correct answer.

1. The study of function is called:

    _____ a. homeostasis.

    _____ b. anatomy.

    _____ c. physiology.

    _____ d. interrelation.

2. The longest bone in the body is the:

    _____ a. humerus.

    _____ b. tibia.

    _____ c. femur.

    _____ d. radius.

3. What type of muscle has the ability to generate its own stimulus to contract?

    _____ a. Skeletal muscle

    _____ b. Smooth muscle

    _____ c. Cardiac muscle

    _____ d. Striated muscle

Emergency Medical Responder Practice

Your patient fell off a ladder while painting his house. He is complaining about back pain.

1. In order from superior to inferior, list the sections of the spinal column.

    _____

    _____

    _____

    _____

You are assisting the athletic trainer at your local high school with an injured volleyball player. The patient was preparing for a regional game and the tensions were high. She landed awkwardly on her left leg and is complaining about pain around her knee and is not able to bend her leg.

2. What type of joint is the knee?

    _____

    _____

    _____

3. What structure that attaches bone to bone might be injured?

    _____

    _____

    _____

4. What structure that attaches muscle to bone might be injured?

    _____

    _____

    _____

Matching

Match the following descriptions with the appropriate term.

1. _____ The study of structure
2. _____ Anatomy that looks at the structures visible to the naked eye
3. _____ Larger, medial bone of the lower leg
4. _____ The study of function
5. _____ Five fused vertebrae forming the posterior pelvic girdle
6. _____ Shoulder blade
7. _____ Bones that form the spinal column
8. _____ Bone of the arm
9. _____ The body's state of balance between all the body processes
10. _____ Anterior portion of the pelvis
11. _____ Medial bone of the lower arm
12. _____ Anatomy that looks at the structures only visible through a microscope
13. _____ Smaller, lateral bone of the lower leg
14. _____ Bone joints that are fused together
15. _____ Connect muscles to bones
16. _____ Major bone of the pelvic girdle; contains the iliac crests
17. _____ Muscle type under conscious control
18. _____ The breastbone
19. _____ Movable bone of the lower jaw
20. _____ Muscle type found only in the heart

a. Anatomy
b. Gross anatomy
c. Microscopic anatomy
d. Physiology
e. Homeostasis
f. Mandible
g. Vertebrae
h. Sacrum
i. Sternum
j. Ilium
k. Pubis
l. Scapula
m. Humerus
n. Ulna
o. Tibia
p. Fibula
q. Immovable joints
r. Tendons
s. Voluntary muscle
t. Cardiac muscle

The Respiratory System

The respiratory system is responsible for bringing air into the lungs, where the needed oxygen is exchanged with the waste product carbon dioxide. **Ventilation** is the mechanical process of moving air in and out of the body. **Respiration** refers to exchange of gases in the cells.

Inspiration, also called inhalation, occurs when the respiratory system takes air into the body. **Expiration**, also called exhalation, occurs when the respiratory system expels air from the body. One cycle of inspiration and expiration is counted as one respiration. The average adult resting respiratory rate is 12–20 breaths per minute. Children have a higher respiratory rate.

Human physiology was once summed up by saying, "The air goes in and out and the blood goes round and round." As simple as this sounds, this statement does sum up the respiratory system (ventilation and respiration), the circulatory system (perfusion), and the general body processes used to support life (metabolism and homeostasis).

ASK YOURSELF

■ What are the structure and functions of the respiratory system?

ventilation the mechanical process of moving air in and out of the body.

respiration movement of air in and out of the lungs.

inspiration movement of air into the lungs.

expiration movement of air out of the lungs.

pharynx   throat.
larynx   the voice box.
trachea   the windpipe.

The airflow during the respiratory process is illustrated in Figure 5-5a ■.

The **pharynx** lies posterior to the oral cavity (Figure 5-5b ■). The **larynx** is at the superior end of the trachea. It is commonly called the voice box because it contains the vocal cords. You can feel the larynx on the anterior neck (also called the Adam's apple). The **trachea** is commonly called the windpipe and contains C-shaped rings of cartilage to keep it open. If you slowly run your finger over the trachea, you can feel the ridges formed by the

■ **Figure 5-5a** The respiratory system diagram.

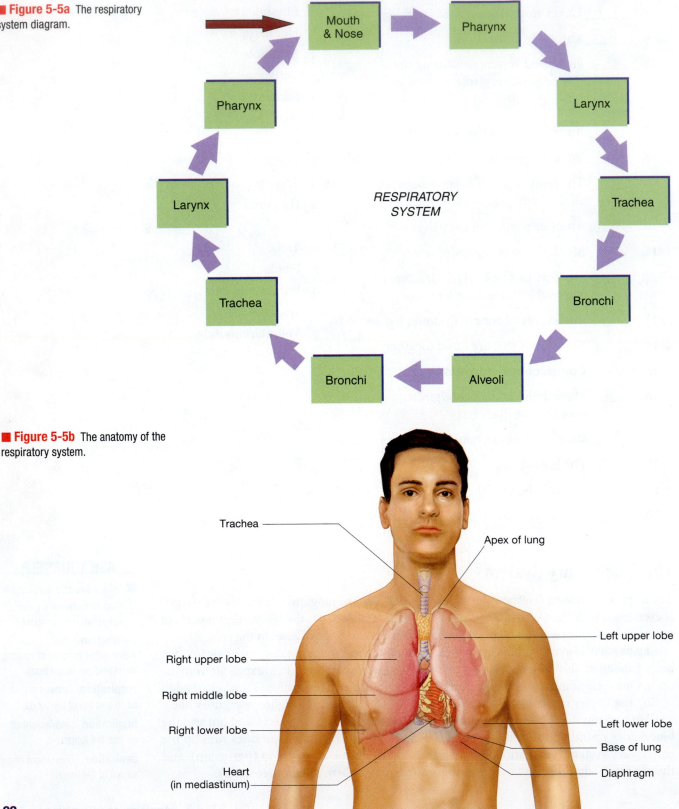

■ **Figure 5-5b** The anatomy of the respiratory system.

cartilage rings. Two main **bronchi** branch off from the trachea and continue to branch off into smaller and smaller bronchi, called bronchioles. The **alveoli** are located at the end of the bronchioles like a cluster of grapes. The exchange of oxygen and carbon dioxide occurs at the alveoli. To help picture the trachea, bronchi, bronchioles, and alveoli, think about a piece of broccoli turned upside down.

The respiratory system must work in conjunction with the muscular and skeletal systems to allow air to move in and out of the lungs. The major muscle of the respiratory system is the **diaphragm**. The diaphragm is a large, flat muscle that divides the thoracic and abdominal cavities. When relaxed, the diaphragm is dome shaped. During inhalation, the diaphragm contracts and flattens and the muscles of the chest wall and those between the ribs (intercostal muscles) work together to expand the size of the thoracic cavity and allow air to enter the lungs. During exhalation, the diaphragm relaxes and the chest wall and intercostal muscles work together to contract the size of the thoracic cavity and force air out of the lungs and airway.

The Cardiovascular System

The cardiovascular system consists of the heart, which pumps the blood throughout the body; the blood vessels, which carry the blood from the heart to the tissues and then back to the heart; and the blood, which carries oxygen and nutrients to the cells and carries carbon dioxide and waste products from the cells for elimination (Figure 5-6a ■). The blood also carries components to help fight infection and cause clotting at the site of an injury.

The blood flow during the circulatory process is illustrated in Figure 5-6b ■.

Physically, the heart consists of two **atria** (singular: *atrium*), superior chambers; and two **ventricles**, inferior chambers. Functionally, the heart works as the right side of the heart (right atrium and right ventricle) receives blood from the body and pumps blood to the lungs, and the left side of the heart (left atrium and left ventricle) receives blood from the lungs and pumps blood to the body (Figure 5-7 ■). On the surface of the heart are the **coronary arteries** that supply the heart muscle with its circulation. When the blood supply in the coronary arteries is diminished, the patient experiences chest pain that may result in a heart attack.

bronchi part of the airway branching off the trachea

alveoli structure at the end of the bronchioles where gas exchange occurs

diaphragm major muscle of the respiratory system

ASK YOURSELF

■ What are the structure and functions of the cardiovascular system?

atria superior chambers of the heart.

ventricles inferior chambers of the heart.

coronary arteries arteries supplying the heart muscle with blood.

■ **Figure 5-6a** The anatomy of the circulatory system.

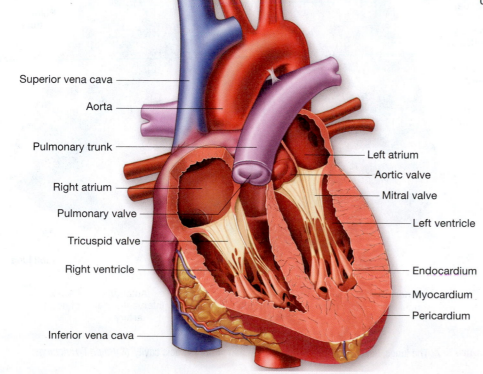

Superior vena cava

Aorta

Pulmonary trunk

Right atrium

Pulmonary valve

Tricuspid valve

Right ventricle

Inferior vena cava

Left atrium

Aortic valve

Mitral valve

Left ventricle

Endocardium

Myocardium

Pericardium

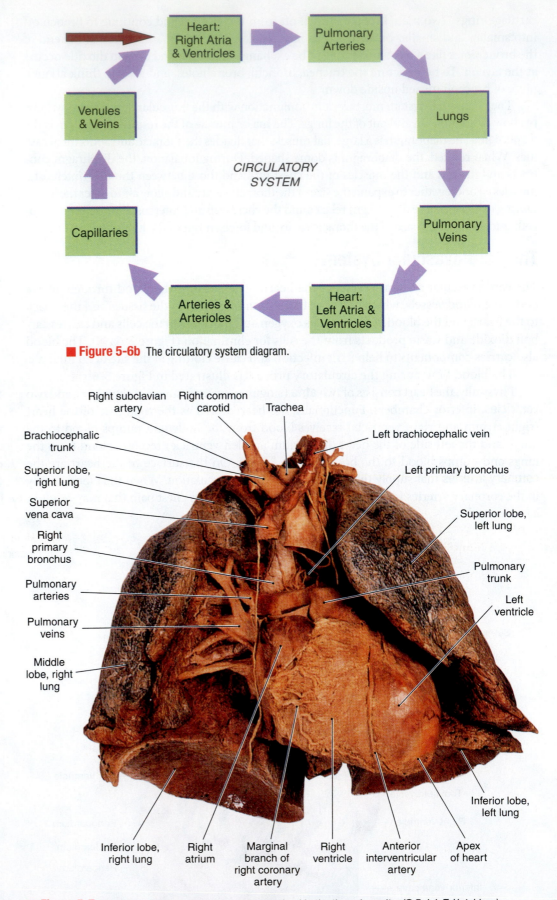

CIRCULATORY SYSTEM

Heart: Right Atria & Ventricles → Pulmonary Arteries → Lungs → Pulmonary Veins → Heart: Left Atria & Ventricles → Arteries & Arterioles → Capillaries → Venules & Veins →

■ Figure 5-6b The circulatory system diagram.

Right subclavian artery
Right common carotid
Trachea
Left brachiocephalic vein
Brachiocephalic trunk
Superior lobe, right lung
Left primary bronchus
Superior vena cava
Superior lobe, left lung
Right primary bronchus
Pulmonary trunk
Pulmonary arteries
Left ventricle
Pulmonary veins
Middle lobe, right lung
Inferior lobe, left lung
Inferior lobe, right lung
Right atrium
Marginal branch of right coronary artery
Right ventricle
Anterior interventricular artery
Apex of heart

■ Figure 5-7 The lungs, heart, and great vessels contained in the thoracic cavity. (©*Ralph T. Hutchings*)

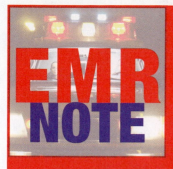
arteries   vessels that carry blood away from the heart.

arterioles   small arteries connected to the capillaries.

capillaries   thin blood vessels where exchange of gases, nutrients, and wastes occurs.

veins   vessels that carry blood back to the heart.

venules   small veins connected to the capillaries.

Blood vessels are responsible for the transportation of the blood to and from the body's cells. **Arteries** carry blood away from the heart. Arteries have a thick muscular wall that allows them to contract and regulate the flow of blood. As arteries become smaller, they are called **arterioles**. **Capillaries** are very thin blood vessels where the exchange of gases, nutrients, and wastes between the blood and the cells occurs. **Veins** carry blood back to the heart. **Venules** are small veins that connect the capillaries to the veins. Veins contain one-way valves that prevent the back-flow of blood (Figures 5-8 ■ and 5-9 ■).

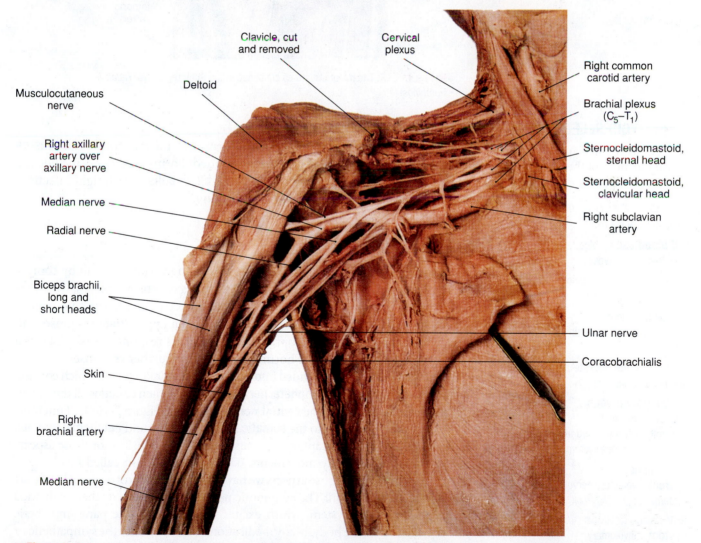

■ **Figure 5-8** The major structures contained in the right axillary region. (© *Ralph T. Hutchings*)

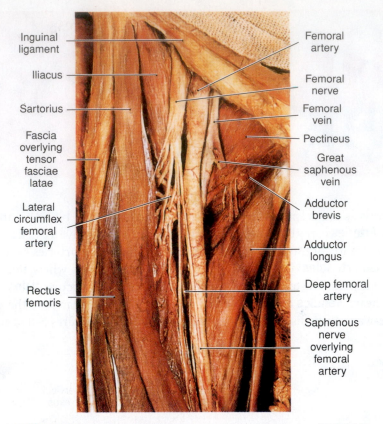

Labels (left, top to bottom): Inguinal ligament, Iliacus, Sartorius, Fascia overlying tensor fasciae latae, Lateral circumflex femoral artery, Rectus femoris

Labels (right, top to bottom): Femoral artery, Femoral nerve, Femoral vein, Pectineus, Great saphenous vein, Adductor brevis, Adductor longus, Deep femoral artery, Saphenous nerve overlying femoral artery

■ **Figure 5-9** The major structures contained in the thigh region. (© Ralph T. Hutchings)

ASK YOURSELF

■ What are the structure and functions of the nervous system?

plasma   yellowish liquid component of the blood.

red blood cells   blood cells that carry oxygen.

white blood cells   blood cells that fight infection.

platelets   blood components that help with clotting.

central nervous system   brain and spinal cord.

peripheral nervous system   nerves that transmit impulses to and from the central nervous system.

somatic nervous system   voluntary nervous system.

autonomic nervous system   involuntary nervous system.

The blood is made of two major components: formed elements and plasma. **Plasma** is the yellowish liquid in which blood cells are suspended. Formed elements include the **red blood cells**, which carry oxygen to the cells; **white blood cells**, which fight infection; and **platelets**, the components that help in blood clotting.

The Nervous System

The nervous system receives, interprets, and responds to the various stimuli by coordinating the activities of the various organ systems. It consists of sensory nerves, which receive the information from various receptors; interconnected or interpretive nerves, which interpret and analyze sensory input and determine an appropriate response; and motor nerves, which carry out the appropriate response. This response usually causes a muscle to contract or a gland to secrete hormones that cause further responses.

Physically, the nervous system is divided into the **central nervous system**, which consists of the brain and spinal cord; and the **peripheral nervous system**, which contains all the nerves that transmit messages to and from the central nervous system (Figure 5-10 ■). Functionally, the nervous system is divided into the **somatic nervous system** and **autonomic nervous system**. The somatic, also called voluntary, nervous system is responsible for those aspects we have control over, such as body movements. The autonomic, also called involuntary, nervous system is responsible for those aspects we have no or little control over, such as heart rate, respiratory rate, and digestion. The autonomic nervous system can further be divided into the sympathetic nervous system, which excites the body, and the parasympathetic nervous system, which slows the body. Many medications work on either the sympathetic or parasympathetic nervous system to help regulate body functions.

THE BRAIN

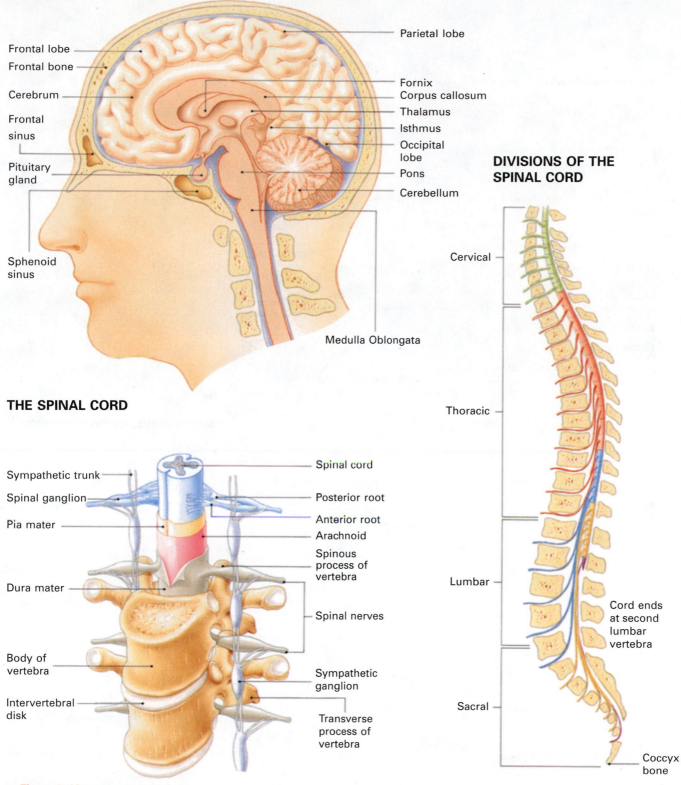

Frontal lobe

Frontal bone

Cerebrum

Frontal sinus

Pituitary gland

Sphenoid sinus

Parietal lobe

Fornix

Corpus callosum

Thalamus

Isthmus

Occipital lobe

Pons

Cerebellum

Medulla Oblongata

THE SPINAL CORD

Sympathetic trunk

Spinal ganglion

Pia mater

Dura mater

Body of vertebra

Intervertebral disk

Spinal cord

Posterior root

Anterior root

Arachnoid

Spinous process of vertebra

Spinal nerves

Sympathetic ganglion

Transverse process of vertebra

DIVISIONS OF THE SPINAL CORD

Cervical

Thoracic

Lumbar

Sacral

Cord ends at second lumbar vertebra

Coccyx bone

■ **Figure 5-10a** The nervous system.

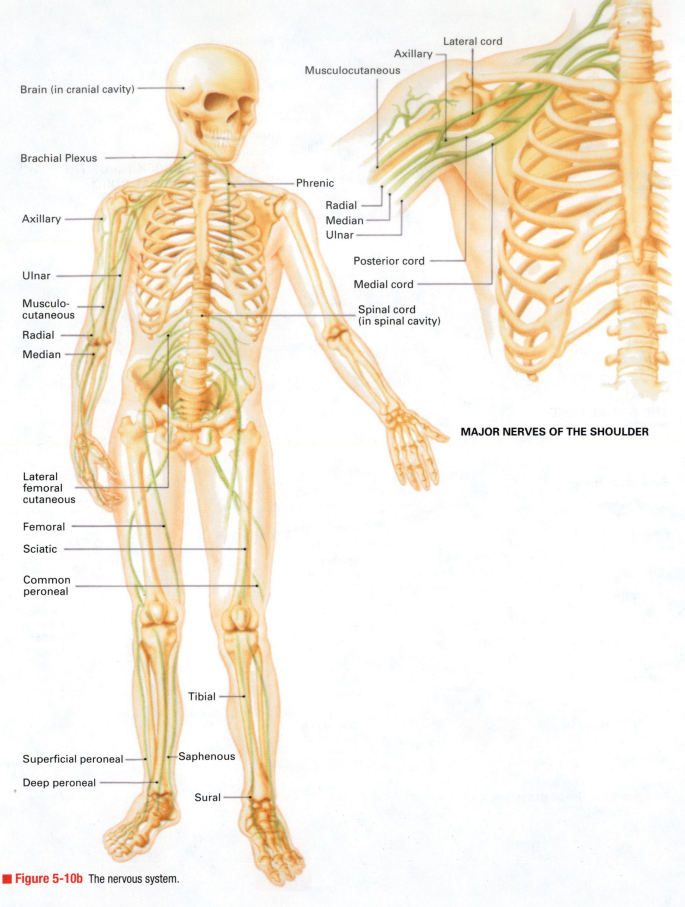

Brain (in cranial cavity)

Brachial Plexus

Axillary

Ulnar

Musculo-
cutaneous

Radial

Median

Lateral
femoral
cutaneous

Femoral

Sciatic

Common
peroneal

Superficial peroneal

Deep peroneal

Phrenic

Spinal cord
(in spinal cavity)

Tibial

Saphenous

Sural

Axillary

Musculocutaneous

Lateral cord

Radial

Median

Ulnar

Posterior cord

Medial cord

MAJOR NERVES OF THE SHOULDER

■ **Figure 5-10b** The nervous system.

While most nervous impulses are processed by the brain, this takes time. When a stimulus, such as touching a hot stove, has a potential for causing injury a different path is used. The impulse only goes to the spinal cord, and an "emergency" response is sent out. This type of response is called a **reflex**.

reflex   emergency nervous system response.

Stop, Review, Remember

Multiple Choice

Place a check next to the correct answer.

1. Gas exchange occurs in the respiratory system in the:

   _____ a. alveoli.

   _____ b. bronchi.

   _____ c. larynx.

   _____ d. trachea.

2. The heart pumps blood into the:

   _____ a. capillaries.

   _____ b. arteries.

   _____ c. veins.

   _____ d. venules.

3. The brain and spinal cord are components of the:

   _____ a. peripheral nervous system.

   _____ b. somatic nervous system.

   _____ c. autonomic nervous system.

   _____ d. central nervous system.

Emergency Medical Responder Practice

Your patient has a large cut on his leg and has lost about a cup of blood.

1. List the four components of the blood and what each does.

   _____

   _____

   _____

   _____

Matching

Match the following descriptions with the appropriate term.

1. _____ Movement of air in and out of the lungs

2. _____ The windpipe

3. _____ Blood cells that carry oxygen

4. _____ At the end of the bronchioles where gas exchange occurs

5. _____ Inferior chambers of the heart

6. _____ Arteries supplying the heart muscle with blood supply

a. Ventilation

b. Inspiration

c. Pharynx

d. Trachea

e. Bronchi

f. Alveoli

g. Diaphragm

h. Ventricles

i. Coronary arteries

j. Arteries

7. _____ Carry blood away from the heart

8. _____ Small veins connected to the capillaries

9. _____ Major muscle of the respiratory system

10. _____ Carry blood back to the heart

11. _____ Throat

12. _____ Yellowish liquid component of the blood

13. _____ Movement of air into the lungs

14. _____ Blood cells that fight infection

15. _____ Small arteries connected to the capillaries

16. _____ Blood components that help with clotting

17. _____ Nerves that transmit impulses to and from the central nervous system

18. _____ Part of the airway branching off the trachea

19. _____ Involuntary nervous system

20. _____ Emergency nervous system response

k. Arterioles

l. Venules

m. Veins

n. Plasma

o. Red blood cells

p. White blood cells

q. Platelets

r. Peripheral nervous system

s. Autonomic nervous system

t. Reflex

ASK YOURSELF

■ What are the structure and functions of the integumentary system?

epidermis outermost layer of the skin.

dermis middle layer of the skin.

subcutaneous layer innermost layer of the skin.

The Integumentary System (Skin)

The integumentary system consists of the skin, hair, and nails. The skin protects the body from the environment. It is our first line of defense against infection and helps regulate our body temperature. The skin contains nerves which allow us to sense heat, cold, touch, pressure and pain and transmit this information to the brain and spinal cord. The hair also helps in protection and temperature regulation. The nails help us to manipulate and pick up objects.

There are three major layers of skin (Figure 5-11 ■). The outermost layer is called the **epidermis**. It gives the skin its color and consists mainly of dead skin cells. The middle layer is the **dermis**. It contains blood vessels, hair follicles, sweat glands, oil glands, and sensory nerves. The innermost layer is called the **subcutaneous layer** (also called the hypodermis). This layer is mainly composed of fat. The thickness of this layer will vary from individual to individual and from body region to body region.

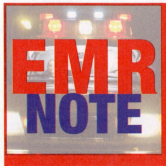

As we age, the thickness of the subcutaneous layer decreases. If you compare the back of the hand of someone in their early 20s to someone in their 50s or 60s, you will see the difference in the thickness of the subcutaneous layer.

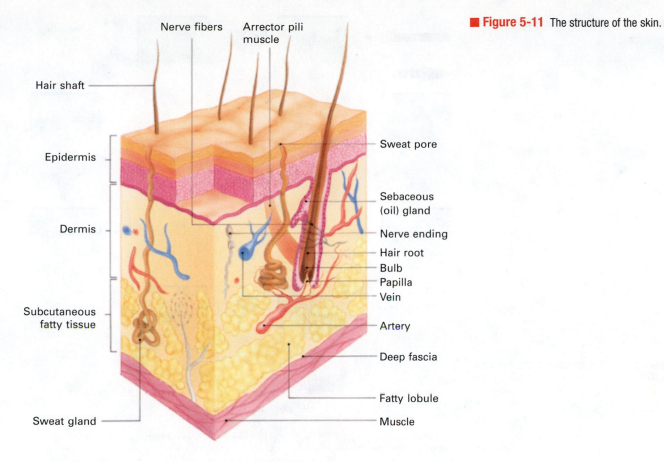

Nerve fibers Arrector pili muscle

Hair shaft

Epidermis — Sweat pore

Dermis — Sebaceous (oil) gland

— Nerve ending

— Hair root

— Bulb

— Papilla

— Vein

Subcutaneous fatty tissue — Artery

— Deep fascia

— Fatty lobule

Sweat gland — Muscle

The Digestive System

The digestive system is responsible for the processing of food, absorption of nutrients, and elimination of wastes. The digestive system consists of essentially a long tube (alimentary canal) and accessory organs of digestion. Digestion incorporates two processes: mechanical and chemical. The mechanical process includes chewing, swallowing, the rhythmic movement of material through the digestive tract (peristalsis), and elimination of wastes (defecation). The chemical process includes the release of various chemicals throughout the digestive tract to assist in the breakdown of material and the absorption of nutrients.

The movement of food through the digestive process is illustrated in Figure 5-12a ■.

As we swallow, food and liquid move from the mouth, through the pharynx, through the esophagus, and into the stomach (Figure 5-12b ■). In the **stomach**, material is churned with various digestive chemicals. Material then moves into the small intestine where additional chemicals are added and further digestion and absorption occurs. The digestive process continues in the large intestine and excess water is removed before elimination of waste.

Additional components of the digestive process include the liver, the gallbladder, the pancreas, and the appendix.

The Urinary System

The urinary system is responsible for the filtration of the blood, removing excess water, salts, minerals, and other waste products. The urinary system also helps in the regulation of blood pressure.

ASK YOURSELF

■ What are the structure and functions of the digestive system?

stomach   organ in the digestive system where material is churned with digestive chemicals.

kidney   organ of the urinary system that filters blood.

ureter   tube that carries urine from the kidney to the urinary bladder.

urinary bladder   organ that stores urine.

urethra   canal that carries urine from the urinary bladder for elimination.

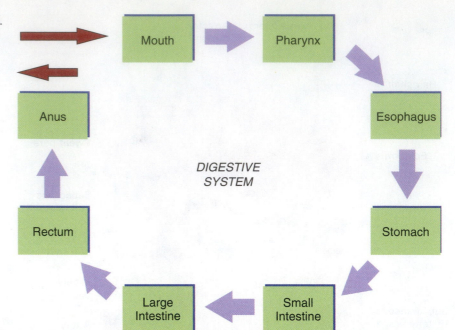

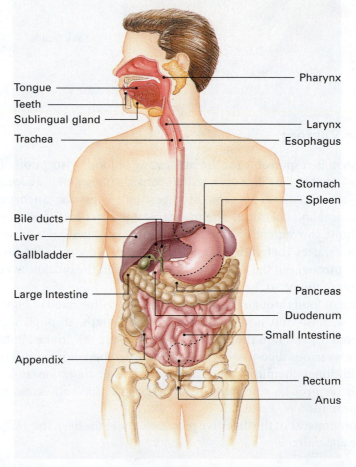

The urinary system consists of two **kidneys**, which serve as filters; two **ureters**, which carry the urine and waste from the kidneys to the **urinary bladder**, which holds the urine until elimination; and the **urethra**, which carries the urine from the urinary bladder for elimination (Figure 5-13 ■).

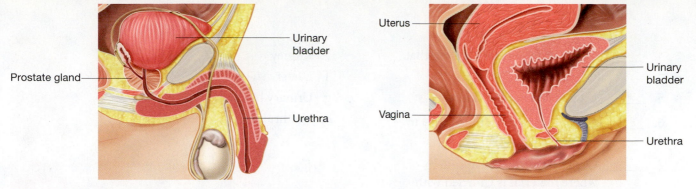

■ **Figure 5-13** The urinary system.

✳ Stop, Review, Remember

Multiple Choice

Place a check next to the correct answer.

1. The outermost layer of the skin is the:

   ____ a. subcutaneous.

   ____ b. dermis.

   ____ c. epidermis.

   ____ d. subdermis.

2. All of the following are organs in the digestive system except the:

   ____ a. liver.

   ____ b. gallbladder.

   ____ c. kidney.

   ____ d. pancreas.

3. Urine is eliminated from the urinary bladder through the:

   ____ a. urethra.

   ____ b. esophagus.

   ____ c. ureter.

   ____ d. jejunum.

Emergency Medical Responder Practice

You are treating a patient who was burned in a house fire. You can see that there is a burn on the patient's leg down to the fatty tissue.

1. If you can see the layer of fatty tissue, what layer or layers of skin have been burned away?

   _____

   _____

   _____

   _____

Matching

Match the following descriptions with the appropriate term.

1. _____ Carries urine from the urinary bladder for elimination

2. _____ Outermost layer of the skin

3. _____ Innermost layer of the skin

a. Epidermis

b. Dermis

c. Subcutaneous layer

d. Stomach

4. _____ Organ of the urinary system that filters blood

5. _____ Middle layer of the skin

6. _____ Carries urine from the kidney to the urinary bladder

7. _____ Organ in the digestive system where material is churned with digestive chemicals

8. _____ Organ that stores urine

e. Kidney
f. Ureter
g. Urinary bladder
h. Urethra

ASK YOURSELF

■ What are the structure and functions of the lymphatic/immune system?

■ What are the structure and functions of the endocrine system?

■ What are the structure and functions of the reproductive (male and female) system?

The Lymphatic/Immune System

The lymphatic/immune system helps defend the body against infection and disease and returns tissue fluids back to the bloodstream.

Excess fluid from the tissues is collected in the lymphatic tissue, then moved through the lymphatic ducts where it reenters the circulatory system. As this fluid moves through the lymphatic ducts, it is filtered through **lymph nodes** where a large number of white blood cells help defend against infection.

You may have noticed swollen lymph nodes, especially in the neck, when you come down with a respiratory infection. This is due to the increased amount of white blood cells in the lymph nodes used to fight the infection. Most likely, you have either had, or know someone who has had, a tonsillectomy (removal of the tonsils). The **tonsils** are a pair of lymph nodes in the posterior oral cavity. Repeated infections and other situations may require the removal of the tonsils.

The Endocrine System

The endocrine system consists of various glands that release chemicals called **hormones**. Hormones help to regulate various body systems and processes. These hormones affect the physical and mental abilities, reproduction, and behavior. The changes that occur during puberty to both boys and girls result from the release of hormones.

Glands of the endocrine system include the hypothalamus, pineal, pituitary, thyroid, parathyroid, thymus, adrenal, pancreas, ovaries, and testes.

The Reproductive System

The reproductive system is responsible for the development of specialized cells and structures designed to create and protect the developing fetus until birth.

The male reproductive system consists of two **testicles**, where the sperm are produced; two vas deferens, which carry the sperm from the testicles; accessory glands; and the penis. Though most of these structures are external, some are internal (Figure 5-14a ■).

The female reproductive system consists of two **ovaries**, where the ovum (or eggs) are stored; two fallopian tubes (also called uterine tubes), which carry the ovum from the ovaries and where fertilization usually occurs; the **uterus**, where the fetus develops; the vagina (or birth canal); and external genitalia (Figure 5-14b ■). The menstrual cycle is a recurring cycle of physiological changes that occurs in females of reproductive age. This cycle lasts about 28 days, ending in menstruation.

lymph node   organ of the lymphatic system where white blood cells filter the blood.

tonsils   lymph nodes in the posterior oral cavity.

hormones   chemicals that help regulate various body systems and processes.

testicles   glands producing sperm.

ovaries   glands storing ovum.

uterus   organ where fetus develops.

Male Reproductive System

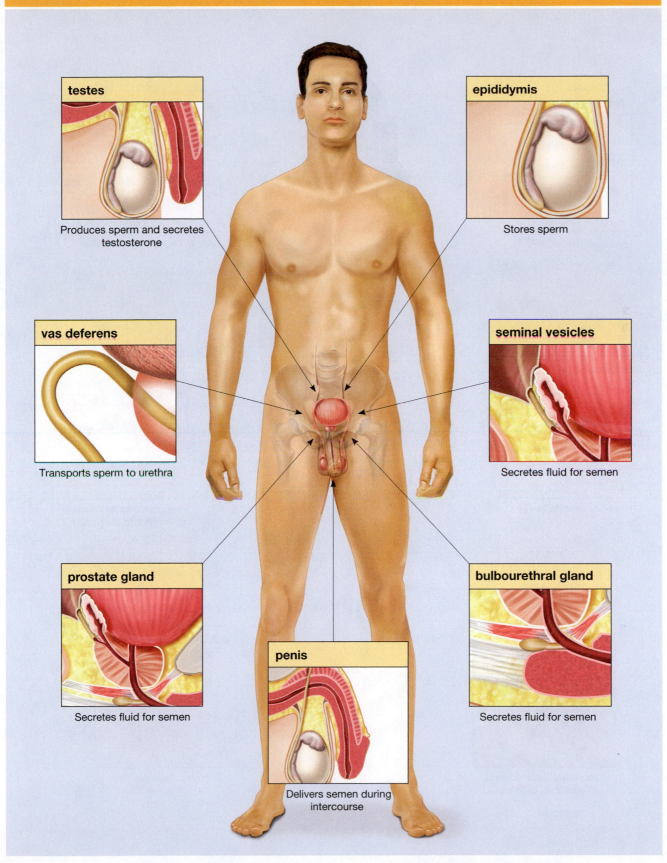

testes

Produces sperm and secretes testosterone

epididymis

Stores sperm

vas deferens

Transports sperm to urethra

seminal vesicles

Secretes fluid for semen

prostate gland

Secretes fluid for semen

penis

Delivers semen during intercourse

bulbourethral gland

Secretes fluid for semen

■ **Figure 5-14a** The male reproductive system.

Female Reproductive System

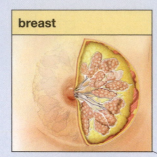

breast

Produces milk

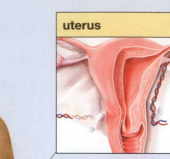

uterus

Site of development of fetus

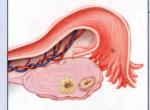

fallopian tube

Transports ovum to uterus

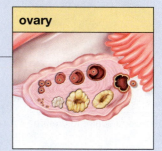

ovary

Produces ova and secretes estrogen and progesterone

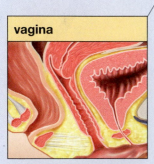

vagina

Receives semen during intercourse; birth canal

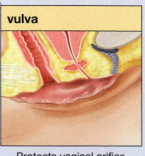

vulva

Protects vaginal orifice and urinary meatus

■ **Figure 5-14b** The female reproductive system.

Life Support Chain

Life, as we know it, is dependent on a consistent chain of events to provide the gases and nutrients our bodies need and to eliminate the carbon dioxide and waste products our bodies do not need (Figure 5-15 ■).

The following factors may interfere with this process, thus causing a breakdown in the system and resulting in a variety of conditions:

ASK YOURSELF
- What is the life support chain?
- What factors can interfere with the life support chain?

- *Composition of ambient air.* Atmospheric air contains approximately 21 percent oxygen. Smoke and other chemicals in the air may decrease the amount of oxygen available to inhale.

- *Condition of the respiratory system.* There must be an adequate flow of air into and out of the lungs. This flow could be diminished by an airway obstruction, an infection causing a fluid buildup in the airways, an allergic reaction causing the airways to constrict, or medical conditions that may cause the alveoli to lose elasticity or fill with fluid thus causing a problem in the exchange of oxygen and carbon dioxide.

- *Condition of the circulatory system.* If the heart is not pumping effectively, blood flow will be diminished. If the amount of blood is diminished (such as bleeding), too thin, or too thick, the carrying of nutrients and wastes to and from the cells will be affected. If the blood vessels are constricted or dilated, blood flow will be affected.

- *Condition of the tissues and cells.* If the tissues and cells are damaged due to a medical or traumatic situation, the ability to exchange gases, nutrients, and wastes will be affected.

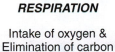

VENTILATION & RESPIRATION

Intake of oxygen & Elimination of carbon dioxide

PERFUSION

Transport of oxygen & carbon dioxide to/from the cells

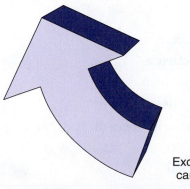

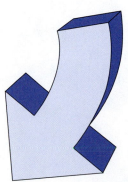

CELLULAR RESPIRATION

Exchange of oxygen & carbon dioxide within the cells

■ **Figure 5-15** Necessary components of life.

THE LAST WORD

The best possible patient outcome occurs when all the components of the response—the lay public, the Emergency Medical Responders, the EMTs/AEMTs/Paramedics, and the emergency physicians, nurses, and support staff—work together for the good of the patient. Likewise, the various body systems must all work together for the good of the body. Any breakdown in the coordination of these body systems may result in injury, illness, or even death.

The body systems include the *skeletal system*, providing support, protection, and blood production; the *muscular system*, providing movement and heat generation; the *respiratory system*, providing gaseous exchange; the *cardiovascular system*, responsible for the transport of gases, nutrients, and wastes; the *nervous system*, responsible for system coordination; the *integumentary system*, responsible for protection and temperature regulation; the *digestive system*, responsible for food processing, nutrient absorption, and waste elimination; the *urinary system*, responsible for filtration and waste elimination; the *lymphatic/immune system*, responsible for protecting against infection; the *endocrine system*, responsible for system and process regulation; and the *reproductive system*, responsible for the continuation of life.

✳ *Chapter Review*

Multiple Choice

Place a check next to the correct answer.

1. The study of structure is called:

_____ a. homeostasis.

_____ b. anatomy.

_____ c. physiology.

_____ d. interrelation.

2. All of the following are components of the pelvic girdle except the:

_____ a. ilium.

_____ b. clavicle.

_____ c. ischium.

_____ d. pubis.

3. How many muscles are in the body?

_____ a. 200

_____ b. 300

_____ c. 400

_____ d. 600

4. In what order does air enter the respiratory system?

_____ a. Pharynx, larynx, trachea, bronchi, alveoli

_____ b. Pharynx, trachea, larynx, bronchi, alveoli

_____ c. Larynx, pharynx, trachea, bronchi, alveoli

_____ d. Trachea, pharynx, larynx, alveoli, bronchi

5. Which of the following blood vessels contain valves?

_____ a. Arteries and arterioles

_____ b. Veins and venules

_____ c. Arteries and venules

_____ d. Veins and arterioles

6. The exchange of gases, nutrients, and waste products occurs in the:

_____ a. arterioles.

_____ b. venules.

_____ c. bronchioles.

_____ d. capillaries.

7. Functionally, the nervous system is divided into the:

_____ a. somatic and parasympathetic nervous systems.

_____ b. autonomic and sympathetic nervous systems.

_____ c. somatic and autonomic nervous systems.

_____ d. autonomic and parasympathetic nervous systems.

8. The layer of the skin that contains the blood vessels, hair follicles, sweat glands, oil glands, and sensory nerves is the:

_____ a. subcutaneous.

_____ b. dermis.

_____ c. epidermis.

_____ d. subdermis.

9. The innermost layer of the skin is the:

_____ a. subcutaneous.

_____ b. dermis.

_____ c. epidermis.

_____ d. subdermis.

10. The urinary system is responsible for all of the following except:

_____ a. filtration of the blood.

_____ b. human perpetuation.

_____ c. removing excess water and substances.

_____ d. help in the regulation of blood pressure.

Emergency Medical Responder Practice

The life support chain includes the intake of oxygen and elimination of carbon dioxide (ventilation and respiration), the transport of oxygen and carbon dioxide to/from the cells (perfusion), and the exchange of oxygen and carbon dioxide within the cells (cellular respiration).

1. List the factors that may interfere with this process and give examples of each.

_____

_____

_____

_____

_____

_____

Label

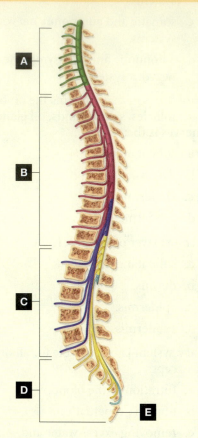

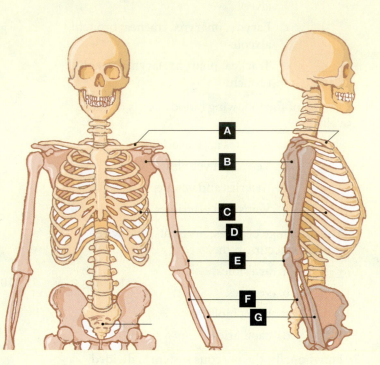

Label the following sections of the spinal column:

1. (A) _____

2. (B) _____

3. (C) _____

4. (D) _____

5. (E) _____

Label the following bones of the skeletal system:

1. (A) _____

2. (B) _____

3. (C) _____

4. (D) _____

5. (E) _____

6. (F) _____

7. (G) _____

Matching

Match the following physiological systems with the appropriate body system.

1. _____ System and process regulation
2. _____ Support, protection, and blood production
3. _____ Protection and temperature regulation
4. _____ Gaseous exchange
5. _____ Transport of gases, nutrients, and wastes
6. _____ Food processing, nutrient absorption, and waste elimination
7. _____ Movement and heat generation
8. _____ System coordination
9. _____ Filtration and waste elimination
10. _____ Protecting against infection

a. Skeletal
b. Muscular
c. Respiratory
d. Cardiovascular
e. Nervous
f. Integumentary
g. Digestive
h. Urinary
i. Lymphatic/immune
j. Endocrine

Matching

Match the following descriptions with the appropriate term.

1. _____ Attach bone to bone
2. _____ Five vertebrae forming the lower back
3. _____ Four vertebrae forming the tailbone
4. _____ Form the loops on the inferior pelvis
5. _____ Collarbone
6. _____ Bone of the leg; largest bone in the body
7. _____ Chemicals that help regulate various body systems and processes
8. _____ Bone joints that have a great range of motion
9. _____ Anatomy that looks at the external surfaces and the shapes given by underlying structures
10. _____ Movement of air out of the lungs
11. _____ The voice box
12. _____ Bone joints that have a limited range of motion
13. _____ Part of the skull containing the brain
14. _____ Superior chambers of the heart
15. _____ Lateral bone of the lower arm
16. _____ Thin blood vessels where exchange of gases, nutrients, and wastes occurs
17. _____ Seven vertebrae forming the neck
18. _____ Brain and spinal cord
19. _____ Muscle type not under conscious control
20. _____ Organ of the lymphatic system where white blood cells filter the blood
21. _____ Lymph nodes in the posterior oral cavity
22. _____ Gland producing sperm
23. _____ Twelve vertebrae forming the upper back
24. _____ Gland storing ovum
25. _____ Organ where fetus develops
26. _____ Cartilage at inferior end of the sternum

a. Topographic anatomy
b. Ligaments
c. Cranium
d. Cervical spine
e. Thoracic spine
f. Lumbar spine
g. Coccyx
h. Xiphoid process
i. Ischium
j. Clavicle
k. Radius
l. Femur
m. Slightly movable joints
n. Freely movable joints
o. Involuntary muscle
p. Expiration
q. Larynx
r. Atria
s. Capillaries
t. Central nervous system
u. Lymph node
v. Tonsils
w. Hormones
x. Testicles
y. Ovaries
z. Uterus

True/False

Indicate whether each of the following is true (T) or false (F) on the line provided.

1. _____ The bones of the skeleton consist of both living tissue and nonliving materials.

2. _____ Muscles are attached to bones by ligaments.

3. _____ The diaphragm is the major muscle of the respiratory system.

4. _____ Arteries carry oxygenated blood.

5. _____ The peripheral nervous system consists of the nerves, which carry information back and forth from the body to the spinal cord and brain.

6. _____ The subcutaneous layer is thicker in older patients than in younger patients.

7. _____ The esophagus connects the pharynx to the stomach.

8. _____ The urethra carries urine from the kidneys to the urinary bladder.

9. _____ Tonsils are lymph nodes at the posterior oral cavity.

10. _____ Hormones are produced by the endocrine system.

11. _____ The fetus develops in the vaginal canal.

EXPLORE **PEARSON mybradykit™**

Please go to **www.bradybooks.com** to access mykit for this text. You will find quizzes, critical thinking scenarios, weblinks, animations, and videos related to this chapter—and much more. Look for online information on identifying body systems as well as animations on the heart and endocrine system.

Register your access code from the front of your book by going to **www.bradybooks.com** and selecting the mykit links.

Life Span Development

NAVIGATION GUIDE

The following items provide an overview to the purpose and content of this chapter. The Education Standard and Competency are from the National EMS Education Standards.

Education Standard Life Span Development

Competency Uses simple knowledge of age-related differences to assess and care for patients.

Objectives After reading this chapter, you should be able to:

1. Define key terms introduced in this chapter.
2. Describe the major physiological and psychosocial characteristics for each of the following stages of life:
   a. Infancy
   b. Toddler phase
   c. Preschool age
   d. School age
   e. Adolescence
   f. Early adulthood
   g. Middle adulthood
   h. Late adulthood
3. Give examples of behavior and communication with patients that show consideration of the patient's stage of life.

Key Terms Page references indicate first major use in this chapter. The Margin Glossary in this chapter provides definitions as you read.

infancy, p. 114	trust vs. mistrust, p. 117	adolescence, p. 120
Moro reflex, p. 115	scaffolding, p. 117	early adulthood, p. 123
palmar reflex, p. 115	temperament, p. 117	middle adulthood, p. 124
rooting reflex, p. 115	toddler phase, p. 117	late adulthood, p. 125
sucking reflex, p. 115	preschool age, p. 118	
bonding, p. 117	school age, p. 119	

Media Resources Please go to **www.bradybooks.com** to access mykit for this text. You will find quizzes, critical thinking scenarios, weblinks, animations, and videos related to this chapter—and much more. Look for online information on the process of aging. You will also find a video clip on pediatric growth and development.

ASK YOURSELF

■ Can you define the key terms introduced in this chapter?

INTRODUCTION

Life span development looks at the physiological (physical) and psychosocial (mental and social) changes that occur from birth to death. In this chapter, we will follow Jamie as she develops through the following stages of life:

- Infancy
- Toddler phase
- Preschool age
- School age

- Adolescence
- Early adulthood
- Middle adulthood
- Late adulthood

CASE STUDY

THE CALL

You are dispatched as an initial response unit to a private residence for an unresponsive teenager. When you arrive at the residence, the mother is frantic and escorts you to her son's basement bedroom where you find a teenage boy lying on the bed.

■ Discussion: *What are the questions you should first ask the parent as you confirm the boy is unresponsive?*

ASK YOURSELF

■ How would you describe the major physiological and psychosocial characteristics of the following stage of life?
  ■ Infancy

infancy stage of life from birth to 1 year of age.

Infancy (Birth to Age 1 Year)

If you have ever spent time around infants, you can attest to the phenomenal changes that occur during this first year of life. This is the period referred to as **infancy**. The infant is a small bundle of joy, totally dependent upon others, and grows to begin walking and developing a unique personality (Figure 6-1 ■).

Physiological

As Jamie ages, her normal pulse rate and respiratory rate will decrease and her blood pressure will increase. Her vital signs are listed in Table 6-1.

At birth, Jamie will weigh 3.0–3.5 kg (6.6–7.7 lb). Her weight will likely double by 6 months and triple by 12 months. Her head will be equal to 25 percent of her total body weight.

While in her mother's uterus, her lungs did not function and she had a different pattern of circulation before birth than after. The transition from fetal circulation to pulmonary circulation occurs within the first few days after birth.

Jamie's airway is shorter, narrower, less stable, and more easily obstructed than at any other stage in her life. She is primarily a "nose breather" until at least 4 weeks of age. Nasal

TABLE 6-1	Vital Signs: Infant	
HEART RATE	**RESPIRATORY RATE**	**SYSTOLIC BLOOD PRESSURE**
120–160/minute	30–60/minute (Drops to 30–40 soon after birth)	70 mmHg at birth to 90 mmHg at 1 year

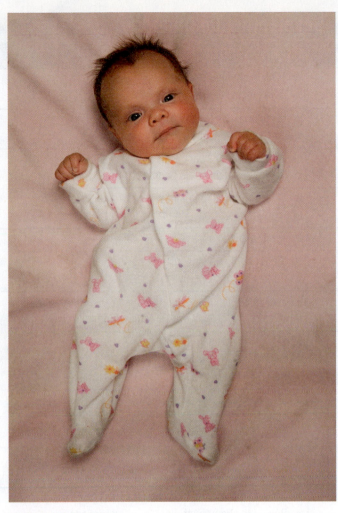

■ Figure 6-1 Infant.

congestion can cause difficulty breathing. She is also a diaphragm breather, thus you may see more movement in her abdomen than the chest.

During pregnancy, certain antibodies that help protect from disease are passed to her from her mother. Jamie is also breast-fed and receives antibodies to many of the diseases her mother has had. This helps protect Jamie until she can produce her own antibodies either from vaccination or exposure to a disease.

Jamie's nervous system includes four reflexes that will diminish over time:

- **Moro reflex**. When you startle her, she throws her arms out, spreads her fingers, and then grabs with her fingers and arms. These movements should be relatively equal on both sides.
- **Palmar reflex**. When you place your finger in her palm, she grasps it. Within a couple of months, this merges with the ability to release an object in the hand.
- **Rooting reflex**. When you touch Jamie's cheek when she is hungry, she turns her head toward the side touched.
- **Sucking reflex**. When you stroke Jamie's lips, she starts sucking. This reflex works in conjunction with the rooting reflex.

Initially, Jamie will sleep from 16–18 hours total throughout the day and night. This will soon change to about 4–6 hours during the day and 9–10 hours during the

Moro reflex when startled, an infant throws his arms out, spreads his fingers, then grabs with his fingers and arms.

palmar reflex when you place your finger in an infant's palm, he will grasp it.

rooting reflex when you touch a hungry infant's cheek, he will turn his head toward the side touched.

sucking reflex when you stroke a hungry infant's lips, he will start sucking.

TABLE 6-2 Developmental Changes

AGE	CHARACTERISTICS
2 months	■ Tracks objects with eyes ■ Recognizes familiar faces
3 months	■ Moves objects to mouth with hands ■ Distinct facial expressions (smile, frown)
4 months	■ Drools without swallowing ■ Begins to reach out to people
5 months	■ Sleeps through the night without waking for feeding ■ Discriminates between family and strangers
5–7 months	■ Teeth begin to appear
6 months	■ Sits upright in high chair ■ Begins making one-syllable sounds
7 months	■ Fear of strangers ■ Moods shift quickly (crying to laughing to crying)
8 months	■ Begins responding to word "no" ■ Can sit alone ■ Can play "peek-a-boo"
9 months	■ Responds to adult anger ■ Pulls himself up to standing position ■ Explores objects by mouthing, sucking, chewing, and biting
10 months	■ Pays attention to his name ■ Crawls well
11 months	■ Attempts to walk without assistance ■ Begins to show frustration about restrictions
12 months	■ Walks with help ■ Knows own name

night. Although each infant varies, usually in 2–4 months the infant will sleep through the night. Even though infants do sleep a lot, they are easy to awaken.

Jamie's extremities grow in length from a combination of growth plates, at the end of each long bone (humerus and femur), and the epiphyseal plates, near the end of the long bones. As mentioned in Chapter 5, "Anatomy and Physiology," the bones at the top of the skull are not fused at birth. The "soft spot" between these bones is called a fontanelle. The posterior fontanelle usually closes in 2 or 3 months, and the anterior one closes between 9 and 18 months. Looking at the anterior fontanelle, you can get a good idea of Jamie's state of hydration. Normally, the fontanelle is level with, or slightly below, the surface of the skull. If the fontanelle is sunken, this indicates dehydration. If the fontanelle is bulging, increased pressure inside the skull should be suspected.

There are certain milestones during Jamie's first year. Some of these are listed in Table 6-2.

Psychosocial

Jamie's primary means of communication is crying. Those close to Jamie will soon learn if she is crying because she is hungry, is tired, needs to be changed, or has some other reason.

Within the first 6 months, Jamie will bond with her caregivers and start displaying the following characteristics:

- **Bonding**. This is her sense that her needs will be met. When she is hungry, she is fed. When she needs to be held, she is.
- **Trust vs. mistrust**. Jamie likes an orderly, predictable environment. When her environment is disorderly and irregular, she develops anxiety and insecurity.
- **Scaffolding**. She learns by building on what she already knows.
- **Temperament**. This is her reaction to her environment.

You will learn more about the pediatric patient in Chapter 25, "Pediatric Emergencies."

Toddler Phase (12–36 Months)

During the **toddler phase**, physical, mental, and social development continues. Body systems continue to grow and refine themselves and the toddler develops more individuality. This age group's curiosity has led to such affectionate terms as "curtain climbers" or "rug rats." Their developing personality is sometimes referred to as the "terrible twos." Like all phases of childhood, these years can be a very rewarding time for both toddler and caregivers (Figure 6-2 ■).

bonding the sense that needs will be met.

trust vs. mistrust concept developed from an orderly, predictable environment versus a disorderly, irregular environment.

scaffolding building on what one already knows.

temperament the infant's reaction to his environment.

toddler phase stage of life from 12–36 months.

ASK YOURSELF

- How would you describe the major physiological and psychosocial characteristics of the following stage of life?
  - Toddler phase

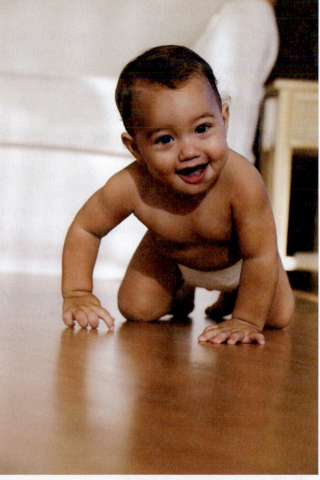

■ **Figure 6-2** Toddler. (© Rick Gomez/Masterfile)

TABLE 6-3 Vital Signs: Toddler

HEART RATE	RESPIRATORY RATE	SYSTOLIC BLOOD PRESSURE
80–130/minute	20–30/minute	70–100 mmHg

ASK YOURSELF

■ How would you explain examples of behavior and communication that show consideration of the patient's stage of life?

Physiological

Jamie's body temperature ranges from 96.8°F–99.6°F (36.3°C–37.9°C). She will gain approximately 2.0 kg (4.4 lb) per year. Her vital signs are listed in Table 6-3.

All her body systems will continue to develop and improve in efficiency. Fine motor skills, the use of hands and fingers to grasp and manipulate objects, begin developing. By 36 months of age, Jamie has all her primary teeth.

Though Jamie is physiologically capable of being toilet trained by the age of 12–15 months, she is not psychologically ready until 18–30 months of age. It is important not to rush toilet training. She will let her parents know when she is ready. The average age for completion of toilet training is 28 months.

Psychosocial

Cognitive development deals with the development of knowledge and thinking. Table 6-4 shows some of the cognitive development Jamie will experience.

ASK YOURSELF

■ How would you describe the major physiological and psychosocial characteristics of the following stage of life?
  ■ Preschool age

preschool age stage of life from 3–5 years.

Preschool Age (3–5 Years)

Preschool age is a time of continued physiological and psychosocial development. This is often a time when preschoolers are put into social interaction situations such as day care or preschools (Figure 6-3 ■).

Physiological

Jamie's body systems continue to develop and refine the various processes. Her vital signs are listed in Table 6-5.

Psychosocial

Jamie attends a preschool where she is involved with various peer groups. Peer groups provide a source of information about other families and the outside world. Interaction with peers offers opportunities for learning skills, comparing herself to others, and feeling part of a group.

TABLE 6-4 Cognitive Developmental Changes

AGE	CHARACTERISTICS
12 months	■ Begins to grasp that words "mean" something
18–24 months	■ Begins to understand cause and effect ■ Develops separation anxiety, clinging and crying when a parent leaves
24–36 months	■ Begins developing "magical thinking" and engages in play-acting, such as playing house
3–4 years	■ Masters the basics of language that will continue to be refined throughout childhood

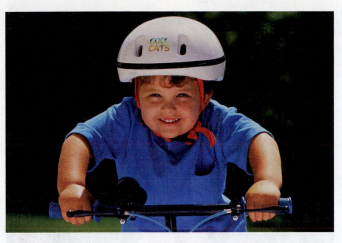

■ **Figure 6-3** Preschool age. (© David P. Hall/Masterfile)

TABLE 6-5 Vital Signs: Preschool Age		
HEART RATE	RESPIRATORY RATE	SYSTOLIC BLOOD PRESSURE
80–120/minute	20–30/minute	80–110 mmHg

School Age (6–12 Years)

Whether attending a public or private school, or being home-schooled, the stage of development referred to as **school age** opens vast opportunities for the child.

Physiological

Jamie's body temperature is approximately 98.6°F (37°C) and she will gain 3 kg (6.6 lb) and grow 6 cm (2.4 in.) per year (Figure 6-4 ■). Her vital signs are listed in Table 6-6.

One of the most obvious changes during this time is the loss of her primary teeth. Replacement with permanent teeth begins.

Psychosocial

This is a transition time for both Jamie and her parents. Her parents spend less time with her than they did during previous age groups and provide more general supervision. Jamie develops better decision-making skills and is allowed to make more decisions on her own.

Self-esteem develops and may be affected by popularity with peers, rejection, emotional support, and neglect. Negative self-esteem can be very damaging to further development.

As Jamie matures, moral development begins when she is rewarded for what her parents believe to be right and punished for what her parents believe to be wrong. With cognitive growth, moral reasoning appears and the control of her behavior gradually shifts from external sources to internal self-control.

TABLE 6-6 Vital Signs: School Age		
HEART RATE	RESPIRATORY RATE	SYSTOLIC BLOOD PRESSURE
70–110/minute	20–30/minute	80–120 mmHg

ASK YOURSELF

■ How would you describe the major physiological and psychosocial characteristics of the following stage of life?
  ■ School age

school age stage of life from 6–12 years.

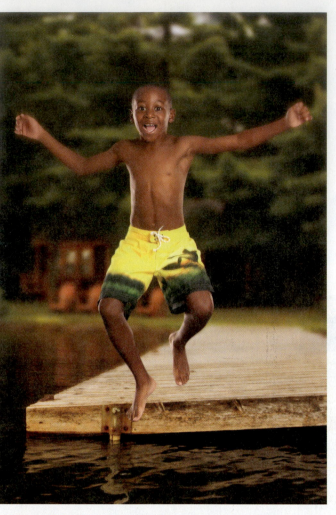

■ **Figure 6-4** School age. *(© Graham French/Masterfile)*

ASK YOURSELF

■ How would you describe the major physiological and psychosocial characteristics of the following stage of life?
■ Adolescence

adolescence stage of life from 13–18 years.

Adolescence (13–18 Years)

While life span development is a continual process, dynamic physiological and psychosocial changes occur during three major age groups: infancy, with the transition from fetal life to life in the world; **adolescence**, with the transition from childhood to adulthood; and late adulthood, with its deterioration of systems (Figure 6-5 ■).

Physiological

During this stage, Jamie will usually experience a rapid 2- to 3-year growth spurt, beginning distally with enlargement of her feet and hands followed by enlargement of her arms and legs. Her chest and trunk enlarge in the final stage of growth. Girls are usually finished growing by the age of 16 and boys by the age of 18. In late adolescence, the average male is taller and stronger than the average female. Jamie's vital signs are listed in Table 6-7.

At this age, both males and females reach reproductive maturity. Secondary sexual development occurs, with noticeable development of the external sexual organs. In females, menstruation begins and breasts develop.

Psychosocial

Adolescence can be a time of serious family conflicts as the adolescent strives for independence and parents strive for continued control.

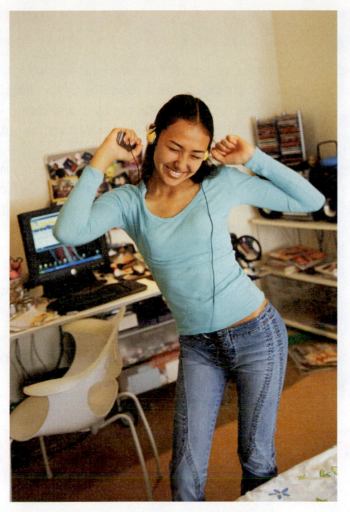

■ **Figure 6-5** Adolescence. (© Raoul Minsart/Masterfile)

TABLE 6-7 Vital Signs: Adolescence		
HEART RATE	**RESPIRATORY RATE**	**SYSTOLIC BLOOD PRESSURE**
55–105/minute	12–20/minute	80–120 mmHg

At this age, Jamie is trying to achieve more independence and develop her own identity. She becomes interested in the opposite sex, and finds this somewhat embarrassing. She not only wants to be treated like an adult but also enjoys the comforts of childhood.

Body image is a great concern at this point in life. This is a time when eating disorders are common. It also is a time when self-destructive behaviors begin, such as use of tobacco, alcohol, illicit drugs, and unsafe driving. Depression and suicide are more common at this age group than in any other.

As adolescents develop their capacity for logical, analytical, and abstract thinking, they begin to develop a personal code of ethics.

THE RESPONSE ✳

The patient is a 16-year-old male who is not responding to stimuli, is breathing, and has a slow, weak pulse. The mother states he has a history of heart problems for which he takes medication. He didn't come upstairs for breakfast, and she found him on his bed but couldn't wake him.

You ensure an open airway, place the patient on oxygen, and continue your assessment. When the paramedics arrive, you give them a verbal report on the patient's condition when you arrived, the treatment rendered, and the response to that treatment.

The paramedics place the patient on a cardiac monitor and establish an intravenous (IV) line. After further assessment, they continue care for an unresponsive patient with an unknown problem.

You assist the paramedics in preparing for transport and accompany them in the ambulance.

■ Discussion: *If the mother had elaborated on the patient's heart problem, would that have changed the care provided?*

✳ Stop, Review, Remember

Multiple Choice

Place a check next to the correct answer.

1. When an infant feels assurance that his needs will be met it is called:

   _____ a. trust.

   _____ b. scaffolding.

   _____ c. temperament.

   _____ d. bonding.

2. Which of the following is the normal heart rate range for a school-age child?

   _____ a. 140–160

   _____ b. 80–130

   _____ c. 70–110

   _____ d. 55–105

Emergency Medical Responder Practice

You are back at the station after responding to a vehicle collision on a rural road. This is the sixth call this summer at the same location where teenage drivers lost control and crashed into the trees.

As the newest member of your department, you ask the senior EMR why this is so common.

1. Why do so many teenagers take these risks?

   _____

   _____

   _____

   _____

Early Adulthood (20–40 Years)

With great pomp and circumstance, the adolescent graduates from childhood to adulthood (Figure 6-6 ■). Some say the best years are behind; some say the best years are ahead. But life is what you make of it and **early adulthood** opens up great opportunities.

Physiological

This is the period of life when Jamie will develop lifelong habits and routines. Her vital signs are listed in Table 6-8.

Peak physical condition occurs between 19 and 26 years of age, when all body systems are at optimal performance levels. At the end of this period, the body begins its slowing process.

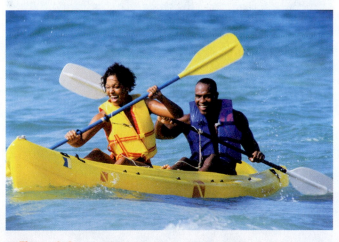

■ **Figure 6-6** Early adulthood. *(© George Shelley/Masterfile)*

TABLE 6-8 Vital Signs: Early Adulthood

HEART RATE	RESPIRATORY RATE	BLOOD PRESSURE
Average 70/minute	16–20/minute	120/80 mmHg

Psychosocial

The highest levels of job stress occur at this point in life, when Jamie is trying to establish her identity. Love develops, both romantic and affectionate. Childbirth is most common in this age group, with new families providing new challenges and stress.

Middle Adulthood (41–60 Years)

For most, **middle adulthood** is a time of reflecting on how far they have come and where they want to go. This internal conflict is often called "midlife crisis."

Physiological

During this stage of development, Jamie has no significant changes in vital signs from the early adulthood group.

She is starting to have some vision problems and is now wearing prescription glasses. Her cholesterol is a little high and she is concerned about health problems. Cancer often develops in this age group, weight control becomes more difficult, and for women in the late 40s to early 50s, menopause commences. Heart disease is the major killer after the age of 40 in all age, sex, and racial groups (Figure 6-7 ■).

ASK YOURSELF

■ How would you describe the major physiological and psychosocial characteristics of the following stage of life?
   ■ Middle adulthood

middle adulthood stage of life from 41–60 years.

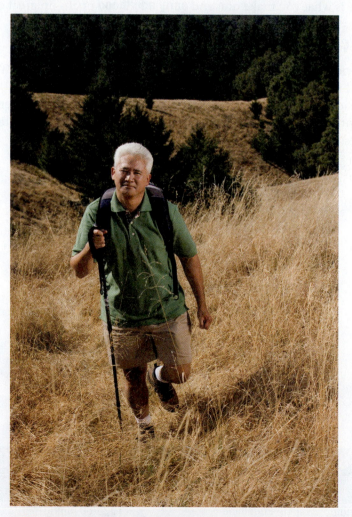

■ **Figure 6-7** Middle adulthood. (© Masterfile/Royalty Free)

Psychosocial

Jamie is becoming more task oriented as she sees the time for accomplishing her lifetime goals diminish. Still, she tends to approach problems more as challenges than as threats. With her children starting lives of their own, she is experiencing "empty-nest syndrome," or the time after the last offspring has left home. This may also be a time of increased freedom and opportunity for self-fulfillment.

She is concerned about her children as they start their new lives, and she is also concerned about caring for aging parents.

Late Adulthood (61 Years and Older)

Late adulthood is often referred to as the "twilight years." This stage of development brings about several physiological and psychosocial changes second only to those seen during infancy or adolescence (Figure 6-8 ■).

Physiological

Jamie's vital signs will be dependent on her physical and health condition.

Her cardiovascular system becomes less efficient, and the volume of blood decreases. She is less tolerant of tachycardia (fast heart rate). Her respiratory system deteriorates and

ASK YOURSELF

■ How would you describe the major physiological and psychosocial characteristics of the following stage of life?
■ Late adulthood

late adulthood stage of life from 61 years and older.

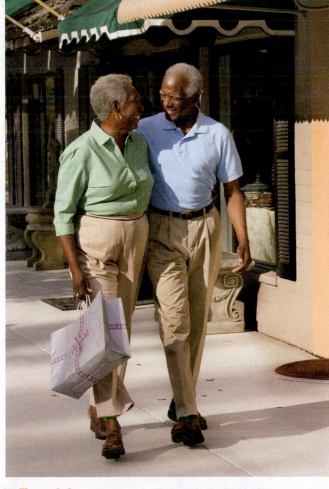

■ **Figure 6-8** Late adulthood. (© Kevin Dodge/Masterfile)

makes her more likely to develop respiratory disorders. Changes in the endocrine system result in decreased metabolism. Her sleep-wake cycle also is disrupted, causing her to have sleep problems. All other body systems are deteriorating as time progresses.

Psychosocial

As Jamie ages she will face many challenges. Motivation, personal interests, and the level of activities will enhance this later time of life. She faces the following challenges:

- *Living environment.* How long can she live at home? Does she need to be in an assisted living facility, or perhaps a nursing home?
- *Self-worth.* Though she has slowed down a bit, she is concerned with producing quality work that benefits herself and others.
- *Financial burdens.* With limited income and increasing expenses, financial concerns weigh heavily on her decisions.
- *Death and dying.* She sees friends and relatives become ill and die. Concerns of her own health condition and mortality often come to mind.

You will learn more about the geriatric patient in Chapter 26, "Geriatric Patients."

CASE STUDY

TRANSITION

Once in the ambulance, the patient responds to treatment and is able to answer questions appropriately. During the patient interview, you learn that the patient took his cardiac medication as prescribed and that he had a beer while out with some friends. He was concerned about his parents finding out.

The patient's condition continues to improve, and he is transferred to the care of emergency department personnel.

While you and the paramedics are completing documentation, you discuss why this patient drank while taking his medication. Your discussions include the aspect that adolescents tend to engage in risk-taking behavior and are often in conflict with their parents.

- Discussion: *Had you thought about the possibility that this patient may have had alcohol?*

THE LAST WORD

Over the course of one's life, there are numerous changes in physical, mental, and social aspects. These range from the drastic changes during infancy as all the body systems develop and the infant learns to interact with society, to the changes during adolescence as the body matures, to the changes occurring during late adulthood as the geriatric patient's body systems, and sometimes mental abilities, deteriorate.

Having an understanding of these life changes will help you to better understand what your patient is experiencing.

Chapter Review

Multiple Choice

Place a check next to the correct answer.

1. What happens to the vital signs over a person's lifetime?
   _____ a. Heart rate decreases, respiratory rate decreases, and blood pressure decreases.
   _____ b. Heart rate decreases, respiratory rate decreases, and blood pressure increases.
   _____ c. Heart rate increases, respiratory rate decreases, and blood pressure decreases.
   _____ d. Heart rate increases, respiratory rate increases, and blood pressure decreases.

2. The anterior fontanelle closes between:
   _____ a. 2–3 months.
   _____ b. 6–12 months.
   _____ c. 9–18 months.
   _____ d. 18–24 months.

3. "Magical thinking" usually begins at:
   _____ a. 12–18 months.
   _____ b. 18–24 months.
   _____ c. 23–36 months.
   _____ d. 36–48 months.

4. At what developmental stage does the individual form peer groups?
   _____ a. Toddler
   _____ b. Preschooler
   _____ c. School-age child
   _____ d. Adolescent

5. Girls are usually finished growing by the age of _____ and boys by the age of _____.
   _____ a. 14, 16
   _____ b. 15, 17
   _____ c. 16, 18
   _____ d. 17, 19

6. Normal systolic blood pressure in an adolescent is:
   _____ a. 80–120 mmHg.
   _____ b. 80–110 mmHg.
   _____ c. 70–100 mmHg.
   _____ d. 70–90 mmHg.

7. The highest levels of job stress occur during:
   _____ a. adolescence.
   _____ b. early adulthood.
   _____ c. middle adulthood.
   _____ d. late adulthood.

8. All of the following usually occur during middle adulthood except:
   _____ a. childbirth.
   _____ b. cancer.
   _____ c. heart disease.
   _____ d. menopause.

9. A person in late adulthood has:
   _____ a. less tolerance of tachycardia and decreased metabolism.
   _____ b. less tolerance of tachycardia and increased metabolism.
   _____ c. more tolerance of tachycardia and decreased metabolism.
   _____ d. more tolerance of tachycardia and increased metabolism.

10. At what three stages do the most dramatic physiological and psychosocial changes occur?
   _____ a. Infancy, school age, late adulthood
   _____ b. Infancy, adolescence, late adulthood
   _____ c. Infancy, early adulthood, late adulthood
   _____ d. Infancy, adolescence, middle adulthood

Emergency Medical Responder Practice

There are many challenges that persons face in late adulthood. Think about the following challenges and list how you or your community might help meet them.

Living environment

_____

_____

_____

_____

Self-worth

_____

_____

_____

_____

Financial burdens

_____

_____

_____

_____

Death and dying

_____

_____

_____

_____

Matching

Match the following characteristics with the appropriate development stage.

1. _____ Develops self-esteem
2. _____ Triples body weight
3. _____ Is concerned with self-worth
4. _____ Forms peer groups
5. _____ Reaches reproductive maturity
6. _____ Reaches peak physical condition
7. _____ Has all primary teeth
8. _____ Experiences empty-nest syndrome

a. Infancy
b. Toddler phase
c. Preschool age
d. School age
e. Adolescence
f. Early adulthood
g. Middle adulthood
h. Late adulthood

EXPLORE **PEARSON mybradykit™**

Please go to **www.bradybooks.com** to access mykit for this text. You will find quizzes, critical thinking scenarios, weblinks, animations, and videos related to this chapter—and much more. Look for online information on the process of aging as well as a video clip on pediatric growth and development.

Register your access code from the front of your book by going to **www.bradybooks.com** and selecting the mykit links.

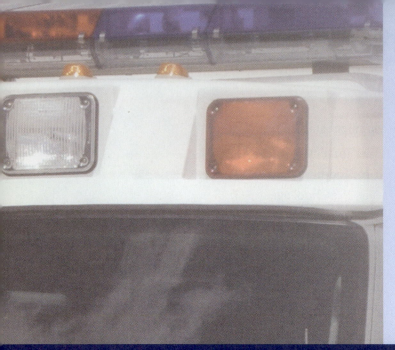

SECTION 1
Review and Practice Examination

Assess what you have learned in this section by checking the best answer for each multiple-choice question. When you are done, check your answers against the key provided in Appendix B.

1. Which of the following best describes the role of EMRs?
   _____ a. Volunteer their time to respond to emergencies
   _____ b. Transport ill and injured patients to the hospital
   _____ c. Work in the emergency department
   _____ d. Provide the first minutes of emergency medical care

2. The EMS providers with the highest level of training are:
   _____ a. Paramedics.
   _____ b. Emergency Medical Technicians.
   _____ c. Advanced Emergency Medical Technicians.
   _____ d. Emergency Medical Responders.

3. A critically injured patient has the best chance of survival if he can be transported to a(n):
   _____ a. emergency department.
   _____ b. trauma center.
   _____ c. intensive care unit.
   _____ d. cardiovascular care center.

4. The required component of an EMS system that exists to continually review and improve an EMS system is:

   _____ a. evaluation.
   _____ b. medical oversight.
   _____ c. regulation and policy.
   _____ d. public information and education.

5. When the ambulance arrives to transport the patient you have been caring for, you state to the EMTs, "Mrs. McEnroe is worried about locking the doors and taking her keys with her." You have just demonstrated the professional trait of:
   _____ a. confident demeanor.
   _____ b. integrity.
   _____ c. motivation.
   _____ d. patient advocacy.

6. A patient tells you what medication he is taking, but you are not sure what the medication is used for, so you take out a pocket reference guide and look it up. Which of the following best describes the significance of this action?
   _____ a. It is an important way of avoiding errors in patient care.
   _____ b. It demonstrates a weakness in your competence as an EMR.
   _____ c. It is outside the scope of practice of EMRs to look up medications.
   _____ d. It will trigger a review by the medical director.

7. Which of the following statements about the relationship between research and care provided by EMRs is true?
_____ a. Once you learn a certain skill, it will always be in your scope of practice.
_____ b. Research is needed to refine the scope of practice of EMRs.
_____ c. EMRs play no role in research to determine the scope of practice.
_____ d. Research is important at higher levels of EMS care, but not at the EMR level.

8. Which of the following situations should make you most concerned about the possibility of violence as you approach the scene of an emergency?
_____ a. A group of eight to ten people is standing outside as you arrive.
_____ b. A sign on the front door indicates oxygen is in use.
_____ c. The call is to a private residence in a rural area.
_____ d. The patient meets you on the front porch of the residence.

9. As you arrive at the scene of a call for an injured person, the front door swings open, revealing a woman holding a shotgun. Which of the following would provide you with the best cover?
_____ a. Ducking behind a leafy bush or shrub
_____ b. Holding a piece of equipment next to your head as you run for your vehicle
_____ c. Moving behind a large tree
_____ d. Diving to the ground and lying flat

10. In which of the following situations would you most highly suspect the presence of a hazardous material?
_____ a. You are responding to a private home for a patient with chest pain who has taken nitroglycerin.
_____ b. You notice that a motor vehicle collision involves a car and a tractor-trailer.
_____ c. You notice that a motor vehicle collision involves a small pickup truck that struck a utility pole.
_____ d. Dispatch reports your patient, the victim of a gunshot wound, has lost a lot of blood.

11. The use of Standard Precautions to protect yourself from communicable disease applies to:
_____ a. only patients who have signs or symptoms of an illness.
_____ b. only patients who are bleeding, vomiting, or coughing.
_____ c. all patient care situations.
_____ d. interactions with all health care providers and patients.

12. Which of the following immunizations is required for health care workers?
_____ a. Tetanus
_____ b. Hepatitis D
_____ c. Tuberculosis
_____ d. Pneumonia

13. While you are caring for a patient with a cut on his forehead, the finger of your glove tears and some of the patient's blood comes in contact with your skin. Which of the following is the best way to prevent contracting a bloodborne disease from this patient?
_____ a. Ask the patient if he has any infectious diseases, including syphilis or hepatitis.
_____ b. Put a new glove over the top of the damaged one.
_____ c. Use an alcohol swab to clean off your finger.
_____ d. Wash your hands with soap and water as soon as possible.

14. Which of the following situations requires the use of eye and face protection equipment?
_____ a. Suctioning the mouth of a patient who is coughing up blood
_____ b. All patient care contact
_____ c. Patients who you suspect have not bathed for a long period of time
_____ d. Bandaging an infected wound on a patient's foot

15. In terms of communicable disease, which of the following would be considered an exposure?
_____ a. Vomit soaks into your pants when you kneel down to assist a sick patient.
_____ b. You are splashed in the face with fluids while assisting with childbirth.
_____ c. You get the blood of a patient with tuberculosis on your hands.
_____ d. As you help move a patient, you notice that his clothes are wet with urine and some of it has soaked into your shirtsleeve.

16. Which of the following situations is most likely to be considered stressful by many EMS personnel?
_____ a. Interacting with law enforcement or fire personnel on the scene
_____ b. Calls involving seriously ill or injured children
_____ c. Having bystanders present at the scene
_____ d. The sight of blood

17. While you are caring for a patient, his adult daughter becomes very upset that the ambulance has not yet arrived. She raises her voice and demands that you do something to hurry up the ambulance. Which of the following would be the best response?
_____ a. Leave the patient's side and immediately call for law enforcement backup.
_____ b. Tell the daughter to calm down and be quiet.
_____ c. Tell the patient you cannot help him if he allows his daughter to yell at you.
_____ d. Assure the patient and his daughter that the ambulance will arrive as soon as possible.

18. You have noticed that you don't feel very motivated to volunteer for shifts with the rescue squad, you get easily irritated by people in general, and you would rather be alone than with your family. Which of the following would be most likely to be helpful?
_____ a. Drink more caffeine to increase your motivation.
_____ b. Drink a cocktail, beer, or some wine to relax.
_____ c. Increase your physical activity to reduce stress.
_____ d. Realize that stress is a fact of EMS life and it will pass on its own.

19. You have responded to a patient whose family fears he is dead. The patient does not respond to you, is not breathing, and does not have a pulse. In which of the following situations would you still need to begin resuscitation?
_____ a. The patient's family tells you they don't want him to be "hooked up to machines."
_____ b. There is a strong odor of decay and the skin is peeling.

_____ c. The body is in an extreme state of rigidity.
_____ d. The patient has a gunshot wound that has destroyed the entire head above the lower jaw.

20. Your patient is an elderly female who was diagnosed with cancer 6 months ago, but refused treatment for the disease. She is now very ill and seems near death. Her husband is calm and seems to be handling the situation well. Which of the following is most accurate in describing the husband's grieving process?
_____ a. He has come to accept his wife's death.
_____ b. He is in denial that his wife is dying.
_____ c. He appears to be depressed.
_____ d. You should anticipate a sudden outburst of anger from him.

21. When you are lifting a patient, which of these principles should you follow?
_____ a. Rotate at the waist to move the patient to your left or right.
_____ b. Bend at the waist and lift with the back muscles.
_____ c. Keep your feet together.
_____ d. Use the muscles of your legs to do the work of lifting.

22. You and one other EMR are on the scene of a motor vehicle collision. The left side of the vehicle is against a building and you can only access the right side. There are two patients in the front seat. The passenger is awake but has severe injuries to her legs and is complaining of abdominal pain. The driver is unresponsive, is slumped over the steering wheel, has severe bleeding from his head, and is making gurgling noises when he breathes. Which of the following statements regarding this situation is most accurate?
_____ a. This requires an urgent move. Wait for additional help before moving the passenger.
_____ b. This requires an emergency move. Carefully remove the passenger with the help you have available so you can get to the driver.
_____ c. This requires an urgent move, but you and the other EMR can handle it.
_____ d. This requires an emergency move, but you should wait for additional help to arrive.

23. You have responded to a patient who states she does not need or want your help, so you contact medical direction by radio for advice. This is an example of _____ medical direction.
    _____ a. on-line
    _____ b. off-line
    _____ c. indirect
    _____ d. protocol-driven

24. Which of the following must be present in order to obtain expressed consent?
    _____ a. The patient is under the influence of drugs or alcohol.
    _____ b. The patient is unresponsive.
    _____ c. The patient is a minor, and a parent or guardian is not available.
    _____ d. The patient has been informed of the risks and benefits of care and refusing care.

25. You have responded to a motor vehicle collision, and notice that there are both empty and full beer cans in the car. The driver's speech is slurred and he is trying to walk away from the scene, even though he has a cut on his forehead. Which of the following statements concerning this situation is most accurate?
    _____ a. You should restrain the patient from leaving and contact law enforcement so that you cannot be sued for abandoning the patient.
    _____ b. You should explain to the patient that you are more concerned about his health than you are with the legality of his actions and ask to look at his injury.
    _____ c. You should let the patient walk away and leave the scene so that you are not charged with battery or false imprisonment.
    _____ d. You should tell the patient you understand his fear of being arrested and offer to drive him to the emergency department.

26. You have arrived at an extended care facility (nursing home) for a patient in cardiac arrest. The nurse tells you that the patient has a DNR order and that you should not provide any emergency care. Which of the following would be the best action?
    _____ a. Advise the nurse that you will need to look at the DNR order.

    _____ b. Get the telephone number of a family member so you can confirm that the patient has a DNR order.
    _____ c. Begin and continue resuscitative measures until a higher-level EMS provider arrives.
    _____ d. Advise the nurse that EMS providers can honor living wills, but not DNR orders.

27. You have arrived at a convenience store where the cashier was shot in an attempted burglary. Law enforcement is on the scene and you can see through the window that the patient has lost a lot of blood. Which of the following is the best approach in this situation?
    _____ a. Ask law enforcement officers to move the patient out of the store so you can care for him.
    _____ b. Enter the scene but take care to avoid unnecessarily touching or moving anything.
    _____ c. Enter the scene and approach as you would any other patient. Crime scene evidence is not the concern of EMS personnel.
    _____ d. Wait for a higher-level EMS provider to arrive before approaching the patient.

28. Your patient, a 77-year-old man, states that his doctor previously diagnosed him with tachycardia. This means the patient has a history of which of the following?
    _____ a. Slow heart rate
    _____ b. Fast heart rate
    _____ c. Slow breathing
    _____ d. Fast breathing

29. When you are assessing the anterior aspect of a patient's body, this is the same as assessing the _____ of the patient's body.
    _____ a. back
    _____ b. front
    _____ c. lower half
    _____ d. upper half

30. The opposite of proximal is:
    _____ a. internal.
    _____ b. superficial.
    _____ c. anterior.
    _____ d. distal.

31. Which of the following structures is contained within the thoracic cavity of the body?
_____ a. Brain
_____ b. Spleen
_____ c. Heart
_____ d. Urinary bladder

32. Your patient has been ejected (thrown) from a vehicle during a high-speed collision. A bruise over the right upper quadrant of the abdomen should lead you to suspect that the patient may have an injury to the:
_____ a. urinary bladder.
_____ b. spleen.
_____ c. esophagus.
_____ d. liver.

33. The state of optimal healthy functioning that all of the body's systems attempt to maintain is called:
_____ a. physiology.
_____ b. microscopic anatomy.
_____ c. homeostasis.
_____ d. gross anatomy.

34. As you arrive on the scene of a motor vehicle collision, a nurse who has stopped to assist the patients tells you he thinks one of the patients has a cervical spine injury. This means the patient may have an injury to the:
_____ a. neck.
_____ b. upper back.
_____ c. lower back.
_____ d. tailbone.

35. The wings of the pelvis are made up of the _____ bones.
_____ a. ischial
_____ b. iliac
_____ c. pubis
_____ d. sacral

36. A patient with a fractured femur has a fracture of the:
_____ a. arm.
_____ b. lower arm.
_____ c. leg.
_____ d. lower leg.

37. The structure and function of the hip joint make it a(n) _____ joint.
_____ a. freely movable
_____ b. hinge
_____ c. immovable
_____ d. gliding

38. The large muscle in the anterior thigh is an example of _____ muscle.
_____ a. smooth
_____ b. involuntary
_____ c. skeletal
_____ d. cardiac

39. You have assessed the respirations of a 40-year-old male and found the respiratory rate to be 16 per minute. You would classify this rate as:
_____ a. slower than expected.
_____ b. faster than expected.
_____ c. normal for his age.
_____ d. abnormal for his age.

40. Medically, the term for the voice box is:
_____ a. larynx.
_____ b. trachea.
_____ c. pharynx.
_____ d. bronchus.

41. Oxygen and carbon dioxide are exchanged at the level of the:
_____ a. alveoli.
_____ b. larynx.
_____ c. trachea.
_____ d. bronchi.

42. In order for inspiration to occur, the diaphragm must:
_____ a. relax to make the thoracic cavity larger.
_____ b. relax to make the thoracic cavity smaller.
_____ c. contract to make the thoracic cavity larger.
_____ d. contract to make the thoracic cavity smaller.

43. The heart muscle receives oxygenated blood from the:
_____ a. carotid arteries.
_____ b. pulmonary arteries.
_____ c. coronary arteries.
_____ d. ventricular arteries.

44. Which of the following can be predicted, based on knowledge of the different jobs of the atria and ventricles and of the right and left sides of the heart?
_____ a. The atria and ventricles need the same amount of strength.
_____ b. The atria need more strength than the ventricles.
_____ c. The right ventricle is stronger than the left ventricle.

_____ d. The left ventricle is stronger than the right ventricle.

45. Your patient tells you her doctor says she has a low platelet count. You should suspect that:
_____ a. the level of glucose in the patient's blood is too high.
_____ b. the level of oxygen delivered to the patient's tissues is low.
_____ c. the patient's blood does not clot normally.
_____ d. the patient cannot fight infection normally.

46. The layer of the skin that consists mostly of fat is the _____ layer.
_____ a. subcutaneous
_____ b. integumentary system
_____ c. epidermis
_____ d. dermis

47. The structure that allows the urinary bladder to empty is the:
_____ a. ureter.
_____ b. gallbladder.
_____ c. bile duct.
_____ d. urethra.

48. Your patient says she has a history of a urinary tract infection. This could include any of the following structures except the:
_____ a. gallbladder.
_____ b. ureter.
_____ c. urethra.
_____ d. kidney.

49. Your patient reports "swollen glands" in his neck. This should lead you to suspect that the patient may have:
_____ a. an autonomic nervous system problem.
_____ b. diabetes.
_____ c. an infection.
_____ d. digestive problems.

50. The structure meant to contain a developing fetus during pregnancy is the:
_____ a. uterus.
_____ b. fallopian tube.
_____ c. ovary.
_____ d. cervix.

51. The specific process by which oxygen and nutrients are delivered to the tissues is called:
_____ a. homeostasis.
_____ b. metabolism.

_____ c. perfusion.
_____ d. respiration.

52. For medical purposes, a child from birth to the age of 1 year is referred to as a(n):
_____ a. newborn.
_____ b. infant.
_____ c. toddler.
_____ d. adolescent.

53. Which of the following is in the normal range for the heart rate (per minute) of a 2-week-old child?
_____ a. 80
_____ b. 100
_____ c. 150
_____ d. 180

54. As you begin to lay a 1-week-old infant on the bed to examine him, he throws out his arms, fingers spread. Which of the following is most accurate concerning this reaction?
_____ a. This is normal in older infants, but not at this age.
_____ b. It is an abnormal reflex that could indicate shaken-baby syndrome.
_____ c. This is normal when infants of this age are startled.
_____ d. This is a normal reflex until adulthood.

55. The "soft spot" of an infant's head is called the:
_____ a. fontanelle.
_____ b. epiphyseal plate.
_____ c. cerebral membrane.
_____ d. xiphoid process.

56. Your patient is a 16-year-old female softball player who was struck in the face by a ball. Her nose looks deformed, she has a loose tooth, and she is bleeding from her nose and a cut lip. She did not lose consciousness; she is oriented to person, time, and place; and she has the following vital signs: heart rate of 92, respiratory rate of 20, and blood pressure of 92/66. Which of the following is most important for you to keep in mind when caring for this patient?
_____ a. You must ask her if she has started menstruating.
_____ b. Her blood pressure is abnormally low for this age group.
_____ c. She will be very concerned about the effects of the injuries on her appearance.
_____ d. She is likely to exhibit "magical thinking" about the injury.

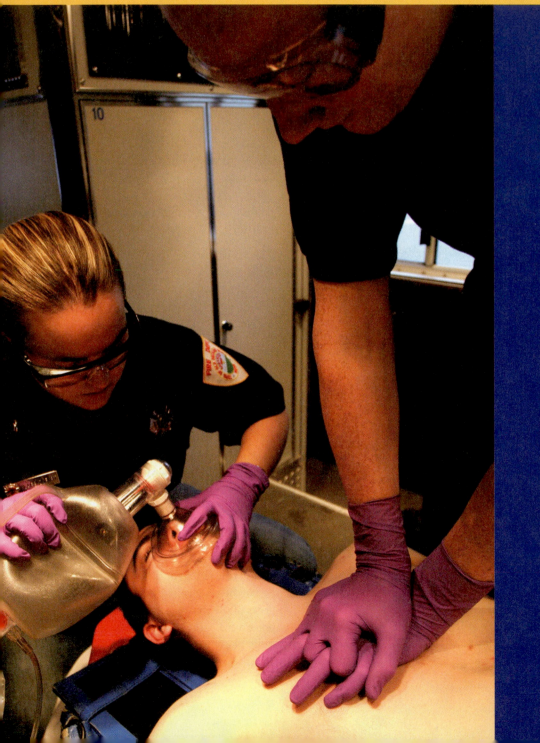

SECTION 2
Airway and Cardiac Resuscitation

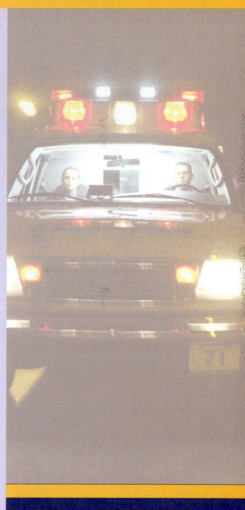

✳ SECTION OUTLINE

In this section, you will cover the following EMS Education Standards:

- ■ Anatomy and Physiology
- ■ Pathophysiology
- ■ Airway Management, Respiration, and Artificial Ventilation
- ■ Shock and Resuscitation

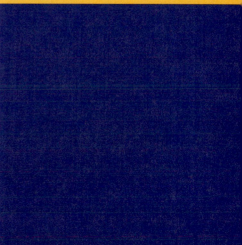

Airway

NAVIGATION GUIDE

The following items provide an overview to the purpose and content of this chapter. The Education Standards and Competencies are from the National EMS Education Standards.

Education Standards Anatomy and Physiology; Airway Management, Respiration, and Artificial Ventilation

Competencies Uses simple knowledge of the anatomy and function of the upper airway, heart, vessels, blood, lungs, skin, muscles, and bones as the foundation of emergency care.

Applies knowledge (fundamental depth, foundational breadth) of general anatomy and physiology to assure a patent airway, adequate mechanical ventilation, and respiration while awaiting additional EMS response for patients of all ages.

Knowledge Areas Airway Management
- Airway anatomy
- Airway assessment
- Techniques of assuring a patent airway
Respiration
- Anatomy of the respiratory system
- Physiology and pathophysiology of respiration
  - Pulmonary ventilation
  - Oxygenation
  - Respiration
    - External
    - Internal
    - Cellular
- Assessment and management of adequate and inadequate respiration
- Supplemental oxygen therapy
Artificial Ventilation
- Assessment and management of adequate and inadequate ventilation
- Minute ventilation
- Alveolar ventilation
- Effect of artificial ventilation on cardiac output

Objectives   After reading this chapter, you should be able to:

1. Define key terms introduced in this chapter.
2. Describe the anatomy and physiology of breathing.
3. Discuss conditions that lead to inadequate breathing.
4. Use assessment findings to differentiate between patients who are breathing adequately, those who are breathing inadequately, and those who are not breathing at all.
5. Explain the concept of oxygen saturation.
6. Explain safety precautions needed when handling oxygen tanks and administering oxygen.
7. Describe the indications, contraindications, precautions, and procedures for performing each of the following skills:
   a. Pulse oximetry
   b. Head-tilt, chin-lift maneuver
   c. Jaw-thrust maneuver
   d. Modified chin lift
   e. Suctioning
   f. Inserting an oropharyngeal (oral) airway
   g. Administering oxygen by mask and nasal cannula
   h. Providing ventilations with a pocket face mask
   i. Providing ventilations with a bag-valve mask
   j. Relieving foreign body airway obstruction in patients of all ages
8. Intervene to establish and maintain the airway and breathing by performing the following skills:
   a. Head-tilt, chin-lift maneuver
   b. Jaw-thrust maneuver
   c. Modified chin lift
   d. Suctioning
   e. Inserting an oropharyngeal (oral) airway
   f. Administering oxygen by mask and nasal cannula
   g. Providing ventilations with a pocket face mask
   h. Providing ventilations with a bag-valve mask
   i. Relieving foreign body airway obstruction in adult patients

Key Terms   Page references indicate first major use in this chapter. The Margin Glossary in this chapter provides definitions as you read.

inhalation, p. 142
exhalation, p. 142
hypoxia, p. 146
patent, p. 146
cyanosis, p. 146
paradoxical motion, p. 147
flail segment, p. 147
pulmonary ventilation, p. 147
oxygenation, p. 147
respiration, p. 148

modified chin lift, p. 150
suction catheters, p. 152
oropharyngeal airway, p. 154
accessory muscle use, p. 158
retractions, p. 158
pulse oximeter, p. 160
oxygen saturation, p. 160
carbon dioxide, p. 161
carbon monoxide, p. 161
regulators, p. 162

liters per minute, p. 162
O ring, p. 162
oxygen supply tube, p. 162
nonrebreather mask, p. 163
Venturi mask, p. 163
ventilation port, p. 171
one-way valve, p. 171
Sellick maneuver, p. 173

Media Resources   Please go to **www.bradybooks.com** to access mykit for this text. You will find quizzes, critical thinking scenarios, weblinks, animations, and videos related to this chapter—and much more. Look for online information on effective BVM ventilations. You will also find a video clip on the two-person BVM technique.

INTRODUCTION

Airway care is arguably the most important skill of all the things you will do for your patients as an Emergency Medical Responder (See The Big Picture: Airway).

The Big Picture
Airway

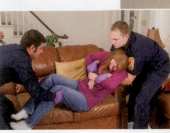

1 Move patient to the floor.

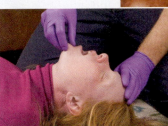

2 Open the airway.

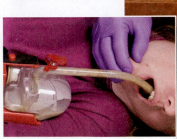

3 Suction if necessary.

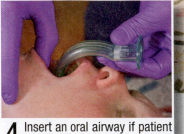

4 Insert an oral airway if patient is unresponsive without gag reflex.

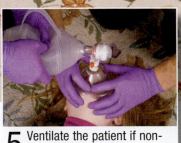

5 Ventilate the patient if non-breathing or breathing inadequately.

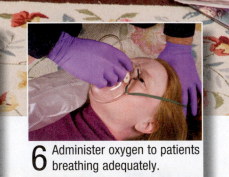

6 Administer oxygen to patients breathing adequately.

You will see a common theme in this chapter. It is that breathing must be present and adequate. It is not an all-or-nothing proposition. It is possible that a patient who appears to be breathing is not actually breathing enough to support life. You will learn, in the order you will assess or care for the airway, how to perform these valuable interventions. Thus, the vital concept to understand is that:

To survive, a patient must breathe deeply enough and at an adequate rate. Without BOTH adequate rate and adequate depth, your patient will die.

Anatomy and Physiology Revisited

Before learning about airway assessment and care, it is important to review the anatomy and physiology of the airway (Figures 7-1 ■ and 7-2 ■).

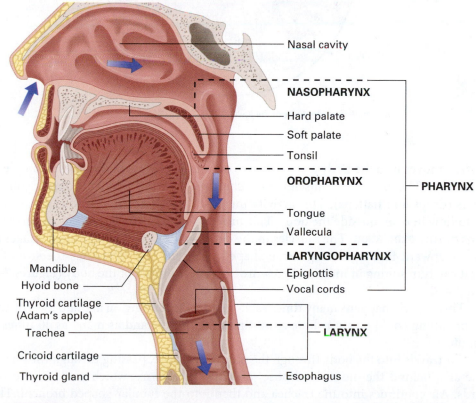

■ **Figure 7-1** Anatomy of the upper airway.

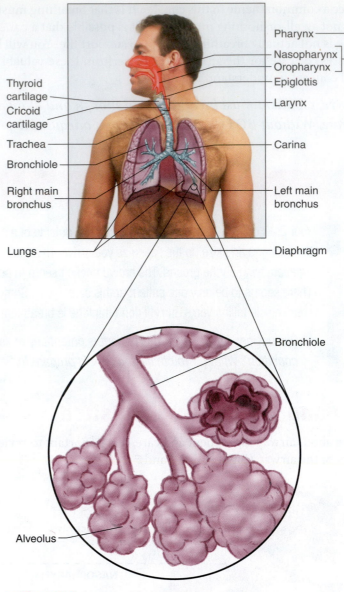

Thyroid cartilage
Cricoid cartilage
Trachea
Bronchiole
Right main bronchus
Lungs

Pharynx
Nasopharynx
Oropharynx
Epiglottis
Larynx
Carina
Left main bronchus
Diaphragm

Bronchiole
Alveolus

■ **Figure 7-2** Anatomy of the lower airway.

Air moves into the body and air moves out of the body. This process is simple, yet vital to life. The intercostal muscles in the chest wall contract while the diaphragm contracts (drops and flattens). This activity increases the size of the chest cavity, causing air to flow in from outside the body. This process is called **inhalation**. The reverse happens during **exhalation**. The muscles in the chest wall relax; the diaphragm relaxes and moves upward into its resting dome-shaped position. This decreases the size of the chest cavity, resulting in increased pressure that forces air out of the body (Figures 7-3 ■ and 7-4 ■).

This process happens many times each minute. Depending on age and level of activity, breathing could occur as little as 10 times per minute and as many as 40 times per minute.

Air travels into the body through the mouth and nose, passing through the pharynx (the area behind the mouth and nose) and into the larynx, which contains the vocal cords. Air continues into the trachea and then into the tubular-shaped bronchi. These bronchi divide into smaller and smaller segments called bronchioles. Bronchioles end at

inhalation the process of bringing air into the chest cavity.

exhalation the process of air moving out of the chest cavity as the muscles used during inhalation relax.

ASK YOURSELF

■ Can you define key terms introduced in this chapter?

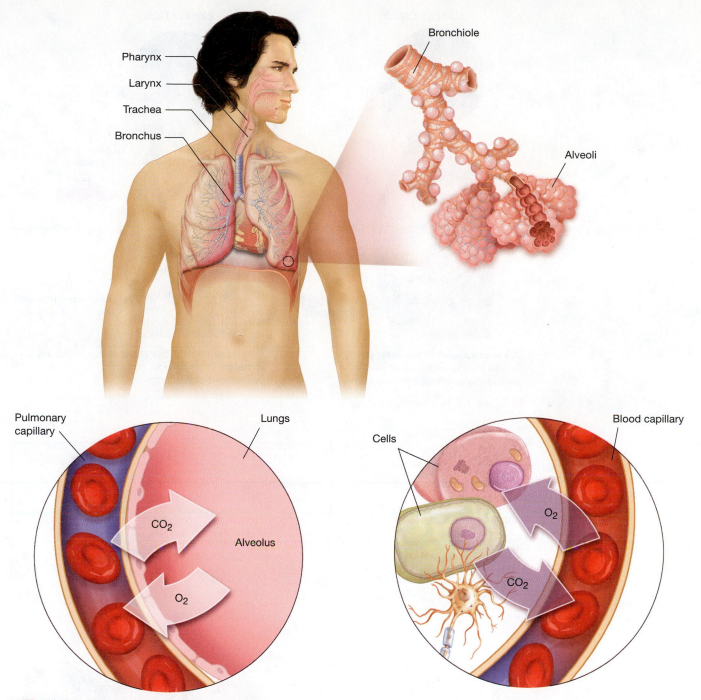

Figure 7-3 The process of inhalation and exhalation.

the alveoli, which is where oxygen is moved from the inhaled air and transferred to the bloodstream (Figure 7-4).

There are anatomy differences between adult and child patients (Figure 7-5 ■). The following differences are important to consider as you assess and treat different age groups:

■ The child patient has a smaller mouth and nose.

■ The tongue of the child patient takes up proportionately more space in the mouth.

■ Airway structures are more easily obstructed in the child.

■ The airway structures may be less developed than in an adult patient.

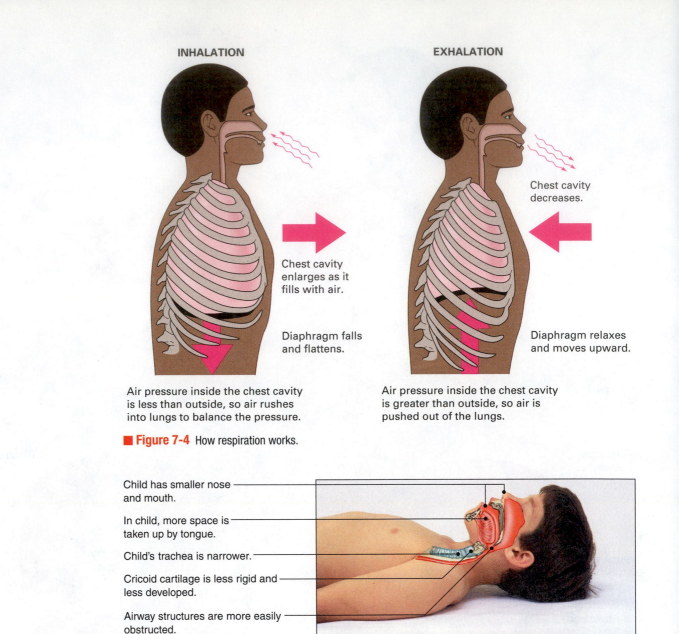

INHALATION

Chest cavity enlarges as it fills with air.

Diaphragm falls and flattens.

Air pressure inside the chest cavity is less than outside, so air rushes into lungs to balance the pressure.

EXHALATION

Chest cavity decreases.

Diaphragm relaxes and moves upward.

Air pressure inside the chest cavity is greater than outside, so air is pushed out of the lungs.

■ **Figure 7-4** How respiration works.

Child has smaller nose and mouth.

In child, more space is taken up by tongue.

Child's trachea is narrower.

Cricoid cartilage is less rigid and less developed.

Airway structures are more easily obstructed.

■ **Figure 7-5** Comparison of the airways of an adult and an infant or child.

ASK YOURSELF

■ What are possible conditions that lead to inadequate breathing?

By understanding the anatomy and physiology of adults and children and how air moves in and out of the body, we can identify four basic reasons why a patient could die from airway problems:

1. No air gets into the body at all. The patient isn't breathing. The chest muscles and diaphragm don't contract.

TABLE 7-1 Respiratory Status

STATUS	SIGNS	EMR CARE	
Breathing adequately	<ul><li>Rate and depth of breathing are normal.</li><li>No abnormal breath sounds.</li><li>Air moves freely in and out of the chest.</li><li>Skin color appears to be normal.</li></ul>	<ul><li>Monitor the patient's breathing for any changes.</li><li>If allowed, also administer oxygen by nonrebreather or nasal cannula.</li></ul>	
Breathing inadequately Patient is moving some air in and out but breathing is slow or shallow and not enough to sustain life.	<ul><li>Rate and/or depth or breathing not within normal range.</li><li>Shallow breathing; diminished or absent breath sounds.</li><li>Noises with breathing such as snoring, gurgling, or gasping.</li><li>Blue or gray skin color (cyanosis)</li><li>Decreased minute volume.</li></ul>	<ul><li>Assist ventilations.</li><li>If allowed, also administer supplementental oxygen during ventilation by way of a pocket face mask or bag-valve mask.</li></ul>	
No breathing at all	<ul><li>No chest rise.</li><li>No evidence of air being moved from the mouth or nose.</li><li>No breath sounds.</li></ul>	<ul><li>Provide ventilations.</li><li>If allowed, also administer supplemental oxygen during ventilation by way of a pocket face mask or bag-valve mask.</li></ul>	

2. No air gets into the body at all. The airway is obstructed by a foreign object, often in the larynx. The patient may have vomited, causing a full or partial obstruction.

3. Breathing is too shallow. The breathing isn't sufficient to bring in the oxygen required by the body. Breathing is minimal; the muscles of the chest and diaphragm contract only slightly.

4. Breathing is too fast or too slow. Breathing that is too slow doesn't bring in enough air. Breathing that is too fast is often shallow. Either case (too slow or too fast) results in not enough inhaled air reaching the alveoli (Table 7-1).

Normal respiratory rates vary from patient to patient based on age, level of physical activity, fever, illness, and injury. Generally, respiratory rates considered normal by age group are:

- Adult   12–20 breaths/minute
- Child   15–30 breaths/minute
- Infant   30–60 breaths/minute

Remember that these rates are a guideline. When the body senses the need for oxygen, such as in the case of a patient having an asthma attack or a patient with chest injuries, the body's usual response is to increase the respiratory rate to bring in more air from which oxygen can be obtained. The condition of low oxygen levels in the body is called **hypoxia**.

The body will also increase the pulse rate in response to hypoxia. This is to pump more oxygen-containing blood throughout the body.

Assessing the Airway and Breathing

While the steps for airway, breathing, and circulation (the ABCs) are considered separate, assessment for one frequently involves the other. This section will discuss assessment of the airway and breathing.

ASK YOURSELF

■ How would you use assessment findings to differentiate between patients who are breathing adequately, those who are breathing inadequately, and those who are not breathing at all?

Once you approach and begin to care for the patient, you must ensure he has an open airway. If the airway is blocked for any reason, you must correct it immediately.

How you assess airway and breathing will depend on your initial observations of the patient. Patients who appear alert and oriented usually have an open airway. Patients who are unresponsive or appear sleepy or lethargic will intuitively require more frequent airway assessment and care.

If you find a responsive and alert patient, talk to him. As he speaks, look for any signs that he may have airway blockages. You might notice coughing, choking, or unusual noises coming from the patient's mouth. Look for signs of vomiting on or around the patient's mouth or clothes, or in the immediate area. Most responsive patients have a **patent** airway and this is easily determined by observing the patient.

patent   an airway that is open and clear.

Patients who have an altered mental status—which may range from confused to fully unresponsive—pose more of a challenge in airway assessment. There is greater likelihood that airway care will be necessary, and you will also need to more frequently assess the airway while the patient is in your care due to the potential for airway problems to develop.

Note the patient's skin color, temperature, and condition. Normal skin is warm, dry, and pink. Take note of whether the skin is pale or gray, or shows signs of **cyanosis** (a blue color). Dark-skinned patients are more difficult to assess in this regard. You will note that their skin may become slightly lighter or grayer, but many times you will find changes in color in the lips and mucous membranes (for example, the mouth and around the eye). Changes in skin color, temperature, and condition indicate hypoxia and/or reduced circulation.

cyanosis   blueness or lividness of the skin, as from imperfectly oxygenated blood.

Assess the patient's airway quickly and efficiently. If the patient is sitting or lying, get down to the patient's level. Unresponsive patients and those who don't appear able to maintain their own airway should be placed supine on a flat surface—preferably the floor—until EMS arrives with a stretcher. Remember that patients who have suspected neck or spine injuries may be worsened with movement. Only move the spine-injured patient if necessary to provide lifesaving airway care.

If you find a patient who has an altered mental status but is breathing adequately and does not have any airway problems, such as requiring suction, he may be placed in the recovery position (Figure 7-6 ■). Place the patient on his side with his head resting on the arm closest to the ground. A knee may be flexed to help keep the patient in that position. The recovery position is used to allow drainage of saliva from the mouth to prevent aspiration. Monitor the patient carefully. If inadequate breathing develops, you will move the patient to a supine position and ventilate.

The first and most important breathing assessment is whether the patient is breathing adequately. Remember that you may find a patient in one of three breathing conditions:

■ Breathing adequately

■ Breathing inadequately

■ Not breathing at all

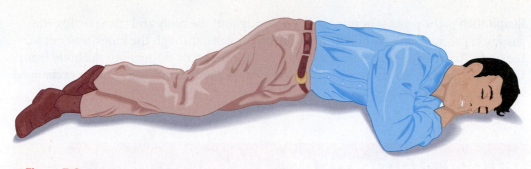

Figure 7-6 The recovery position.

Assessing the patient's breathing will vary slightly depending on whether the patient is responsive. Patients who are talking give an important sign of how they are breathing. If the patient speaks easily and effortlessly, without having to frequently catch his breath every few words, he is breathing well and has minimal distress. If he can only speak a few words before he is out of breath, this is an indication of significant distress.

The airway may also be swollen as a result of trauma, infection, or an allergic reaction. Observe for swelling, blotchiness, or discoloration around the lips, mouth, and throat. Listen for unusual sounds such as wheezing or stridor. These sounds indicate airway obstruction. Wheezing is usually caused by narrowed airways in the lungs. Stridor is often found with obstruction or swelling of the upper airway. Both create sounds that are described as "musical" because of their varying pitches. Ask the patient or family if the patient's voice has any unusual qualities (such as raspy).

Other observable signs of respiratory distress include:

- Noisy breathing (such as wheezes, bubbling, or gurgling sounds).
- Use of accessory muscles in the neck and chest.
- Anxiety or restlessness.
- Poor skin color (pale, gray) or cyanotic (blue—a late sign).
- Chest trauma—especially to the sternum and ribs. You may see **paradoxical motion** in the chest cavity. This is when a segment of detached, broken ribs (called a **flail segment**) moves in the opposite direction of the remainder of the chest cavity. This is a late sign.

Use your senses to evaluate the airway:

- Observe for vomit around the scene—especially around the patient's face and clothes. Look into the patient's mouth for vomit, secretions, blood, teeth, or anything that doesn't belong there.
- Listen for sounds that indicate obstruction. Gurgling noises generally indicate fluid such as saliva, vomit, or blood in the airway. Snoring sounds frequently indicate mechanical obstruction—most commonly by the patient's own tongue.
- Observe for signs of hypoxia, which also indicate the patient may need airway care. The brain uses a significant portion of the oxygen taken in by the body. Any reduction in oxygen to the brain results in immediate symptoms. Anxiety or agitation is a common and early sign.

There are several terms that are important in this chapter. They include the following:

Pulmonary ventilation is the process of moving air in and out of the lungs.

Oxygenation refers to the levels of oxygen in the blood that will be carried to the body.

---

paradoxical motion
movement opposite of the normal; in the chest, a section of ribs moving in the opposite direction of the majority of ribs.

flail segment   a section of ribs that have been broken and detached from the chest cavity.

pulmonary ventilation
the process of moving air in and out of the lungs.

oxygenation   the levels of oxygen in the blood that will be carried to the body.

respiration the process of using oxygen throughout the body and transporting the gas waste product carbon dioxide in and out of the body's cells, through the lungs, and out of the body.

Respiration is the process of using oxygen throughout the body and transporting the gas waste product carbon dioxide from the body's cells, through the lungs, and out of the body. Respiration is a vital series of processes that occur throughout the body from the cells to the capillaries to the alveoli where oxygen and carbon dioxide are exchanged in and out of the bloodstream.

✴✴ Stop, Review, Remember

Multiple Choice

Place a check next to the correct answer.

1. The muscles used in the chest to allow the body to inhale and exhale are the:

    _____ a. intercostal muscles.

    _____ b. diaphragmatic muscles.

    _____ c. retro-sternal muscles.

    _____ d. trapezius muscles.

2. At what location does the actual exchange of oxygen from inhaled air to the blood occur?

    _____ a. Bronchiole

    _____ b. Bronchus

    _____ c. Alveoli

    _____ d. Trachea

3. What is the most important thing to check when doing an assessment of breathing?

    _____ a. Number of breaths in a minute

    _____ b. Inspiratory volume

    _____ c. Color of airway

    _____ d. Adequacy of breathing

4. To assess the airway of an unresponsive person, the EMR should position him:

    _____ a. supine on the floor.

    _____ b. prone on the floor.

    _____ c. left lateral recumbent on the floor.

    _____ d. sitting in a chair.

True/False

Mark whether each of the following statements is true (T) or false (F).

1. _____ It is possible for someone to be breathing and still be dying from lack of oxygen.

2. _____ The patient who appears awake and alert will most likely have an open airway.

3. _____ Cyanosis is an early sign of respiratory distress.

4. _____ Swelling in the airway can only be a result of an allergic reaction.

Critical Thinking

An unresponsive male is found nearly face down in a public restroom. You note vomit on the floor near him, and he is gurgling when he breathes. Upon closer assessment, you see that he also has a frothy, clear sputum around his mouth. He is wearing a medical alert bracelet.

1. With this limited information, would you say his airway is open or in jeopardy?

    _____

    _____

    _____

    _____

2. What is the best first step the EMR can take to further assess this patient?

_____

_____

_____

_____

3. If his skin color was found to be gray and his lips cyanotic (blue), would these be early or late signs of respiratory distress?

_____

_____

_____

_____

Opening the Airway

When a patient is alert and responsive, he will maintain his own airway. That means he will clear secretions and keep the passage between his mouth and nose through to the larynx open. If the patient has an altered mental status—especially if he is unresponsive—the airway is in peril.

The most common airway obstruction is the tongue. When a patient is unresponsive in a supine position, the muscles holding the tongue in place relax and it falls posteriorly against the back of the throat, effectively closing off the airway. Air will no longer move in or out. Unless this is corrected, the patient will die. Fortunately the process to correct this is relatively easy.

The tongue can be moved away from the back of the throat by tilting the head back. This section will instruct you how to tilt the head safely and effectively. Since this procedure involves movement of the neck, you will learn a different procedure to use on patients who are suspected of having an injury to the neck or spine.

Head-Tilt, Chin-Lift Maneuver

The head-tilt, chin lift maneuver is the procedure you will use to open the airway of an unresponsive patient unless you suspect a spine injury (Scan 7-1). To perform this procedure, take a position on the side of the patient alongside the head. Place one hand on the patient's forehead and the other at the tip of the jaw (chin). Move the jaw up and toward the top of the patient's head. Use the hand on the forehead to assist in tilting the head back.

Be sure the fingers you use to lift the jaw press against the jawbone (mandible) itself rather than against the soft tissues underneath.

If you are treating a patient who is unresponsive and requires a technique such as the head-tilt, chin-lift maneuver, remember that you will not be able to perform any other care activities unless you have help on scene or until EMS arrives. The airway will require your constant attention either opening it, clearing it, or ventilating the patient. These are your first and most important priorities.

ASK YOURSELF

- What are the indications, contraindications, precautions, and procedures for performing each of the following skills?
  - Pulse oximetry
  - Head-tilt, chin-lift maneuver
  - Jaw-thrust maneuver
  - Modified chin lift
  - Suctioning
  - Inserting an oropharyngeal (oral) airway
  - Administering oxygen by mask and nasal cannula
  - Providing ventilations with a pocket face mask
  - Providing ventilations with a bag-valve mask
  - Relieving foreign body airway obstruction in patients of all ages

ADULT

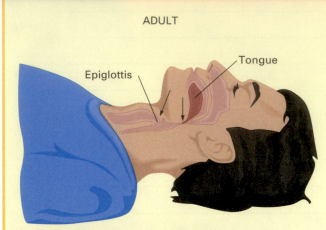

7-1a An adult airway occluded by the tongue.

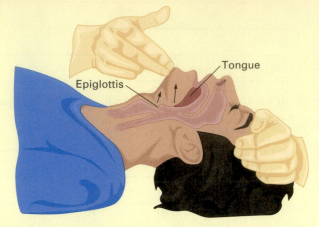

7-1b Opening the airway by tilting the head back and lifting the chin.

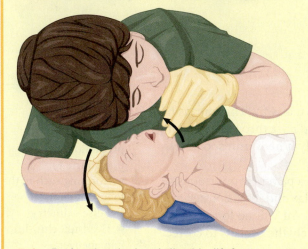

7-1c Performing the head-tilt, chin-lift for an infant.

Jaw-Thrust Maneuver

When you suspect your patient may have a spinal injury, tilting the head back could cause further injury. In this case the jaw-thrust maneuver is recommended. This maneuver opens the airway without tilting the head back.

Take a position at the top of the patient's head. Place your fingers behind the angle of each side of the mandible. Your elbows will be against the surface the patient is lying on. Your thumb may be placed against the cheekbones for leverage or against the mandible to open the mouth. Lift the mandible with your fingers. This will lift the tongue from the back of the throat (Scan 7-2).

The **modified chin lift** is an alternative to the techniques already mentioned. By lifting the chin alone and not tilting the head back, the airway may be opened with less aggravation of spine injury.

modified chin lift the chin lift used without the head tilt designed to minimize spinal movement while opening the airway.

Suction

After you open the airway you will examine it for secretions such as vomit, blood, or excessive saliva as well as solid obstructions such as food or teeth. Any materials you find

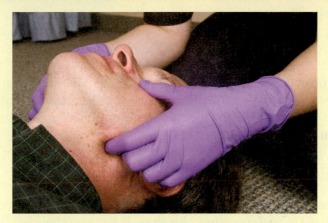

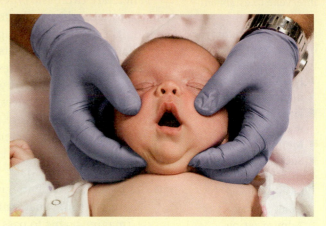

7-2a Jaw-thrust maneuver view of EMR's finger position at angle of the jaw just below the ears.

7-2b Infant jaw thrust.

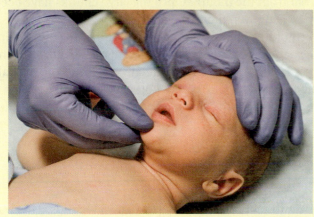

7-2c Infant chin lift.

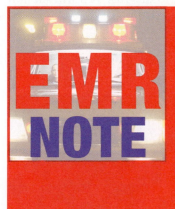

A Few Words of Caution: Jaw-Thrust Maneuver

The jaw-thrust maneuver is difficult to do. It can be tiring to perform for prolonged times, and in some patients it may not be as effective as the head-tilt, chin-lift maneuver. Carefully evaluate how well you are able to open and maintain the airway using the jaw-thrust maneuver. If you aren't able to keep the airway open—or if you are unable to ventilate the patient—you should immediately switch to the head-tilt, chin-lift maneuver. Even though it may aggravate spinal injury, the alternative to not opening the airway is death.

must be removed quickly and efficiently. If items enter the larynx, trachea, or lungs, airway obstruction is likely.

Long-term complications of airway infection and irritation also result when foreign matter enters the lungs. This is often fatal, meaning you may "save" the patient on the scene only to have him die later in the hospital from airway complications. Making sure

- How would you intervene to establish and maintain the airway and breathing by performing the following skills?
  - Head-tilt, chin-lift maneuver
  - Jaw-thrust maneuver
  - Modified chin lift
  - Suctioning
  - Inserting an oropharyngeal (oral) airway
  - Administering oxygen by mask and nasal cannula
  - Providing ventilations with a pocket face mask
  - Providing ventilations with a bag-valve mask
  - Relieving foreign body airway obstruction in patients of all ages

suction catheters

devices that attach to a suction unit and are inserted into the pharynx to remove solids and liquids from the airway.

the airway is *both* open and clear is essential. Suctioning is the procedure used to clear the airway (Figures 7-7a and 7-7b ■).

There are two basic types of suction units. One is manually (hand or foot) powered and the other is electric (battery or electricity from another power source). Electric powered units are generally thought to be more efficient but are also larger and more expensive. Manually powered units are less expensive and may be more easily transported in small medical kits used by responders.

These devices are used with **suction catheters** to clear the airway. The most commonly used suction catheters are rigid, wide-bore catheters such as the Yankauer, "tonsil tip" or Hi-D catheters. These are made of rigid plastic and are easily maneuvered through the pharynx to remove secretions.

Flexible catheters are rarely used by EMRs. They are small bore and aren't able to suction thick secretions. Many flexible catheters are used by Advanced EMTs and Paramedics to suction patients' airways through advanced airway devices.

There are times that patients will vomit a very thick mixture of partially digested foods. Imagine trying to pass a bowl of beef stew through a straw. It just won't happen. In cases such as this you will roll the patient to his side and use a gloved hand and a gauze pad if available to sweep the material from the mouth. Once the large chunks have been removed, you can use a large-bore catheter to remove the rest.

Many times you will be either holding the airway open or ventilating the patient when you see secretions or hear the patient begin vomiting. You will then begin suctioning. While you are suctioning, the patient will not be getting any oxygen. You have already learned that patients can die from a lack of oxygen. You have also learned that a patient can die from foreign material and stomach acid entering the airway. This provides the guidelines for suctioning:

Suction as quickly and efficiently as you can to remove the material from the pharynx so you can again begin ventilations and maintain the open airway.

An older guideline for suctioning was to suction for no longer than 15 seconds. This was a general guideline designed to ensure that EMS providers suction as quickly and efficiently as possible. Unfortunately, patients sometimes vomit for longer than 15 seconds or vomit material that takes longer than 15 seconds to clear. In this case you will suction until the airway is clear and then resume your other airway care duties.

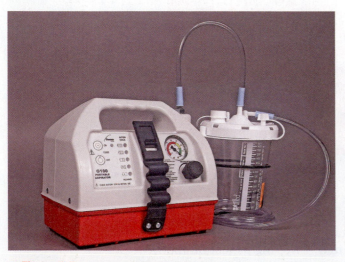

■ **Figure 7-7a** An example of a suction unit.

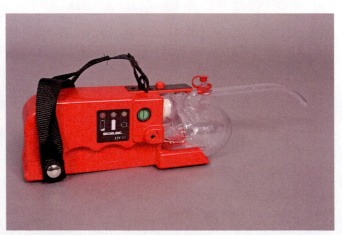

■ **Figure 7-7b** An example of a handheld suction unit.

To suction, follow these guidelines (Scan 7-3):

1. Reconsider the Standard Precautions determination you made earlier. You must wear gloves and face protection while suctioning.
2. Roll the patient to his side.
3. Open the mouth if it isn't open.

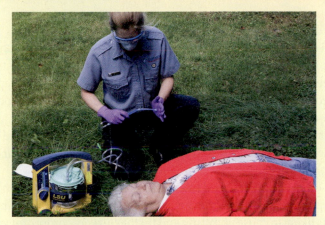

7-3a Prepare suction unit.

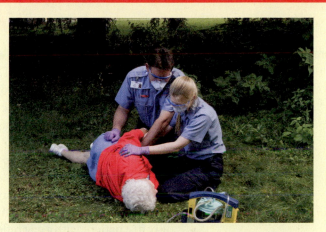

7-3b Roll the patient to his/her side.

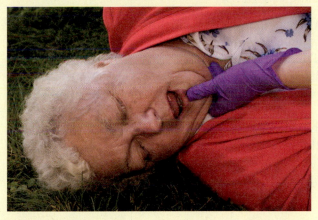

7-3c Open mouth.

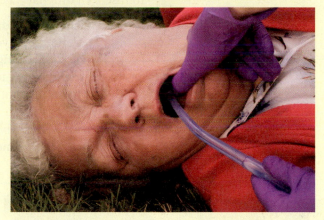

7-3d Place tip in the mouth only as far as you can see.

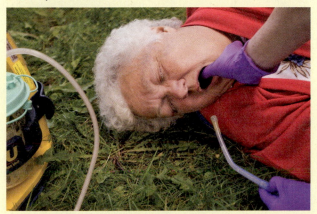

7-3e Suction while moving the tip out.

4. Insert the suction catheter into the mouth with the suction off. Insert the catheter only as far as you can see.
5. When the catheter is in place, apply suction by placing your finger over the hole in the proximal tip of the catheter.
6. Withdraw the suction catheter as you suction. Move the catheter from side to side or in a twisting fashion as you withdraw.
7. Limit your suction time to the minimum necessary to clear the airway.
8. Continue airway care including maintaining an open airway and applying oxygen or ventilation (discussed later in the chapter).

Oropharyngeal Airways

Now that the airway is open and clear, you may decide to place an **oropharyngeal airway** (Figures 7-8a and 7-8b ■). This is a curved device that is placed in the mouth and rests in the oropharynx. It helps to keep the tongue away from the back of the throat and keep the airway open. It is also referred to as an airway adjunct because it is an adjunct method to assist in keeping the airway open.

The device alone will not maintain the airway. You will still need to perform a head-tilt, chin-lift maneuver or the jaw-thrust technique and monitor the airway carefully during the entire time you care for the patient.

The oropharyngeal airway—often simply referred to as an "oral airway" or OPA—is indicated in patients who are unresponsive and do not have a gag reflex. Inserting an oral airway in a patient with a gag reflex is likely to cause vomiting and further airway compromise.

To insert an oropharyngeal airway (Scan 7-4):

1. Reevaluate the Standard Precautions determination you made during the size-up. At a minimum, you should be wearing gloves. Face protection is required in the event splashing of fluids is likely.
2. Measure the airway to determine the appropriate size. It should measure from the center of the mouth to the earlobe or from the corner of the mouth to the angle of the jaw.
3. Have suction available in the event of vomiting.
4. Open the patient's mouth.

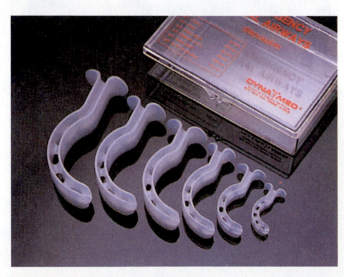

■ **Figure 7-8a** Oropharyngeal (oral) airways.

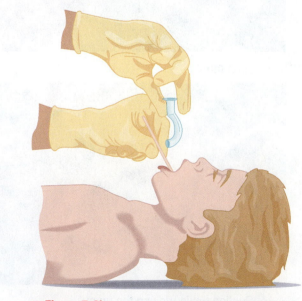

■ **Figure 7-8b** Inserting an oropharyngeal airway in an infant or child.

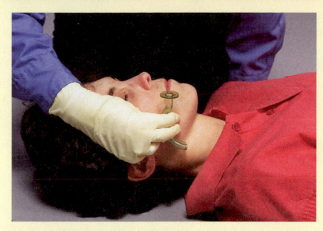

7-4a Measure to ensure correct size.

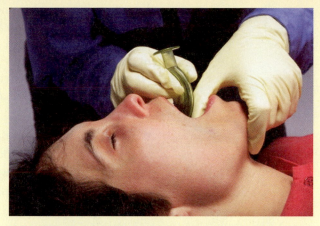

7-4b In an adult, insert with top pointing up toward the roof of the mouth.

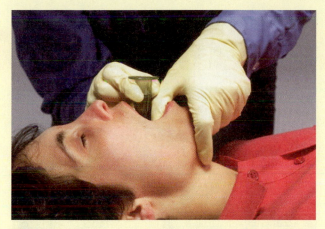

7-4c Then gently rotate it until it reaches the proper position.

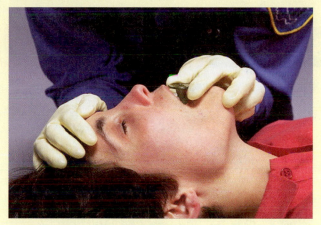

7-4d Continue until the flange rests on the patient's teeth.

5. Insert the airway with the end pointed up (toward the roof of the mouth). This prevents pushing the tongue back into the throat. If you hear gagging or retching sounds at any time as you advance the airway, the patient has an intact gag reflex. Do not continue to insert the airway. Remove it and maintain the airway without the use of this adjunct.

6. If the patient does not have a gag reflex, continue to insert the airway. Rotate the airway 90 degrees so it follows the curve of the base of the tongue. The flange of the airway will rest against the patient's teeth. Some protocols also allow the oral airway to be inserted 45 degrees (to the side) and rotated into place.

EMR Patient Assessment: Breathing

After you assess the airway for patency and correct any problems you find, you will next assess and care for breathing problems. As mentioned earlier, breathing may range from normal to absent with a wide variety of conditions in between.

You must assess breathing quickly but accurately. An understanding of the respiratory anatomy and physiology mentioned earlier is vital.

It can't be said enough: *Without adequate breathing, your patient will die.* Your initial evaluation will revolve around determining whether the patient is breathing or not. You may find some patients who are not breathing at all. These patents have no chest rise and fall and no air moving in and out of the mouth. They often have poor skin color, no movement, and other signs that will help your decision.

If you look at your patient and find he is breathing, you must next determine if the patient is breathing *adequately*. Consider the following examples of patients you may encounter (Scans 7-5 and 7-6):

- You are called for a patient with chest pain. He is sitting in a chair and looks alert as you arrive. When you ask him how you can help, he explains his pain while speaking in full sentences.

- You are called for a patient who, according to relatives, complained of a headache before passing out. She is on the ground and unresponsive. You notice her breathing seems slow and irregular. A gurgling sound comes from her throat. Her color is poor.

SCAN 7-5   Assessing Breathing—Responsive Patient

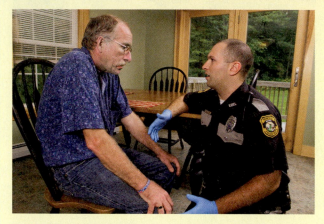

7-5a Observe patient's general appearance. Note signs of distress or anxiety. Observe skin color and accessory muscle use.

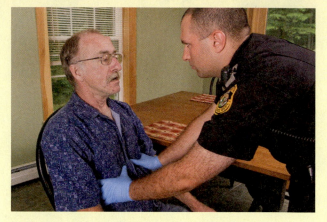

7-5b Spread your fingers over the ribs with thumbs near the sternum. Assess rate and depth of respirations.

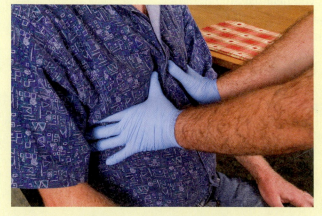

7-5c Feel for equal and adequate chest expansion.

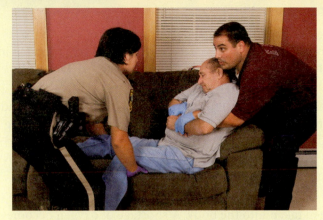

7-6a Unresponsive patient moved to floor.

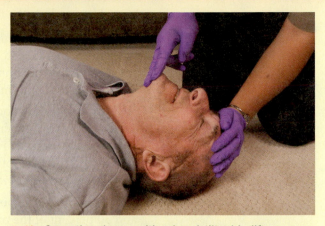

7-6b Open the airway with a head-tilt, chin lift.

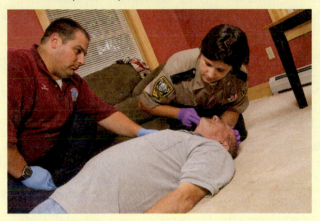

7-6c Observe rate of breathing.

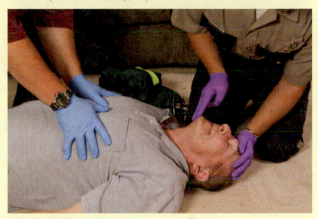

7-6d EMR places hand over each side of patient's chest to feel for adequate/equal expansion.

If the patient appears lifeless without breathing (or only with agonal breathing) begin with a pulse check as part of the C-A-B approach.

- You are called for a patient who fell down two or three stairs. He is holding a badly broken lower leg. His breathing is rapid but deep. He is screaming because of the pain.
- You are called to a patient who was thrown from a car after a rollover collision. His color is poor. He is not moving or talking. You don't see his chest rise. No air appears to be moving in and out of his mouth.

These patients are a small sampling of what you might see in the field. The first patient has a potentially serious condition: chest pain. His alertness, lack of anxiety, ability to speak full sentences, and sitting position are signs that his breathing is likely adequate.

The second patient is not breathing adequately. You may have guessed this because of the slow, irregular breathing, unresponsiveness, and poor color. She also requires suction. Not all unresponsive patients will be breathing inadequately, but this patient clearly is.

The third patient is breathing adequately. While many would think the screaming is a bad sign (it does indicate severe pain), it means that the patient is moving air in and out. Patients who are in pain, excited, or agitated will be breathing more rapidly. Ensure the breathing is deep enough to indicate adequate breathing.

The fourth patient is not breathing at all. You will need to ventilate him. Providing artificial ventilation will be taught later in this chapter. You must also remember to use the jaw-thrust maneuver when opening the airway because of the potential for spine injury.

These four scenarios have illustrated many factors you will use to evaluate a patient's breathing. They include the following:

- *Rate and depth of breathing.* To be breathing adequately, a patient must have both adequate rate and depth. You may have noticed how much this is repeated in the chapter. It's that important. Normal respiratory rates are listed in Table 7-1. Remember that rates may vary for a variety of reasons.

- *Abnormal sounds.* You may hear stridor (an almost musical high-pitched sound indicating partial upper airway obstruction), wheezing (a high-pitched whistling sound indicating narrowed air passages as in asthma), snoring (caused by upper airway obstruction—often from the tongue), and gurgling (usually indicating liquid in the upper airway and the need for suction).

- *Mental status.* The body needs oxygen to function. The brain uses between 25 and 30 percent of the oxygen taken into the body. A shortage of oxygen becomes evident quickly in the patient's mental status. Patients who are hypoxic experience anxiety or restlessness as an early sign. They may become agitated as hypoxia gets worse.

- *Increased or decreased pulse and respiratory rate.* When the body needs oxygen, the respiratory rates and pulse will increase. This is the body's attempt to distribute more oxygen. As the hypoxia becomes severe and the patient is near death, these rates frequently slow down. This is especially true in infants and children. This slowing is a late and serious sign.

- *Movement of the chest.* As explained earlier, the rise and fall of the chest and diaphragm are required to move air in and out of the body. Look for this rise and fall as a means to evaluate the presence and depth of breathing.

- *Effort or work of breathing.* Breathing should be relatively effortless. When it appears that the patient must work very hard to breathe, it is a sign of distress. You may see this as **accessory muscle use** (using muscles in the neck and abdomen to assist breathing), **retractions** (appearance of the skin "sucking in" between the ribs, around the clavicles, and above the sternum), gasping, or using the abdominal muscles to breathe.

accessory muscle use the use of muscles in the neck, shoulder, and abdomen to assist in breathing.

retractions the appearance of skin being "sucked in" between the ribs, over the clavicle, and above the sternum; indicates difficulty breathing.

✳ Stop, Review, Remember

Multiple Choice

Place a check next to the correct answer.

1. What is the most common airway obstruction?

    _____ a. Raw steak

    _____ b. Water

    _____ c. Tongue

    _____ d. Nasal secretions

2. What is the preferred method for opening the airway of the unresponsive adult without suspected spinal injury?

    _____ a. Head-tilt, chin-lift maneuver

    _____ b. Jaw-thrust maneuver

    _____ c. Modified chin lift

    _____ d. Anterior tongue displacement

3. What is the preferred type of suction catheter for use by the EMR?

_____ a. Soft

_____ b. Rigid

_____ c. Flexible

_____ d. Firm

4. An oropharyngeal airway is inserted _____ so that the tongue doesn't become an airway obstruction.

_____ a. along the natural curvature of the tongue

_____ b. backward and then flipped inside the mouth

_____ c. upside down or toward the cheek

_____ d. quickly before the tongue contracts

5. Mental status is an important sign to assess when determining breathing adequacy because:

_____ a. the brain responds to hypoxia by displaying disorientation.

_____ b. hypoxia causes rapid eye movements thus creating a stagger.

_____ c. the barrier between the airway and brain thins during a hypoxic event.

_____ d. less blood is created during a hypoxic state.

Matching

Match the following descriptions with the correct term.

_____ 1. Used in patients with possible spinal injury who cannot have a jaw-thrust maneuver

_____ 2. Rigid suction catheter used to clear secretions

_____ 3. Used in patients without signs of trauma to open the airway

_____ 4. Most often used to open the airway of patients involved in traumatic events with spinal compromise

_____ 5. Rigid device used to displace the tongue and open the airway

a. Head-tilt, chin-lift

b. Jaw-thrust maneuver

c. Modified chin lift

d. Oropharyngeal airway

e. Yankauer catheter

Critical Thinking

An adult female is found in an alley following a fight. She is unconscious and bleeding from the face. You hear her groaning when you roll her over to her back. Upon opening the airway, you find blood and teeth in her throat. She is breathing two times a minute.

1. What is the first thing you should do to facilitate clearing the airway?

_____

2. After that, what should you do to allow assisted ventilations to reach the lungs?

_____

EMR Emergency Care: Breathing

When patients have breathing problems, there are two things we can do to help them. We can help increase oxygen levels by giving them oxygen. When they aren't breathing enough, or at all, we can help by moving air in and out of the lungs for them. This is called ventilation. You will be trained to perform both of these lifesaving interventions. But first we will discuss oxygen and how to administer it.

ASK YOURSELF

■ What is the concept of oxygen saturation?

Oxygen

Oxygen is a gas that is present in inhaled air. About 21 percent of the air we breathe in is oxygen. The human body has an amazing system in which the air we inhale reaches the alveoli deep in the lungs where oxygen is removed from inhaled air and delivered to the bloodstream. Capillaries pick up that oxygen from the alveoli and deliver it via the bloodstream to tissues throughout the body. When there is a problem anywhere along that system, the amount of oxygen delivered to the tissues of the body is decreased. This is called hypoxia.

When oxygen is transported through the alveoli into the capillaries, oxygen is picked up by a substance called hemoglobin in the bloodstream. Hemoglobin is found in red blood cells and is responsible for carrying the oxygen throughout the body. A device called a **pulse oximeter** (Figure 7-9 ■) can measure how much of the hemoglobin is actually carrying oxygen at any given time. This is called **oxygen saturation**.

The oximeter presents the reading as a percentage. This indicates the percentage of hemoglobin that is saturated with oxygen. Applied to a finger, a probe assesses saturation by sending a light through the finger.

If you apply a pulse oximeter to a patient who is breathing well and distributing oxygen throughout the body, you would expect to see a pulse oximetry reading above 96 percent. Lower readings (90 to 95 percent) may indicate hypoxia. Below 90 percent is very serious hypoxia.

pulse oximeter a device to measure the amount (percentage) of oxygen saturation in the blood.

oxygen saturation the percentage of hemoglobin in the red blood cells that are saturated with oxygen.

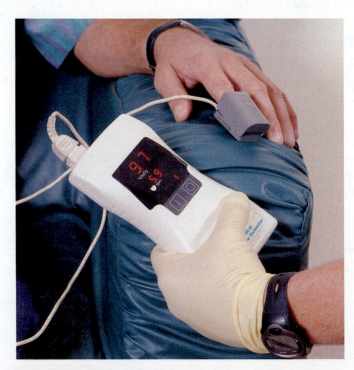

■ **Figure 7-9** Pulse oximeter.

Experienced EMRs are aware of certain cautions. First, the pulse oximeter is a device. It can malfunction or give an improper reading. You should never assume a patient is "OK" or doesn't need oxygen because of a good reading when the patient looks hypoxic. Likewise you may see some patients with a low reading when they look just fine. Wise EMRs use the pulse oximeter as one source of information—not the only fact in their decision making.

Hemoglobin not only carries oxygen to the body's tissues, it also carries **carbon dioxide** back to the lungs so it can be removed from the body. In the case of **carbon monoxide** poisoning (for example, from car exhaust or faulty heating systems), hemoglobin will also carry this substance. Some oximeters are capable of measuring how much oxygen and carbon monoxide are being carried by the hemoglobin.

Pulse oximetry is mentioned here because newer protocols for oxygen administration may be based on pulse oximeter readings. It will be discussed in greater detail in Chapter 11, "Patient Assessment: History and Vital Signs." For example, you may have a protocol where suspected heart attack patients will receive a small amount of oxygen (or sometimes no oxygen) if they have a pulse oximetry reading of 95% or greater AND show no other signs of hypoxia. The patient would receive greater amounts of oxygen if the oximetry reading was lower or if there were signs of hypoxia.

carbon dioxide a waste product of metabolism.

carbon monoxide a colorless, odorless gas that is a poisonous result of incomplete combustion.

Oxygen Delivery to Patients

Oxygen is carried in cylinders (Figure 7-10 ■). Most of the cylinders today are made of aluminum. Some part of the cylinder will be green, which is one indication that the content of the cylinder is oxygen. The cylinder will also have a stem that will only accept regulators designed to deliver oxygen.

ASK YOURSELF

■ What are the safety precautions needed when handling oxygen tanks and administering oxygen?

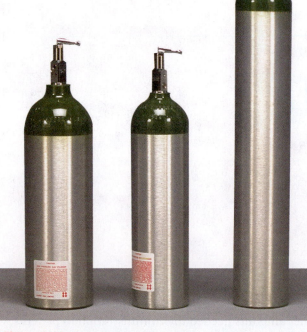

■ **Figure 7-10** Jumbo D, D and E cylinders.

Since these cylinders contain a compressed gas, it is important to store and transport the cylinders carefully. Do not drop them or allow them to be placed or used anywhere there is flame. Oxygen will fuel fires and can be dangerous around sparks or flame. No one should be allowed to smoke where oxygen is present or in use.

The cylinders most frequently carried in first response vehicles or by response teams are identified by letters. As the letters move through the alphabet, the amount of oxygen contained in the cylinders increases. A "D" cylinder, when full, contains 350 liters of oxygen. An "E" cylinder contains 625 liters of oxygen.

Regulators are used to allow the compressed oxygen to leave the cylinder in a controlled and measured fashion. The regulators provide a gauge that measures the oxygen in **liters per minute** (lpm).

The regulators for oxygen have a three-pin system. To place a regulator on a tank, align the pins from the regulator (one large pin on top, two smaller pins below) with the holes on the side of the stem. Once the regulator is seated in the holes, secure the regulator by tightening the knob on the side of the regulator. Tighten it firmly and only by hand. Do not use tools or wrenches.

The oxygen tank will have a valve at the top that must be opened after the regulator is attached. Opening the tank before the regulator is applied will result in oxygen being released under high pressure. If you turn on the tank with the regulator attached and you hear a loud hissing, the regulator isn't fitted tightly. Turn the tank off and reapply the regulator. Some recommend opening and closing the valve very quickly before attaching the regulator to remove dust and debris. A small **O ring** is applied over the large pin in the regulator to maintain this seal and keep debris out. This should be changed when you change the regulator. Follow the instructions given by your service or oxygen supplier.

The gauge on the cylinder will read 2,000 pounds per square inch (psi) when full. Do not let a cylinder go below the safe residual pressure of 200 psi. Switch to a new tank before that point. When performing a daily check or restocking your emergency kit, most agencies advise replacing the cylinder when it reaches 500 psi so as not to run out on the next call.

regulator a device that is attached to an oxygen cylinder to provide a measured flow of oxygen from the cylinder to the patient.

liters per minute the measure of oxygen delivery to a patient.

O ring a circular ring placed between an oxygen cylinder and a regulator to maintain a firm seal.

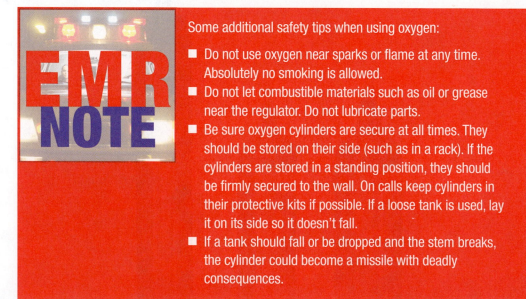

Some additional safety tips when using oxygen:

- Do not use oxygen near sparks or flame at any time. Absolutely no smoking is allowed.
- Do not let combustible materials such as oil or grease near the regulator. Do not lubricate parts.
- Be sure oxygen cylinders are secure at all times. They should be stored on their side (such as in a rack). If the cylinders are stored in a standing position, they should be firmly secured to the wall. On calls keep cylinders in their protective kits if possible. If a loose tank is used, lay it on its side so it doesn't fall.
- If a tank should fall or be dropped and the stem breaks, the cylinder could become a missile with deadly consequences.

oxygen supply tube tubing that runs between a regulator and a device such as a pocket face mask to supply oxygen.

Oxygen regulators reduce the high pressures inside the tank to a level that can be regulated to the smaller amounts needed for administration to patients. Oxygen can be administered directly to patients using masks or a nasal cannula. An **oxygen supply tube** may also be connected to a pocket face mask or bag-valve mask to add additional oxygen while ventilating a patient.

There is an important difference between oxygen delivery devices and those used to ventilate patients. The oxygen mask and nasal cannula require the patient to be breathing adequately. These devices are placed on the patient and require the patient to breathe the oxygen deep into the lungs to reach the alveoli. Ventilation devices such as the bag-valve mask and the pocket mask deliver oxygen to the patient by actively pushing air into the alveoli. The pocket face mask actually moves the air into the patient by your breath, whereas the bag-valve mask moves air into the lungs by a squeeze of the bag. Oxygen masks and nasal cannulas should never be used on a patient with inadequate breathing because the oxygen they deliver will likely not reach the alveoli in adequate amounts to sustain life.

There are two types of masks used in EMS. The more common mask is the **nonrebreather mask** (Figures 7-11a to 7-11c ■). Some systems also use the **Venturi mask** in certain patient situations (Figure 7-12 ■).

nonrebreather mask an oxygen delivery device that consists of a reservoir and a mask; designed to provide up to 90 percent concentration of oxygen to the patient.

Venturi mask a mask that mixes room air with oxygen to create specific oxygen concentration percentages; often used in patients with chronic obstructive pulmonary disease (COPD) or on long-term oxygen therapy.

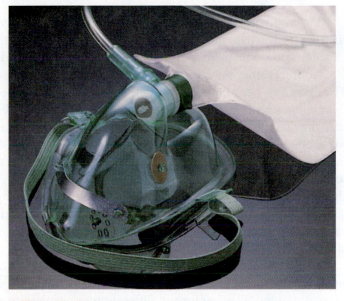

■ **Figure 7-11a** Nonrebreather mask.

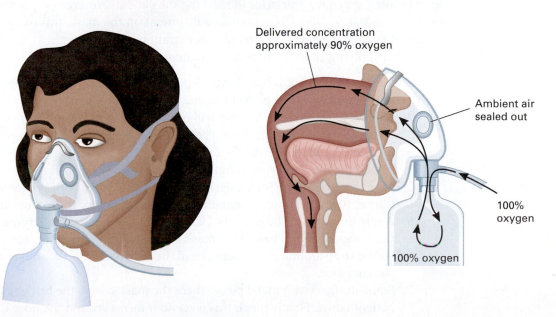

■ **Figure 7-11b** Nonrebreather mask applied to a patient. ■ **Figure 7-11c** Showing oxygen percentages delivered through mask.

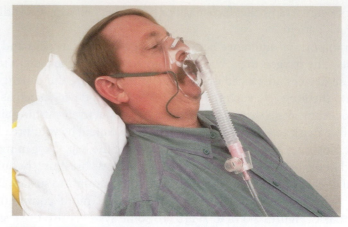
■ **Figure 7-12** Venturi mask.

The nonrebreather mask delivers up to 90 percent oxygen when well fitted to the patient's face. The patient breathes oxygen from a reservoir bag so he receives it at this high concentration. The patient exhales through ports on the side of the mask.

Nonrebreather masks are connected to oxygen and run at approximately 10–15 lpm. The exact liter per minute flow is determined by the status of the reservoir bag. If the patient collapses the bag and it doesn't refill before the next breath, you must increase the liter flow so the bag remains inflated. Usually, 15 lpm is the maximum you would need to accomplish this task.

Because the nonrebreather mask forms a tight seal on the patient's face and flapper valves are present on the surface of the mask to ensure oxygen is delivered only through the reservoir bag, it is essential to always monitor the attached oxygen tank to make sure it does not run out of oxygen. A patient on a nonrebreather mask can potentially suffocate if the oxygen source is allowed to run out. This is especially true in patients with an altered mental status.

The Venturi mask delivers oxygen at lower concentrations. It is often used when patients have certain chronic lung conditions and with some patients who are on long-term oxygen therapy. There are many different types of Venturi masks that use different systems to mix oxygen with air prior to reaching the patient. For example, oxygen may flow into the mask at 6–8 lpm. By setting an adjustment on the mask, this oxygen is blended with air to give the patient a delivered concentration of 30 percent.

When applying an oxygen mask to a patient (Scan 7-7):

1. Be sure the patient is breathing adequately. If he is breathing inadequately, you must ventilate with a pocket face mask or bag-valve mask.
2. Explain to the patient that you will be applying an oxygen mask.
3. Turn the valve on top of the oxygen cylinder on. Observe the gauge to verify there is enough oxygen in the cylinder.
4. Attach the mask's oxygen tubing to the regulator.
5. Turn the regulator to set the desired amount of oxygen. For nonrebreather masks, start at 10 lpm. Follow the manufacturer's guidelines for the Venturi mask.
6. Apply the mask to the patient's face. The reservoir bag on the nonrebreather mask should be full before the mask is applied to the patient's face. Place the elastic strap around the patient's head. Be sure the mask fits snugly around the patient's face.
7. Some masks have a metal piece where the mask covers the bridge of the patient's nose. Gently pinch this piece so it forms around the nose to hold the mask in place.

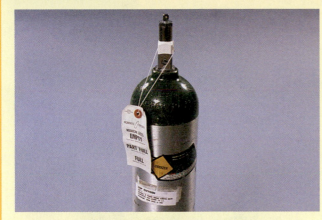

7-7a Select the correct cylinder. Check for the label "Oxygen USP."

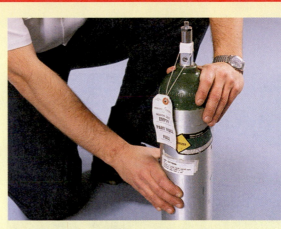

7-7b Place the cylinder in an upright position and stand to one side.

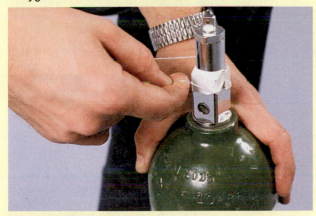

7-7c Remove the plastic wrapper or cap protecting the cylinder outlet.

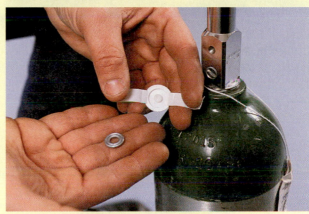

7-7d Retain the plastic washer.

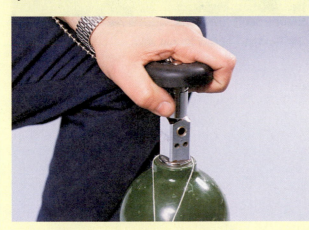

7-7e Crack the main valve for one second.

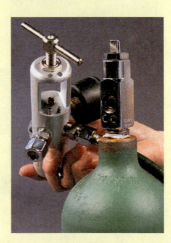

7-7f Select the correct pressure regulator and flowmeter.

(continued)

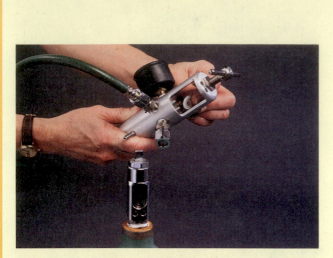

7-7g Place the cylinder valve gasket on the regulator oxygen port.

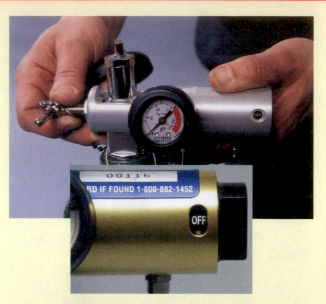

7-7h Make certain that the pressure regulator is closed.

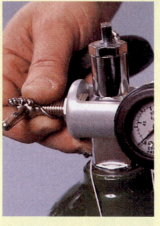

7-7i Align pins.

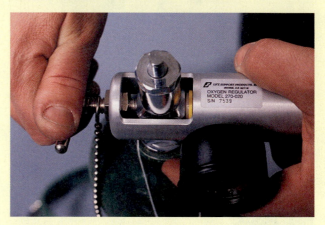

7-7j Tighten T-screw for pin yoke.

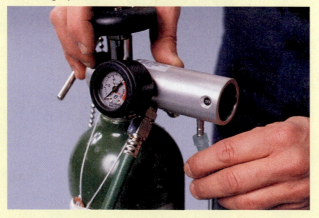

7-7k Attach tubing and delivery device.

8. Monitor the patient carefully:
   a. Observe for changes in the patient's condition after administration of oxygen. Look for overall patient condition (including mental status); changes in breathing rate, depth, or effort; skin color; and pulse rate changes.
   b. The patient may experience increased anxiety after a mask is placed on his face. The patient may perceive the mask as smothering or suffocating rather than helping him. Remember that the patient may be anxious to begin with. Reassure and try to calm him.
   c. Note the level of your oxygen tank to be sure it doesn't run out. Make sure the reservoir bag in the nonrebreather mask remains inflated. Be sure the oxygen tubing stays nonkinked and attached to the mask and the regulator so oxygen is being delivered.

Nasal Cannula

The nasal cannula is used when a lower concentration of oxygen is warranted (Figure 7-13 ■). This may be because the patient has an acceptable pulse oximetry reading and does not appear to be in respiratory distress or because your protocols recommend a lower concentration of oxygen in certain patients (such as those with

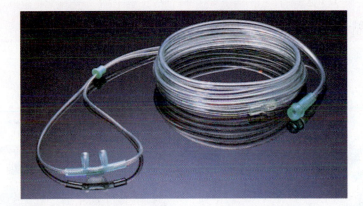

■ **Figure 7-13a** Nasal cannula.

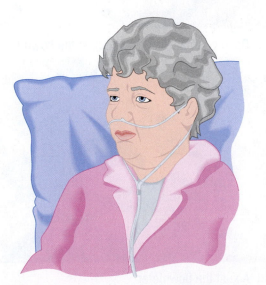

■ **Figure 7-13b** Nasal cannula applied to a patient.

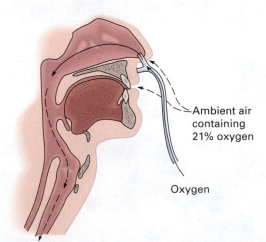

Ambient air containing 21% oxygen

Oxygen

24% to 44% oxygen concentration delivered

■ **Figure 7-13c** Oxygen percentages through cannula.

chronic lung diseases and some heart attack and stroke patients). Cannulas are also used sometimes when the patient is too anxious to wear an oxygen mask. However, it is always important to carefully assess such patients for hypoxia because patients may present with restlessness or anxiety as a sign of hypoxia.

Sometimes called nasal prongs, the cannula has two small prongs, one of which is inserted into each nostril. The tubing is looped behind the patient's ears and then secured under the chin. Oxygen is run at a much lower flow rate than masks, usually 2–4 lpm. Anything faster than 6 lpm creates an uncomfortably forceful flow of oxygen from the prongs and can also dry out the nasal mucosa.

To apply the nasal cannula (Scan 7-8):

1. Be sure the patient is breathing adequately. If he is breathing inadequately, you must ventilate with a pocket face mask or bag-valve mask.
2. Explain to the patient that you will be applying a nasal cannula and tell him that two small parts of the cannula will rest painlessly in the nostrils. The patient may also note a smell of plastic. This is normal.
3. Turn the valve on top of the oxygen cylinder on. Observe the gauge to ensure there is enough oxygen in the cylinder.
4. Attach the cannula's oxygen tubing to the regulator.

SCAN 7-8 Administering Oxygen

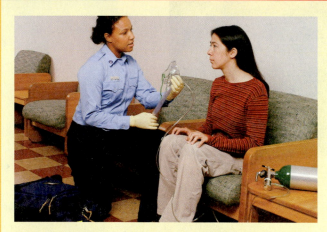

7-8a Explain to the patient the need for oxygen.

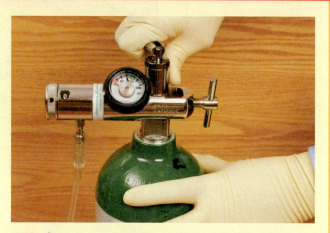

7-8b Open the main valve and adjust the flowmeter.

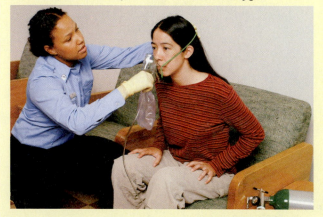

7-8c Place the oxygen delivery device on the patient.

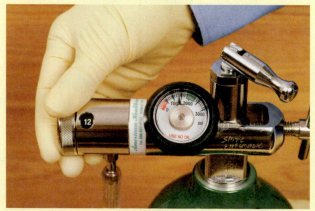

7-8d Adjust the flowmeter.

5. Turn the regulator to set the desired amount of oxygen. Generally oxygen administered through a cannula is run at 2–4 lpm. The maximum flow rate is 6 lpm.
6. Begin by placing one prong in each nostril. Wrap the tubing back up and over the ears. Then bring it down and tighten gently around the patient's chin.
7. Monitor the patient carefully. Observe for:
   a. Changes in the patient's condition after administration of oxygen. Look for overall patient condition (including mental status); changes in breathing rate, depth, or effort; skin color; and pulse rate changes.
   b. Note the level of your oxygen tank to be sure it doesn't run out. Make sure the cannula doesn't become displaced out of the patient's nostrils. Be sure the oxygen tubing stays attached to the regulator so oxygen is being delivered.

To discontinue the use of oxygen, reverse the preceding steps (Scan 7-9). Remove the device from the patient's face. Turn the oxygen flow from the regulator off. Turn off the oxygen tank and bleed the regulator by turning the oxygen on. You will watch the gauge drop to zero. Turn the oxygen off again. Dispose of the mask or cannula.

SCAN 7-9 Discontinuing Oxygen

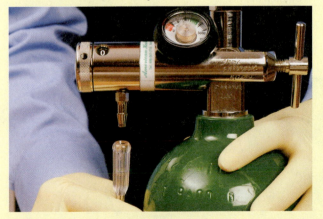

7-9a Remove the delivery device.

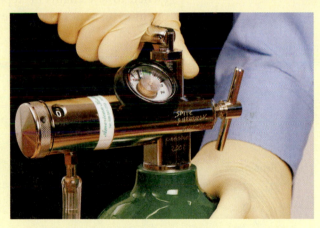

7-9b Close the main valve.

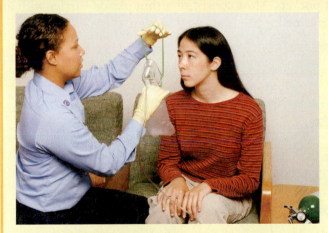

7-9c Remove the delivery tubing.

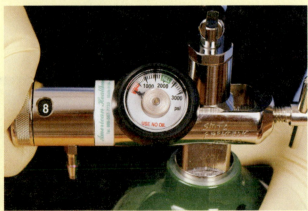

7-9d Bleed the flowmeter.

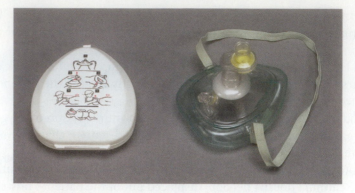

Figure 7-14 A pocket face mask with one-way valve and carrying case.

Ventilating Patients

When a patient is not breathing—or is breathing inadequately—you will provide ventilations. This procedure is vital to provide both the ventilation and the oxygen the patient will need to survive.

Ventilation moves air (and oxygen) into the lungs when the patient is unable to do it himself. The EMR is able to provide ventilation with two devices: the pocket face mask (Figure 7-14 ■) and bag-valve mask (Figure 7-15 ■). Both devices allow air and supplemental oxygen to be moved into the lungs. Other types of barrier devices are available (Figure 7-16 ■). Many of these are designed for personal or off-duty use and may be attached to key chains or kept in pockets. Most consist of a thin plastic barrier with an opening for ventilation to be performed.

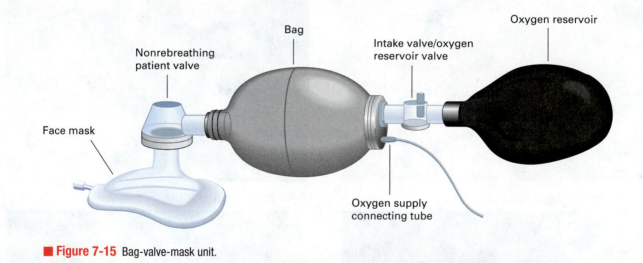

Nonrebreathing patient valve

Bag

Intake valve/oxygen reservoir valve

Oxygen reservoir

Face mask

Oxygen supply connecting tube

Figure 7-15 Bag-valve-mask unit.

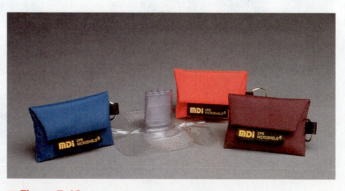

Figure 7-16 An example of a barrier device.

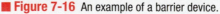

Bag-Valve-Mask Ventilation—Nonbreathing Patient

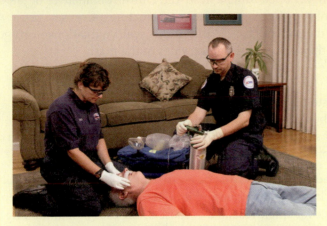

7-10a Open the patient's airway. Then select the correct mask size.

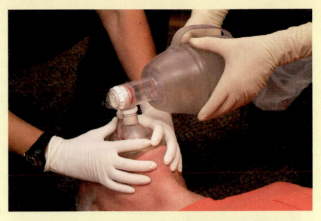

7-10b Side view of positioning of the mask and your hands.

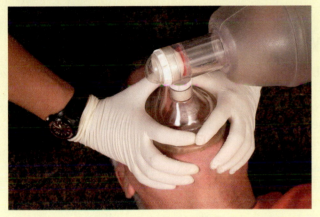

7-10c Top view of positioning of the mask and your hands.

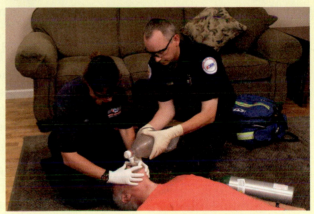

7-10d After the mask is in position, connect the oxygen and begin to ventilate the patient.

Note that we don't use the term "force" to describe how we move air into the lungs. While we do use increased pressure, introducing air into the lungs is done carefully and strategically to avoid complications.

The procedure of ventilation may be performed on patients who are responsive or unresponsive (Scan 7-10a to 7-10d).

Ventilation with the Pocket Face Mask

The pocket face mask fits over the patient's mouth and nose. It has a **ventilation port** with a **one-way valve**. This valve protects you from contact with secretions by allowing air in but does not allow the breath or other substances to come back to your mouth.

The pocket face mask is clear and allows you to see through the mask to determine if the patient requires suctioning. A strap is provided that goes around the patient's head to hold the mask in place. Many masks come with a valve that allows you to administer supplemental oxygen with your breaths.

To ventilate a patient with the pocket face mask:

1. Take appropriate Standard Precautions.
2. Open the airway. Provide suction if necessary. Insert an oral airway if the patient is unresponsive and without a gag reflex.

ventilation port the portion of the pocket face mask that protrudes up from the mask away from the patient; the site where the one-way valve is connected.

one-way valve a device that inserts into the ventilation port of a pocket face mask to prevent air and secretions from the patient from coming in contact with a rescuer.

3. If you have oxygen, connect it to the port on your face mask. Turn it to 15 lpm.
4. Place the mask on the patient's face. Place the strap around the patient's head.
5. Continue to keep the airway open using a head-tilt, chin-lift maneuver or jaw-thrust method while holding the mask in place and creating a firm seal between the mask and the patient's face. Without this seal, ventilations won't go into the lungs. Instead they will escape out the sides of the mask.
6. Seal your lips around the ventilation port and blow a steady, firm breath that lasts about a second. Breaths that are delivered too forcefully will bypass the trachea and instead go into the stomach. This will cause vomiting and result in hypoxia.
7. Deliver these breaths about 10–12 times/minute (every 5–6 seconds).
8. Monitor the patient for signs your ventilations are effective. Check the patient's pulse. If a pulse is not present, you will begin CPR.

The pocket face mask has advantages over the bag-valve mask. It is small and easily stored in a personal first-in kit. It is less expensive and is easier to constantly deliver ventilations. It is the device of choice for single rescuers because of the ease of maintaining a face seal while providing ventilations.

With the pocket face mask you will get closer to the patient's face, which is sometimes considered unpleasant when the patient is vomiting.

Ventilation with a Bag-Valve-Mask (BVM) Device

The bag-valve mask is a device that uses air moved into the lungs when the EMR squeezes a bag that is attached to a mask—hence the name bag-valve-mask device. The device has a reservoir that gathers oxygen so each time the bag is squeezed a high concentration of oxygen is delivered. It can be used on both breathing and nonbreathing patients.

To use the bag-valve mask (Scan 7-10 and 7-11):

1. Take appropriate Standard Precautions.
2. Open the airway. Provide suction if necessary. Insert an oral airway if the patient is unresponsive and does not have a gag reflex.
3. If you have oxygen available, connect it to the reservoir on your bag-valve mask. Turn it to 15 lpm.
4. When two responders are available, one responder will open the airway using the head-tilt, chin-lift maneuver or the jaw-thrust technique and while doing so, the second responder will hold the mask to the patient's face creating a seal. If using the bag-valve mask by yourself, one hand will secure the mask and open the airway simultaneously.
5. To create the seal, use your fingers to seal the mask with the chin. Wrap one or both thumbs around the port at the center of the mask. Use the side of your hands to seal the sides of the mask to the cheek. Be sure you tilt the head back to keep the airway open while you do this. If the patient has a spine injury, perform the jaw thrust using your fingers to move the jaw forward while your thumbs press the mask against the face to create a seal.
6. Squeeze the bag to move air into the patient. As with the breaths you provide with the face mask, you will squeeze the bag firmly and evenly. Avoid squeezing too hard and too fast initially. This could force air into the stomach and cause vomiting.
7. Ventilate 10–12 times per minute (about every 5–6 seconds). Make sure you maintain a face seal with the mask to ensure adequate ventilations. If you are unable to deliver adequate ventilations, switch to a pocket face mask.

Properly ventilating a patient with a bag-valve mask with a good mask seal is an EMR skill that takes considerable practice in order to become proficient.

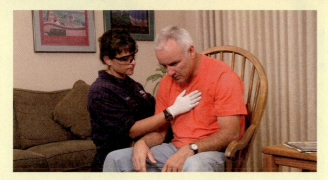

7-11a Assess the patient's respirations.

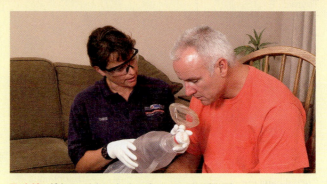

7-11b If breathing is inadequate, calm the patient and explain what you are about to do.

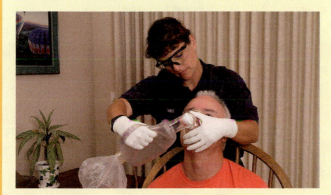

7-11c Squeeze the BVM when the patient attempts to breathe and between the patient's own respirations.

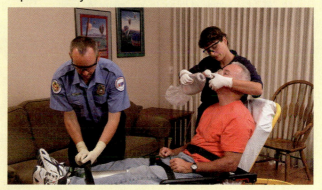

7-11d Continue ventilating and transport promptly.

CASE STUDY

THE RESPONSE

You bring your equipment to the patient. Someone yells, "Look, he is breathing!" You look at the patient and notice some slight gasping respiratory efforts. The patient's skin looks pale and he is not moving at all.

■ Discussion: *Is this adequate or inadequate breathing? What would you do? What would you communicate via radio to incoming units?*

The **Sellick maneuver** is sometimes used during ventilation to reduce vomiting that may occur when air enters the stomach.

With the Sellick maneuver (Figures 7-17a and 7-17b ■) the EMR places the thumb and index finger over the cricoid cartilage and applies backward pressure. The cricoid cartilage is immediately below the Adam's apple in the neck. This pressure helps to close the esophagus, which is believed to reduce vomiting. It may also be used to assist advanced EMS providers during the placement of a tube in the trachea.

Do not perform the Sellick maneuver if the patient is actually vomiting or if the patient is responsive. Do not compress the carotid arteries on the side of the neck.

Sellick maneuver
pressure applied to the cricoid cartilage that may prevent regurgitation and assist in the placement of advanced airway devices.

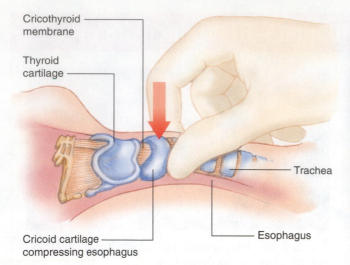

Cricothyroid membrane

Thyroid cartilage

Trachea

Cricoid cartilage compressing esophagus

Esophagus

■ **Figure 7-17a** Anatomy of throat to emphasize the location of cricoid cartilage.

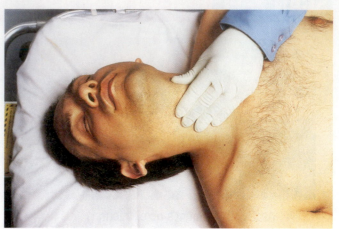

■ **Figure 7-17b** An EMR locates the cricoid cartilage.

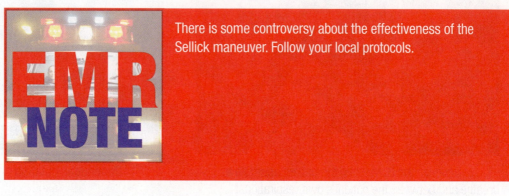

EMR NOTE

There is some controversy about the effectiveness of the Sellick maneuver. Follow your local protocols.

Many providers prefer the bag-valve mask because of the distance it provides from the patient. However, the bag-valve mask is a more difficult procedure. For a single responder, the pocket face mask remains the preferred device. The bag-valve mask is more expensive and larger to store in a kit.

Both the bag-valve mask and pocket face mask can be connected to oxygen. It is believed to be better for the patient when this is done.

When your patient is breathing but doing so inadequately and requires ventilation, the bag-valve mask is the preferred device. Patients who are breathing inadequately may be responsive, unresponsive, or somewhere in between. Since the patient may be responsive, placing a mask over the face may significantly increase anxiety. Remember that hypoxia itself causes anxiety. It is possible that you will be called to ventilate a person who is trying to pull the mask off his face because he feels like he is being suffocated. It is important to continue to ventilate the patient and try to calm him down with a soft, reassuring voice.

When ventilating a breathing patient, the following additional steps will help you perform this challenging task:

1. Explain the procedure to the patient.
2. Apply the mask to the patient's face as described earlier. The patient may be sitting or semisitting. In this case, get behind the patient to ventilate him.
3. Squeeze the bag as the patient breathes. If the patient is breathing very rapidly, you will initially squeeze the bag with each of his breaths. The hope is that the increased volume will slow the patient's respirations to a more normal rate. If you have difficulty doing this or the patient's respirations do not slow, squeeze 10–12 times per minute, each time with the patient's breath, trying to get adequate volume into the lungs.

4. This is a difficult procedure but very valuable. By assisting ventilations, you may be able to keep the patient breathing when he would have stopped breathing altogether. If it is difficult to develop timing of the breaths or if the patient struggles, keep trying. It is vitally important.

Foreign Body Airway Obstruction

Foreign body airway obstruction (FBAO) can occur from a variety of objects, the most common of which is food. This section will provide a review of procedures to remove foreign bodies from the airway. As part of your EMR class, you will likely complete a CPR course. The standards you learn in that course provide the definitive steps to removing airway obstructions. Procedures for pediatric patients will be covered in Chapter 25.

Patients with airway obstruction fit into two broad categories:

- Patients with a mild obstruction will be able to talk and make sounds. They will often cough vigorously in an attempt to expel the object. You will see signs that they are able to move air in and out despite the obstruction.

- Patients with a severe obstruction are totally or almost totally obstructed. They will move no or minimal air in or out. They are not able to talk or cough. These patients often clutch their throat as a sign of choking.

If you encounter a patient with a mild obstruction, you should monitor the patient. If it hasn't already been done, activate EMS. As long as the patient is able to speak and cough forcefully, he should continue to try to expel the object himself. Do not act unless the obstruction worsens and becomes severe.

If you encounter a conscious patient who has a severe obstruction, you must take immediate action (Scan 7-12). Advise the patient that you are trained to help and perform abdominal thrusts (Figure 7-18 ■) until the object is expelled.

Abdominal thrusts are performed by standing behind the patient and reaching around to the front in the area of the abdomen between the lower ribs and the umbilicus (belly button). Use the thumb side of one fist against the abdomen with the other hand

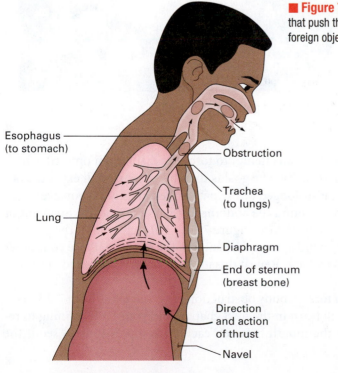

■ **Figure 7-18** The effect of abdominal thrusts that push the diaphragm up, forcing air to expel the foreign object.

Esophagus (to stomach)

Obstruction

Trachea (to lungs)

Lung

Diaphragm

End of sternum (breast bone)

Direction and action of thrust

Navel

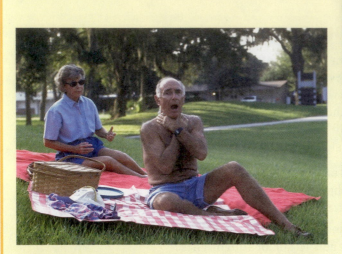

7-12a Universal sign of choking.

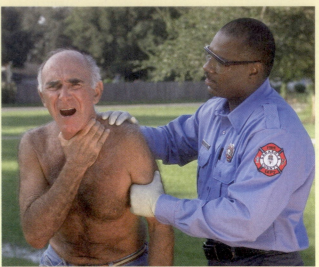

7-12b Determine if patient can speak.

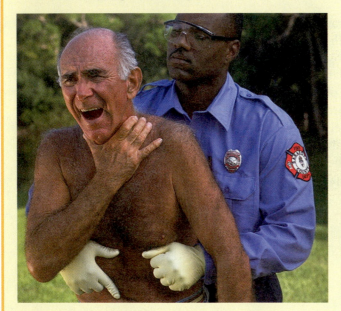

7-12c Perform Heimlich maneuver.

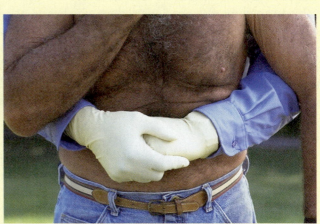

7-12d Hand position for Heimlich.

over the fist. Pull sharply in and up in an attempt to force the diaphragm upward, which increases the pressure in the chest cavity. The goal is that this pressure will expel the object. Repeat this until the object is dislodged or the patient becomes unresponsive.

You may not be able to reach around the abdomen of patients who are pregnant or obese. In this case you will do a chest thrust (Figure 7-19 ■). Reach around the patient's chest. Use the thumb side of one hand against the center of the sternum. Place your other hand over the fist. Squeeze directly back. Repeat this until the object is expelled or the patient loses consciousness.

Unresponsive patients with foreign body obstruction are given CPR (Scan 7-13). Follow the CPR procedures you will learn in the next chapter and your CPR training to relieve the obstruction. Look in the mouth between each 30 compressions to see if the object has become dislodged.

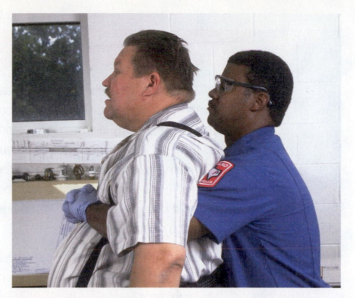

■ **Figure 7-19** Demonstration of chest thrusts on a standing obese patient with an FBAO.

SCAN 7-13 | Foreign Body Airway Obstruction—Unresponsive Adult

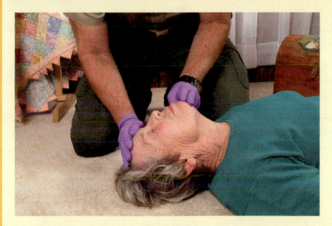

7-13a Open airway.

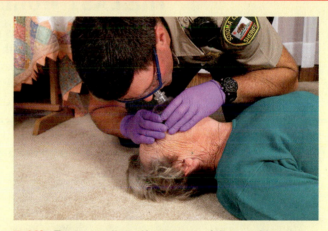

7-13b Try to ventilate. If unsuccessful, reposition the head and try again.

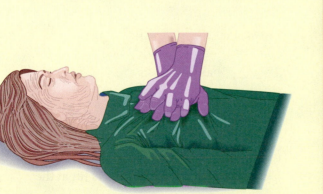

7-13c If still unsuccessful, perform 30 chest compressions.

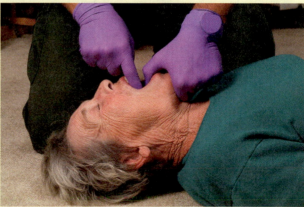

7-13d Remove any visible object, and repeat until successful attempted ventilation, chest compressions, and removal of any visible objects.

TRANSITION

You suction and ventilate the patient. He has a pulse but is breathing minimally. You have already radioed the incoming units to tell them the patient is a high priority in very serious condition. The ambulance crew arrives, pulls out their equipment, and approaches.

They ask you what you have. You tell them that you have an approximately 60-year-old male patient who collapsed suddenly according to family members. He has no history and no complaints before losing responsiveness.

■ Discussion: *Will the ambulance personnel be upset because you haven't done a head-to-toe physical exam and don't know more? Why or why not?*

THE LAST WORD

The material learned in this chapter is at the core of what an Emergency Medical Responder does when first at the scene. The assessments and skills learned in this chapter are the most important lifesaving skills you will perform.

The decisions you make when assessing and caring for the airway truly mean the difference between life and death. Think about what you have learned: opening the airway, suctioning, identifying inadequately breathing or nonbreathing patients, and administering oxygen. There is no chapter in this book with more core lifesaving skills. These skills are foundational for each call—and for the practice of the Emergency Medical Responder.

✳ Chapter Review

Multiple Choice

Place a check next to the correct answer.

1. A pulse oximeter displays a percentage of oxygen in the blood carrying element called:

_____ a. hematocrit.

_____ b. hemoglobin.

_____ c. mononuclei.

_____ d. mitochondria.

2. What term is used to describe the bluish discoloration of the lips in the early stages of hypoxia?

_____ a. Cyanosis

_____ b. Myolosis

_____ c. Steatosis

_____ d. Chondritis

3. When performing a head-tilt, chin-lift maneuver, it is important that the fingers lift at the:

_____ a. soft palate.

_____ b. jawbone.

_____ c. tracheal rings.

_____ d. tongue directly.

4. The area behind the nose and mouth that air passes through first on its journey to the lungs is the:

_____ a. larynx.

_____ b. pharynx.

_____ c. hypopharynx.

_____ d. trachea.

5. When properly fitted to a patient's face, what percentage of oxygen will a nonrebreather mask deliver?

_____ a. 70

_____ b. 80

_____ c. 90

_____ d. 100

6. When ventilating a patient using a bag-valve mask, pushing air quickly into the patient will most likely deliver it to the:

_____ a. bronchioles.

_____ b. alveoli.

_____ c. stomach.

_____ d. trachea.

7. A patient with an airway obstruction who is able to cough and gag is said to have a:

_____ a. complete obstruction.

_____ b. partial obstruction.

_____ c. lower obstruction.

_____ d. dorsal obstruction.

8. Paradoxical chest wall movement during breathing is a fracture of the ribs creating a(n):

_____ a. flail segment.

_____ b. spinous fracture.

_____ c. forced pneumothorax.

_____ d. occlusive segment.

9. Patients who are found to not be breathing adequately should be given oxygen via:

_____ a. nonrebreather mask.

_____ b. Venturi mask.

_____ c. nasal cannula.

_____ d. bag-valve mask.

10. Gas exchange occurring at the alveoli is primarily between oxygen and:

_____ a. carbon monoxide.

_____ b. carbon dioxide.

_____ c. hydrogen.

_____ d. nitrogen.

True/False

Indicate whether each of the following is true (T) or false (F) on the line provided.

1. _____ An O ring is required when using a regulator to deliver oxygen to a patient.

2. _____ The nonrebreather mask will deliver the highest concentration of oxygen to a patient.

3. _____ One must use oxygen when ventilating via a bag-valve mask or it will not function.

4. _____ When suctioning a patient's airway, you should be able to clear all secretions within 15 seconds.

5. _____ It is permissible to assume that the alert patient who speaks to you has an open airway.

Critical Thinking

You are dispatched to the scene of a male in seizure. Upon your arrival, you find him out of his seizure and not responsive. You notice that he has vomited. His wife tells you that he is a diabetic and said he felt his diabetes was "acting up" right before the seizure.

1. Is it likely that he is "securing" his own airway at this point?

_____

_____

_____

2. With suctioning, he begins to breathe deeply and regularly. Should you attempt to place an oropharyngeal airway?

_____

_____

_____

_____

3. What device should you use to deliver oxygen to this patient?

_____

_____

_____

_____

4. If he begins to seize and vomit again, what should you do?

_____

_____

_____

_____

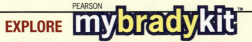

EXPLORE PEARSON **mybradykit**™

Please go to **www.bradybooks.com** to access mykit for this text. You will find quizzes, critical thinking scenarios, weblinks, animations, and videos related to this chapter—and much more. Look for online information on effective BVM ventilation as well as a video clip on the two-person BVM technique.

Register your access code from the front of your book by going to **www.bradybooks.com** and selecting the mykit links.

Cardiac Resuscitation and Defibrillation

NAVIGATION GUIDE

The following items provide an overview to the purpose and content of this chapter. The Education Standards and Competencies are from the National EMS Education Standards.

Education Standards Pathophysiology; Shock and Resuscitation

Competencies Uses simple knowledge of shock and respiratory compromise to respond to life threats.
Uses assessment information to recognize shock, respiratory failure or arrest, and cardiac arrest based on assessment findings, and manages the emergency while awaiting additional emergency response.

Objectives After reading this chapter, you should be able to:

1. Define key terms introduced in the chapter.
2. Describe the role of the heart in maintaining adequate perfusion to the cells of the body.
3. Describe the consequences of cardiac arrest.
4. Given a series of scenarios, perform primary assessments to differentiate between patients who are in cardiac arrest and those who are not.
5. Demonstrate the modifications of technique required to check for a pulse in infants.
6. Explain the urgency of beginning resuscitation for patients in cardiac arrest.
7. Explain each of the links in the chain of survival of cardiac arrest.
8. Demonstrate one-rescuer and two-rescuer CPR for infants, children, and adults.
9. Explain why the lone EMR should begin resuscitation in infants and children prior to calling for EMS.
10. Discuss the modifications in techniques that are necessary for successfully maintaining an open airway and providing ventilations and chest compressions in children and infants during CPR.
11. Describe each of the four arrhythmias that cause cardiac arrest.
12. Explain the importance of early defibrillation in cardiac arrest.
13. Discuss safety considerations in the use of automated external defibrillators (AEDs).
14. Demonstrate safe and effective use of an AED.
15. List reasons that an AED may not deliver a shock to a patient in cardiac arrest.
16. Explain the importance of continuous quality assurance programs for the use of AEDs.
17. Given a series of cardiac arrest scenarios involving infants, children, and adults, demonstrate appropriate assessment and resuscitative techniques, including the integrated use of AEDs (automated and semiautomated), ventilation, and CPR.

18. Demonstrate the steps in caring for a patient who has a return of spontaneous circulation following CPR and defibrillation.

19. Identify situations in which it may not be advisable to begin, or to continue, CPR.

Key Terms Page references indicate first major use in this chapter. The Margin Glossary in this chapter provides definitions as you read.

atria, p. 184

ventricles, p. 184

pulse, p. 184

cardiac arrest, p. 184

apnea, p. 185

agonal breathing, p. 185

cyanosis, p. 185

automated external defibrillator (AED), p. 188

cardiopulmonary resuscitation (CPR), p. 189

xiphoid process, p. 198

arrhythmia, p. 203

defibrillation, p. 203

public access defibrillation (PAD), p. 204

rigor mortis, p. 209

dependent lividity, p. 209

Media Resources Please go to www.bradybooks.com to access mykit for this text. You will find quizzes, critical thinking scenarios, weblinks, animations, and videos related to this chapter—and much more. Look for online information on using an AED. You will also find video clips demonstrating adult CPR with two rescuers and infant CPR.

INTRODUCTION

Each day approximately 850 Americans die from sudden cardiac arrest. That means about every 2 minutes a patient dies, most without ever seeing a hospital. As an emergency responder, your immediate actions to restore minimal circulation play a critical role in changing a potentially tragic outcome. In this chapter we will review the critical interventions necessary to support the cardiovascular system and convert deadly heart rhythms. It is important to remember that your actions fit within a larger system designed to improve success and maximize the chances of resuscitation. This "chain of survival," as the American Heart Association calls it, requires all its components to work together to improve outcomes. The actions that you will undertake may be the most important part (See The Big Picture: Cardiac Resuscitation and Defibrillation).

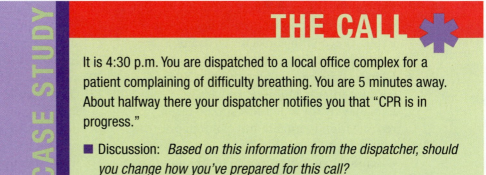

CASE STUDY

THE CALL

It is 4:30 p.m. You are dispatched to a local office complex for a patient complaining of difficulty breathing. You are 5 minutes away. About halfway there your dispatcher notifies you that "CPR is in progress."

■ Discussion: *Based on this information from the dispatcher, should you change how you've prepared for this call?*

The Big Picture
Cardiac Resuscitation and Defibrillation

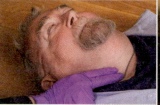

1 If patient is unresponsive, and appears lifeless and not breathing, check pulse.

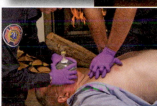

2 If no pulse, begin compressions while preparing the AED.

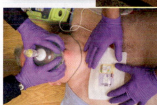

3 Apply the defibrillator and follow prompts.

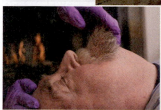

4 Continue CPR at 30:2 ratio.

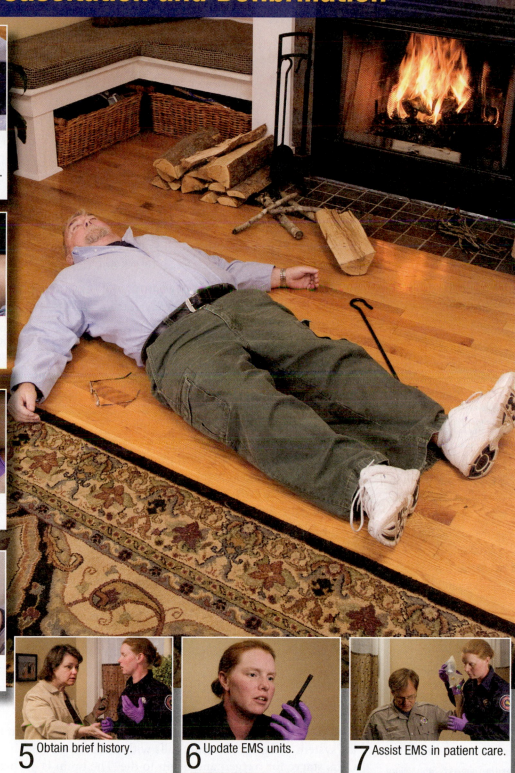

5 Obtain brief history.

6 Update EMS units.

7 Assist EMS in patient care.

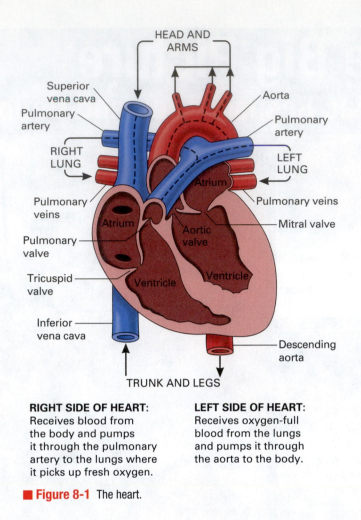

RIGHT SIDE OF HEART: Receives blood from the body and pumps it through the pulmonary artery to the lungs where it picks up fresh oxygen.

LEFT SIDE OF HEART: Receives oxygen-full blood from the lungs and pumps it through the aorta to the body.

■ **Figure 8-1** The heart.

ASK YOURSELF

- What is the role of the heart in maintaining adequate perfusion to the cells of the body?
- Can you define key terms introduced in this chapter?
- What are the consequences of cardiac arrest?

atria the two upper chambers of the heart.

ventricles the two lower chambers of the heart.

pulse the sensation of a change in pressure (a beat) in the arteries created by contraction of the heart.

cardiac arrest the failure of the heartbeat; loss of all pumping action of the heart.

The Heart

In many ways the heart is a simple organ. It has one job, and that is to pump blood. The heart is divided into four chambers: two upper chambers called **atria** and two lower chambers called **ventricles**. The right atrium receives deoxygenated blood returning from the body, and the right ventricle pumps it to the lungs where it picks up oxygen. The left atrium then receives the newly oxygenated blood from the lungs, and the left ventricle pumps that blood out again to the body. This pumping action pressurizes the cardiovascular system and allows blood to perfuse the cells of the body. You can feel the change in pressure, caused by the heart forcefully pumping blood into the arteries, by feeling for your patient's **pulse** (see Chapter 12). The movement of blood through the arteries, capillaries, and veins is essential to staying alive. This perfusion brings oxygen and essential nutrients to the cells and removes carbon dioxide and other waste products. If this exchange were to stop, your patient would quickly die (Figure 8-1 ■).

Cardiac Arrest

Cardiac arrest occurs when the heart stops beating. Without the pump, the cardiovascular system collapses. Pressure falls within the blood vessels, and blood does not move. Cells starve for oxygen and begin to die. The brain is particularly sensitive to a lack of oxygen. Brain cells begin to die after 4–6 minutes, and irreversible damage occurs after 8–10 minutes. Cardiac arrest can be caused by a variety of problems and disorders. Heart disease and trauma are the most common causes in adults, and respiratory problems are the most common causes in infants and children.

EMR Patient Assessment: Cardiac Arrest

Because prompt and immediate interventions are critical to patient survival, you must learn to rapidly recognize cardiac arrest (Scan 8-1). Signs of cardiac arrest include:

- ■ Unresponsive mental status. Tap the patient on the shoulder and shout, "Are you OK?" Does he respond?
- ■ No breathing (**apnea**) or minimal gasping respirations known as **agonal breathing**.
- ■ **Cyanosis** or a bluish tint to skin especially around lips and fingernail beds.
- ■ No pulse.
- ■ No movement by the patient.

Pulselessness is the ultimate finding to confirm cardiac arrest. It is important to remember that not everyone who has cyanosis or who is not breathing is in cardiac arrest. Rather, these symptoms are common findings associated with cardiac arrest and should emphasize to you the need to assess for a pulse. Always complete a thorough primary assessment.

Checking for a Pulse

In a suspected cardiac arrest in an adult or a child at least 1 year old, you should check for a pulse over the carotid artery. To locate the carotid artery, place two fingers on your patient's Adam's apple (larynx), then slide your fingers to the side and stop in the groove between the larynx and large neck muscle (Figures 8-2a and 8-2b ■). Feel for the pulse with gentle pressure for 10 seconds. Do not apply too much pressure as excessive force may actually occlude the artery and hide the pulse. Do not use your thumb as you may feel your own pulse. A pulse may be slow or hard to feel, so you must pay close attention. If you are ever unsure, it is best to assume there is no pulse and begin resuscitative efforts.

ASK YOURSELF

- ■ Given a series of scenarios, what are the primary assessment steps to help you differentiate between patients who are in cardiac arrest and those who are not?

apnea   no breathing.

agonal breathing infrequent, irregular gasping respirations, usually associated with respiratory/cardiac arrest.

cyanosis   a bluish tint to skin, especially around lips and fingernail beds, resulting from hypoxia.

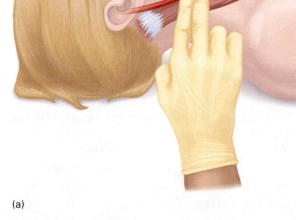

(a)

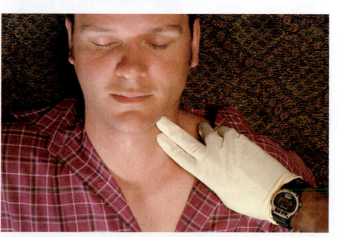

(b)

■ **Figure 8-2** Locating the carotid artery.

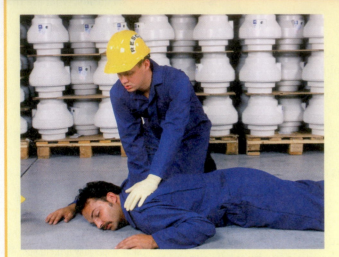

8-1a Check for signs of life (moving, moaning, etc.) as well as performing a quick scan for breathing. Quickly verify no breathing or only agonal breathing.

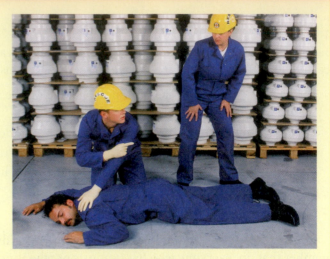

8-1b Activate the EMS system and send someone for an AED.

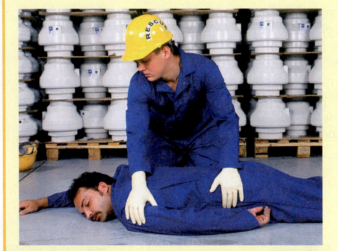

8-1c Place the patient in a supine position on a firm, flat surface.

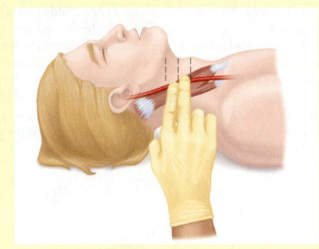

8-1d Check the pulse for no longer than 10 seconds. If no pulse, begin compressions immediately.

Checking for a Pulse in an Infant (0–1 year)

In a suspected cardiac arrest in an infant, you should check for a pulse over the brachial artery. You can locate the brachial artery by placing two or three fingers on the inside of the upper arm between the infant's elbow and shoulder. Then gently feel for a pulse for at least 5 seconds and no more than 10 seconds. In a very small infant such as a newborn, it may also be helpful to assess for a pulse using a stethoscope and listening over the chest for a heartbeat. The American Heart Association has identified the key components to improving outcomes of sudden cardiac arrest in children and has called them the "pediatric chain of survival" (Figure 8-3 ■).

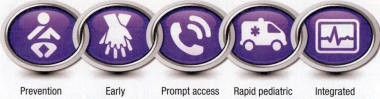

Prevention   Early cardiopulmonary resuscitation (CPR)   Prompt access to the emergency response system   Rapid pediatric advanced life support (PALS)   Integrated post–cardiac arrest care

■ **Figure 8-3** Pediatric Chain of Survival. Reprinted with permission 2010 American Heart Association Guidelines for Cardiopulmonary Resuscitation and Emergency Cardiovascular Care, Part 13: Pediatric Basic Life Support Circulation. 2010; 122[suppl 3]: S862-875 © American Heart Association, Inc.

The Chain of Survival

Successful resuscitation of a patient in cardiac arrest most often comes about through teamwork. When critical components of a larger system work together the patient is afforded the best chance of survival. The American Heart Association has identified the key components to improving outcomes of sudden cardiac arrest and has called them the "chain of survival" (Figure 8-4 ■). The links in the chain include:

- *Immediate recognition and activation.* This includes awareness training and early activation of the EMS system. You and your department may play a part in this through training or public information campaigns. Typically this link would mean early recognition of cardiac arrest and an immediate 911 call (or other appropriate emergency number) by bystanders.

- *Early CPR.* This includes training laypeople to perform bystander CPR before the arrival of emergency responders. It also includes your role as an Emergency Medical Responder in initiating CPR as soon as possible.

- *Rapid defibrillation.* This includes putting **automated external defibrillators (AEDs)** in the hands of emergency responders and the early application of these devices in the instance of sudden cardiac arrest. This may include you as an emergency responder using an AED, but it also includes bystanders using a public access defibrillator such as those found in airports and malls.

ASK YOURSELF

■ What are the modified techniques required to check for a pulse in infants?

■ Why is it urgent to begin resuscitation for patients in cardiac arrest?

■ What are the links in the chain of survival of cardiac arrest?

automated external defibrillator (AED) a device designed to recognize fatal heart rhythms and send an electrical current through the chest to correct the problem.

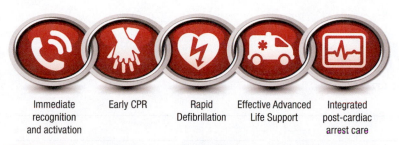

Immediate recognition and activation   Early CPR   Rapid Defibrillation   Effective Advanced Life Support   Integrated post–cardiac arrest care

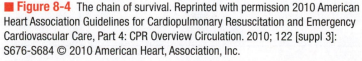

■ **Figure 8-4** The chain of survival. Reprinted with permission 2010 American Heart Association Guidelines for Cardiopulmonary Resuscitation and Emergency Cardiovascular Care, Part 4: CPR Overview Circulation. 2010; 122 [suppl 3]: S676-S684 © 2010 American Heart, Association, Inc.

- *Effective advanced life support.* This includes early access to a higher level of care such as Paramedics or an emergency department and the advanced medications and equipment they can provide. You will play an important role in this link by requesting advanced life support (ALS) early and by making appropriate transport arrangements

- *Integrated post-cardiac arrest care.* Coordinated on-going care including therapeutic hypothermia enhances chances for survival.

All the links in the chain improve survival, but when they work together, outcomes are improved at a greater rate. The best chance of a successful resuscitation comes as a result of all four components being in place and working as one. As an EMR, you should understand your important role within this system and take seriously your potential impact both before (prevention) and during a cardiac arrest situation.

✳ Stop, Review, Remember

Multiple Choice

Place a check next to the correct answer.

1. The upper chambers of the heart are called _____.
   - _____ a. ventricles
   - _____ b. atria
   - _____ c. uvula
   - _____ d. septum

2. The left _____ pumps oxygenated blood out to the body.
   - _____ a. ventricle
   - _____ b. atrium
   - _____ c. septum
   - _____ d. uvula

3. Another term for a stoppage of the heart is:
   - _____ a. respiratory arrest.
   - _____ b. apnea.
   - _____ c. tachycardia.
   - _____ d. cardiac arrest.

4. For an adult patient in suspected cardiac arrest, the most reliable place to assess for a pulse is the _____ artery.
   - _____ a. femoral
   - _____ b. brachial
   - _____ c. coronary
   - _____ d. carotid

5. A bluish tint to skin, especially around lips and fingernail beds, is known as _____.
   - _____ a. cyanosis
   - _____ b. jaundice
   - _____ c. diaphoresis
   - _____ d. cirrhosis

Emergency Medical Responder Practice

1. List at least four signs of cardiac arrest.

   a. _____

   b. _____

   c. _____

   d. _____

2. List the five links that make up the American Heart Association chain of survival.

a. _____

b. _____

c. _____

d. _____

e. _____

Short Answer

1. Compare the five links of the American Heart Association chain of survival to the existing resources in your community. How does your response area meet or fall short of the chain?

_____

_____

_____

_____

EMR Emergency Care: Cardiac Arrest

For a patient in cardiac arrest, your immediate actions are critical. Be decisive and act quickly.

Activate the EMS System

The fact that you have responded makes it likely that someone has already activated the EMS system. However, you should never assume this to be the case. Recall that the chain of survival emphasizes early access to advanced care. In addition to accessing the system in general, you may need to make a specific request for advanced assistance. In the case of suspected cardiac arrest, ensure that you will have access to defibrillation (if you do not have it already) and that you have access to advanced care. Remember that the closest advanced care may be the nearest hospital.

The exception to this rule is a pediatric cardiac arrest. In this case, the most likely causes of the arrest are airway and breathing problems; therefore, immediate corrective actions are your priority. That does not mean you should not call for advanced care, but rather that the call should never delay your immediate airway and breathing interventions.

Adult Cardiopulmonary Resuscitation

Cardiopulmonary resuscitation (CPR) consists of timed compressions and ventilations to provide a minimal level of circulation to a person whose heart has stopped (Scan 8-2). CPR may provide roughly one-quarter to one-third of normal circulation. Although that is significantly less than what a normally functioning cardiovascular system provides, it may be enough to support life until the heart can be prompted to resume normal pumping. Circulation is achieved through artificial ventilations and chest compressions. These compressions change the pressure inside the chest and mechanically force blood to flow. However, this is a very different process than the body uses, so you must be cautious to allow full recoil of the chest and time for proper exhalation. (This will be explained further in the next section.)

It is important to remember that CPR can cause serious complications and should never be started on a patient with a pulse. Take care to verify pulselessness and to assure there are no signs of life present prior to beginning compressions (review Scan 8-1a to 8-1d).

cardiopulmonary resuscitation (CPR)
timed artificial ventilations and chest compressions designed to maintain minimal circulation in a patient with cardiac arrest.

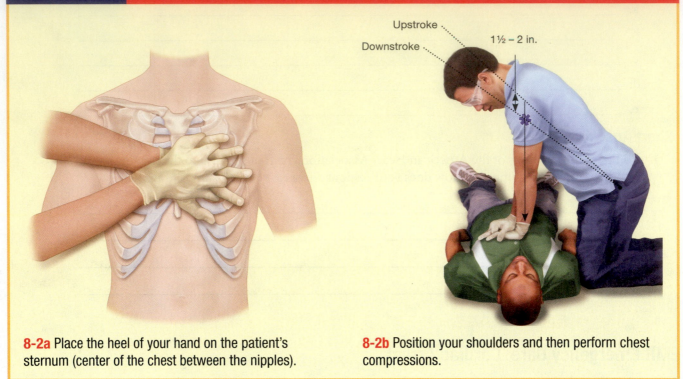

8-2a Place the heel of your hand on the patient's sternum (center of the chest between the nipples).

8-2b Position your shoulders and then perform chest compressions.

Adult Compressions

CPR is accomplished by compressing the chest and changing the internal pressure to move blood. Important components of performing chest compressions are patient position, hand position, provider position, depth, and rate:

■ *Patient position.* Move the patient to a firm surface. Chest compressions require the chest to actually be compressed. If your patient is lying on a soft surface (like a bed) the full effect of compressions will be lost. You should immediately move your patient to the floor, a rigid spine board, or a similarly firm surface.

■ *Hand position.* Expose the chest. Remove clothing and anything that will interfere with hand-to-chest contact. Locate your compression site. In an adult, you will place the heel of one hand on the center of your patient's chest between the nipples and then place the other hand on top of the first.

■ *Provider position.* Kneel at the patient's side. After finding the appropriate hand position, you will straighten your arms and position your shoulders so they are directly over your hands. When compressing, you will want to be positioned squarely over the patient's chest (Scan 8-2a and 8-2b).

■ *Depth.* You will compress the patient's sternum hard and fast. Keep your elbows locked and let the weight of your upper body assist you with the compression. Compress the chest straight down approximately 2 inches and then allow full recoil. You should not remove your hands, but be sure your weight does not limit chest movement as this will limit blood flow with compressions.

■ *Rate.* You will compress at a rate of 100 compressions per minute. That means you should complete 30 compressions in about 23 seconds.

Adult Ventilations

After completing 30 compressions, you will provide initial ventilations. We have already discussed artificial ventilation in Chapter 7. You will use those skills in CPR. Important points to review include the following:

- Protect yourself from the transmission of infectious disease by ventilating with a barrier device (such as a pocket mask) or a bag-valve mask.
- Ventilations should be given over 1 second with enough air to make the chest rise. Supplemental oxygen should be attached if available.
- You will time your ventilations with compressions, but be sure to allow adequate exhalation time. Remember that in this situation, your patient is dependent mostly on relaxation of the chest and gravity to exhale. Ventilations that are administered too rapidly do not allow time for proper exhalation and therefore may not allow for the complete ventilation of waste products.

One-Rescuer Adult CPR Sequence (Scan 8-3)

1. Check for responsiveness. If the patient is unresponsive and shows no signs of life, you will begin a C-A-B approach.
2. Activate the EMS system if this has not already been done. Request advanced life support assistance.
3. Move the patient to a firm surface and position yourself.
4. Check for a pulse for 10 seconds. If there is no pulse, begin CPR.
5. Give 30 compressions. Compressions should be given hard and fast at a rate of at least 100 per minute, allowing full recoil of the chest between compressions.
6. Give two ventilations, ensuring chest rise with each breath.
7. Repeat the 30:2 cycle until an AED arrives, ALS takes over, or the patient begins to move (Scan 8-3a to 8-3d).

ASK YOURSELF

- How would you describe the steps of the one-rescuer and two-rescuer CPR for infants, children, and adults?

A Second Rescuer Arrives

If another rescuer arrives, you will want to be sure the EMS system has been activated before he joins the resuscitation effort. Also, that rescuer should obtain an AED if one is nearby. Once both of those steps are accomplished, the second rescuer should assist with CPR.

Studies have shown that the provider doing compressions will tire quickly and the force of compressions will decrease (even though this may not be perceived by the rescuer doing compressions). Therefore, the second rescuer should position himself on the opposite side of the patient so that he will be ready to take over compressions at the end of the cycle. When 30 compressions are complete, the first rescuer should move to the airway and the second rescuer should resume compressions after the two breaths are administered. Both rescuers should communicate so as not to interrupt the CPR cycle with the switch.

Any additional rescuers should be detailed to obtain a patient history, retrieve additional equipment, and prepare for transport of the patient.

Two-Rescuer Adult CPR Sequence (Scan 8-4)

1. Check for signs of life. Scan the chest for breathing.
2. One rescuer should activate the EMS system if this has not already been done and retrieve an AED if possible while the other begins CPR.
3. Move the patient to a firm surface.

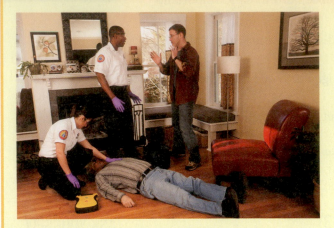

8-3a If a patient appears lifeless and without breathing (or with only agonal breathing) begin C-A-B approach.

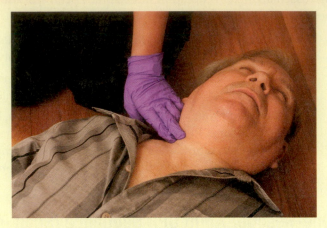

8-3b Check pulse for no longer than 10 seconds.

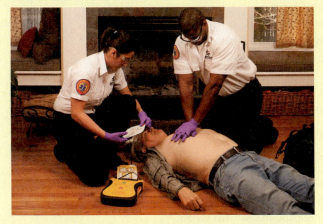

8-3c Perform cycles of 30 compressions followed by 2 ventilations. Integrate defibrillation when an AED is available.

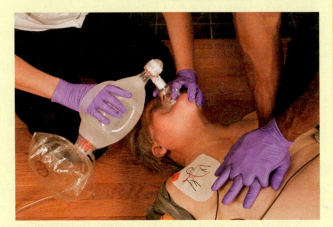

8-3d Continue cycles of 30 compressions and two ventilations. Limit pulse checks during resuscitation to maximize continuous compression.

4. Position the rescuers. With two rescuers, one provider will do compressions (kneeling at the patient's side) and the other will ventilate (kneeling above the patient's head). It will be important to switch these roles every 5 cycles or 2 minutes to prevent compressor fatigue.

5. Give 30 compressions. The compression rate does not change with two rescuers. Compressions should be given hard and fast at a rate of at least 100 per minute, allowing full recoil of the chest between compressions. The provider doing compressions should count his compressions out loud so the provider doing ventilations can anticipate the timing of ventilations.

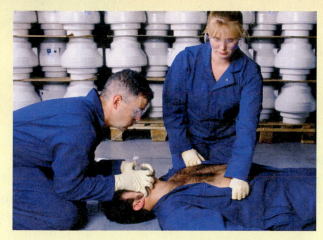

8-4a Two rescuers get in position, one at the head and one at the patient's side.

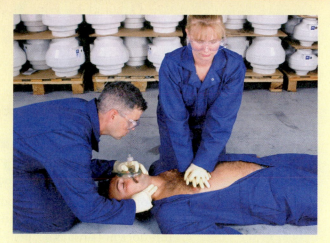

8-4b The rescuer at the side performs 30 compressions at a rate of 100 per minute.

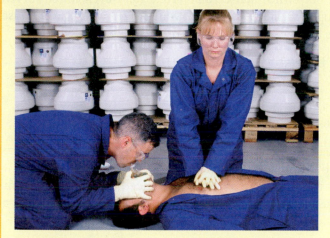

8-4c After every 30 compressions, the rescuer at the head delivers two breaths.

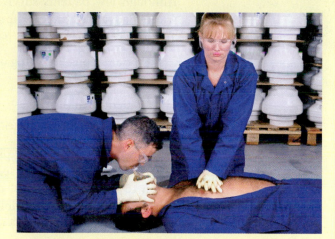

8-4d Repeat cycles of 30 compressions and 2 ventilations for 5 cycles then switch positions. Observe the patient for movement or breathing during resuscitation. Pulse checks delay CPR and should not be performed frequently.

6. Give two ventilations ensuring chest rise with each breath.
7. Repeat the 30:2 cycle for 5 cycles or 2 minutes and then switch roles. Continue until an AED arrives, ALS takes over, or the patient begins to move (Scan 8-4a to 8-4d).

When switching roles, the compressor should "call for the switch." That is, he should let the ventilator know that after the current cycle, the switch will occur. After the 30 compressions, the ventilator will administer two breaths and then quickly move to the patient's side, locate his hand position, and begin the next round of 30 compressions. The compressor simultaneously will move to the airway position and prepare to ventilate at the end of the cycle.

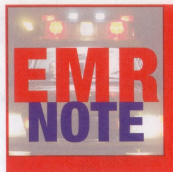

Monitoring the Quality of CPR

Effective CPR can be monitored by feeling for a carotid pulse during compressions. Quality compressions should produce a faint pulse. The chest should also rise with each ventilation. Additionally, the patient's skin color may improve with effective CPR (although this does not always occur).

Return of Spontaneous Circulation

Although few patients survive out-of-hospital cardiac arrest (and even fewer survive without advanced cardiac life support), it is possible that your patient will regain a pulse. You may recognize that this has happened if you see any of the following signs:

- Spontaneous breathing or gasping
- Patient movement
- Patient swallowing
- Return of patient consciousness (unlikely)

Out-of-hospital CPR typically has very poor outcomes. Remember that your goal may not be to regain a pulse, but rather to stimulate a minimal level of blood circulation to keep your patient perfusing while awaiting advanced care. Although improvement may not be visible, good CPR may be the best chance the patient has at survival.

Complications of CPR

Although your technique may be perfect, some complications may arise from CPR. Fractured ribs and separated rib cartilage, a fractured sternum, and even collapsed lungs are possible as a result of CPR. Although we try to prevent such complications by using good technique, the overall benefit of CPR clearly outweighs the risk of complications in a person without a pulse.

Adult CPR Key Points

- Activate the EMS system early. Get advanced care to the patient as soon as possible.
- Push hard and fast. Quality compressions are the key to good CPR.
- Switch often to avoid fatigue.
- Limit interruptions in compressions. If absolutely necessary to interrupt compressions, limit the interruption to no more than 10 seconds. CPR takes several compressions to achieve minimal blood flow. Every time you stop, it takes several more compressions to regain that flow.

THE RESPONSE

You arrive in front of the office building and see several people waiting for you at the front door. They frantically wave you in. Your dispatcher has informed you that CPR is in progress, so you and your partner decide to bring in the portable suction and a backboard as well as the usual jump bag.

The bystanders lead you to an area of cubicles. You see two bystanders performing CPR on a 58-year-old man. You notice that he is cyanotic.

You assess the scene. Many of the patient's coworkers have gathered and they are saddened and distressed over the situation. They tell you the patient had been feeling "sick" all day and passed out at his desk. Coworkers witnessed the episode and noted he just slumped over in his chair. They tell you he was not breathing when they approached him.

Their employer had hosted a CPR training class a few months ago and, therefore, many of them were prepared to begin a resuscitation. They began CPR immediately.

At the end of their next cycle your partner assesses for a pulse and tells you he cannot find one. You allow one of the bystanders to continue compressions while you attach the AED.

■ Discussion: *For how long should you allow the bystanders to continue compressions? Why?*

✴ Stop, Review, Remember

Multiple Choice

Place a check next to the correct answer.

1. The appropriate volume of air to administer to a patient while doing CPR ventilations is:

    _____ a. 1,000 mL.

    _____ b. 5,000 mL.

    _____ c. enough to make the chest rise.

    _____ d. enough to make the abdomen rise.

2. The appropriate hand position for CPR compressions on an adult is:

    _____ a. over the sternum at the nipple line.

    _____ b. on the nipple line, just to the right of the sternum.

    _____ c. on the nipple line, just to the left of the sternum.

    _____ d. over the point where the sternum ends and the abdomen begins.

3. The appropriate rate of compressions for adult CPR is _____ per minute.

_____ a. 30

_____ b. 60

_____ c. 80

_____ d. 100

4. When performing adult CPR, one cycle means _____ compressions to two ventilations.

_____ a. 30

_____ b. 15

_____ c. 10

_____ d. 5

5. When performing two-rescuer adult CPR, it is recommended that you switch compressors every _____ cycles or 2 minutes.

_____ a. 4

_____ b. 5

_____ c. 6

_____ d. 7

Emergency Medical Responder Practice

1. You are alone and approaching a patient with suspected cardiac arrest. Assuming the scene is safe, list the first four steps you would take.

a. _____

b. _____

c. _____

d. _____

2. List at least two signs of quality CPR.

a. _____

b. _____

Short Answer

1. Explain the steps involved with switching compressors during adult two-rescuer CPR.

_____

_____

_____

_____

2. You are doing one-rescuer adult CPR and a second rescuer arrives. What responsibilities need to be addressed prior to that rescuer assisting with CPR?

_____

_____

_____

_____

3. List at least two "key points" of adult CPR and discuss why they are so important.

_____

_____

_____

1. You are walking in the local park and witness a man collapse and go into what you believe to be cardiac arrest. The nearest phone is at least 5 minutes away and there is no one else near you. Discuss the steps you would take to assist this patient.

_____

_____

_____

_____

Pediatric CPR

CPR changes slightly when dealing with children and infants. Although the principles remain the same, certain adjustments must be made to account for the differences in anatomy and for the different reasons pediatric patients go into cardiac arrest. You will also start CPR on pediatric patients sooner than on adults. *When you encounter a heart rate of less than 60 beats per minute in an infant or child patient (up to 8 years of age) with signs of poor perfusion you must begin CPR, even though the child still may have a pulse!*

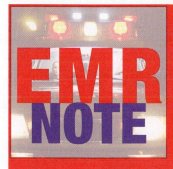

EMR NOTE

The American Heart Association groups pediatric patients into the following categories:

Neonate (newborn): 0–1 month
Infant: 1 month–1 year
Child: 1 year– 8 years

Some CPR courses for professional rescuers use the onset of puberty as the point a child is considered an adult.

Resuscitate Now; Call Later

Because the most common reasons for pediatric arrest are airway and breathing issues, calling for assistance and ALS help is secondary to initiating resuscitative steps. That does not mean you should not call right away. If resources allow, the EMS system should be activated and advanced care should be requested immediately. Only if you are forced to choose between accessing the system and starting CPR should you choose to start CPR. Research tells us that if there is any chance of a successful resuscitation in a pediatric patient, it will most likely be the result of the basic airway and ventilatory management you will perform immediately. Although advanced care is still important, it may be less important in this population than in adults. If you must leave the patient to access the EMS system, you should perform at least 5 cycles of CPR before leaving. Depending on the size of the child and the distances involved, you may be able to take the patient with you when you call for assistance and continue CPR immediately after the phone call.

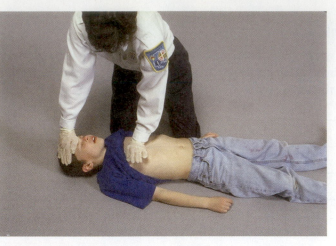

■ **Figure 8-5** Compressions on a larger child.

ASK YOURSELF

■ What modifications in techniques are necessary for successfully maintaining an open airway and providing ventilations and chest compressions in children and infants during CPR?

xiphoid process the small protrusion at the end of the sternum.

Pediatric Compressions

The principles of chest compressions in pediatrics are the same as in adults. Push fast and hard and allow complete recoil of the chest. However, due to smaller anatomy, certain modifications must be made (Figure 8-5 ■):

■ *Patient position.* Move the patient to a firm surface. Remember that infants and newborns usually need padding behind their shoulders to prevent airway occlusion when lying flat.

■ *Hand position.*

■ *Child.* Expose the chest. Locate your compression site. The hand position in a child is the same hand position as for an adult; you will place the heel of one hand on the center of your patient's chest between the nipples. Depending on the size of the child, you may need to use only one hand to compress or you may place the other hand on top of the first.

■ *Infant.* Draw an imaginary line between the nipples. Place two fingers on the sternum just below this line. Do not compress on the small protrusion at the end of the sternum called the **xiphoid process**. We will discuss an alternative hand position for compressions on an infant later in this chapter.

■ *Depth.* You will compress the patient's sternum hard and fast. Compress the chest of a pediatric patient (infant and child until the age of puberty) straight down approximately one-third to one-half the front-to-back depth of the chest and then allow full recoil. You should not remove your hands, but be sure you allow full chest movement.

■ *Rate.* You will compress at a rate of 100 compressions per minute. That means you should complete 30 compressions in about 23 seconds.

Pediatric Ventilations

After your first set of compressions, you will deliver ventilations. Pediatric airway management and ventilation are discussed in greater detail in Chapter 7; however, there are a few important concepts to keep in mind:

■ When opening the airway, you may have to account for a larger head especially in newborns and infants. Often placing 2–4 cm of padding behind the shoulders will prevent flexing the neck and occluding the airway when laid flat (Figure 8-6 ■).

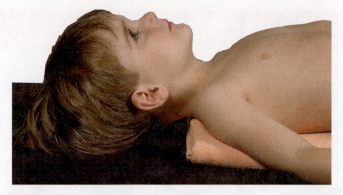

■ **Figure 8-6** To keep the airway aligned, place folded towel under the shoulders.

■ Protect yourself from the transmission of infectious disease by ventilating with a barrier device (such as a pocket mask) or a bag-valve mask. If you only have an adult pocket mask, you may be able to turn the mask upside down to obtain a seal. In this case the point of the mask that you would typically seat on the bridge of an adult's nose would be placed on the chin of a small pediatric patient. Consider size-appropriate bag-valve masks.

■ Even though you will be using significantly less volume, the measurement used to determine adequate ventilation in pediatrics is the same as the one used in adults: chest rise. Ventilations should be given slowly over 1 second with enough air to make the chest rise. Supplemental oxygen should be attached if available.

■ You will time your ventilations with compressions, but be sure to allow adequate exhalation time.

One-Rescuer Pediatric (Infant and Child) CPR Sequence (Scan 8-5)

1. Patient appears lifeless and has no breathing or agonal breathing.
2. Move the patient to a firm surface and position yourself.
3. Check for a pulse. If there is no pulse, begin CPR.
4. Give 30 compressions. Compressions should be given hard and fast at a rate of at least 100 per minute, allowing full recoil of the chest between compressions.
5. Give two ventilations, ensuring chest rise with each breath.
6. Repeat the 30:2 for 5 cycles or 2 minutes and then activate the EMS system or call for advanced help if this has not already been done.

Two-Rescuer Pediatric (Infant and Child) CPR Sequence

1. Check for responsiveness.
2. One rescuer should activate the EMS system if this has not already been done and retrieve an AED if possible while the other begins CPR.
3. Move the patient to a firm surface.
4. Position the rescuers. With two rescuers, one provider will do compressions (kneeling at the patient's side) and the other will ventilate (kneeling above the patient's head). Even in pediatric CPR, it is important to switch these roles every 5 cycles or 2 minutes to prevent compressor fatigue.
5. Check for a pulse. If there is no pulse, begin CPR.
6. The compression to ventilation ratio is different in pediatric two-rescuer CPR. When two rescuers are present, you will give 15 compressions and then two breaths. As in adults, compressions should be given hard and fast at a rate of at least 100 per minute, allowing full recoil of the chest between compressions.

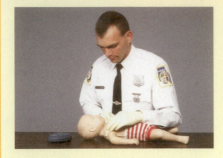

8-5a Determine unresponsiveness with a shake-and-shout method.

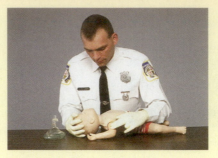

8-5b Determine pulselessness at the brachial artery in an infant or carotid artery in a child.

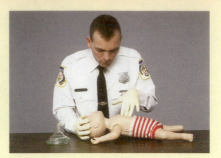

8-5c Locate the correct hand position.

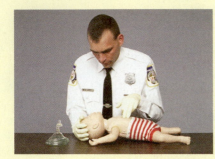

8-5d Provide chest compressions at a rate of 100 per minute.

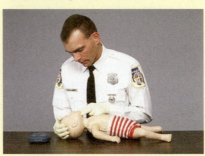

8-5e Gently open the airway.

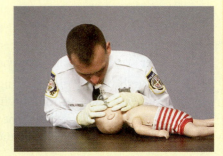

8-5f Cover the infant's mouth and nose with a pocket mask. Ventilate until the chest rises.

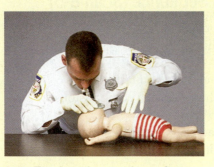

8-5g Two breaths are given after every 30 compressions.

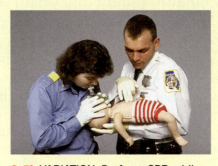

8-5h VARIATION: Perform CPR while a second person is carrying the baby.

The provider doing compressions should count his compressions out loud so the provider doing ventilations can anticipate the timing of ventilations.

7. Repeat the 15:2 cycle for 10 cycles or 2 minutes and then switch roles. Continue until an AED arrives, ALS takes over, or the patient begins to move.

Alternative Compression Technique for Newborns and Small Infants

The American Heart Association recommends that you use the "thumbs-encircling" technique when the size of the infant allows you to do so and when you are performing two-rescuer CPR. See Figure 8-7 ■. They suggest that this technique allows for better blood flow and consistently results in a better force of compression.

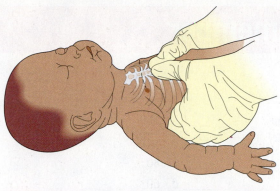

Figure 8-7 Thumbs-encircling compression technique.

This technique can be achieved with the following steps:

- Draw an imaginary line between the nipples and place both of your thumbs side by side over the infant's sternum, just below the imaginary line. Avoid compressing the xiphoid process. Note your thumbs may overlap on very small infants.
- Encircle the infant's chest and support the infant's back with the fingers of both hands.
- With your hands encircling the chest, use your thumbs to compress the sternum one-third to one-half the front-to-back depth of the chest. As you push down with your thumbs, squeeze the infant's chest with your fingers.
- Allow complete recoil of the chest between compressions.

Complications of Pediatric CPR

Many of the same complications of CPR exist in the pediatric population as well. However, you should specifically consider hypothermia as a major complication with infants and children. Always take steps to keep your pediatric patient warm while the resuscitation is ongoing. See Table 8-1 for a CPR Summary.

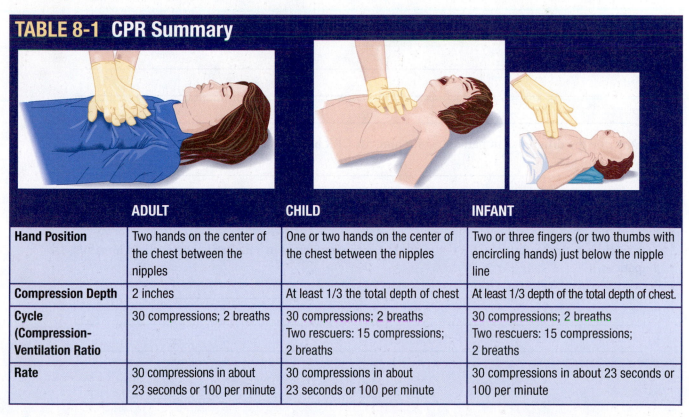

TABLE 8-1 CPR Summary

	ADULT	CHILD	INFANT
Hand Position	Two hands on the center of the chest between the nipples	One or two hands on the center of the chest between the nipples	Two or three fingers (or two thumbs with encircling hands) just below the nipple line
Compression Depth	2 inches	At least 1/3 the total depth of chest	At least 1/3 depth of the total depth of chest.
Cycle (Compression-Ventilation Ratio	30 compressions; 2 breaths	30 compressions; 2 breaths Two rescuers: 15 compressions; 2 breaths	30 compressions; 2 breaths Two rescuers: 15 compressions; 2 breaths
Rate	30 compressions in about 23 seconds or 100 per minute	30 compressions in about 23 seconds or 100 per minute	30 compressions in about 23 seconds or 100 per minute

Multiple Choice

Place a check next to the correct answer.

1. Which of the following age groups does the American Heart Association consider to be an infant?

   _____ a. 2–5 years

   _____ b. 2–8 years

   _____ c. 1–5 years

   _____ d. 0–1 year

2. The appropriate volume of air to use while ventilating an infant is:

   _____ a. 100 mL.

   _____ b. 200 mL.

   _____ c. enough to see the chest rise.

   _____ d. the entire volume of an appropriately sized infant bag-valve mask.

3. The appropriate compression rate for infants and children is _____ compressions per minute.

   _____ a. 100

   _____ b. 120

   _____ c. 80

   _____ d. 60

4. When performing compressions on an infant, you should avoid the _____ process.

   _____ a. brachial

   _____ b. apical

   _____ c. xiphoid

   _____ d. ischial

5. The American Heart Association recommends the _____ compression technique for newborns and small infants.

   _____ a. abdominal thrust

   _____ b. head tilt

   _____ c. thumbs-encircling

   _____ d. fingers-flexing

Short Answer

1. If you were alone, why would you activate EMS before starting CPR in an adult, but not in a child?

   _____

   _____

   _____

2. Describe the difference in patient positioning for CPR between an adult and an infant.

   _____

   _____

   _____

3. Explain a complication of CPR that would be more important in a pediatric patient than an adult patient.

   _____

   _____

   _____

1. How could the major emotional components of a pediatric arrest call (both family and crew) affect your care?

_____

_____

_____

_____

Automated External Defibrillators (AEDs)

The majority of cardiac arrest is not caused by a mechanical stoppage of the heart, but rather a lethal electrical rhythm called an **arrhythmia** that causes the heart to beat so abnormally that it cannot pump blood. In many cases, this type of arrhythmia can be resolved by a process called defibrillation. In **defibrillation**, the heart is shocked with electricity to "reset" the rhythm in the hopes that the new rhythm is a normal one that promotes a regular, perfusing beat of the heart.

An automated external defibrillator or AED is designed to recognize lethal arrhythmias and deliver an external defibrillation through pads placed on the patient's chest. There are two basic types of AEDs available: fully automated and semiautomated. After being placed on a patient and turned on, a fully automated AED analyzes the heart rhythm and shocks without any prompting from its operator. A semiautomated device requires its operator to press a button to analyze and then to shock if necessary. Semiautomated AEDs are more commonly found. AEDs come in many shapes and sizes and can be found everywhere from fire trucks to airport terminals. Although there are many different manufacturers, most designs follow a similar pattern. Most AEDs have an "on-off" button and a "shock" button used to deliver the shock. AEDs analyze and deliver the shock through adhesive pads you attach to the patient's chest. Most also utilize voice prompts to instruct the user to perform the steps of operation. This sequence of operation is preprogrammed to reflect local and/or national protocols for defibrillation (Figures 8-8a and 8-8b ■).

arrhythmia an abnormal electrical heart rhythm.

defibrillation an electrical shock applied to the heart to correct lethal heart arrhythmias.

Lethal Arrhythmias

There are four arrhythmias that cause cardiac arrest:

1. Asystole (or "flatline") is a condition where there is no electrical activity in the heart and therefore no pumping.
2. Pulseless electrical activity (PEA) is a condition where the rhythm (the electrical component) of the heart is working fine but yet the mechanical aspect is not. In this case the cardiac rhythm would look normal on an ECG monitor, but the patient would not have a pulse.
3. Ventricular tachycardia is a very fast and inefficient rhythm. Although in some situations it can result in a pulse, often it is associated with cardiac arrest.
4. Ventricular fibrillation is a completely disorganized heart rhythm that causes the heart to stop pumping.

Of these arrhythmias, only ventricular tachycardia and ventricular fibrillation respond to defibrillation. AEDs are designed to recognize both of these rhythms and deliver a shock

ASK YOURSELF

■ What are the four arrhythmias that cause cardiac arrest?

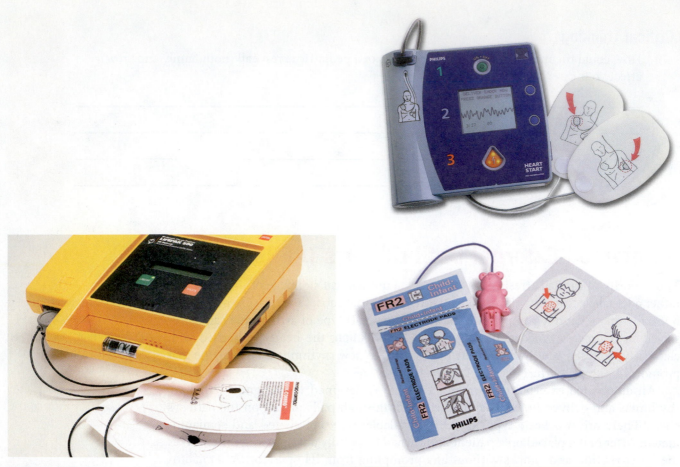

■ **Figure 8-8a** Adult AED.

■ **Figure 8-8b** AED with adult and child pads.

ASK YOURSELF

■ What is the importance of early defibrillation in cardiac arrest?

public access defibrillation (PAD) a program to distribute AEDs to lay rescuers especially in areas of high public use such as malls and airports.

when they are found. AEDs use a microprocessor to recognize these arrhythmias and are very good at sorting them out from other nonshockable rhythms. That said, an AED cannot determine the presence or lack of a pulse in your patient. It is up to you to determine the appropriate situation to attach and operate your machine.

The American Heart Association chain of survival states that early defibrillation is one of the links to improving outcomes in sudden cardiac arrest. Research has shown that the sooner defibrillation is administered to a cardiac arrest patient suffering from one of the shockable arrhythmias, the more likely it is that the patient will survive. Because of this, an effort has been made to distribute AEDs not just to responders, but to the public as well. **Public access defibrillation (PAD)** is a program designed to put AEDs in the hands of the lay rescuer and is the reason you will often find AEDs in malls, airports, and schools.

As a rescuer, you play an essential role in making this link a reality. Lives can be saved by the early use of an AED. You must recognize when to use it and learn the operating steps of your particular machine.

Each AED is slightly different. Be sure to learn your machine's specifications and your department's policies on routine maintenance, operation, and resupply.

AED Safety

Although AEDs are very successful at differentiating lethal arrhythmias from normal rhythms, you should never attach an AED unless you have confirmed your patient has no pulse.

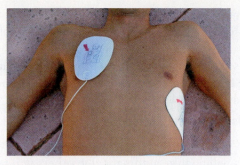

■ Figure 8-9 The AED monitors heart rhythms and delivers shocks through its adhesive pads.

AEDs are, in general, very safe. However, they are designed to perform a high-energy defibrillation under the right circumstances. This defibrillation can seriously harm people who are accidentally in contact with the patient when the shock is delivered. Be sure to appropriately "clear" your patient to make sure no one is in contact with the patient prior to delivering the defibrillation.

Attaching an AED

There has been considerable discussion in the scientific community about whether an AED should be attached immediately or after performing some CPR. Research has not provided a definite conclusion. There are several factors to consider including whether an AED is immediately available, if CPR was in progress prior to your arrival and how long the patient is believed to have been down prior to your arrival. The American Heart Association recommends applying the AED immediately if you have one available. If you don't have an AED immediately available, or if there are multiple rescuers present, CPR should be begun while retrieving or preparing the AED. Always follow your local protocols (Figure 8-9).

Operating an AED

Before operating any AED be sure to review the manufacturer's instructions for that individual machine. Also consult local protocol for specific guidelines as to application and use (Scan 8-6).

The American Heart Association recommends the following steps for deploying an AED:

- *Turn the AED on.*
  - Sometimes this is done simply by opening the device. Other units have specific on-off buttons. Typically, powering on the device will also activate the voice prompts that will instruct you on further steps.
- *Attach the machine's pads to the patient's bare chest.*
  - Follow the manufacturer's recommendation as to pad placement. Remember that left and right refer to the patient's left and right, not yours. On an adult, one pad is typically placed on the upper right chest to the right of the sternum, just below the clavicle. The other pad is placed on the patient's side, to the left of the nipple a few inches below the left armpit.
  - Wipe the chest to clear water or sweat prior to attaching pads. If you find medication patches on the patient's chest, you should remove them and wipe off any remaining medication before attaching pads.
  - If you notice a pacemaker or internally implanted defibrillator under the skin, move the pads to avoid these objects.

ASK YOURSELF

- What are the safety considerations in the use of automated external defibrillators (AEDs)?
- How would you demonstrate safe and effective use of an AED?
- What are the reasons that an AED may not deliver a shock to a patient in cardiac arrest?

- An extremely hairy chest may interfere with pad contact. Often the AED will prompt you to "check electrodes." You should carry a safety razor with your AED to quickly shave away excessive hair. If you do not have a razor and excessive hair is interfering with contact, remove the pads and with them will go much of the troublesome hair. Replace the original pads with new ones and the problem may be resolved.
  - If the AED pads are not connected to the AED, connect them now.
- *Clear the patient and analyze the rhythm.*
  - Some machines will analyze automatically; others will require you to press a button. The AED may take up to 15 seconds to analyze.
  - Be sure to stop CPR and clear the patient during analysis.
  - Once the analysis is complete, the AED will advise "shock" or "no shock advised."
- *If the machine announces "shock advised," clear your patient.*
  - Clearing a patient involves three steps:
    1. Clear yourself. Visually make sure any part of your body (including equipment) is not in contact with the patient.
    2. Verbally instruct all members of your team to clear. Use a loud voice and an unmistakable tone.
    3. Visually inspect that all members are clear of the patient.
  - Only when you have completed all three steps should you administer the shock.
- *Press the shock button to administer the defibrillation.*
  - Typically the patient will display a full body muscle contraction in response to the shock.
- *Immediately after the shock, resume CPR.*
  - After 2 minutes the AED will prompt you to repeat the "analyze and shock" steps again.

AED Use with Pediatric Patients

ASK YOURSELF

- Given a series of cardiac arrest scenarios involving infants, children, and adults, what are the appropriate assessment and resuscitative techniques, including the integrated use of AEDs (automated and semiautomated), ventilation, and CPR?
- What is the importance of continuous quality assurance programs for the use of AEDs?

The American Heart Association states that an AED should be attached to any patient in cardiac arrest. Although it is less likely to find a shockable rhythm in children, if it is found, it can be corrected. Many AEDs come equipped with pediatric pads that adjust the energy levels to appropriate pediatric doses. If the AED is equipped with such pads, they should be used on pediatric patients less than 8 years old. However, if only adult pads are available, you should use them.

Follow the manufacturer's recommendations as to pad placement. Many pediatric pads will be attached in a "front and back configuration." That is, one pad will be applied to the anterior chest and the other will be applied to the back. *Never* overlap pads.

Continuing Quality Assurance and Call Review

Any call that uses an AED should be reviewed (preferably with involvement of your service's medical director). Many AEDs are equipped to transfer data about the call (sometimes even voice recordings). This information should be used to improve future performance and device guidelines to aid success in similar situations. Be sure call review also includes postcall inspection and service of your equipment. Any service that is equipped with an AED should develop standard operating guidelines for the routine checking, use, and postcall evaluation of the AED.

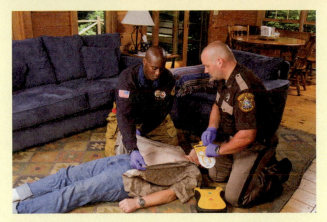

8-6a If patient appears lifeless, use a C-A-B approach.

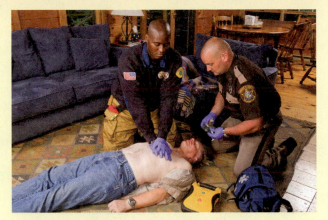

8-6b Perform CPR while preparing the AED.

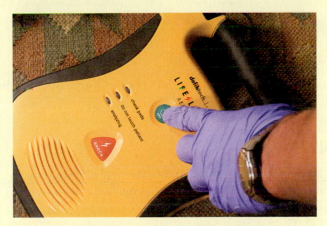

8-6c Turn on device and follow voice prompts.

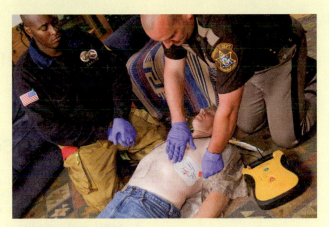

8-6d Apply pads.

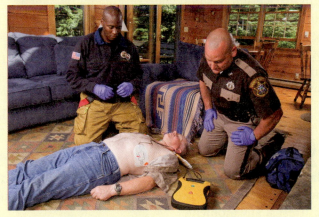

8-6e Analyze.

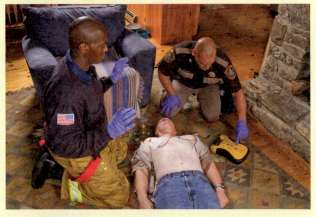

8-6f Clear patient and defibrillate if advised to do so.

(continued)

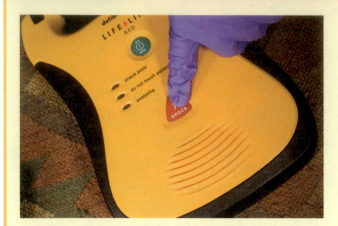

8-6g Push the shock button to defibrillate.

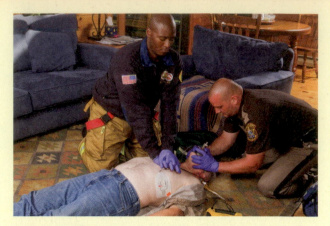

8-6h Begin CPR and follow device prompts.

Putting It All Together

Now that you have reviewed the procedure for AED use, let's review how it fits into the total resuscitation picture.

Adult Resuscitation Sequence

1. Observe the patient for signs of lifelessness. Scan the chest for breathing.
2. Activate the EMS system if this has not already been done. Request advanced life support assistance.
3. Send someone for an AED if one is not present.
4. Move the patient to a firm surface and position yourself.
5. Check the pulse for up to 10 seconds.
6. If there is no pulse, attach the AED or begin compressions. (Remember that rescuers may work together to do both at the same time.)
7. Perform 30 compressions then two ventilations.
8. Continue CPR and follow prompts on the AED. If the AED delivers a shock, continue compressions for at least 2 minutes.

ASK YOURSELF

■ How would you demonstrate the steps in caring for a patient who has a return of spontaneous circulation following CPR and defibrillation?

Return of Spontaneous Circulation

In some cases CPR and defibrillation may return a pulse to your patient. You may find a pulse or more likely notice spontaneous breathing. However, this patient is extremely unstable and may return to cardiac arrest at any moment.

■ Although your patient may have a pulse, he may not be breathing or breathing adequately. Be sure to continue rescue breathing if necessary and always apply high-concentration oxygen.

- Monitor the pulse carefully (especially if your patient is unconscious). Although he has regained a pulse, there is no guarantee he will continue to have it. Constantly reassess.
- Some local protocols allow you to keep the AED pads attached to the patient. Always follow local guidelines.

Ethical Considerations of Cardiac Arrest

Ethical dilemmas can arise both before and after starting CPR. Often the question will arise as to whether to begin resuscitative efforts. You should always follow local protocols, but as a rule, signs of obvious death include **rigor mortis**, or stiffening of the body after death; **dependent lividity**, or the pooling of blood in the lower areas of the body after death; and decapitation or other injuries incompatible with life. As an EMR, you may be in a position to evaluate for such signs and decide if resuscitation is indicated. You may also need to consider the presence of do not resuscitate (DNR) orders. If the patient has a valid DNR order, CPR should not be started. Finally you may need to consider termination of CPR. You should always follow local protocols, but in general, CPR should be continued until the rescuer is exhausted, the patient is turned over to another provider of equal or higher level, the patient is resuscitated, or the patient has been declared dead by a proper authority. Remember that the outcome of cardiac arrest is more often than not a tragedy for family and friends of the patient. Often emotional support to your patient's loved ones will be as valuable as any technical skill.

ASK YOURSELF
- What are some situations in which it may not be advisable to begin, or to continue, CPR?

rigor mortis   stiffening of the body after death.

dependent lividity   the pooling of blood in the lower areas of the body after death.

CASE STUDY

TRANSITION

You attach the AED and turn it on. It commands, "shock advised." You clear yourself and your team and press the shock button. The patient convulses and CPR is resumed. There is no obvious change in your patient.

Moments later the paramedics arrive. You give them a full report as CPR is continued. They attach their defibrillator and shock the patient again. They start an IV and administer cardiac medications.

- Discussion: *Do you assume that the second shock resulted in the patient having a pulse? Why?*

THE LAST WORD

As an EMR, you play a crucial role in the chain of survival. Early activation of the EMS system, early CPR, early defibrillation, and early access to advanced care are all links reliant upon your action. Remember also the core concepts of resuscitation: push hard and fast, and limit interruptions. Use your AED quickly and appropriately, and do not forget the emotional component to a cardiac arrest call.

Chapter Review

Multiple Choice

Place a check next to the correct answer.

1. Another term for no breathing at all is:
   - _____ a. apnea.
   - _____ b. dyspnea.
   - _____ c. asystole.
   - _____ d. aphasia.

2. The correct depth of compressions for adult CPR is:
   - _____ a. 1.5–2 inches.
   - _____ b. 0.5–1 inch.
   - _____ c. 3/4 the front-to-back depth of the chest.
   - _____ d. 1/8 the front-to-back depth of the chest.

3. To prevent compressor fatigue a switch should occur every ____.
   - _____ a. 2 cycles or 5 minutes
   - _____ b. 3 cycles or 7 minutes
   - _____ c. 4 cycles or 1 minute
   - _____ d. 5 cycles or 2 minutes

4. The appropriate rate of compressions for one-rescuer CPR is ____ per minute.
   - _____ a. 40
   - _____ b. 60
   - _____ c. 80
   - _____ d. 100

5. According to the American Heart Association, AEDs should not be used on patients younger than .
   - _____ a. 1 year
   - _____ b. 5 years
   - _____ c. 8 years
   - _____ d. AEDS may be used on patients of any age.

Short Answer

1. List at least three problems associated with attaching AED pads.
   - a. _____
   - b. _____
   - c. _____

2. With regard to the previous question, describe the steps you would take to resolve those problems.
   - a. _____
   - b. _____
   - c. _____

3. List the two shockable arrhythmias.
   - a. _____
   - b. _____

4. List three reasons to stop CPR once it has been initiated.
   - a. _____
   - b. _____
   - c. _____

Critical Thinking

1. You have two rescuers at the scene of an apparently lifeless patient. You have all of your equipment including an AED. How should you proceed?

   _____

   _____

   _____

   _____

2. Your patient has a DNR order, but the family on scene wants you to "do everything you can." What actions would you take?

   _____

   _____

   _____

   _____

Case Study

You are the Emergency Medical Responder called to assist a "woman down" in the mall. You arrive to find a 72-year-old patient unconscious, unresponsive, and cyanotic. Bystanders state they "just found her, but do not know how long she has been here."

1. Assuming the scene is safe, what would be your immediate actions?

   _____

   _____

   _____

2. If this patient has no pulse, would you immediately apply an AED or begin CPR first? Why?

   _____

   _____

   _____

3. What assessment findings might prevent you from starting resuscitative efforts?

   _____

   _____

   _____

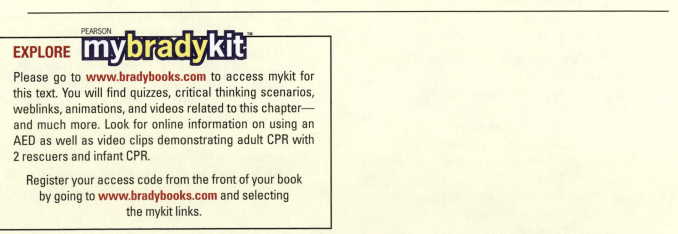

EXPLORE PEARSON **mybradykit**™

Please go to **www.bradybooks.com** to access mykit for this text. You will find quizzes, critical thinking scenarios, weblinks, animations, and videos related to this chapter—and much more. Look for online information on using an AED as well as video clips demonstrating adult CPR with 2 rescuers and infant CPR.

Register your access code from the front of your book by going to **www.bradybooks.com** and selecting the mykit links.

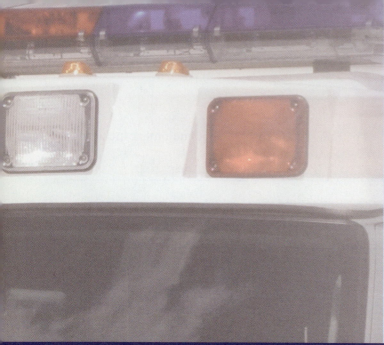

SECTION 2
Review and Practice Examination

Assess what you have learned in this section by checking the best answer for each multiple-choice question. When you are done, check your answers against the key provided in Appendix B.

1. When the intercostal muscles of the chest contract and the diaphragm drops, which of the following occurs?
   _____ a. Inhalation
   _____ b. Air is forced out of the lungs
   _____ c. Decreased size of the chest cavity
   _____ d. Increased pressure of the chest cavity

2. The vocal cords are contained within the:
   _____ a. pharynx.
   _____ b. trachea.
   _____ c. bronchi.
   _____ d. larynx.

3. Oxygen is moved from the lungs to the bloodstream when air reaches the:
   _____ a. bronchi.
   _____ b. bronchioles.
   _____ c. alveoli.
   _____ d. pharynx.

4. Which of the following is an expected body response to hypoxia?
   _____ a. Increased respiratory rate, decreased heart rate
   _____ b. Decreased respiratory rate, decreased heart rate
   _____ c. Decreased respiratory rate, increased heart rate
   _____ d. Increased respiratory rate, increased heart rate

5. Upon arriving at the scene of a medical emergency, you see a patient who is unresponsive and snoring. Which of the following should you do first?
   _____ a. Check the carotid pulse.
   _____ b. Begin bag-valve-mask ventilations.
   _____ c. Use a head-tilt, chin-lift to open the airway.
   _____ d. Apply oxygen using a nonrebreather mask.

6. You have arrived at the home of a 72-year-old patient whose wife called 911 because she couldn't wake him up. The patient is slumped to the side in his recliner and does not respond to your voice or a pinch to his shoulder. Which of the following should you do next?
   _____ a. Apply oxygen by nonrebreather mask.
   _____ b. Tilt the recliner all the way back and open the patient's airway.
   _____ c. Move the patient to the floor and look for breathing and signs of life.
   _____ d. Advise incoming EMS units that the patient is in cardiac arrest.

7. A 14-year-old male patient with a history of asthma is wheezing, but he is agitated with you. He does not want you to place an oxygen mask on his face. Which of the following should you assume?

_____ a. The patient may be hypoxic and needs your help, even though he appears to be refusing oxygen.

_____ b. The patient does not need oxygen by mask and you should respect his wishes.

_____ c. Whoever called 911 was mistaken about the cause of the emergency.

_____ d. You could be sued if you try to get the patient to accept oxygen when he does not want it.

8. A patient who was struck several times in the face during a barroom fight is lying on his back and you can hear gurgling noises when he breathes. Which should you do first?

_____ a. Perform the head-tilt, chin-lift maneuver.

_____ b. Begin ventilations with a bag-valve-mask device.

_____ c. Stabilize the spine and suction the airway.

_____ d. Insert an oral airway.

9. Your patient is a 17-year-old female who has consumed an excessive amount of alcohol at a party. She is unresponsive and vomiting. Which of the following is the best course of action?

_____ a. Turn the patient on her side and suction until the airway is clear.

_____ b. Preoxygenate the patient using a bag-valve-mask device and then suction until the airway is clear.

_____ c. Preoxygenate the patient using a bag-valve-mask device and then suction for 15 seconds.

_____ d. Place the patient supine and suction for 15 seconds before applying oxygen with a nonrebreather mask.

10. A patient with a history of depression was found lying in bed and his wife was unable to wake him. When you enter the room you hear loud snoring. Which of the following are the most likely explanation and course of action?

_____ a. The patient is choking on a foreign body; you should perform abdominal thrusts (the Heimlich maneuver).

_____ b. The patient has adequate breathing since you can hear him snore with every breath; you should apply oxygen.

_____ c. The patient's tongue is obstructing his airway; you should perform a head-tilt, chin-lift maneuver.

_____ d. The patient has vomited; begin suctioning immediately.

11. Your patient is a 30-year-old man who fell from his second-story roof as he was cleaning out his gutters. On your arrival, the patient was unresponsive and had inadequate breathing. You have attempted to perform a jaw-thrust maneuver, but are unable to ventilate the patient. What should you do next?

_____ a. Suction the mouth to remove secretions.

_____ b. Place the patient on his side and await the incoming EMS crew for further instructions.

_____ c. Apply an oxygen mask with a flow rate of at least 10 liters per minute.

_____ d. Perform a head-tilt, chin-lift.

12. As you are ventilating a patient, she vomits a large amount of undigested food. Which of the following is the best course of action?

_____ a. Turn the patient on her side, manually remove as much material as you can from the airway, and then suction the rest with a rigid suction catheter before resuming ventilations.

_____ b. Use a flexible suction catheter to remove the material as you continue to ventilate.

_____ c. Suction using a rigid suction catheter for no more than 15 seconds before resuming ventilations. Reoxygenate the patient before suctioning again.

_____ d. Suction using a rigid suction catheter for as long as it takes to remove the material, applying suction both while inserting and withdrawing the catheter.

13. Which of the following best describes the depth of insertion of a rigid suction catheter to remove fluids from the airway?

_____ a. It is used only between the cheek and gums.

_____ b. It is inserted until you feel resistance.

_____ c. It is inserted only as far as you can see.

_____ d. It is inserted to the level of the epiglottis.

14. Which of the following statements regarding oropharyngeal airways is true?
_____ a. Once inserted, it is no longer necessary to use a head-tilt, chin-lift or jaw-thrust maneuver to maintain the airway.
_____ b. It is used to help keep the tongue away from the back of the airway.
_____ c. It is a convenient piece of equipment because one size fits all.
_____ d. It can be inserted in any patient with a diminished level of responsiveness.

15. You have begun to insert an oropharyngeal airway into a patient when you hear retching sounds. Which of the following is the best course of action?
_____ a. Remove the device and maintain the airway without it.
_____ b. Pause until the patient stops gagging, then continue advancing the device.
_____ c. Rotate the device 90 degrees to reduce stimulation of the gag reflex.
_____ d. Use a device that is one size smaller than the one that stimulated the gag reflex.

16. Your patient is a 50-year-old female with a long history of emphysema related to smoking. She began having difficulty breathing about 3 hours ago, but has worsened over the past hour. On your arrival, the patient responds only to a painful stimulus, and is taking a gasping breath about every 10 seconds. Which of the following is most likely?
_____ a. The patient is exhausted and in a deep sleep.
_____ b. If the patient were hypoxic, her respiratory rate would be increased.
_____ c. Severe hypoxia and impending death have resulted in a slowing of the respiratory rate.
_____ d. The patient's claim of difficulty breathing was obviously exaggerated.

17. A pulse oximeter is used to measure the amount of _____ in a patient's blood.
_____ a. carbon dioxide
_____ b. carbon monoxide
_____ c. oxygen
_____ d. oxygen and carbon monoxide

18. Which of the following statements is most accurate concerning pulse oximetry?
_____ a. A reading of above 90 percent is adequate for most patients.
_____ b. Patients with a reading higher than 96 percent do not need supplemental oxygen.
_____ c. Patients with carbon monoxide poisoning may have a normal pulse oximetry reading.
_____ d. Pulse oximetry is a better indicator of respiratory status than either respiratory rate or respiratory depth.

19. An oxygen cylinder will always be, or be marked with, the color:
_____ a. yellow.
_____ b. green.
_____ c. blue.
_____ d. orange.

20. Which of these devices is used to control the amount of oxygen delivered to a patient?
_____ a. Regulator
_____ b. O ring
_____ c. Compressor
_____ d. Supply tubing

21. Which device is used to oxygenate patients with inadequate breathing?
_____ a. Bag-valve mask
_____ b. Venturi mask
_____ c. Nonrebreather mask
_____ d. Nasal cannula

22. The oxygen flow rate needed to adequately deliver oxygen using a nonrebreather mask is _____ liters per minute.
_____ a. 2–6
_____ b. 4–6
_____ c. 6–10
_____ d. 10–15

23. When using a nasal cannula, the oxygen flow rate should not be greater than _____ liters per minute.
_____ a. 2
_____ b. 4
_____ c. 6
_____ d. 8

24. When providing ventilations by pocket face mask or bag-valve-mask device, the rate of ventilation for adult patients should be one breath every _____ seconds.
_____ a. 2–3
_____ b. 5–6

_____ c. 8–10
_____ d. 10–12

25. Which of the following is most accurate regarding devices used to ventilate patients who are not adequately breathing?

_____ a. Pocket face masks are more convenient, but cannot provide supplemental oxygen.

_____ b. Pocket face masks are safer than bag-valve-mask devices because they prevent forceful ventilation that distends the stomach.

_____ c. A Venturi mask is preferred because it fatigues the rescuer less than either a pocket face mask or bag-valve mask.

_____ d. An adequate seal between the mask and the patient's face is required with both a pocket face mask and a bag-valve-mask device.

26. Without perfusion, brain cells begin to die in _____ minutes.

_____ a. 1–2
_____ b. 3–5
_____ c. 4–6
_____ d. 8–10

27. The most common cause of cardiac arrest in infants and children is:

_____ a. respiratory problems.
_____ b. congenital heart defects.
_____ c. trauma.
_____ d. heart disease.

28. Cardiac arrest is confirmed when the patient is determined to be:

a. _____ unresponsive.
b. _____ not breathing.
c. _____ cyanotic.
d. _____ pulseless.

29. You have arrived on the scene of a 4-year-old child who was reported to be choking. The patient is cyanotic, unresponsive, and not breathing. You should:

_____ a. check the brachial pulse for 5 to 10 seconds.

_____ b. check the carotid pulse for 5 to 10 seconds.

_____ c. listen for heart sounds by placing your stethoscope on the chest.

_____ d. begin chest compressions.

30. Which of the following would demonstrate the first link in the chain of survival from cardiac arrest?

_____ a. A police officer arrives on the scene with an AED.

_____ b. Paramedics arrive within 10 minutes of the cardiac arrest.

_____ c. Bystanders recognize cardiac arrest and call 911.

_____ d. A trained layperson begins CPR.

31. During your morning run you pass a yard where an elderly man has just collapsed. His wife is frantic and has not yet called for help. The patient is unresponsive, not breathing, and pulseless. Which of the following should you do to give the patient the best chance of survival?

_____ a. Check the pulse for 1 minute to verify cardiac arrest.

_____ b. Call 911, then begin CPR.

_____ c. Begin rescue breathing, then call 911.

_____ d. Perform 2 minutes of CPR, then call 911.

32. Which of the following best explains the purpose of CPR?

_____ a. It may provide enough circulation to support life until the heart can resume normal pumping.

_____ b. It will cause a heart that has stopped beating to start pumping again.

_____ c. It is used to relieve foreign body airway obstruction.

_____ d. It is used in adults to ventilate the lungs until breathing resumes.

33. When performing CPR in an adult patient, you should provide chest compressions at a rate of about _____ compressions per minute.

_____ a. 30
_____ b. 60
_____ c. 100
_____ d. 150

34. Which of the following is an important principle in performing CPR on adults?

_____ a. Remove your hands from the chest after each compression to ensure full recoil of the chest wall.

_____ b. Perform each ventilation hard and fast.

_____ c. When working alone, use a cycle of 30 compressions to 2 ventilations.

_____ d. Straddle the patient's hips, facing the patient's chest, and place one hand over the other at the lower end of the patient's sternum.

35. Your patient is a 75-year-old female who collapsed at home. While performing chest compressions, you feel a "popping" sensation when you press down on the sternum. What should you do?

_____ a. Continue chest compressions and ventilations normally.

_____ b. Discontinue chest compressions, but ventilate the patient every 6 to 8 seconds.

_____ c. Stop CPR and inform the incoming EMS crew.

_____ d. Perform chest compressions at a depth of 1/2 to 3/4 inches and ventilate normally.

36. You have arrived at a residence for a report of a sick child. The patient is a 7-month-old female who has had a respiratory infection for several days. She is limp and does not respond to you. Her color is grayish, and she is not effectively moving air through her mouth or nose after you open her airway. The patient has a brachial pulse of 40. What should you do?

_____ a. Begin ventilations and chest compressions.

_____ b. Perform ventilations and keep the patient warm.

_____ c. Notify the incoming EMS unit of your assessment findings, then begin CPR.

_____ d. Apply oxygen and continue to monitor the pulse.

37. Your patient is a 12-month-old male who has had progressive difficulty breathing over the past several hours. He is now lethargic with poor skin color and labored, grunting respirations at a rate of 60 per minute. His brachial pulse is 140 per minute. Which of the following will be most beneficial in the management of this patient?

_____ a. Perform a head-tilt, chin-lift and begin ventilations.

_____ b. Perform a jaw-thrust maneuver and begin ventilations.

_____ c. Begin CPR.

_____ d. Place a small folded towel under the shoulders and begin ventilations.

38. When performing chest compressions on a 2-month-old infant, the correct technique is to:

_____ a. place the heel of one hand on the sternum and place your other hand on top of the first; push hard and push fast with a depth of 1 1/2 to 2 inches.

_____ b. use the heel of one hand to press over the lower half of the sternum; use a rate of 120 compressions per minute.

_____ c. place the tips of two fingers over the sternum on an imaginary line between the nipples; compress the chest about one-third of its depth at a rate of 100 per minute.

_____ d. encircle the chest with your hands, placing the thumbs over the sternum between the nipples and compress hard and fast without allowing the chest to completely recoil between compressions.

39. The correct ratio of chest compressions to ventilations in one-rescuer child CPR is:

_____ a. 5:1.

_____ b. 15:1.

_____ c. 15:2.

_____ d. 30:2.

40. Which of the following arrhythmias may be successfully shocked by an AED?

_____ a. Asystole

_____ b. Pulseless electrical activity

_____ c. Ventricular tachycardia

_____ d. Atrial fibrillation

41. Which of the following is a function of an AED?

_____ a. Determining whether a patient is in cardiac arrest

_____ b. Determining whether a patient in cardiac arrest has a shockable rhythm

_____ c. Delivering a shock to all patients in cardiac arrest

_____ d. Displaying a tracing of the cardiac rhythm for interpretation by the EMR

42. You have arrived at a remote area of a large automobile manufacturing plant, where a 50-year-old male collapsed 10 minutes ago. Which of the following should you do first?

_____ a. Apply the AED and determine whether the patient is in a shockable rhythm.

_____ b. Begin CPR, and then apply the AED.

_____ c. Open the airway, assess breathing, and check for a pulse.

_____ d. Determine whether the patient has a history of heart disease.

43. Which of the following is the typical placement of defibrillation pads in the adult patient?

_____ a. One under the left nipple and the other over the left shoulder blade

_____ b. One to the left of the left nipple, just below the armpit, and the other to the right of the right nipple, just below the armpit

_____ c. One directly over the sternum, and the other on the center of the patient's back, exactly opposite the first pad

_____ d. One just below the right clavicle and the other to the left of the nipple, below the armpit

44. As you are applying AED pads, you note an object about half the size of a deck of cards under the skin of the chest on the left side. The patient's son says it is a pacemaker that was implanted a few years ago. How should you proceed?

_____ a. Use the AED, but avoid placing a pad directly over the device.

_____ b. Ensure pad placement is exact, even if one is placed over the device.

_____ c. Call for medical direction before proceeding with CPR or AED placement.

_____ d. Begin CPR but do not use the AED in this patient.

45. You have applied an AED to a pulseless patient and pressed the "analyze" button. The machine announces, "no shock advised." This means:

_____ a. the patient is not in cardiac arrest.

_____ b. the AED has malfunctioned and you must proceed with CPR.

_____ c. the patient is in cardiac arrest but the rhythm causing it will not respond to a shock.

_____ d. the machine has detected that it would be dangerous to deliver a shock. You should check to make sure no one is in contact with the patient and analyze again.

46. Which of the following is true concerning the use of AEDs in children?

_____ a. Cardiac arrest in children is rarely due to a shockable rhythm, but an AED can be used on a patient of any age.

_____ b. Adult pads must never be used on children under 8 years old.

_____ c. Pediatric pads must be used on infants less than 1 year old.

_____ d. Only one defibrillation pad should be used on children to reduce the amount of electricity delivered to the heart.

47. You have delivered a shock to a patient in cardiac arrest. After performing 2 minutes of CPR, a pulse check reveals that the patient has a weak carotid pulse of 58 per minute. You should:

_____ a. resume CPR.

_____ b. push the "analyze" button.

_____ c. assess ventilations.

_____ d. place the patient in the recovery position until EMS arrives.

48. You have responded to a report of a possible suicide. Your patient is a 70-year-old man who has a self-inflicted shotgun wound to the face and head, with a large portion of the skull and brain missing. The patient is not breathing and does not have a pulse. You should:

_____ a. begin CPR.

_____ b. notify the incoming EMS unit.

_____ c. attach the AED.

_____ d. determine if the patient has a DNR order.

49. You have applied the AED and pushed "analyze." After 10 seconds, the AED has neither shocked nor indicated that no shock is advised. You should:

_____ a. turn the machine off, then turn it back on to reset it.

_____ b. turn the machine off, remove the pads, and begin CPR.

_____ c. continue to wait for the machine to analyze.

_____ d. remove the pads, shave hair from the chest if necessary, and apply fresh pads.

50. Which of the following statements is true regarding the safety of the EMR during defibrillation?

_____ a. The EMR may be shocked if he is in contact with the patient when a shock is delivered.

_____ b. A provider using a bag-valve mask does not have to clear the patient; the rubber in the BVM will insulate him from being shocked.

_____ c. The EMR is not in danger of being shocked as long as he is not in contact with any metal on the patient's body or clothing.

_____ d. Only the patient can be shocked as long as the AED is working properly.

SECTION 3
Patient Assessment

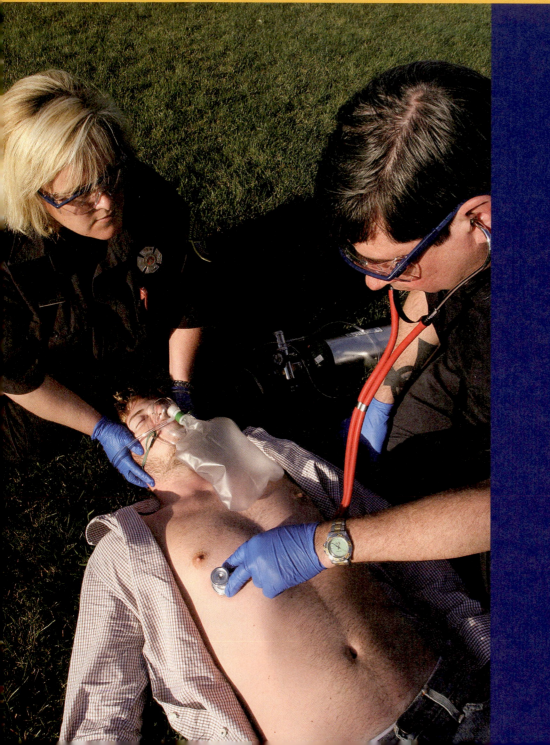

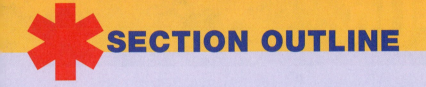

SECTION OUTLINE

In this section, you will cover the following EMS Education Standard:
- Assessment

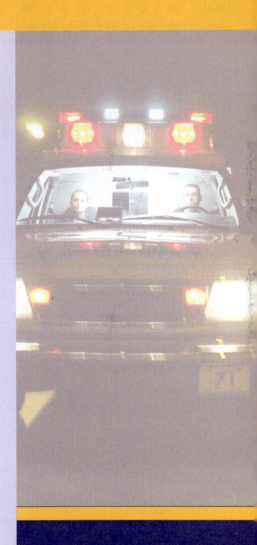

Patient Assessment: Scene Size-Up

✳ NAVIGATION GUIDE

The following items provide an overview to the purpose and content of this chapter. The Education Standard and Competency are from the National EMS Education Standards.

Education Standard Assessment (Scene Size-Up)

Competency Uses scene information and simple patient assessment findings to identify and manage immediate life threats and injuries within the scope of practice of the EMR.

Knowledge Area Scene Size-Up
- Scene safety
- Scene management
  - Impact of the environment on patient care
  - Addressing hazards
  - Violence
  - Need for additional or specialized resources
  - Standard Precautions

Objectives After reading this chapter, you should be able to:

1. Define the key terms introduced in this chapter.
2. Describe the unique responsibilities of the EMR who arrives first on the scene.
3. Describe each of the following five components of the scene size-up:
   a. Scene safety
   b. Standard Precaution determination
   c. Resource determination
   d. Number of patients
   e. Mechanism of injury/nature of illness
4. Explain why scene size-up must continue throughout the call.
5. Anticipate the hazards associated with specific types of calls.

6. Recognize indications of violence.
7. Given a scenario involving scene violence, use cover, concealment, and retreat as ways to maintain your safety.
8. Recognize indications of hazardous materials and environmental hazards on the scene of an emergency.
9. Survey the scene to determine the patient's mechanism of injury or nature of illness.
10. Survey the scene to determine the number of patients present and additional resources needed.
11. Determine what Standard Precautions are needed to protect yourself when caring for specific patients.

NAVIGATION GUIDE *(continued)*

Key Terms Page references indicate first major use in this chapter. The Margin Glossary in this chapter provides definitions as you read.

scene size-up, p. 221
index of suspicion, p. 230
head-on collision, p. 231
velocity, p. 231

rear-end collision, p. 232
side impact collision, p. 232
rollover collision, p. 232
ejection, p. 232

rotational collision, p. 232
motorcycle collision, p. 233
Standard Precautions, p. 238

Media Resources Please go to **www.bradybooks.com** to access mykit for this text. You will find quizzes, critical thinking scenarios, weblinks, animations, and videos related to this chapter—and much more. Look for online information from the NHTSA on scene safety as it relates to vehicles and hazards.

INTRODUCTION

The EMR is usually the first to arrive on the scene. This fact brings special responsibilities—and can also place the EMR in the path of danger.

This chapter deals with important issues such as violence and dangers at the scene as well as how to prevent injury to yourself and your patients. You will also learn to protect yourself from diseases and to make observations of the scene that will help you make decisions that affect the care of your patient (See The Big Picture: Scene Size-Up).

The **scene size-up** is the first part of the patient assessment process and is generally considered to have five major components:

1. Scene safety
2. Standard Precaution determination
3. Resource determination
4. Number of patients
5. Mechanism of injury/nature of illness

Although the size-up is performed as the first part of your assessment, it is reconsidered frequently throughout the call. A scene may suddenly become unsafe after you have been there for a period of time or a patient may become unresponsive and suddenly require suction—and you must take additional precautions from spraying fluids.

Some call the scene size-up concepts "scene management" when placed together. The scene size-up provides a foundation for the success of the remainder of the call.

scene size-up the responder's impression of the overall scene

ASK YOURSELF

- Can you define the key terms found in this chapter? What are the unique responsibilities of the EMR who arrives first on the scene?

- What are the five components of the scene size-up and can you describe them in detail?

- Why must scene size-up continue throughout the call?

CASE STUDY

THE CALL ✳

You receive a call for a man who has fallen ill in the paint shop where you work. You are an Emergency Medical Responder for your local fire department and your employer usually comes to you when something happens. Today is no different.

- Discussion: *What do you think your first question will be regarding the scene?*

The Big Picture
Scene Size-Up

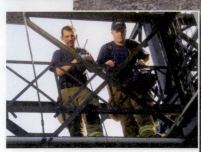

1 Assess for scene safety.

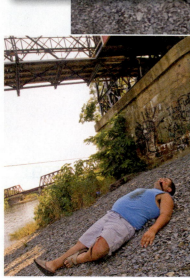

2 Examine the mechanism of injury and determine the number of patients.

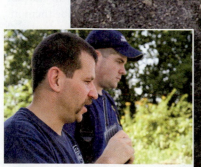

3 Radio for additional resources if needed.

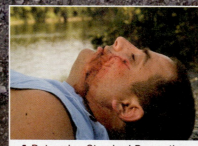

4 Determine Standard Precautions.

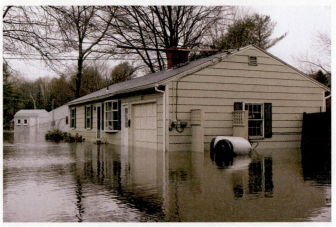

Figure 9-1b There may be hazardous materials; look for signs of danger.

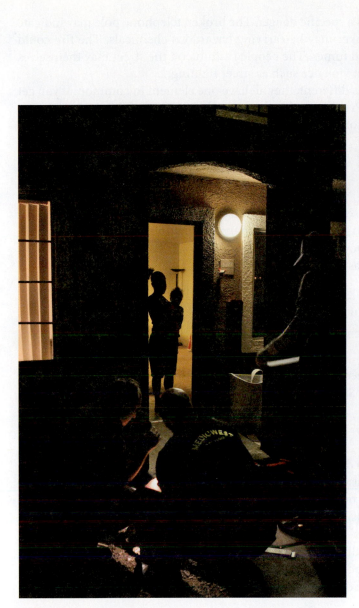

Figure 9-1a Be cautious when approaching the scene.

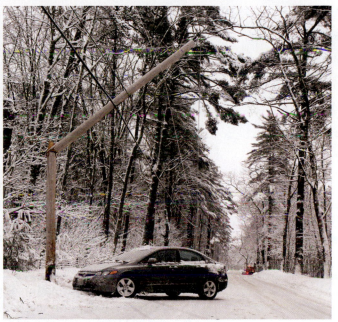

Figure 9-1c Electrical wires may soon come down.

Scene Safety

As the first person from the EMS system to arrive on scene, you must carefully scrutinize the scene for dangers. Dangers can come from a variety of sources such as people, chemicals, unstable vehicles or surfaces, and fire (Figures 9-1a to 9-1c ■).

Most calls go by uneventfully and safely. Unfortunately, it is likely that at some time in your EMS experience you may encounter danger. Most scenes give signs of danger beforehand. The alert EMR spots these clues before coming in contact with the danger.

Your size-up will begin with the dispatch information and continue from a distance as you approach the scene. Consider the following situations you may see as you approach:

■ You see a telephone pole apparently snapped and is hanging on the wires.

■ You see some sort of tanker truck rolled over in a ditch.

■ You see a fire inside a large warehouse.

■ You turn the corner onto the street where your call is and you observe dozens of people running from the scene.

ASK YOURSELF

■ How do you anticipate the hazards associated with specific types of calls?

Each of these scenes indicates a specific danger. The broken telephone pole may indicate downed power lines. The tanker may be carrying hazardous chemicals. The fire could produce dangerous smoke and fumes. The people running on the street may themselves be fleeing from danger—often violence such as street fighting.

While each of the scenes is different, they all have one element in common: If you get too close, you are in danger. Preventing this danger is the purpose of the size-up.

This section will discuss some of the common signs of danger and ways you can protect yourself on scene.

Identifying Violence

ASK YOURSELF

■ What are the indications of violence on a scene?

It may seem to be common sense to protect yourself from violence. Yet the nature of emergency calls is for things to happen fast and unexpectedly. Your observations and tactics heading into the emergency scene and while you are on scene are vital.

Begin your observations as you approach. Look for:

■ Any signs of fighting or violence (loud voices, weapons, broken glass, and so on)

■ Signs that alcohol or drugs are present or in use

■ Unusual silence (emergencies are often active scenes, "too quiet" may actually be a sign of danger)

While you may feel the need to rush to the scene, it is prudent—both for safety as well as patient care—not to hurry. Stay focused and observant as you approach.

Response to Violence

It is not your job as an EMR to disarm violent people or place yourself in harm's way. Your first and best option is to spot violence early and avoid it. You are not required to enter any violent scene until it has been secured by the police. (As a police officer/EMR you may jointly have these responsibilities.)

If you observe signs of violence before reaching the scene or patient, retreat to a position of safety and notify the dispatcher that the police will be required at the scene. Provide as much information as possible to assist the police in quickly and safely controlling the scene. Enter only after the dispatcher has told you that the scene is safe and has been secured by the police.

There may be times when the dispatcher has determined the scene isn't safe for you to respond to. You may be dispatched but staged at a safe location close to the scene until the police have made the scene secure. If you are told to stage but aren't given a specific location, be sure you stage several blocks from the scene or in a position that is not within direct sight of the scene—and in a position that those fleeing from the scene won't pass by and involve you in the danger.

ASK YOURSELF

■ Given a scenario involving scene violence, how do you use cover, concealment, and retreat as ways to maintain your safety?

Other times you will be assessing or treating a patient and you will suddenly be faced with violence. Safety is a concern throughout the call—not just during the initial size-up. You should always be aware of your surroundings in the event tempers flare, a violent person enters or emerges, a weapon is produced, or the patient becomes hostile. As discussed and demonstrated in Chapter 2, the following tactics can be used to help you retreat from the danger safely:

■ *Distraction* is the tactic of using EMS equipment or other items at the scene (such as chairs) to create distance between you and an aggressor. This is done in conjunction with retreat. For example, suppose you are treating a patient in a living room or bedroom, and he becomes aggressive. You turn to exit the room. As the patient moves in your direction, you throw your EMS kit in his direction to slow his approach. Alternatively, tip over a small object as you leave the room. This blocks the door temporarily to give you extra time to retreat.

- *Cover* is the principle of taking a position behind an object that hides your body and provides protection. The ideal protection is one that will stop bullets. (Fortunately, it is rare that people shoot at EMS providers.) This may be a large tree, a dumpster, or the engine block of a vehicle.

- *Concealment* hides your body but doesn't offer protection. Examples of concealment may include bushes or shrubs, the interior walls of houses or businesses, and car doors. Concealment should be used when cover can't be found and it benefits you to be out of sight of an aggressor.

- *Retreat* is the preferred response when you observe or encounter danger. It is best when used strategically with cover, concealment, and distraction. Move swiftly and decisively away from the danger, integrating cover when possible as you move. Do not stop moving away from the danger until you are safe. This may mean moving back to your vehicle and driving from the scene or moving a considerable distance away and maintaining a safe position of cover.

Remember to use a radio or cell phone to update incoming units so they do not fall victim to the same violence you avoided (Figures 9-2a to 9-2e ■).

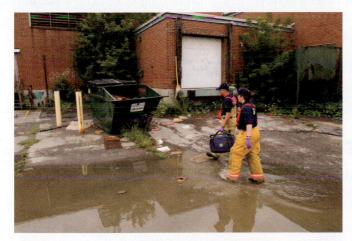

■ **Figure 9-2a** You must observe the scene and approach carefully.

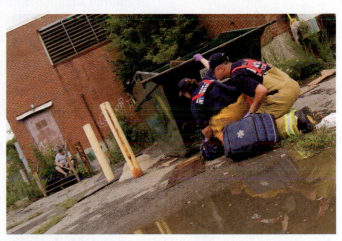

■ **Figure 9-2b** Demonstrate proper cover behind a solid object.

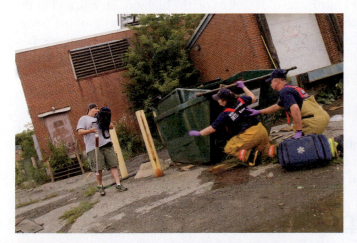

■ **Figure 9-2c** Use available equipment as a distraction.

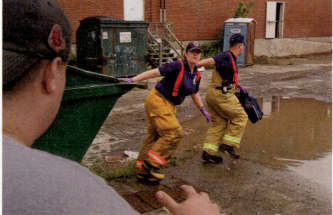

■ **Figure 9-2d** Always continue to observe your surroundings while you retreat from a scene.

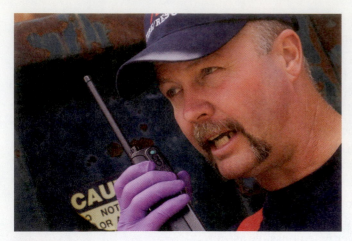

Figure 9-2e Use your radio or cell phone to call for help. Make sure you remain in a safe position with cover.

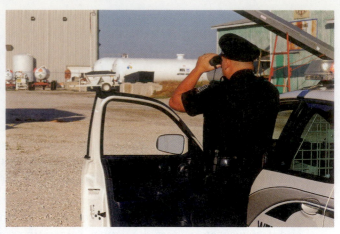

Figure 9-3 Evaluate a hazmat incident from a safe distance.

As an EMR, you will be looked upon to help protect the safety of the patient, family, and bystanders as well as yourself—although not while putting your life in danger. There are times when you will shout instructions to those at a scene to immediately leave a dangerous area.

In another situation, a family member might begin threatening an EMS crew because he feels responders are taking too long on the scene. In this case, you may be able to move the patient closer to transportation by working with the ambulance crew to safely resolve the situation.

Scenes are dynamic and can occasionally be dangerous. In the event of a real or perceived threat, your responses using the concepts learned in this section are vital to you and your patient.

Physical Hazards at the Scene

Violence is not the only hazard at an emergency scene. Anything from extremes in temperature to the terrain to hazardous materials may pose a danger to you. This section will discuss some of these hazards.

Hazardous Materials

ASK YOURSELF

■ What are indications of hazardous materials and environmental hazards on the scene of an emergency?

Hazardous materials are present in structures as well as on the highway, on rail, and in the air. It is likely you will encounter these substances on a call at some point. You may be required to have additional training through your agency in reference to hazardous materials.

The key to hazardous material response is to maintain a safe distance from the start. Your dispatch information may have given you an idea that hazardous materials are involved by the location of the call (such as a rail yard or highway) or the types of vehicles involved (such as a tank truck).

Emergency vehicles generally carry binoculars to allow responders to observe the scene from a safe distance (Figure 9-3 ■). If you suspect hazardous materials are involved, ask your dispatcher to contact a specialized hazardous material response team. Maintain a safe position, generally uphill and upwind from the incident. The Department of Transportation *Emergency Response Guidebook* can be used to determine safe distances both for emergency personnel and for the evacuation of businesses or residences.

Emergency Medical Responders today must also be prepared for a response to terrorist incidents. These incidents may result from domestic or international terrorists and involve a number of methods including chemical, biological, nuclear, explosive, and others.

As an EMR, you have the potential to get there very early in the call. Although these incidents are usually dramatic and large scale, the principles of scene size-up still apply. Specifically in terrorist incidents:

- There is a potential for a large number of patients to be injured or killed.
- The scene may extend for large areas.
- You will need to think and evaluate carefully before entering the scene to avoid the substance or scene that has injured others.
- You will be functioning within a large-scale operation and must follow the incident management system.
- You will have to use extreme caution while responding and on the scene due to the risk of *secondary devices,* such as delayed detonation of a second explosive device designed to injure rescuers such as yourself.

Additional information on handling hazardous material emergencies can be found in Chapter 30. Substances that may be used in terrorist incidents will be discussed further in Chapter 31.

Environmental Hazards

Emergency scenes can be found anywhere from city street corners to farm silos. It is up to the EMR to evaluate each scene for hazards.

Motor vehicle collisions can pose a danger from spilled gasoline and jagged metal. Perhaps one of the most deadly hazards is the traffic that is passing the scene. Although required to wear protective clothing when working in or near the roadway, several EMRs are killed each year while providing care in that setting.

Motorists driving by emergency scenes often pay more attention to "rubbernecking" the crash than driving carefully and attentively. Intoxicated drivers, those with poor vision, and those who drive too fast approaching the scene pose a significant hazard.

Do not work in the highway without protection from traffic hazards. This protection may include a properly positioned police cruiser with warning lights activated or ideally a large piece of apparatus or equipment (fire engine or highway department dump truck) physically blocking the scene from oncoming traffic. On the interstate highway system, specialized vehicles that block the scene and provide directional arrows and traffic control may be available.

Regardless of the protection in place at the scene, remember to be observant and monitor traffic at all times.

Extremes in weather also pose a potential danger for you and your patient (Figure 9-4 ■). Look at the scene and the time it will take until the patient will be placed in the climate-controlled ambulance. Will cold or heat at the scene negatively affect the patient or responders? If so you may need to take action to protect those on scene from the environment.

If you are working at night you may need to call for assistance to provide lighting at the scene. You may consider calling the fire department or highway crews. Calls such as motor vehicle collisions with entrapment, those with multiple patients and off-road calls are examples of when lighting may be necessary. When working at night, remember that it will be more difficult for others to see you which could cause a hazard at scenes such as motor vehicle accidents.

Other environmental hazards such as steep slopes, fire, and unstable vehicles must be addressed before approaching the patient. They pose a substantial risk of injury or death to both patients and responders. Call for the appropriate resources, including the fire department and specialty rescue teams (such as high angle, low angle, trench, and structural collapse teams).

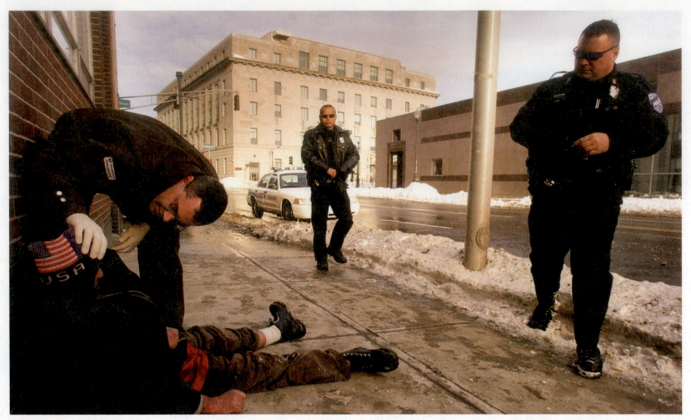

■ Figure 9-4 Extremes in weather can pose a danger to you and your patient. (© Mark C. Ide)

✴ Stop, Review, Remember

Multiple Choice

Place a check next to the correct answer.

1. Which of the following situations poses the least danger to the properly prepared responder?

   _____ a. Snapped utility pole with hanging power lines

   _____ b. Tanker truck rolled over and leaking

   _____ c. Patient with an infectious disease that is spread only by direct contact

   _____ d. A fire in an industrial warehouse building

2. What is the term used to describe a position that hides the body and provides it protection?

   _____ a. Cover

   _____ b. Concealment

   _____ c. Retreat

   _____ d. Camouflage

3. If there is a suspicion that hazardous materials may be involved in a call, the EMR should:

   _____ a. respond directly to the scene to verify the hazard.

   _____ b. send the newest member of the crew to confirm the hazard.

   _____ c. retreat to a safe distance and use tools such as binoculars to gain more information.

   _____ d. taste the powdery substance next to the patient to decide if it's salt or sugar.

True/False

Mark whether each of the following statements is true (T) or false (F).

1. _____ Hazards at the scene of a call are limited to hazardous materials and other chemicals.

2. _____ When working on a highway, a responder is required to wear highly visible and reflective clothing for protection.

3. _____ Weather can be considered a hazard to a patient.

Critical Thinking

You approach a call for a domestic-related incident. Your dispatcher has requested that you stage out of the area to await police arrival. Nothing appears to be going on as you drive in the area of the scene.

1. Should you disregard the dispatcher and approach the scene to find a patient? Why or why not?

   _____

   _____

   _____

   _____

2. A person comes running at you in your response unit bleeding with what appears to be a weapon. What should you do?

   _____

   _____

   _____

3. Once the scene is safe for you to operate in, you are treating a patient who you find to have a concealed knife. What is your best course of action?

   _____

   _____

   _____

   _____

Mechanism of Injury and Nature of Illness

Your initial observations of the scene can be used for more than determining if hazards are present. These observations can also affect your initial patient care determinations. For example:

- You observe a man at the bottom of a long flight of stairs. He appears to be unresponsive and contorted. He is bleeding from his head.
- You observe a man slumped over in a chair unresponsive. It looks like he has vomited.
- You see a person in a vehicle that has massive damage from a crash.
- A person is sitting on her front step holding her ankle.

ASK YOURSELF

- What is the best way to survey the scene to determine the patient's mechanism of injury or nature of illness?

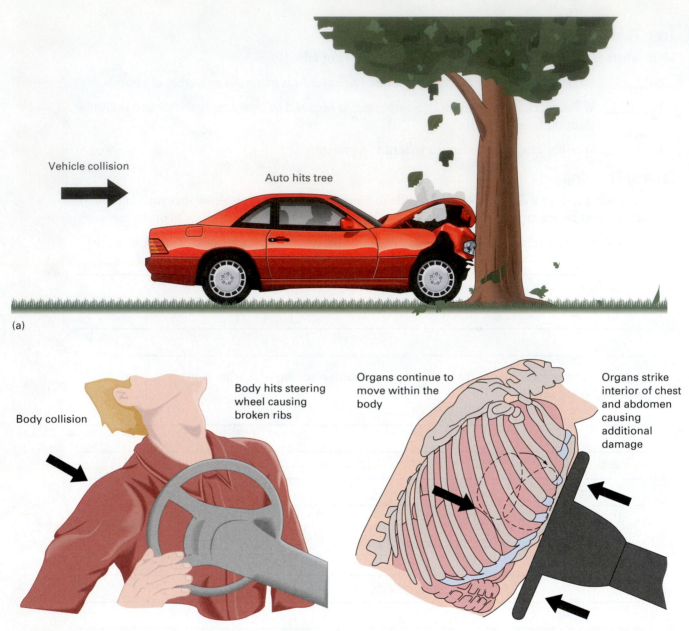

(a)

Vehicle collision → Auto hits tree

Body collision

Body hits steering wheel causing broken ribs

Organs continue to move within the body

Organs strike interior of chest and abdomen causing additional damage

(b) *Then, the occupant impacts the interior of the car.*

(c) *Finally, the occupant's organs impact the internal surfaces of the body.*

■ **Figure 9-5** Three basic impacts involved in any car crash can cause injury to the patient.

Each of these situations gives information on the scene—and the patient. The first patient appears as if he could be seriously injured. The second patient appears very ill. Both of these patients will require you to take certain Standard Precautions.

The third patient may require a special team to extricate him from the vehicle—but that same observation also indicates you should suspect he is seriously injured. The last patient may not be as seriously injured based on what you see.

Mechanism of injury is the physical forces that caused the patient's injuries. You will examine these to develop an idea of the potential for injury. It is a potential for injury because it is not a guarantee the patient is injured, but rather a likelihood. This is sometimes referred to as developing an **index of suspicion** for injury (Figure 9-5 ■).

A general rule for mechanism of injury is that the faster the speeds involved in the injury—or the greater the height—the more injury you have the potential to see.

index of suspicion when a responder believes there is a high likelihood a person is injured based upon the mechanism present.

Motor Vehicle Collisions

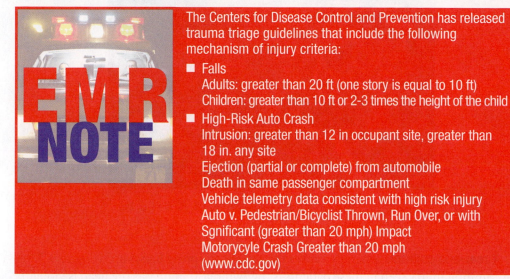

There are several factors that you will use to determine mechanism of injury in a motor vehicle collision. The first is the type of collision. Each has certain predictable injury patterns.

The **head-on** (or front-end) **collision** thrusts occupants forward in the vehicle. The level of injury greatly depends on the speed of the collision and the restraints used by the occupants. The greater the speed (or **velocity**) in a collision, the greater the potential for injury. The restraints used by the occupants will generally reduce the injuries you see. Seat belts and air bags greatly reduce injury in head-on collisions by preventing impact with the steering wheel and dashboard.

In head-on collisions the forces will drive front seat occupants forward in one of two general paths: up and over or down and under. The up-and-over pathway brings the driver's chest into the steering wheel and the head to the windshield (Figure 9-6 ■). The down-and-under pathway brings the body down under the steering wheel, causing injury to the legs and hips from striking the dash below the steering wheel. Injuries sustained through these energy pathways are significantly diminished by the use of vehicle restraints and air bags.

head-on collision vehicle struck from/at the front.

velocity speed of an object.

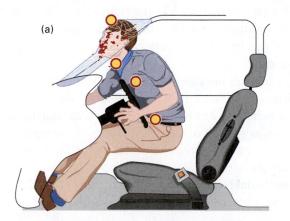
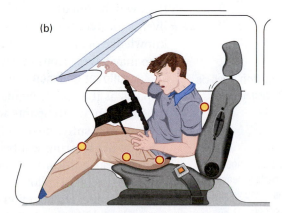

■ **Figure 9-6**   In a head-on crash, the patient can be forced in either (a) an up-and-over pathway of motion or (b) a down-and-under pathway of motion. The yellow dots indicate areas of potential injury due to these mechanisms.

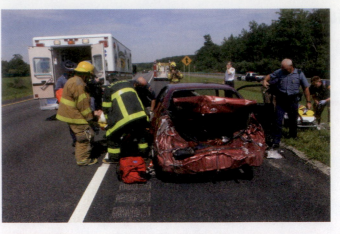

■ **Figure 9-7** Motor vehicle accident—rear impact. *(© Mark C. Ide)*

A **rear-end collision** generally causes the patient to spring backward (Figure 9-7 ■). The common injury seen in these patients is the "whiplash" injury as the head is violently thrown back, injuring the neck. Many vehicles have high headrests that help to reduce—but not totally eliminate—whiplash injuries. After the body is thrown backward it may then fly forward, which can cause injuries similar to those seen in the head-on collision. Since the impact is from the rear, air bags will not deploy to protect the occupant from these injuries.

A **side-impact** (also called t-bone or broadside) **collision** can also cause serious injuries. The lateral impact can cause head and neck injuries. The force of the side impact can also directly impact a patient in the passenger compartment. Imagine sitting in the driver's seat when a car strikes your door and pushes it into you. You could expect chest and abdominal injuries in anyone (driver or passenger) who took impact directly where they were sitting.

As a general rule, patients struck on the "near side" (on the side of the car where they are sitting) are at greater risk for serious injury than those who are struck "far side" (on the opposite side of the car from where they are sitting). Recent crash data have shown a significant reduction in death and injuries when near-side collision vehicle occupants are protected by side-impact air bags with integrated head air bag protection.

Your knowledge of anatomy and physiology from Chapter 5 will help you predict injuries. The driver of the vehicle who is struck by the side impact will be struck in the left side, which contains the spleen. The passenger will be struck in the right side, where the liver is located. Both of these organs cause serious internal bleeding when injured. Your knowledge of anatomy and observations of mechanism of injury can help identify those who may have serious injuries early in the call.

A **rollover collision** can cause multiple injuries because the vehicle sustains multiple impacts as it rolls. Items inside the vehicle also become airborne and strike occupants, causing injury. Occupants who wear seat belts and remain inside the vehicle during a rollover may suffer no or only minor injuries as a result of the crash. However, occupants who are not wearing seat belts face the risk of **ejection** from the vehicle, which is associated with a significant risk of serious injury and death.

Recognize the rollover collision as a potential hazard to you if the vehicle is found on its roof or side. Do not enter or work around a vehicle in these positions until it has been properly stabilized.

In a **rotational collision**, a vehicle is struck, usually in a corner, and spun (Figure 9-8 ■). This frequently results in secondary collisions with other vehicles or inanimate objects such as light poles. As with rollover collisions, multiple injury patterns are likely.

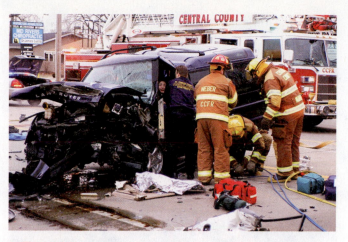

■ **Figure 9-8** Motor vehicle accident—rotational collision (corner impact). *(© Ray Kemp/911 Imaging)*

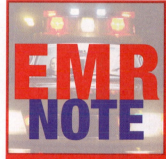

Passenger Restraint Systems

There are vehicles of all types and ages on the road today. Some vehicles have the most up-to-date safety features while others have none. In addition to examining the vehicle for the amount and location of damage, assess for the use of safety devices. These devices can both prevent and cause injury.

Air bags deploy from the steering wheel or the dash and frequently damage the windshield. Don't assume that all windshield damage is from the patient's head or torso when air bags deploy. Air bags and seat belts can in some cases also cause injury themselves, although usually much less than would be caused by the collision.

Air bags only deploy in certain types of crashes. For the air bag to deploy, sensors are activated by impact in a certain location in the vehicle (the front bumper for front-impact air bags and the doors for side-impact air bags). You will not see air bag deployment in very low-speed collisions or rear-end collisions, or if the front bumper is not directly involved in the crash. The use of child restraint seats has caused a dramatic reduction in injuries to children during collisions. Note whether children involved in collisions were restrained in a car seat—and if it appears they were restrained properly.

A **motorcycle collision** can cause serious injuries (Figure 9-9 ■). Currently less than half of the states require that all motorcycle riders wear helmets. Determine if the patient was wearing a helmet or not. There are several patterns you may see including:

■ Ejection over the handlebars, which occurs in front-end collisions. The ejection often results in leg and hip injuries from striking the handlebars as the rider is thrown over them. Other injuries may occur as the patient strikes the ground or other objects.

■ Side impact, which often causes injuries to the rider's hip and legs from direct contact with the vehicle. Other injuries may occur during subsequent impacts until the bike and rider come to rest.

■ Laying the bike down, which is a method of avoiding collisions. The rider will turn the bike sideways and bring it down to the ground to avoid the frontal

motorcycle collision
crash that involves a motorcycle and is especially dangerous due to lack of protection.

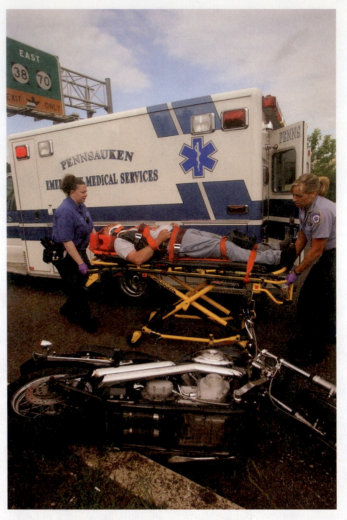

■ **Figure 9-9** Motorcycle crash. *(© Mark C. Ide)*

impact. This results in lacerations, abrasions, and burns but is usually less severe than the impact would have been.

Injuries from Falls

Falls may range from simply tripping to a fall from significant heights—and will surely be a reason you will be called as an EMR (Figure 9-10 ■). The factors you should look for when evaluating the mechanism of injury in a fall include:

- The height the patient fell from. Greater than 2–3 times the patient's height is (20 ft for adults) usually considered a significant mechanism of injury.
- The part of the patient that struck the surface (head first, feet first).
- The surface the patient fell on (pavement versus sand or grass).
- Whether anything broke the fall or caused additional injuries during the fall (falling through bushes might reduce the impact, but striking a concrete ledge during a fall would likely cause additional injuries).

You may see a few specific patterns. Patients who jump from a height and land feet first often sustain heel fractures as well as fractures of the legs. The energy is transmitted up through the lower body and could result in spinal fractures. Patients who trip and fall often try to catch themselves with an outstretched arm. This results in a fracture of the distal

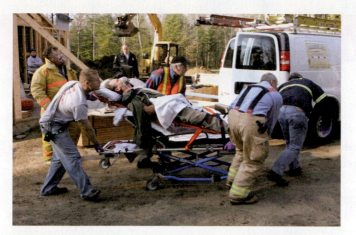

■ Figure 9-10 Falls can cause injury to many parts of the body.

forearm and a deformity called the "silver fork deformity," because the deformity of the wrist resembles the shape of a fork.

Mechanism of injury is important because patients often concentrate on only one injury at a time. You may come upon a patient who is holding his arm which he believes is broken. That same patient may also have a head or chest injury or internal bleeding he is unaware of. By examining the forces involved in the trauma, you may come to believe more injuries are likely and perform additional examinations to find those injuries (Table 9-1).

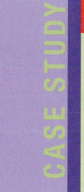

CASE STUDY

THE RESPONSE

You begin observing from a distance and notice a man on the ground. You know there are several drums of solvent and chemicals in the area normally. As you get near the door, another man comes outside "to get some fresh air." Then he vomits.

■ Discussion: *Should you go in? What else could you look for or ask before you approach the scene to determine why people are sick?*

TABLE 9-1 Scene Size-Up

COMPONENT	ACTIONS
Scene safety	Observe for violence, hazardous materials, environmental factors, and other things at the scene that may pose a hazard to you, the patient, family members, and bystanders. Call for assistance from departments (e.g., police, fire) and teams (hazmat) as necessary.
Standard Precaution determination	Take appropriate precautions to prevent exposure to blood and body fluids.
Resource determination	Do you have all the help you need at the scene? Do you need specialty teams, vehicle extrication, or utility companies because of downed wires? Call for the help you need at this point.
Number of patients	Be sure to call for additional patient care assistance early. Call for additional ambulances and personnel in proportion to the potential number of patients.
Mechanism of injury or nature of illness	Observe the scene for factors that may have contributed to a patient's injuries (e.g., falls, damage to vehicles). In the case of medical patients, scan the scene for clues to the patient's medical problem or condition.

Multiple Choice

Place a check next to the correct answer.

1. When a responder believes there is a high likelihood a person is injured based upon the mechanism present, it is referred to as:

    _____ a. head-on collision.

    _____ b. index of suspicion.

    _____ c. velocity.

    _____ d. proximate causation.

2. An automobile crash that propels occupants forward in a vehicle is referred to as a:

    _____ a. head-on collision.

    _____ b. rear-impact collision.

    _____ c. side-impact collision.

    _____ d. rollover.

3. What type of automobile crash causes a "direct" impact to the passengers due to the close proximity of the passenger compartment to the striking forces?

    _____ a. Head-on collision

    _____ b. Rear-impact collision

    _____ c. Side-impact collision

    _____ d. Rollover

4. In a motorcycle crash, what type of injuries should the EMR suspect if it was an "over the handlebar" ejection?

    _____ a. Leg and hip

    _____ b. Head and neck

    _____ c. Chest and abdomen

    _____ d. All of the above

True/False

Mark whether each of the following statements is true (T) or false (F).

1. _____ The greater the speed or velocity in a crash, the potential for injury decreases.

2. _____ In a rollover collision where the vehicle occupant is unrestrained, there can be multiple injury patterns due to the multiple points of impact.

3. _____ The surface that a fall patient lands on is an important factor to consider in determining mechanism of injury.

Critical Thinking

You arrive on the scene of a rolled over vehicle, still resting on its roof. Two occupants are reported to have been in the vehicle. No one is visible and no noises are heard.

1. What should your first and primary concern be?

    _____

    _____

    _____

2. When access is gained, what types of injuries may be present?

    _____

    _____

    _____

3. As the occupants had not been wearing seat belts and are not present in the vehicle, what has likely happened and where are they likely to be found?

_____

_____

_____

_____

Resource Determination and Number of Patients

Resource determination involves all of the elements presented in this chapter so far. Before you get to the patient's side it is critical to make sure that all hazards have been addressed and that all necessary help has been summoned. Experience in emergency situations over the years has shown that once rescuers get involved in individual patient care they tend to focus on that patient and may lose track of time—and forget to make necessary notifications.

Table 9-2 provides examples of situations an individual EMR may observe and the appropriate resources to call for.

Number of Patients

Perhaps once or twice in your career, you may encounter a call with dozens or hundreds of patients. More frequently you will encounter calls with two or three patients who will pose logistical challenges to care for (Figure 9-11 ■).

ASK YOURSELF

■ How do you survey the scene to determine the number of patients present and additional resources needed?

TABLE 9-2 Scene vs. Response	
WHAT YOU SEE	**WHAT YOU CALL FOR**
A crash on the interstate highway with four patients.	■ Adequate protection from traffic (fire engine, police cruiser, or highway truck with markings). ■ Additional ambulances. If all patients are severely injured, you may need four ambulances if available.
A crash on the interstate highway with four patients. You observe heavy damage to the vehicles with possible entrapment.	Resources listed above **plus:** ■ Fire department for vehicle extrications. ■ Consider air medical evacuation of patients if allowed in local protocols.
A patient and two family members who feel dizzy and weak in their home. They had been unable to afford heat so they were using a kerosene heater indoors.	Fire department to safely enter the scene with self-contained breathing apparatus. Ensure that multiple ambulances have been dispatched to the scene.
A worker who was sickened when he unknowingly mixed cleaning chemicals together.	Fire department and hazardous materials units. Even though only one patient is currently ill, if any other patients were in the area additional assistance may be needed.
A man was cutting down a tree that fell unexpectedly across power lines and knocked them down. The patient is injured but very close to the wires.	Call for the power company to deal with wires before approaching the patient. Fire department will provide additional resources for dealing with the tree or equipment the patient used at the scene as well as additional personnel.

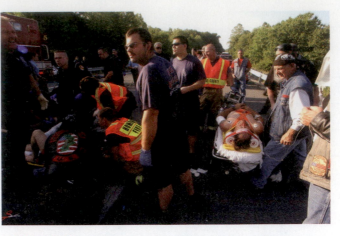

■ **Figure 9-11**   Multiple-casualty incident. *(© Mark C. Ide)*

Many consider the term MCI to stand for "mass-casualty incident." In fact, it is a *multiple*-casualty incident. The difference? The latter term is more realistic because two or three seriously injured patients—or ten nonseriously injured patients—pose challenges to assess and treat with limited rescuers. Even when faced with one patient who requires CPR, it would be helpful to have others available to help. Call for additional ambulances and personnel before you begin patient care.

Remember, the earlier you call for help the earlier the help will arrive to assist you and the patients on the scene.

Standard Precautions

To prevent the transmission of disease, you will keep the body fluids of others from coming in contact with you. This concept is referred to as **Standard Precautions**, as you learned in Chapter 2.

The scene size-up is where you will make decisions about what precautions you must take. The precautions required differ from call to call. At some calls you may need no precautions whereas you will require extensive precautions at other scenes.

As you approach the scene you will look for hazards, mechanism of injury, or nature of illness; determine the number of patients; and determine if any resources are necessary. These are performed from a distance. Once you have determined the scene is safe, you move closer to your patient where you can observe what precautions are necessary.

Many EMRs are taught to take Standard Precautions before leaving the vehicle or before seeing the patient. Caution is advised when using this practice for two reasons: (1) the gloves you put on early may be damaged while you carry your equipment to the scene and (2) if you believe you have already taken Standard Precautions before you reach the patient, you may fail to take additional necessary precautions at the scene.

As you approach the patient, you will make several quick but important determinations that will help you to decide what precautions are necessary. Remember that you can't determine what precautions to take until you see the situation. Table 9-3 presents common situations and the precautions you should take.

You should carry equipment for Standard Precautions on your person when you are on duty. You should also have equipment immediately available when you open your kit at the patient's side. You may have to change your gloves when they become soiled. Make sure you have multiple sets of gloves and alternative protection available.

TABLE 9-3 Standard Precautions Decisions

IF YOU SEE THIS IN THE SCENE SIZE-UP:		YOU SHOULD TAKE THE FOLLOWING PRECAUTIONS:
Minor bleeding.	→	Gloves.
Severe bleeding and/or spurting bleeding.	→	Gloves, eye protection, and protection for clothing if likely to become soiled. Patient care activity: bleeding control.
Unresponsive patient. Blood or secretions in or around the mouth.	→	Gloves and eye protection. Patient care activity: suction.
A patient who does not appear to have open wounds but has an odor of urine or feces.	→	Gloves to begin. Eye protection in the event you believe material may spray or spatter. Patient care activity: patient assessment, lifting and moving.
A car crash with broken glass and a patient who does not appear to have open wounds.	→	Gloves and specialized clothing (such as turnout gear) to protect you from the broken glass as well as gloves to protect you from the potential injuries caused by broken glass you may not be able to see. Patient care activity: spinal immobilization, potential for bleeding control, lifting and moving the patient.

CASE STUDY

TRANSITION

A woman just inside the door comes to you and asks what is wrong. She feels dizzy. You direct a manager to call for additional ambulances and the fire department with their hazardous material team. Then you call for everyone to exit the area and come outside the building. You keep people in a designated area to prevent contamination and make sure no one wanders off.

The man who was on the ground inside had been overcome by some sort of fumes or chemical reaction. He remains in critical condition. The people you directed to come outside received limited exposure and are treated and released at the hospital. In all, 14 people were decontaminated and treated. Experts will try to determine which chemicals may have combined to cause the reaction. One thing is clear, your scene size-up prevented you from becoming a patient and put a safe plan in place that quickly and efficiently treated over a dozen patients.

■ Discussion: *What would have happened if you had become a patient? How would you have helped your patients?*

THE LAST WORD

The elements of the scene size-up are critical to the call because they are critical to your safety and the safety of your patient. You will also make important determinations early—when they make the greatest difference. These include determining the number of patients and identifying things you will need assistance with early in the call and calling for help right away.

Chapter Review

Multiple Choice

Place a check next to the correct answer.

1. When approaching a scene, you note the following things. Which is a sign that there is something wrong that is not readily visible?

   _____ a. Broken glass at an automobile crash

   _____ b. Unusual silence at a call for a cardiac arrest

   _____ c. Medication patches on the floor of a nursing home

   _____ d. Black tire marks on the pavement of an interstate

2. What term describes the action of moving swiftly away from danger?

   _____ a. Cover

   _____ b. Concealment

   _____ c. Retreat

   _____ d. Camouflage

3. Terrorist incidents pose a particular new set of response hazards, including:

   _____ a. a large number of patients injured or killed.

   _____ b. a scene that encompasses a large area.

   _____ c. the potential for exposure to chemical, biological, radiological, nuclear, and electrical hazards.

   _____ d. all of the above.

4. What scene hazard listed is considered to be one of the deadliest?

   _____ a. Spilled gasoline

   _____ b. Passing traffic

   _____ c. Jagged metal

   _____ d. Steep inclines

5. An automobile crash that causes occupants to spring backward is a:

   _____ a. head-on collision.

   _____ b. rear-end collision.

   _____ c. side-impact collision.

   _____ d. rollover.

Short Answer

1. List six sources of personal danger to emergency responders.

   _____

   _____

   _____

   _____

2. When evaluating a fall patient, what are the four factors to include in your primary assessment?

   _____

   _____

   _____

   _____

3. What do the initials "MCI" stand for and what is the primary concern?

_____

_____

_____

_____

Critical Thinking

A rollover collision has occurred on the local interstate. You, as an EMR, are the first person to arrive at the scene and are therefore tasked with incident command.

1. What is the first thing you should determine to ensure you have adequate units to handle the incident?

_____

_____

_____

_____

2. In order to protect responders and patients, who else besides additional medical units should you contact?

_____

_____

_____

3. As other units arrive, you take a more active role in patient care. Who among the vehicle's occupants should be required to sign a refusal and who must be transported and why?

_____

_____

_____

EXPLORE PEARSON mybradykit™

Please go to www.bradybooks.com to access mykit for this text. You will find quizzes, critical thinking scenarios, weblinks, animations, and videos related to this chapter—and much more. Look for online information on scene safety as it relates to vehicles and hazards from the NHTSA.

Register your access code from the front of your book by going to www.bradybooks.com and selecting the mykit links.

Patient Assessment: The Primary Assessment

✳ NAVIGATION GUIDE

The following items provide an overview to the purpose and content of this chapter. The Education Standard and Competency are from the National EMS Education Standards.

Education Standard Assessment (Primary Assessment)

Competency Uses scene information and simple patient assessment findings to identify and manage immediate life threats and injuries within the scope of practice of the EMR.

Knowledge Area Primary Assessment
- Level of consciousness
- ABCs
- Identifying life threats
- Assessment of vital functions
- Begin interventions needed to preserve life

Objectives After reading this chapter, you should be able to:

1. Define key terms introduced in this chapter.
2. Describe the purpose of the primary patient assessment.
3. Explain the importance of scene safety and using personal protective equipment.
4. Identify patients for whom you should take spinal precautions.
5. Explain each of the eight basic components of a primary patient assessment.
6. Determine patients' chief complaints.
7. Perform each of the following components of the primary patient assessment:
   a. Form a general impression of the patient.
   b. Determine level of consciousness.
   c. Assess the airway status.
   d. Assess adequacy of breathing.
   e. Assess adequacy of circulation.
   f. Assess for disability.
   g. Expose the patient to assess for pertinent findings.
   h. Update the incoming EMS units with pertinent information from your assessment.
8. Use primary assessment findings to identify patients who are in serious, or potentially serious, condition.
9. Intervene as necessary in the primary assessment to maintain airway, breathing, and circulation.

NAVIGATION GUIDE *(continued)*

Key Terms Page references indicate first major use in this chapter. The Margin Glossary in this chapter provides definitions as you read.

general impression p. 246   *level of consciousness* p. 247   *agonal* p. 254

chief complaint p. 246   *patent* p. 248

Media Resources Please go to **www.bradybooks.com** to access mykit for this text. You will find quizzes, critical thinking scenarios, weblinks, animations, and videos related to this chapter—and much more. Look for online information on patient assessment techniques. You will also find video clips on assessment of pain and conducting a detailed physical exam.

INTRODUCTION

Once you have completed the scene size-up, you will perform a primary assessment. The primary assessment is the most important part of patient care because it must identify and correct life threats the patient may be experiencing. It is worth repeating: the primary assessment is about identifying and correcting conditions that can kill your patient. You must perform it before you do anything else.

Not every patient will have life-threatening conditions. Some will have a minor illness or injury, others will be in serious condition, and others will fall somewhere in between. Your assessment will help you identify how to treat each patient. (See The Big Picture: Primary Assessment of the Medical Patient and The Big Picture: Primary Assessment of the Trauma Patient.)

ASK YOURSELF
- What is the purpose of the primary patient assessment?
- How would you explain the importance of scene safety and using personal protective equipment?
- How would you explain each of the eight basic components of a primary patient assessment?

CASE STUDY

THE CALL

You are the Emergency Medical Responder called to assist a 36-year-old male who has cut his leg badly with a chain saw while cutting trees. You arrive to find him seated with his leg wrapped in a blood-soaked T-shirt. There is a great deal of blood on the ground. As you approach him, he calls out to you for help.

- Discussion: *There are several immediate concerns for this patient. How should you begin your assessment?*

Eight Components of the Primary Assessment

The primary assessment has eight basic components:

- General impression
- Level of consciousness
- Airway
- Breathing
- Circulation
- Disability
- Expose
- Update incoming EMS units

The Big Picture

Primary Assessment of the Medical Patient

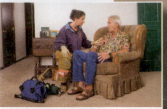

1 Develop a general impression.

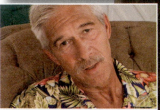

2 Assess the patient's level of responsiveness.

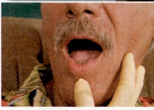

3 Assess ABCs.

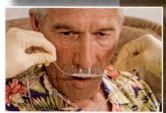

4 If indicated based on the patient's condition, apply oxygen.

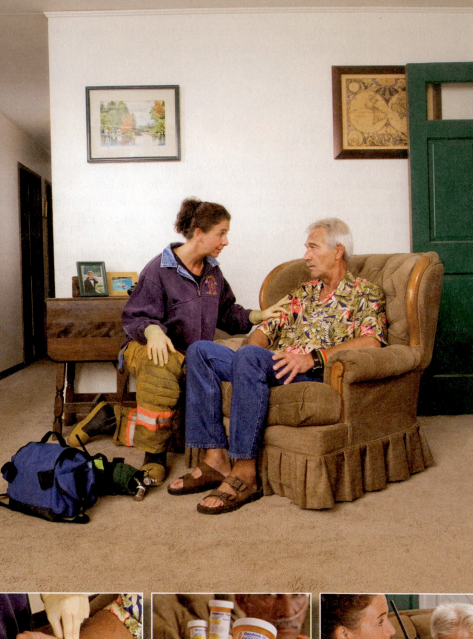

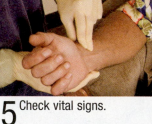

5 Check vital signs.

6 Obtain a medical history and check medications.

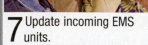

7 Update incoming EMS units.

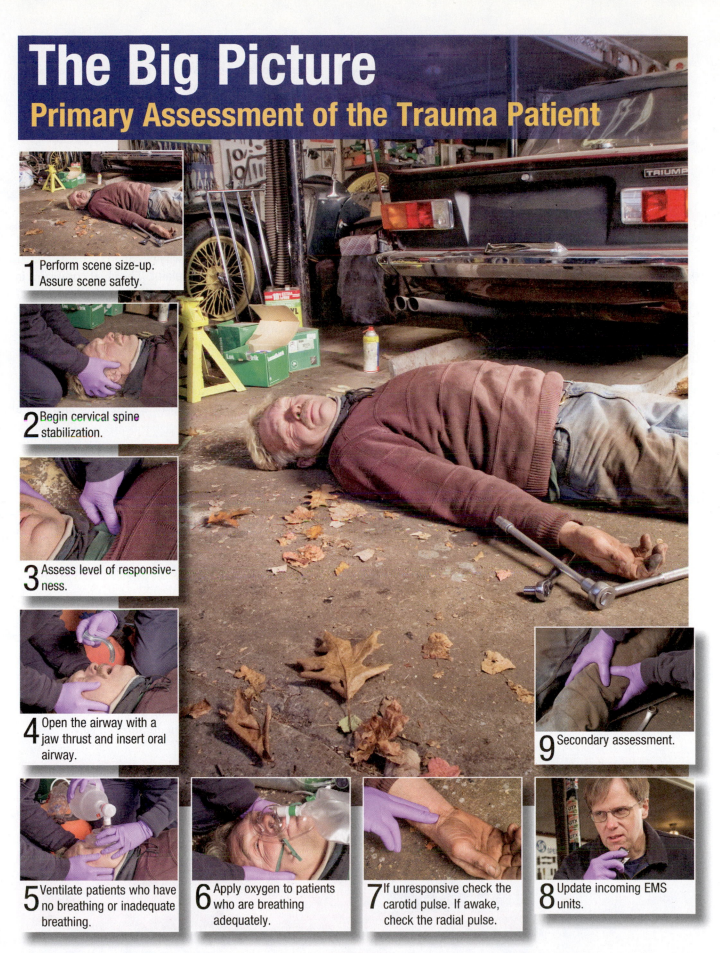

The Big Picture
Primary Assessment of the Trauma Patient

1 Perform scene size-up. Assure scene safety.

2 Begin cervical spine stabilization.

3 Assess level of responsiveness.

4 Open the airway with a jaw thrust and insert oral airway.

5 Ventilate patients who have no breathing or inadequate breathing.

6 Apply oxygen to patients who are breathing adequately.

7 If unresponsive check the carotid pulse. If awake, check the radial pulse.

8 Update incoming EMS units.

9 Secondary assessment.

General Impression

general impression how the patient looks to you as you approach.

chief complaint the patient's response to your question about how he is feeling or what is wrong.

The **general impression** is how the patient looks to you as you approach. This step is not technical and does not involve any equipment. Experienced EMRs—and experienced EMS providers at all levels—can look at a patient from a distance and gain important information that will set a foundation for their initial actions.

It has been said that a first impression may be the most important. In EMS, the general impression is your first impression. It's vitally important and sets a foundation for the remainder of the call. Your general impression should help you answer an important question: Is this a serious patient where I will have to get to work on lifesaving treatments right away (or within the first few minutes), or do I have time to casually ask a few questions about what is wrong because the patient initially seems OK?

When you get to a patient's side, you will ask him if he wants your help. This is a method of gaining consent as discussed in Chapter 3. You will also ask why he called for help or what is wrong. The answer to this question is called the **chief complaint**. The chief complaint is usually documented in the patient's own words. For example, "I fell." Or, "My chest hurts." This valuable information will help guide your assessment. Unresponsive patients will not be able to provide a chief complaint. In this case look to family members, coworkers, or bystanders for information on what happened leading up to the call for help.

Scenarios

Consider the following patient scenarios you could encounter. As you read each one, look for clues as to whether the patient will require a lot of help or a little help and if the condition is immediately life threatening or not.

1. A patient at the mall tripped getting off the escalator. She is awake, sitting on the floor, and holding her ankle.
2. A patient fell several stories from the roof of a construction site. He appears to have a few extremities that are at an unnatural angle. He looks unresponsive and has blood coming from his mouth.
3. An older woman flags you down and excitedly yells, "Oh, please, please help! I think my husband may be dying. He fell over mowing the lawn and he isn't moving."
4. A woman asks for your help because she is weak. She has had the flu for 3 days and is vomiting.

Did you get any ideas about which patients are more serious? The second and third patients are potentially the most serious based on early information (Table 10-1).

Serious or not? Now let's look at each of the cases and examine what we can learn from what appears to be basic information (see Table 10-1). Remember that the scene size-up and primary assessment may flow together. For example, you may begin airway care and spinal stabilization on the man who fell from the roof while asking a coworker how far the patient fell. The exception is safety. *Never enter a scene until you are sure it is safe.*

ASK YOURSELF

- What are the steps you take to perform a primary assessment?
- Can you find and define key terms introduced in this chapter?
- How do you determine a patient's chief complaint?
- How do you identify patients for whom you should take spinal precautions?

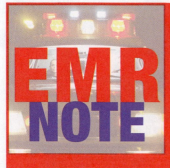

EMR NOTE

You will learn the patient assessment skills in a step-by-step manner. This will help ensure a structured and thorough approach to your patient assessment. When you encounter a serious patient in a stressful situation, your knowledge of these steps will help you provide lifesaving care. You will also find unusual situations and patients with varied problems. The same steps will apply, but you will have to adapt them to each situation you encounter.

TABLE 10-1 Initial Response to Different Types of Patients

SCENARIO	SCENE SIZE-UP CONSIDERATIONS	PRIMARY ASSESSMENT OBSERVATIONS
A patient at the mall tripped getting off the escalator. She is awake, sitting on the floor, complaining of pain, and holding her ankle.	Are there any hazards from the escalator? Did she fall from the last step or from the top? Is her ankle injury open or bleeding?	You see the patient sitting and complaining of pain. You know she is responsive and in pain.
A patient fell several stories from the roof of a construction site. He appears to have a few extremities that are at an unnatural angle. He looks unresponsive and has blood coming from his mouth.	The mechanism of injury is significant. You will have to take Standard Precautions of (at least) gloves and eye/face protection because of blood in the mouth. Make sure there is no risk from falling objects or other construction hazards. Will additional assistance be required to extricate the patient or move him to the ambulance?	The patient does not appear to be responsive. He may have a spine injury and will require cervical spine stabilization. He will require airway care including opening, suction, and possibly ventilation.
An older woman flags you down and excitedly yells, "Oh, please, please help me! I think my husband may be dying. He fell over mowing the lawn and he isn't moving."	Although you haven't seen the patient, you should prepare for the worst in the equipment you bring and Standard Precautions you take.	Something happened that made a patient suddenly become unresponsive and appear as if he was dead. Even if he simply passed out and then got better, it is best to be prepared.
A woman appears alert and asks for your help because she is weak. She has had the flu for 3 days and is vomiting.	You should be prepared to keep vomit from your face, skin, and clothes.	Although the woman appears alert, you should watch the airway in the event she becomes weaker and can't protect her airway during an episode of vomiting. Ready your suction unit.

The following are early signs that a patient is in serious or potentially serious condition:

- Unresponsive or altered mental status
- Anxious, agitated, or sleepy appearance
- Cool, sweaty skin
- A position indicating chest pain or difficulty breathing
- Severe pain (Figure 10-1a ■)

Early signs that a patient may not be in serious condition (although you'll always check in greater detail later) include the following:

- Patients who appear awake and alert
- No apparent difficulty breathing and no chest pain (can talk without having to catch his breath)
- Normal skin color and condition, and relaxed appearance (Figure 10-1b ■)

Level of Consciousness

Determining the patient's **level of consciousness**, or responsiveness, is very important. As you approach the patient and make a general impression, you begin this determination.

ASK YOURSELF

- How do you use primary assessment findings to identify patients who are in serious, or potentially serious, condition?

level of consciousness a patient's responsiveness.

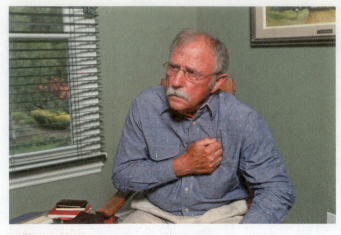

■ **Figure 10-1a** Your general impression will be that this man is in pain.

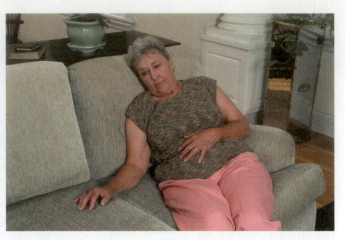

■ **Figure 10-1b** Your general impression may be of an altered mental status.

There are four widely accepted levels of responsiveness: alert, verbal, painful stimulus, and unresponsive. The mnemonic AVPU will help you to remember these four levels:

Alert—The patient is awake and aware of what is going on around him. He knows where he is and what he is doing there.

Verbal—The patient will talk or make some noise, but he is not alert. Something is wrong. There are many patient conditions that fit this category, ranging from the patient who appears OK but is confused as to what day it is or where he is, to someone who simply moans or mumbles.

Pain—This person does not respond to speaking, shouting, or even light shaking. He only responds to a painful stimulus (see the following information on how to apply a painful stimulus).

Unresponsive—This patient is unresponsive such that he does not respond to a voice, gentle shaking, or a painful stimulus. He truly doesn't respond to anything.

To test for level of responsiveness, you will take information learned in your size-up and general impression and do one of two things:

- If the patient appears awake, you will talk with him to see if he is oriented (knows where he is, his purpose, and the date and time).
- If the patient appears unresponsive, scan quickly for signs of life and breathing. If none, begin the C-A-B approach. If the patient does appear to be breathing, attempt to get a response by a pinch or gentle shake.

To apply a painful stimulus, pinch the muscle at the base of the neck where it meets the shoulder. You may also put pressure on a fingernail using a pen or pinch the webbing between the finger and thumb. Note any response from the patient, including moaning or movement that is caused by the painful stimulus.

Airway

Chapter 7 discussed techniques and procedures you will use to assess and care for a patient's airway and breathing. This is the beginning point where your skills will be put to use.

The purpose of the airway portion of the primary assessment is to be sure the airway is open and will remain open if you divert your attention somewhere else during the patient assessment. This is often called a **patent** airway. If for any reason the airway isn't

ASK YOURSELF

■ What are some ways you will intervene as necessary in the primary assessment to maintain airway, breathing, and circulation?

patent an open airway that appears it will remain open.

	OBSERVATION	ACTION
Level of Responsiveness # AV # PU	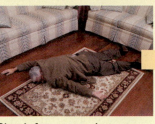 Check for responsiveness.	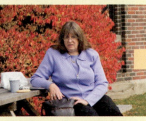 If apparently lifeless, use C-A-B approach.
	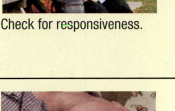 Check for responsiveness.	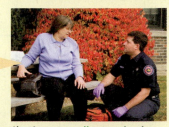 Alert patients generally require less urgent action, but be alert for potentially unstable patients.
Airway # A	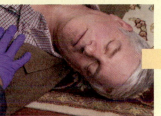 Patient is unresponsive. You don't suspect trauma.	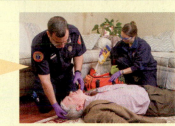 Open the airway using the head-tilt, chin-lift maneuver. If spine injury is suspected, use the jaw-thrust maneuver.
	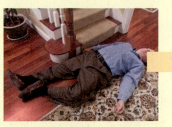 Patient is responsive. Trauma is suspected and spine injury is possible.	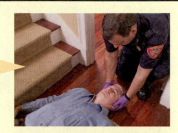 If trauma is suspected, use the jaw thrust maneuver to open the airway.
	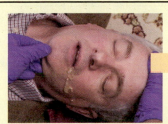 Examination of the airway reveals vomit or secretions.	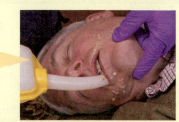 Roll the patient to the side and suction.

	OBSERVATION	ACTION
Breathing **B**	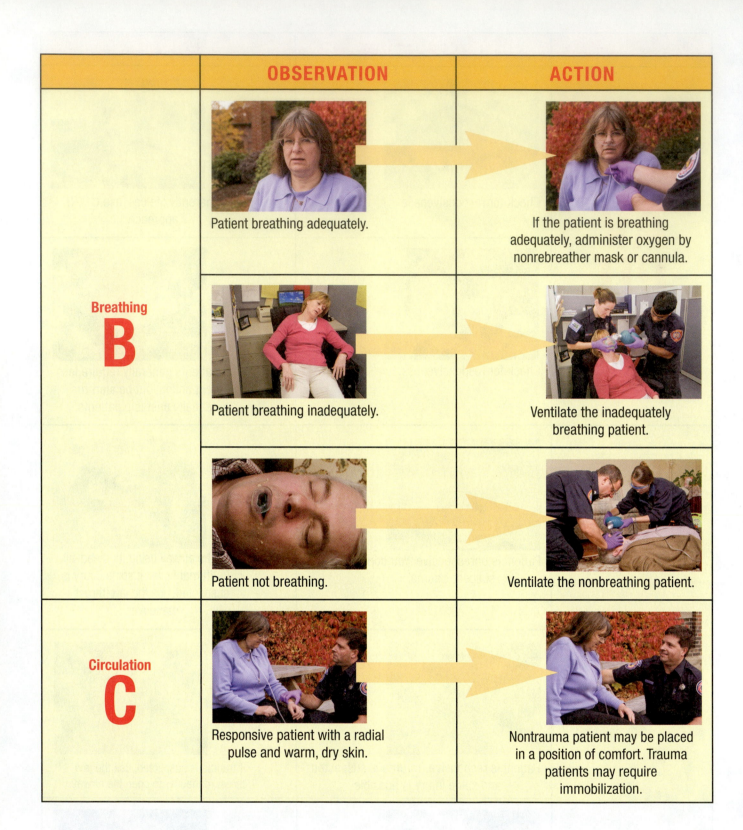 Patient breathing adequately.	If the patient is breathing adequately, administer oxygen by nonrebreather mask or cannula.
	Patient breathing inadequately.	Ventilate the inadequately breathing patient.
	Patient not breathing.	Ventilate the nonbreathing patient.
Circulation **C**	Responsive patient with a radial pulse and warm, dry skin.	Nontrauma patient may be placed in a position of comfort. Trauma patients may require immobilization.

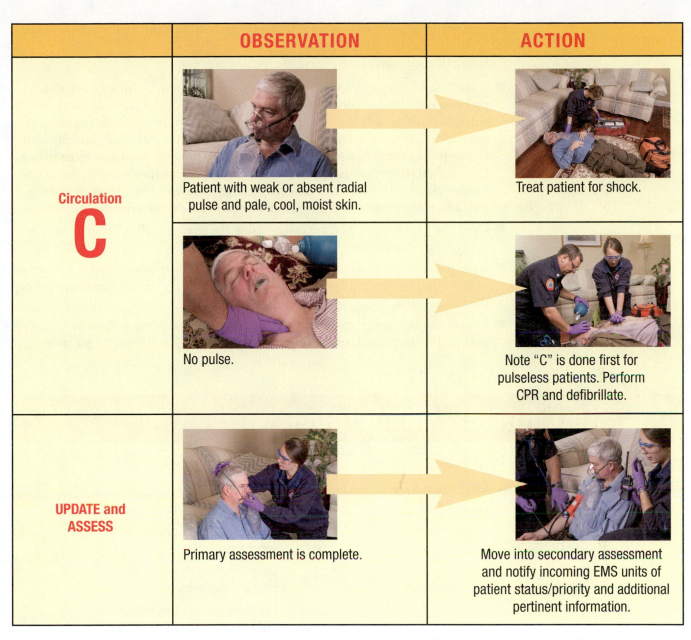

	OBSERVATION	ACTION
Circulation **C**	Patient with weak or absent radial pulse and pale, cool, moist skin.	Treat patient for shock.
	No pulse.	Note "C" is done first for pulseless patients. Perform CPR and defibrillate.
UPDATE and ASSESS	Primary assessment is complete.	Move into secondary assessment and notify incoming EMS units of patient status/priority and additional pertinent information.

A-B-C may be done in any order based on the patient's injuries and priorities.

open—or won't remain open—prompt action is required. Remember, the primary assessment identifies and treats life threats.

During this segment of the patient assessment process:

- If you believe the patient will have problems maintaining his airway—or if the problem may develop soon—move the patient to a position (such as the floor) where you will be able to perform the techniques listed in the following steps. If the patient has a suspected spinal injury, move the patient carefully, usually with two or more Emergency Medical Responders, keeping the head and spine in line. Of course, if the patient isn't breathing or requires immediate suction, this is the highest priority. If you do not have help present, move the patient as carefully as possible, but promptly, and provide airway care. This is the priority.

- Open the patient's airway if necessary, using the head-tilt, chin-lift maneuver or the jaw-thrust maneuver.

- If the patient is unresponsive and can't maintain his own airway, you will insert an oral or nasal airway and use the head-tilt, chin lift or jaw-thrust maneuver to keep the airway open.

- If there are any foreign materials in the airway, you will remove them by positioning the patient, suctioning, and for larger visible objects, finger sweeps.

✱ Stop, Review, Remember

Multiple Choice

Place a check next to the correct answer.

1. The mnemonic for remembering the levels of consciousness is:
   _____ a. SAMPLE.
   _____ b. ABC.
   _____ c. 4-CONS.
   _____ d. AVPU.

2. The patient who responds only to a pinch of the muscles near the neck is responsive to:
   _____ a. voice.
   _____ b. pain.
   _____ c. carotid stimulation.
   _____ d. pressure.

3. Which of the following steps is NOT part of the "A" or airway portion of the primary assessment?
   _____ a. Inserting an oral airway
   _____ b. Suctioning
   _____ c. Checking a pulse
   _____ d. Jaw-thrust maneuver

4. The general impression is best described as:
   _____ a. how the patient looks as you approach.
   _____ b. the patient's status after the primary assessment.
   _____ c. key information you will call or radio to the incoming EMS units.
   _____ d. a check of the patient's mental status.

5. Which of the following would indicate a potentially serious patient? Each of these patients is alert and oriented.
   _____ a. A patient who is complaining of a broken arm
   _____ b. A patient who was punched in the nose with moderate bleeding
   _____ c. A patient who was involved in a minor car crash and complains of neck pain
   _____ d. A patient who complains of abdominal pain and has cool, moist skin

Emergency Medical Responder Practice

For each of the following patients, determine whether you should use a head-tilt, chin-lift maneuver or the jaw-thrust maneuver to open the patient's airway:

1. Your patient was found unresponsive on the couch.

   _____

   _____

   _____

2. Your patient was raking leaves and collapsed.

   _____

   _____

   _____

3. Your patient was working on scaffolding and fell about 8 feet.

   _____

   _____

   _____

4. Your patient was taking a nap. Her husband couldn't wake her up.

   _____

   _____

   _____

5. Your patient was the victim of an assault. He was hit in the head with a pipe or bat.

   _____

   _____

   _____

Short Answer

1. Define chief complaint.

   _____

   _____

   _____

2. What are spinal precautions? What sort of patient should they be applied to?

   _____

   _____

   _____

3. If you find a patient to be responsive to verbal stimulus, do you need to check painful stimulus? Why or why not?

_____

_____

_____

Breathing

You must ensure all patients are breathing—and breathing adequately—in order for them to survive. In practice, you will approach responsive and unresponsive patients differently when you make this determination.

Responsive patients will likely be breathing. It is your job to determine if the patient is breathing adequately. As you approach the patient, you will notice important signs and symptoms including skin color, how many words the patient can speak before catching his breath, and his level of responsiveness. Hypoxia (low oxygen levels in the blood) can cause anxiety, restlessness, and occasionally frantic or combative behavior.

As you examine the patient more closely, look for deep, equal chest expansion and note an approximate respiratory rate. Remember that breathing must be of a normal rate and depth (volume) to be considered adequate. Breathing that is very fast or very slow is likely inadequate breathing to sustain life for long periods of time. Patients in distress may also use accessory muscles in their neck and chest to help breathe. This alone doesn't indicate inadequate breathing, but since it is taking extra work to breathe, the patient could fatigue and begin breathing inadequately at any time. Be careful not to mistake **agonal** (occasional, gasping) respiration with adequate breathing.

When assessing the unresponsive patient, get to the patient's level. You will not be able to use observations such as the patient's speech in this case so your assessment will be more hands-on. Feel the chest for expansion. The chest will rise noticeably when the patient is breathing adequately. Expansion will be minimal (and may be unequal if the chest is injured) when the patient is breathing inadequately. You will also look for signs and symptoms including skin color and condition, respiratory rate, and accessory muscle use. Refer back to the beginning of this chapter, which shows the Big Picture of assessment.

Patients who are experiencing respiratory distress or chest pain, who have traumatic injury, or who appear unstable should receive oxygen if you have it available. Patients who are breathing inadequately or not at all should receive oxygen via assisted ventilations with a pocket face mask or bag-valve mask.

Oxygenation and ventilation, if necessary, should start immediately. If two EMRs are on scene, one may place oxygen on the patient who is breathing adequately while the other continues the assessment process. If the patient is unresponsive but breathing adequately and does not have a suspected spine injury, administer oxygen and place him in the recovery (or lateral recumbent) position. This will facilitate drainage of secretions. Monitor the patient carefully.

Circulation

The key elements of checking circulation are to ensure there is a pulse, to observe for obvious, severe bleeding, and to begin to determine if the patient is in shock. If the patient is unresponsive and does not appear to have respirations, check the carotid pulse at the neck. If the carotid pulse is absent and the patient has no other signs of life, begin CPR and prepare an AED. Check a responsive patient's radial pulse at the wrist.

agonal occasional and gasping, when referring to respiration.

If a patient is responsive and breathing, he obviously has a pulse. But this is not the only reason you check the pulse. In addition to checking for the presence or absence of a pulse, you will also look for signs of inadequate circulation, also called hypoperfusion or simply "shock." A person in shock may demonstrate a weak and rapid pulse.

When the body's tissues aren't getting enough blood—and therefore not getting enough oxygen—the body responds in a predictable fashion. The pulse and respiratory rates rise and the skin becomes pale, cool, and clammy. To look for these important findings you will need to touch the patient, and feeling for a radial pulse in the responsive patient is an effective means of doing so. Simply reasoning that the patient has a pulse because he is breathing isn't enough.

In addition, abnormal electrical activity in the heart can often produce an abnormally slow, rapid, or irregular pulse. These are all key items to look for in the circulation portion of the primary assessment.

Scenario

Consider a patient in a car crash. You stop to assist and you find the patient up, walking, and oriented. It was a substantial crash with a significant mechanism of injury. The patient tells you she is fine. She speaks in full sentences without distress although she appears a little out of breath. You insist on doing an assessment and she agrees. While someone stabilizes her head and spine, you perform a primary assessment. You confirm that her breathing is a bit rapid, as is her pulse. Her skin is cool and a bit moist. As you continue to talk with her, she becomes a little anxious. This condition could be caused by the stress of the crash—or it could be the beginning signs and symptoms of shock.

The ambulance arrives. You tell the EMTs of your findings. They say they'll keep an eye on it. You run into one of the crew members a few days later who tells you, "Good call on that patient." It turns out the patient had internal bleeding and was rushed to surgery. You realize that following procedure and not taking shortcuts or making assumptions is very important.

Another critical step in the circulation phase of the primary assessment is to check the patient for external bleeding. In this step you should identify and control severe (life-threatening) bleeding. Severe bleeding is not always obvious. Patients who have heavy clothes or are lying on carpeting can lose a surprisingly large amount of blood before it becomes visible. You should wear gloves anytime you check for blood by reaching where you can't see.

Responsive patients will likely be able to tell you if they are injured and bleeding. If the patient has an altered mental status or is unresponsive, you will do a brief hands-on check to look for bleeding in places you can't see such as the small of the back and beneath coats or heavy clothing.

Disability

The disability check, used primarily in trauma patients, is designed to test the central nervous system (the brain and spinal cord). When the central nervous system is injured, the body usually has serious—and predictable—consequences.

The patient's mental status is one of the most significant indicators of central nervous system function. You have already done a determination using the AVPU scale of responsiveness. As you continue to examine the patient, look to see if his eyes open spontaneously, upon stimulus, or not at all. Does the patient speak? If so, does his speech make sense or is it confused or unintelligible?

The ability to move the extremities and sensation are also important indicators of central nervous system function. Responsive patients should be asked to move each extremity. Ask your patient to wiggle his fingers, then his toes. Watch each for movement. Then touch or gently squeeze a finger on each hand to determine if the patient can feel the squeeze or touch. Ask the patient if he can feel the touch. It is generally best not to let the patient see you touch the extremity to ensure accurate results. Do the same with each extremity. The patient should be able to move each extremity when asked as well as feel the touch or squeeze. If the patient does not have these responses, you should suspect serious injury or illness.

✹✹ Stop, Review, Remember

Multiple Choice

Place a check next to the correct answer.

1. Which of the following is not part of the circulation check?

   ____ a. Pulse

   ____ b. Bleeding

   ____ c. Blood pressure

   ____ d. Skin color

2. Hypoxia is defined as:

   ____ a. low blood sugar levels.

   ____ b. low blood oxygen levels.

   ____ c. low blood pressure.

   ____ d. low blood volume.

3. Agonal respirations are:

   ____ a. occasional and gasping.

   ____ b. rapid and deep.

   ____ c. slow and labored.

   ____ d. rapid and labored.

4. The main purpose of the disability portion of the primary assessment is to determine:

   ____ a. whether the patient will be disabled as a result of his injuries.

   ____ b. whether the patient can wiggle his toes.

   ____ c. whether the patient has serious central nervous system problems.

   ____ d. the overall status of the patient.

5. Which of the following patients is more likely to be stable?

   ____ a. A man fell off his bike and hit his head. He is confused.

   ____ b. A man has had vomiting and diarrhea for 3 days. His skin is cool and moist.

   ____ c. A man was involved in a car crash. There is significant impact into the door where the patient was sitting. He has bruising on his side.

   ____ d. A man fell off a step ladder while stocking shelves at a grocery store. He thinks he may have broken his leg. He is alert and in pain.

Emergency Medical Responder Practice

Determine if the patient in each situation is breathing adequately, has inadequate breathing, or isn't breathing at all. Describe what you would do for each patient to ventilate and administer oxygen.

1. Your patient has a chronic lung disease and tripped on a curb at the mall. He is alert and slightly anxious. His respiratory rate is 24. He can speak four- or five-word sentences.

   _____

   _____

   _____

   _____

2. You come upon a car crash on the way home from work. It is a bad crash. A man has been ejected from his vehicle and thrown about 30 feet. You see him take shallow gasping breaths every 10 seconds or so.

   _____

   _____

   _____

   _____

3. You stop by a family holiday party with your first response vehicle when you see your uncle clutching his chest. He is pale and sweaty. He is breathing about 20 times per minute and speaks full sentences between breaths.

   _____

   _____

   _____

   _____

4. You are called to a fight. A man was struck in the chest with a baseball bat. You see he is breathing very rapidly. Palpation of his chest reveals deformity. The left side is deformed. The breaths are very shallow.

   _____

   _____

   _____

   _____

Critical Thinking Questions

1. What is the difference between adequate and inadequate breathing? How can you tell the difference in your patients?

   _____

   _____

   _____

   _____

2. You are performing the disability portion of the primary assessment on a trauma patient and you find he is unable to wiggle or feel in both of his feet. He is able to move and feel with both hands. Is this a serious condition? What might it mean?

_____

_____

_____

3. You are treating a patient who was in a bad car crash. He is responsive to loud verbal stimulus, and his skin is pale, cool, and sweaty. You can't feel a pulse in either wrist but you can feel one at the carotid artery in the neck. What does this mean?

_____

_____

_____

Expose

To fully perform a primary assessment, you should expose all pertinent areas of the patient. You may have already exposed an area such as the chest to assess breathing or to look for blood. The amount you expose will depend on the location and suspected severity of the injury. You will also factor in patient modesty and environmental conditions, such as cold temperatures, into your decision to expose the patient.

Priority/Updating Incoming EMS Units

At the completion of the primary assessment, you will evaluate the information you obtained and update incoming EMS units. You can do this by radio if you have contact, or you may have someone else call 911 and provide additional information.

You will update incoming units with the following information:

- Patient's age and sex
- Chief complaint
- Level of consciousness
- Pertinent information from ABCs
- Other brief, pertinent information that may affect the ambulance's response or preparation for the scene

A sample EMS update may sound like this:

> "EMS 24, we are on the scene with an alert 24-year-old female patient who was a driver in a motor vehicle collision. She is in the car and complains of neck pain. Her ABCs are good. She has sensation and movement in all extremities. We are stabilizing her c-spine and continuing the assessment. She is the only patient at this crash."

THE LAST WORD

You should now have enough information to determine if your patient is potentially seriously ill or injured or if he seems more stable. Seriously ill or injured patients will require additional assessment and care, usually at a rapid pace. More stable patients require further care that can be done at a more relaxed pace.

TRANSITION ✳

The ambulance arrives on scene. You have only been able to complete the primary assessment and didn't get to do a history, blood pressure, or any further examinations. You update the EMS units.

■ Discussion: *Do you think the incoming EMS units will be upset because you only did a primary assessment? Would you tell the incoming EMS units that the patient was stable or unstable?*

✳ Chapter Review

Multiple Choice

Place a check next to the correct answer.

1. How do your findings in the general impression affect the rest of the patient assessment?

   _____ a. The general impression tells you whether further assessment is necessary.

   _____ b. The general impression helps determine the priority of the patient and a general direction for assessment techniques and speed.

   _____ c. The general impression determines if the scene is safe and if any additional resources are necessary.

   _____ d. The general impression helps you determine whether Standard Precautions are necessary.

2. Suction would first be performed in the _____ part of the primary assessment.

   _____ a. general impression

   _____ b. airway

   _____ c. breathing

   _____ d. circulation

3. The radial pulse is located at the:

   _____ a. neck.

   _____ b. groin.

   _____ c. upper arm.

   _____ d. wrist.

4. When exposing the patient, you will expose:

   _____ a. the upper torso.

   _____ b. the lower extremities.

   _____ c. all relevant areas.

   _____ d. only the chest.

5. You are caring for a patient who fell a considerable distance. You suspect a neck and/or spine injury is likely. You are unable to open the airway enough with a jaw thrust to assist breathing. You should:

   _____ a. continue trying the jaw thrust.

   _____ b. place a towel under the patient's head and try the jaw thrust again.

   _____ c. use the head-tilt, chin-lift maneuver instead.

   _____ d. wait for the paramedics to use advanced airway techniques.

Short Answer

1. What are the differences between the scene size-up and the primary assessment?

   _____

   _____

   _____

2. Can a patient who is breathing not have a pulse?

   _____

   _____

   _____

3. Why do you expose a patient as part of the primary assessment?

   _____

   _____

   _____

Critical Thinking

1. It has been said that the primary assessment is the most important part of the patient assessment process. Do you agree? Why or why not?

   _____

   _____

   _____

2. You are alone caring for a patient until EMS responds. Your patient is breathing inadequately. You are assisting ventilations when you notice a leg that is badly angulated (bent) and looks broken. What should you do?

   _____

   _____

   _____

3. What can pulse rate, skin color, skin temperature, and skin condition tell you about a patient?

   _____

   _____

   _____

Case Study

You are an Emergency Medical Responder at a high school where a student is believed to have consumed alcohol. You arrive at the health office and find the patient will only respond to loud verbal stimulus by moaning. You observe stains on the front of his shirt where he appears to have vomited before you arrived.

1. What would your assessment and care for his airway be?

_____

_____

_____

2. How would you assess the patient's breathing?

_____

_____

_____

You are checking the patient's pulse when you hear a gurgling sound. The patient begins to vomit a considerable amount of liquid and solid material.

3. What Standard Precautions should you be taking?

_____

_____

_____

4. How would you care for the vomiting patient?

_____

_____

_____

The patient stops vomiting. You notice that he can no longer be aroused with loud voice commands. He doesn't respond to pain either.

5. How would you classify this patient on the AVPU scale?

_____

_____

_____

6. What would you advise the incoming ambulance personnel?

_____

_____

_____

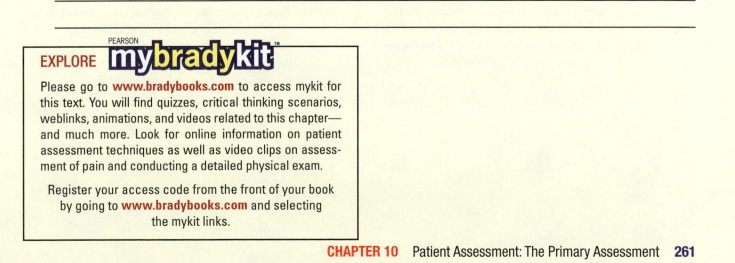

EXPLORE PEARSON **mybradykit**™

Please go to **www.bradybooks.com** to access mykit for this text. You will find quizzes, critical thinking scenarios, weblinks, animations, and videos related to this chapter—and much more. Look for online information on patient assessment techniques as well as video clips on assessment of pain and conducting a detailed physical exam.

Register your access code from the front of your book by going to **www.bradybooks.com** and selecting the mykit links.

Patient Assessment: History and Vital Signs

NAVIGATION GUIDE

The following items provide an overview to the purpose and content of this chapter. The Education Standard and Competency are from the National EMS Education Standards.

Education Standard Assessment (History Taking)

Competency Uses scene information and simple patient assessment findings to identify and manage immediate life threats and injuries within the scope of practice of the EMR.

Knowledge Area History Taking
- Determining the chief complaint
- Mechanism of injury/nature of illness
- Associated signs and symptoms

Objectives After reading this chapter, you should be able to:

1. Define key terms introduced in this chapter.
2. Prioritize the history and vital signs with scene safety and the primary assessment.
3. Describe principles of good communication with patients.
4. Determine a patient's chief complaint, symptoms, nature of illness or mechanism of injury, and pertinent medical history.
5. Summarize the patient's history in communication with other health care providers.
6. Measure a patient's blood pressure, pulse, respirations, and pulse oximetry value.
7. Record a patient's vital signs.
8. Compare a patient's vital signs with the expected values for his age.
9. Assess a patient's skin color, temperature, quality, and capillary refill time.
10. Relate abnormal findings in assessment of the skin to possible problems, such as poor perfusion or oxygenation.
11. Assess a patient's pupils to determine their equality, reaction to light, and size.

NAVIGATION GUIDE *(continued)*

Key Terms Page references indicate first major use in this chapter. The Margin Glossary in this chapter provides definitions as you read.

chief complaint, p. 264

symptom, p. 265

sign, p. 265

mechanism of injury (MOI), p. 267

sphygmomanometer, p. 270

pulse, p. 272

capillary refill, p. 273

systolic pressure, p. 273

diastolic pressure, p. 273

hemoglobin, p. 275

Media Resources Please go to **www.bradybooks.com** to access mykit for this text. You will find quizzes, critical thinking scenarios, weblinks, animations, and videos related to this chapter—and much more. Look for online information on blood pressure and taking a pulse. You will also find a video clip on vital signs assessment.

INTRODUCTION

ASK YOURSELF

- What are the principles of good communication with patients?

- Can you define key terms introduced in this chapter?

Once you have completed the primary assessment, you will need more information to ensure the immediate well-being of the patient and to plan a course of treatment. You will use basic communication skills you have already learned to talk with your patient and find out the reason he called for help and to better explore any medical problems he may have had in the past. At the same time you will obtain the patient's vital signs and look at certain findings that best demonstrate how the body is meeting the basic functions of life. History taking and the findings of your physical examination are combined to ensure that no immediate life threats are missed, to predict changes in patient status, and to complete a thorough patient assessment.

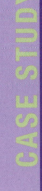

CASE STUDY

THE CALL

On a cold winter evening you are called to a middle-class neighborhood for a woman complaining of difficulty breathing. Your EMR team has been to this address before and knows that this patient often has serious bouts of respiratory problems. Before you arrive, the dispatcher updates you that this patient is not doing well.

- **Discussion:** *What else do you want to know? If your team has been to this address before, what other information may be available?*

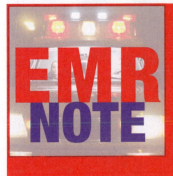

EMR NOTE

Remember the steps in patient assessment. Your scene size-up and primary assessment must come before any secondary assessment or history taking (see Chapter 10). Although it is often easy to forget the first steps (especially with a patient who does not look outwardly sick), the findings of the scene survey focus on your safety and the findings of the primary assessment are the immediate life threats to your patient. Always be thorough and approach patient assessment in an ordered fashion.

■ How do you prioritize the history and vital signs with scene safety and the primary assessment?

■ How do you determine a patient's chief complaint, symptoms, nature of illness or mechanism of injury, and pertinent medical history?

chief complaint the main problem the patient is experiencing; why the patient has called you today.

Patient History

In most cases obtaining a patient history means just talking and listening to your patient. Using good communication skills will make your patient assessment more accurate. Think of how you would like someone to speak to you. Speak clearly and directly, loud enough for patients to hear you but not so loud that it hurts their ears. Allow patients to retrieve their hearing aids or glasses. Bring your body down to their level so you can look them in the eye. Use simple language and don't put words in their mouth. Open-ended questions, questions that require the patient to give more of an answer than "yes" or "no," always provide more accurate information. Instead of asking, "You are having chest pain, right?" consider asking, "What's wrong today?" Instead of asking, "Is the pain sharp?" ask the patient to describe the pain. Letting patients put their complaints in their own words will help differentiate what is actually wrong from what you may assume is wrong.

Chief Complaint

As you learned in Chapter 10, probably the most important question you can ask is "What's wrong?" This simple question allows you to find out why the patient called for emergency help. The **chief complaint** is, in the patient's own words, what is bothering him today (Figures 11-1a and 11-1b ■).

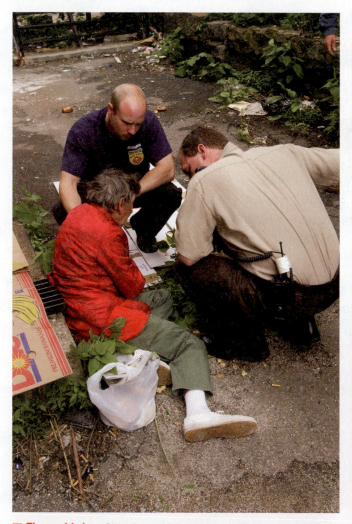

■ **Figure 11-1a** Obtaining a chief complaint from a trauma patient.
(© Mark C. Ide)

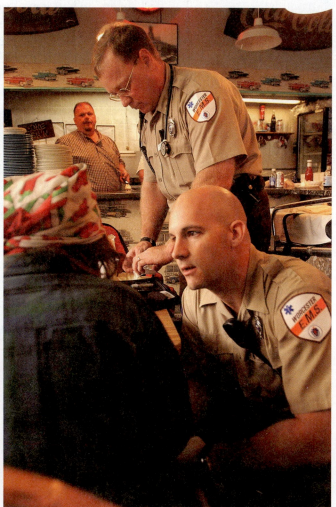

■ **Figure 11-1b** Obtaining a chief complaint from a medical patient.
(© Mark C. Ide)

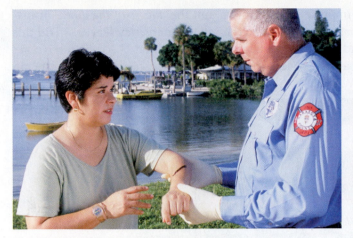

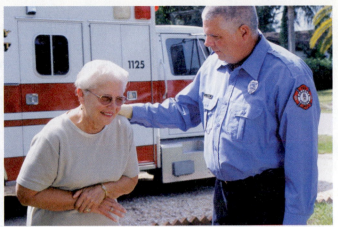

■ Figure 11-2a A sign can be observed by the EMR.

■ Figure 11-2b A symptom is as told to you by the patient.

Most commonly you will obtain the chief complaint from the patient himself. However, there will be times when the patient cannot communicate this to you directly. Young children and unconscious patients are examples of situations where you may have to obtain the chief complaint from family members, bystanders, medical alert jewelry, or even your physical findings. That said, never trust what others tell you if you can communicate with the patient directly.

What a patient tells you or complains of is called a **symptom**. A symptom is a finding relayed to you from the patient and it cannot be observed or measured. "I'm having a pain in my left arm" would be an example of a symptom. Something you observe or measure is a **sign**. Objective findings such as angulated fractures, severe bleeding, or a patient's blood pressure are considered signs (Figures 11-2a and 11-2b ■).

The patient's chief complaint may be specific or vague. In some cases the patient may tell you exactly what is going on. "I'm having an asthma attack" is a good example of a specific complaint. Other times it may be much less specific, for example, "I'm having belly pain." Either way, the chief complaint will help you focus your assessment and treatment.

When the patient cannot communicate with you directly, look for clues from the scene in general. Family members and caregivers often are a great source of information. Use clues from the patient, including medical alert jewelry, medications he is taking, and other physical findings. Also consider scene clues. How warm or cold is the environment? Is there home oxygen, drug paraphernalia, or alcohol on the scene? Are there strong odors or the possibility of poisons or toxins? All of these findings can help you define a chief complaint even when the patient may be unable to communicate directly (Figure 11-3 ■).

symptom a finding relayed to you from the patient; cannot be observed or measured.

sign a finding that is an objective or specific indication of a disease that can be observed.

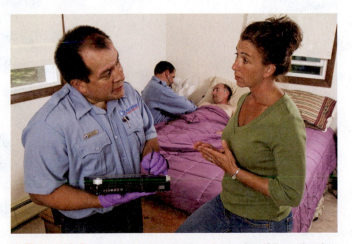

■ Figure 11-3 Get history from family or bystanders if the patient is unresponsive or unable to convey information.

In a medical patient, it is important to inquire about the *nature of the illness* or history of the present illness. What events led up to the call to emergency services? Did this problem develop rapidly or did it occur over a long period of time? Has it gotten worse? Is it a problem associated with a larger disease? For example, if the complaint is chest pain

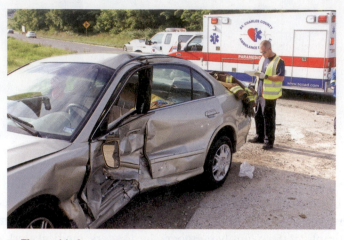

■ **Figure 11-4a** Examine the mechanism of injury to determine the potential for serious injury. (© *Ray Kemp/911 Imaging*)

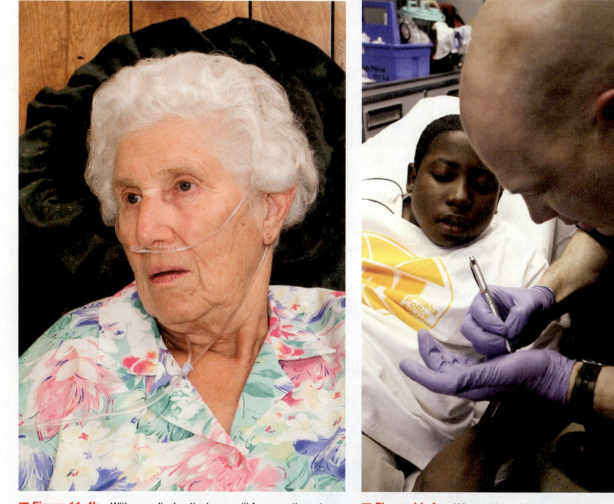

■ **Figure 11-4b** With a medical patient, you will focus on the nature of illness.

■ **Figure 11-4c** When taking a history, speak to the patient at his level.

you might ask, "How long has the pain been going on? Have you had chest pain before?" The patient might tell you that he recently had open heart surgery and he has chest pain every day.

In a trauma patient, you will want to examine the **mechanism of injury (MOI)**. The MOI is the force that was applied to the patient to cause the trauma. In a car versus pedestrian accident, the MOI would be the car striking the patient. Consider aspects such as the height of falls, or the size and speed of the object that struck the patient. How did the patient land, and what did he land on? This information can help you predict the injuries you may be dealing with (Figure 11-4a ■). In a medical patient, you will focus on the nature of the illness (Figures 11-4b and 11-4c ■).

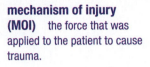

mechanism of injury (MOI) the force that was applied to the patient to cause trauma.

SAMPLE History

Your patient's history does not end with just the chief complaint. Finding more information about the current problem is essential to ruling out life threats and predicting problems to come. The SAMPLE mnemonic may help you remember the key components of a thorough history:

- *S—Signs and Symptoms.* Essentially, this is the chief complaint. What's wrong? What hurts? Again be sure to keep it in the patient's own words.

- *A—Allergies.* Allergies to drugs, food, or other things may be the cause of today's problem or just good information to know to avoid problems in further care. Advanced providers will need this information to avoid administering inappropriate medications.

- *M—Medications.* Record the medications the patient is taking. This may help identify ongoing medical issues. For example, a patient taking insulin would have a history of diabetes. Medications may also give us clues as to what is going on in this particular circumstance. For example, if the patient taking insulin was unconscious, there is a good chance it may be diabetic related (Figure 11-5 ■).

- *P—Past Medical History.* This would include any past medical problems such as diseases or surgeries. Past issues can help identify current problems. The patient may also be wearing a medical alert bracelet or necklace (Figure 11-6 ■). Asking questions like, "Do you see a doctor or have you ever been hospitalized?" may help identify past conditions patients don't recall immediately. Remember that the past medical history can also be confirmed by knowing what medications the patient is taking.

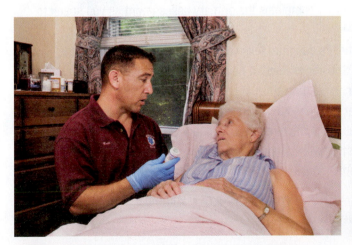

■ **Figure 11-5** Patient medications are a source of information.

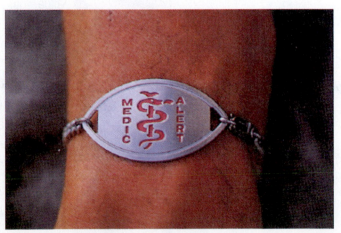

■ **Figure 11-6** Medical alert bracelet.

- L—*Last Oral Intake.* "When was the last time you had anything to eat or drink?" This information may be pertinent to the current condition (accidentally eating peanuts with a peanut allergy) or pertinent if surgery is required.
- E—*Events.* "What led up to calling? What were you doing when this began?" Events help us paint the picture of how the patient got to the point of calling EMS. Often this is extremely important information. Appearances may be deceiving. Chest pain can result from a heart attack or being struck in the chest with a heavy object. A fall can result from slipping on the ice, or getting dizzy and passing out. The history of the present illness will provide essential information to help us draw conclusions.

EMR NOTE

OPQRST

The mnemonic OPQRST is used to help remember what to ask about the patient's signs and symptoms—especially when they involve pain or distress.

Onset—What were you doing when the condition began?
Provocation—Does anything you do make it better or worse (e.g., changing position, movement)?
Quality—Can you describe your pain to me?
Region/**R**adiation—Can you point to where the pain hurts the most? Does the pain seem to move to any other part of your body?
Severity—On a scale of 1–10 with 10 being the worst pain you have ever felt, how would you rate the pain you have now?
Time—How long have you had this pain?

CASE STUDY

THE RESPONSE

You arrive to find the patient sitting up in bed, in obvious respiratory distress. She is awake, but cannot speak. You notice accessory muscle use in her chest and neck. You also notice that her lips are slightly blue. Your partner completes the primary assessment as you speak to the family.

The patient's daughter tells you the patient was "sick all day yesterday." She complained of being tired and nauseated. Tonight just before bed she became short of breath and "got worse fast." You ask if this has ever happened before and the daughter states that it has. She has had multiple bouts of acute pulmonary edema in the past.

Your history will continue later as now your partner tells you he is assisting ventilations.

- Discussion: *What does this history tell you regarding the care your partner begins providing?*

Remember that the history you take is important not just to you, but to all the levels of health care this patient may see. The findings you obtain from the scene such as mechanism of injury, odors, or drug paraphernalia may not be obvious to the doctor in the emergency department. If a patient becomes unresponsive before reaching the hospital you will be the only one to obtain this valuable medical information. Be sure to summarize and give a thorough report of history findings when you transfer care of the patient and always document well.

ASK YOURSELF

- How would you summarize the patient's history in communication with other health care providers?

Stop, Review, Remember

Multiple Choice

Place a check next to the correct answer.

1. Which of the following is an example of an open-ended question?

   _____ a. Are you having chest pain?

   _____ b. Is your chest pain sharp?

   _____ c. What's wrong today?

   _____ d. Do you have high blood pressure?

2. Which of the following would be considered a symptom?

   _____ a. The patient tells you he is having chest pain.

   _____ b. The patient's blood pressure is 120/80.

   _____ c. Your partner notes severe bleeding.

   _____ d. Your partner tells you the patient stopped breathing.

3. The "S" in SAMPLE history stands for:

   _____ a. signs and symptoms.

   _____ b. seriousness and severity.

   _____ c. situation.

   _____ d. single patient.

4. The "A" in SAMPLE history stands for:

   _____ a. alert.

   _____ b. aggravation.

   _____ c. alleviation.

   _____ d. allergies.

5. Which of the following answers would best fit in the "Events" section of the SAMPLE history?

   _____ a. "I was raking leaves and began to have difficulty breathing."

   _____ b. "I had a heart attack 4 years ago."

   _____ c. "I take insulin."

   _____ d. "I'm having chest pain."

Emergency Medical Responder Practice

Define the SAMPLE mnemonic:

1. S _____

2. A _____

3. M _____

4. P _____

5. L _____

6. E _____

Short Answer

1. Explain the term *chief complaint*.

   _____

   _____

   _____

2. Explain how you could obtain a chief complaint if your patient was unable to speak.

   _____

   _____

   _____

3. Explain the term *mechanism of injury*.

   _____

   _____

   _____

   _____

ASK YOURSELF

■ How do you record a patient's vital signs?

■ How do you compare a patient's vital signs with the expected values for his age?

sphygmomanometer
a blood pressure cuff.

Vital Signs

Assessing the patient's vital signs gives you a window into the vital functions that sustain life. Checking a pulse confirms a heartbeat and at least minimal pressure in the cardiovascular system. Assessing respirations examines your patient's effort of breathing. Checking a blood pressure confirms the heart is pumping with enough force and pressure to move blood out to the extremities. Of course there is more information to be found and other measurements to check, but the principle is to determine, at this moment, how well these basic functions are performing. A set of baseline vital signs also allows you to see change over time. Taking multiple sets of vital signs over time (also known as trending) is important because it demonstrates improvement or potential decline. Please see Table 11-1.

For the most part, vital signs are assessed using the basic senses of sight, hearing, and touch. Specialized tools such as a stethoscope, **sphygmomanometer** (otherwise known as a blood pressure cuff), and penlight can give you even more information.

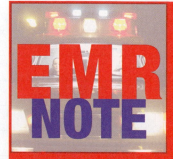

EMR NOTE

Although certain vital signs may be included in the primary assessment, it is extremely important to thoroughly complete that primary assessment before moving on to a baseline set of vital signs. Always beware of letting technology take the place of good assessment skills and common sense.

TABLE 11-1 Vital Signs in Infants and Children

There are significant differences in vital signs between adults and children. These include:

- The size of infants and children make it difficult to locate pulses. When you do locate the pulse, it may be very rapid making it challenging to count and multiply to obtain a proper result.
- Blood pressure is also difficult to obtain and isn't recommended in children under 3.
- Children have the ability to maintain an adequate blood pressure for a long time when they are in shock. Rapid pulse and respirations are early and more reliable indicators of a seriously ill child.
- Mental status is also very valuable as an indicator of patient condition. An infant or child patient that is screaming and wanting to be held by a parent is a good sign while limp, lethargic children who don't seem to care about comfort by their parents are often very seriously ill children.

Additional material on assessing and caring for pediatric patients can be found in Chapter 25.

Respirations

To assess respirations you will count how many times the patient breathes in and out over the course of a minute. This is commonly shortened to count how many times the patient breathes in 30 seconds and then that number is multiplied by 2. However, accuracy is important. If you must assess respirations over 1 minute to ensure an accurate count, then you should do just that. Respirations can be assessed by simply watching the patient's chest or abdomen rise and fall or by placing a hand over the chest or abdomen to feel the rise and fall. Be aware, however, that if the patient realizes you are counting his respirations often he will unconsciously change his rate. It is best to observe breathing without the patient knowing you are watching (Figures 11-7a and 11-7b ■). See Table 11-2.

Respirations should be assessed for both a number and quality. *Rapid, labored, fatigued, shallow,* and *gasping* are all terms you might use to describe the quality of respirations.

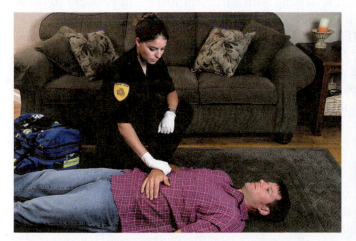

■ **Figure 11-7a** Assessing respirations in a supine patient.

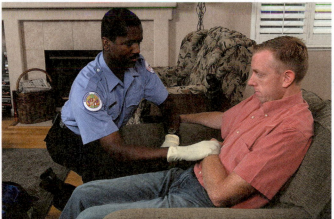

■ **Figure 11-7b** Assessing respirations in a sitting patient.

TABLE 11-2 Normal Respiratory Rates

■ Infant	25–50 breaths per minute
■ Child	15–30 breaths per minute
■ Adult	12–20 breaths per minute

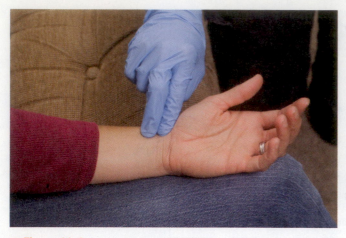

■ **Figure 11-8** Assessing the radial pulse.

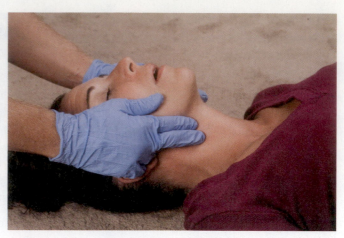

■ **Figure 11-9** Assessing the carotid pulse.

Stridor, snoring, and gurgling are all sounds of upper airway obstruction and should be addressed immediately. Rapid/slow breathing, difficulty speaking, pain with breathing, and wheezing are all ominous signs of respiratory distress.

Pulse

pulse a single pulsation, or beat or throb, of the arteries or heart.

The squeeze of the heart ejects blood into the arteries. This creates a wave of pressure that can be felt in arteries throughout the body. This palpable pressure is called a **pulse**. A pulse can be found anywhere an artery is near the surface of the skin or where it crosses over a bone. Typically the easiest pulse points to feel are over the carotid artery in the neck, the radial artery in the wrist, the brachial artery in the upper arm, and the femoral artery in the groin (there are many other locations to feel for a pulse). The radial pulse is often the most useful pulse point because a pulse there indicates that not only is the heart beating, but it is beating with sufficient force and pressure to move blood out to the distal arm. Often your patient will lose a radial pulse due to low blood pressure in shock situations (Figure 11-8 ■). In taking a pulse, you will assess the number of times the heart beats in 1 minute.

To palpate a pulse, use gentle pressure with your fingers over the area of the artery. Be careful not to use too much pressure as you can actually cut off flow through the artery and lose the pulse. Do not use your thumb as often you can feel your own pulse. Count the number of beats that occur over a minute. Typically, beats are counted for 15 seconds and then multiplied by 4. However, especially in irregular pulses, it may be more accurate to count beats for 30 seconds and multiply by 2 or to count beats over the full minute (Table 11-3 and Figure 11-9 ■).

In addition to the actual rate, you will assess regularity and quality. A pulse can be regular or irregular. Common terms used to describe quality include *strong, weak, bounding,* and *thready* (weak and rapid).

ASK YOURSELF

■ How do you measure a patient's blood pressure, pulse, respirations, and pulse oximetry value?

TABLE 11-3 Normal Pulse Rates	
■ Infant	120–150 beats per minute
■ Child	80–150 beats per minute
■ Adult	60–80 beats per minute

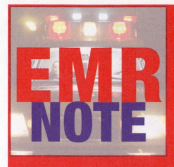

It is difficult to assess a radial pulse in an infant. The small anatomy may make finding this site challenging. Most commonly the brachial artery can be assessed by palpating the space between the bicep and tricep muscle on the upper arm.

Skin

You will assess the color, temperature, quality, and capillary refill time of your patient's skin. These findings can relate a great deal of information about how well your patient is perfusing.

- Color—Normal skin has a pinkish hue and demonstrates good blood flow. Check the skin of dark-skinned patients on the palm of the hand or sole of the feet.
  - Pale skin is a sign of poor blood flow and may indicate poor perfusion. This could be caused by blood loss, but it also could be caused by the peripheral blood vessels constricting away from cold temperatures. Be sure to look at the big picture.
  - Cyanosis is a bluish tint to skin, particularly around the lips and fingernail beds. Cyanosis is a sign of severe hypoxia and should cause you immediate concern.
  - Redness or flushing is caused by dilation of peripheral blood vessels in the skin. This can be caused by certain types of shock, heatstroke, and fever.
  - Yellowish skin is typically caused by liver disease.
- Temperature—Skin is normally 98.6°F (37°C). You can quickly assess skin temperature by feeling it with the back of your hand. Although this is a fairly inaccurate measurement of body temperature, it can quickly alert you to major abnormalities.
  - Cool skin may be a sign of shock.
  - Hot skin may be a sign of fever or heatstroke.
- Condition—Skin is normally dry. Moist skin may be a sign of shock or distress.
- **Capillary refill** time—This test is considered most accurate in children under 6 years of age and sometimes inaccurate in adults. Capillary refill time assesses the length of time it takes to refill the capillary beds of the skin after pressure forces the blood out of them. This can be done by squeezing the fingernail of an adult or the forearm or leg of a child. This gentle squeeze should turn the skin white. When the squeeze is released, blood and a pink color should return to that area. In a healthy person this return should take no more than 2 seconds. Delays could indicate blood loss and shock (Figure 11-10 ■).

Blood Pressure

When the heart squeezes, it exerts pressure. This pressure is the force that drives blood to where it needs to go. Inside the arteries there are two stages of pressure: **systolic**, or the pressure of the contraction of the heart; and **diastolic**, or the pressure of the relaxation of the heart. Measuring these pressures can help us assess how well blood is moving through the cardiovascular system. However, you should remember that a normal blood pressure does not always mean a normal perfusion status in your patient. Just because the pressure inside the vessels is normal, there is no guarantee that the blood is getting where it needs to go.

capillary refill the length of time it takes to refill the capillary beds of the skin after pressure forces the blood out of them; normal is less than 2 seconds.

systolic pressure the pressure of the contraction of the heart.

diastolic pressure the pressure of the relaxation of the heart.

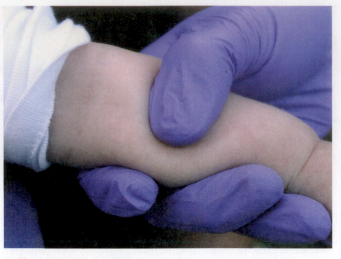

■ **Figure 11-10** Assess capillary refill in children under age 6.

Blood pressure can be measured using a sphygmomanometer or blood pressure cuff. A correct sized cuff should always be used. In general the width of the cuff should cover roughly two-thirds the length of the upper arm and should be large enough that the Velcro can firmly grip when closed. Using a poorly sized cuff can lead to inaccurate readings. There are two ways to assess blood pressure: by auscultation (listening with a stethoscope) or by palpation (feeling). Auscultation is the more accurate of the two but can be difficult in the noisy environment of prehospital medicine.

Blood pressure varies greatly between individuals. "Normal" blood pressure is not a very accurate term. The range will vary depending on the individual and the age of the patient. It is calculated as follows:

■ Child: 80 + (2 × patient's age in years) for systolic and 50–80 mmHg for diastolic
■ Adult: 100 + patient's age in years (up to 150 mmHg) for systolic and 65–90 mmHg for diastolic

You may consider certain "points of concern" when measuring blood pressure in adults. Although you should always look at the larger picture, a systolic blood pressure of less than 90 or greater than 180 should be cause for concern. Remember that it is not always the single number that causes concern, but rather the trend as it reflects changes going on in the body.

Because it may be difficult to properly size a blood pressure cuff in children, there is less emphasis on the need to obtain one. Generally it is not recommended to obtain a blood pressure in children less than 3 years. Even in older children, blood pressure is a notoriously inaccurate measurement of perfusion status.

How to Auscultate a Blood Pressure

1. Select an appropriately sized blood pressure cuff and wrap it around the patient's upper arm. Ideally, shirtsleeves should be removed prior to application. The cuff should rest approximately ½ to 1 inch above the crease in the patient's elbow and the bladder should be centered above the brachial artery (note: some cuffs have markings noting proper placement over the artery). The cuff should be snug, but not too tight. You should be able to easily place one finger under the bottom edge.
2. Find the brachial artery (assess for the pulse) and place the bell of your stethoscope gently over it.

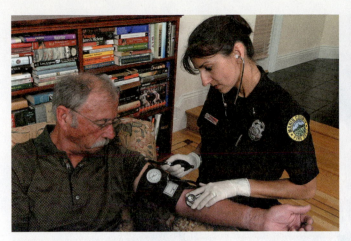

Figure 11-11a Obtaining blood pressure by auscultation.

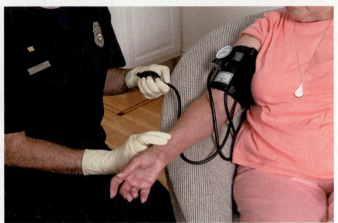

Figure 11-11b Obtaining blood pressure by palpation.

3. Inflate the cuff and listen for pulse sounds. As you continue to inflate, you will lose that pulse. Once you lose the pulse, inflate the cuff 30 mmHg more.
4. Deflate the cuff slowly (approximately 2 mmHg per second) and listen.
5. When you hear two consecutive pulse beats return, record the systolic pressure.
6. Continue deflating and listening to the pulse. When you once again lose the pulse, record the diastolic pressure.
7. Fully deflate and remove the cuff. Record your findings and the limb and position of your patient (Figure 11-11a ■).

If you are unable to hear a blood pressure, you may need to palpate one. Be aware, however, that at times the reason you cannot hear a blood pressure is because it is too low to hear. Always look at the big picture.

Palpating a Blood Pressure

1. Select an appropriately sized blood pressure cuff and wrap it around the patient's upper arm. Ideally, shirtsleeves should be removed prior to application. The cuff should rest approximately ½ to 1 inch above the crease in the patient's elbow and the bladder should be centered above the brachial artery (note: some cuffs have markings noting proper placement over the artery). The cuff should be snug, but not too tight. You should be able to easily place one finger under the bottom edge.
2. Find the patient's radial pulse. Palpate the pulse as you inflate the cuff.
3. Inflate the cuff and palpate the radial pulse. As you continue to inflate, you will lose that pulse. Once you lose the pulse, inflate the cuff 30 mmHg more.
4. Deflate the cuff slowly (approximately 2 mmHg per second) and continue to palpate the radial pulse.
5. When you feel a return of the radial pulse, record the systolic pressure.
6. You will not record a diastolic pressure when palpating. Your documentations will read 120/P (for example). The "P" indicates the blood pressure was palpated. (Figure 11-11b ■)

Pulse Oximetry

A pulse oximeter is a device that measures the amount of oxygen carried on the red blood cells (**hemoglobin**) in your patient's blood. Pulse oximetry can be an accurate way to assess the level of oxygenation in your patient and display trends of improvement or failure.

hemoglobin red blood cells.

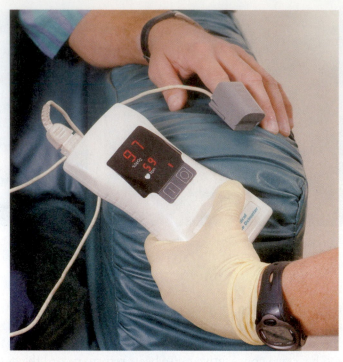

■ **Figure 11-12**   Pulse oximeter.

A pulse oximeter displays oxygen on the hemoglobin in the form of saturation. This is a numeric value displayed as a percentage. Normal oxygen saturation in a healthy person would be 95 to 100 percent. A reading below 95 percent can indicate low levels of oxygen in the blood. Remember that a pulse oximeter is limited to measuring oxygen in the blood. It does not measure oxygen in other tissues. As such, a normal pulse oximetry reading may hide poor oxygenation at the cellular level. Consider the entire patient picture when making a decision about oxygenation (Figure 11-12 ■).

Most pulse oximeters use a probe, or a clamplike device that surrounds a finger or earlobe and transmits infrared light. Although most modern pulse oximeters are very accurate, measurements can be interfered with by nail polish, cold temperatures, and poor circulation, as in shock.

Follow the manufacturer's recommendations for use, but in general the probe is attached to a finger or ear and the machine is turned on. Most pulse oximeters also measure a pulse. If the measured pulse matches with the pulse of your patient, it is reasonable to assume you have a relatively accurate reading. If it does not, assume your reading is inaccurate.

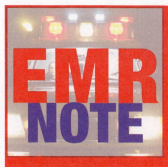

Carbon monoxide (CO) poisoning can give a false normal reading on a pulse oximeter. The CO molecule occupies the same space on the hemoglobin that oxygen would and may trick a pulse oximeter into reporting a higher percentage of oxygen. Because the hemoglobin is fully saturated, the oximetry reading may be normal or even high although the patient may be profoundly hypoxic.

Pupils

Normal pupils react to light by getting smaller when light is present and bigger in low light situations. This predictable reaction can provide information as to the function of the central nervous system and the health of the brain in general.

Use a penlight to shine light into your patient's pupil. (Note: A bright light shining in the eye may be uncomfortable to your patient. Be sure to prepare the patient and limit the amount of time shining a light directly in the eye.) Assess for a constriction of the pupil in response to the light. Pupils should react equally on both sides. If you are in a bright environment it may not be necessary to use a penlight. Simply cover one eye and then expose it to the light of the room. Constriction should occur (Figure 11-13 ■).

Abnormal Pupil Findings

Although many people have pupils of different shapes and sizes, in a patient with acute illness or injury, changes in pupils or in the way pupils react to light can indicate significant problems within the brain (Table 11-4).

ASK YOURSELF

■ How do you assess a patient's pupils to determine their equality, reaction to light, and size?

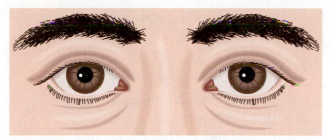

(a) *Normal pupils*

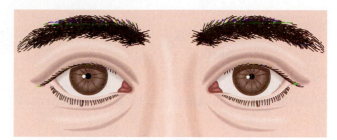

(b) *Constricted pupils*

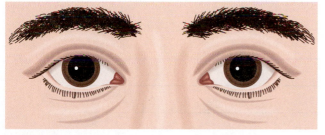

(c) *Dilated pupils*

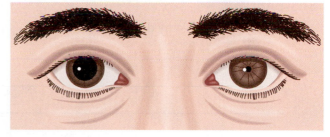

(d) *Unequal pupils*

■ **Figure 11-13** Unequal pupils.

TABLE 11-4	Abnormal Pupil Findings
No reaction	Hypoxia, brain injury
Dilation	Hypoxia, shock
Constricted	Narcotic overdose, stroke
Unequal	Brain injury, stroke, glaucoma, cataract (Note that unequal pupils are a normal finding in some healthy people.)

Stop, Review, Remember

Multiple Choice

Place a check next to the correct answer.

1. If you take a radial pulse for 30 seconds you would multiply your result by _____ to get the pulse rate.

    _____ a. 1

    _____ b. 2

    _____ c. 4

    _____ d. 10

2. Which of the following is NOT a term used to describe respirations?

    _____ a. Grunting

    _____ b. Bounding

    _____ c. Shallow

    _____ d. Gasping

3. To assess the skin of a dark-skinned patient you should check the:

    _____ a. blood pressure

    _____ b. palm of the hands

    _____ c. forehead

    _____ d. back of the neck

4. The top number in the blood pressure is called _____ and represents the _____ of the heart.

    _____ a. systolic/contraction

    _____ b. systolic/relaxation

    _____ c. diastolic/contraction

    _____ d. diastolic/relaxation

5. The pulse oximeter reading represents:

    _____ a. the amount of blood circulating in the body.

    _____ b. the amount of oxygen in the cells.

    _____ c. the percentage of hemoglobin that contains oxygen.

    _____ d. the percentage of blood taken in by the lungs measured against the amount reaching the tissues.

Short Answer

1. What is a pulse? Why do you feel it?

    _____

    _____

    _____

    _____

2. What is the difference between taking a blood pressure by auscultation vs. palpation?

    _____

    _____

    _____

    _____

3. Are gasping respirations adequate? Why or why not?

    _____

    _____

    _____

    _____

Critical Thinking

1. List two reasons a pulse oximeter may provide a normal reading for a patient who is actually in serious condition.

   _____

   _____

   _____

   _____

2. You are on an athletic field at noon assessing a patient's pupils. They appear constricted when you shine your light into them. Why? What can you do to make your exam more accurate?

   _____

   _____

   _____

   _____

CASE STUDY

TRANSITION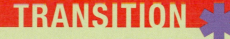

Your partner is successfully bagging the patient and the ambulance is soon to arrive. While your partner controls the airway, you check a radial pulse. Your patient's pulse is rapid (124), regular, and weak. Her skin is cool and wet with perspiration. You notice her fingernails are blue. You next auscultate a blood pressure (92/50). As you are doing this you continue to obtain history from the family. "What was her complaint before this episode?" "Does she have any allergies?" "What was her last oral intake?" As the Paramedics arrive and take over airway management, you report to them your assessment findings. The Paramedics attach continuous positive airway pressure (CPAP) to support the patient's breathing and treat the acute pulmonary edema. They administer nitroglycerine and rapidly transport the patient to the hospital.

■ Discussion: *Why do you think the patient's fingernails are blue?*

THE LAST WORD

History and vital signs provide you with further detail to complete a thorough patient assessment. They pick up where the primary assessment left off and, in conjunction with a complete secondary assessment, identify any additional findings and potential life threats. In addition, they provide a valuable baseline to help identify future trends and transfer potentially critical information to those health care providers who treat the patient but are not on the scene. The key to a useful patient assessment is completeness. Practice a consistent approach to all patients and you will be less likely to miss important findings and more likely to predict potential problems.

Chapter Review

Multiple Choice

Place a check next to the correct answer.

1. Which of the following would be considered a sign?

    _____ a. Chest pain

    _____ b. Nausea

    _____ c. Vertigo

    _____ d. Cyanosis

2. The "P" in SAMPLE history stands for:

    _____ a. pertinent findings.

    _____ b. provocation.

    _____ c. past medical history.

    _____ d. persistence.

3. Another term for a blood pressure cuff is:

    _____ a. sphygmomanometer.

    _____ b. oximeter.

    _____ c. diasystometer.

    _____ d. opthameter.

4. A normal respiratory rate for an adult would be _____ breaths per minute.

    _____ a. 25–50

    _____ b. 15–30

    _____ c. 5–10

    _____ d. 12–20

5. The preferred pulse point to use when assessing the pulse of an infant is the _____ artery.

    _____ a. femoral

    _____ b. brachial

    _____ c. coronary

    _____ d. popliteal

Short Answer

1. Explain the effect carbon monoxide would have on a pulse oximeter reading.

    _____

    _____

    _____

    _____

2. Explain how you would assess capillary refill and what a normal reading would be.

    _____

    _____

    _____

    _____

3. List an abnormal pupil finding and explain what it might indicate.

    _____

    _____

    _____

    _____

Critical Thinking

1. What value is there in trending vital signs?

   _____

   _____

   _____

2. Why is blood pressure an unreliable sign of perfusion?

   _____

   _____

   _____

Case Study

You are tasked with obtaining a history from the family of an unconscious/unresponsive patient.

1. Describe how you could determine the chief complaint prior to the patient becoming unconscious.

   _____

   _____

   _____

2. What other elements of a history might be important with regard to this patient?

   _____

   _____

   _____

Your crew asks you to help obtain a blood pressure. They note they have had trouble auscultating over the loud background noise in the room.

3. Is there an alternative to auscultating a blood pressure? If so, describe the steps you would take.

   _____

   _____

   _____

EXPLORE PEARSON **mybradykit**™

Please go to **www.bradybooks.com** to access mykit for this text. You will find quizzes, critical thinking scenarios, weblinks, animations, and videos related to this chapter—and much more. Look for online information on blood pressure and taking a pulse as well as a video clip on vital signs assessment.

Register your access code from the front of your book by going to **www.bradybooks.com** and selecting the mykit links.

Patient Assessment: Secondary Assessment

NAVIGATION GUIDE

The following items provide an overview to the purpose and content of this chapter. The Education Standard and Competency are from the National EMS Education Standards.

Education Standard Assessment (Secondary Assessment)

Competency Uses scene information and simple patient assessment findings to identify and manage immediate life threats and injuries within the scope of practice of the EMR.

Knowledge Area Secondary Assessment
- Performing a rapid full body scan
- Focused assessment of pain
- Assessment of vital signs

Objectives After reading this chapter, and referring back to Chapter 11, you should be able to:

1. Define key terms introduced in the chapter.
2. Describe the purpose of obtaining a patient's history and vital signs.
3. Explain where obtaining a patient's history and vital signs fits into the patient assessment process.
4. Explain the relationship between good communication skills and obtaining a patient's history.
5. Given several examples of patients' statements, identify the chief complaint.
6. Differentiate between signs and symptoms with respect to the patient assessment and history.
7. Given several scenarios, determine the nature of the patient's illness or mechanism of injury.
8. Explain how the use of the mnemonic SAMPLE can help you obtain a thorough patient history.
9. Given several scenarios, obtain a patient history.
10. Describe the importance of obtaining a baseline set of vital signs and comparing them to later sets of vital signs.
11. Explain the assessment of respirations, pulse, and blood pressure.
12. Obtain complete sets of vital signs from patients of various ages.
13. Compare a patient's vital signs to the normal vital signs for a patient of his age.
14. Relate abnormal skin colors and temperatures to their potential causes, including:
    a. Pale skin
    b. Cyanosis
    c. Redness or flushed skin
    d. Yellowish skin
    e. Cool skin
    f. Hot skin

NAVIGATION GUIDE *(continued)*

Key Terms Page references indicate first major use in this chapter. The Margin Glossary in this chapter provides definitions as you read.

Media Resources Please go to **www.bradybooks.com** to access mykit for this text. You will find quizzes, critical thinking scenarios, weblinks, animations, and videos related to this chapter—and much more. Look for online information on performing patient assessments. You will also find a video clip on conducting a detailed physical exam.

INTRODUCTION

Once you have completed a scene size-up and primary assessment you will begin the **secondary assessment**. The earlier components were centered around dangers and life threats. Consider the secondary assessment as an investigation. It is your job to systematically assess the patient to figure out what else may be wrong.

Depending on your EMS system, you may have only a few minutes until the ambulance arrives—or you may have quite a bit of time. The secondary assessment will be performed during that time and is critical in determining the care you give—as well as gathering vital information for you to hand off to the ambulance crew (Figures 12-1a and 12-1b ■) (See The Big Picture: Assessment of the Medical Patient and The Big Picture: Assessment of the Trauma Patient).

secondary assessment
a second investigation to systematically assess the patient to determine what else may be wrong.

ASK YOURSELF

- Can you define key terms introduced in the chapter?

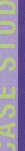

CASE STUDY

THE CALL

Your response unit is dispatched to a patient who "is not feeling well." As you respond to the scene you wonder more about the patient and the variety of conditions that could cause a patient to "not feel well."

- Discussion: *Even though the complaint is vague, what will be your first priorities on the scene?*

The Big Picture
Assessment of the Medical Patient

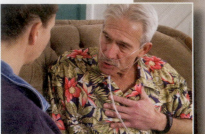

1 Assess based on chief complaint.

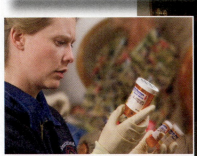

2 Obtain history. Check medications.

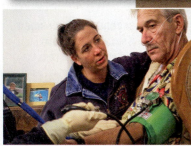

3 Check vital signs. Maintain a positive demeanor.

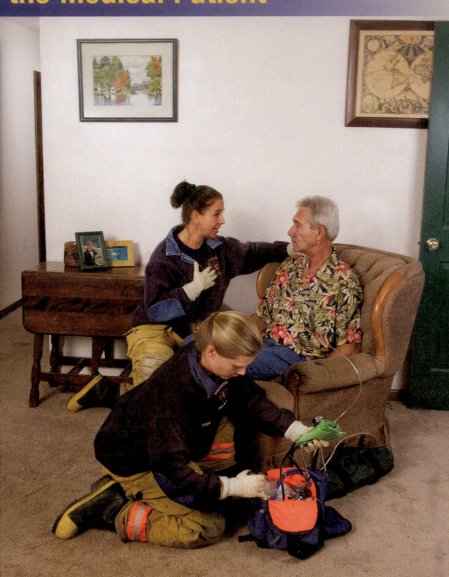

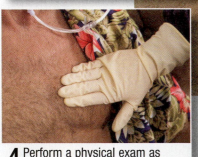

4 Perform a physical exam as appropriate.

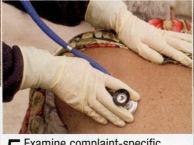

5 Examine complaint-specific areas.

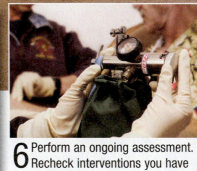

6 Perform an ongoing assessment. Recheck interventions you have performed.

The Big Picture

Assessment of the Trauma Patient

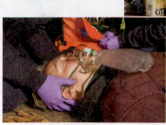

1 Determine patient priority based on MOI, complaint, primary assessment.

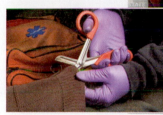

2 Expose the patient as appropriate.

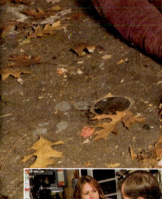

3 Perform a head-to-toe exam.

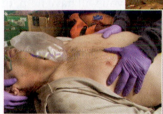

4 Perform vital signs.

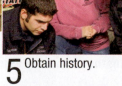

5 Obtain history.

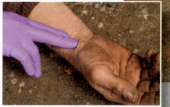

6 Monitor the patient. Continue reassessment until ambulance arrives.

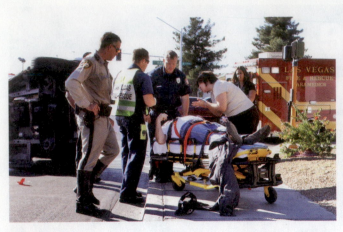

Figure 12-1a You will be assessing two types of patients: medical and trauma. This patient is a trauma patient.

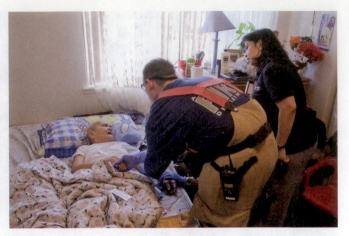

Figure 12-1b Each patient receives a similar primary assessment, but the secondary assessment differs for each patient type. This patient is a medical patient.

General Principles of Assessment

ASK YOURSELF

- What is the purpose of obtaining a patient's history and vital signs?
- How does obtaining a patient's history and vital signs fit into the patient assessment process?

The secondary assessment is a process where you will take a history, perform a hands-on assessment, and take vital signs. You learned about history and vital signs in Chapter 11.

This section discusses general principles of assessment. The first of these is priority. Since you will arrive on scene first, you will have many important priority decisions to make. The most important is making sure the scene is safe and that life threats have been addressed first.

You may be called to a scene where a patient is not breathing. Perhaps another patient will be unresponsive and vomiting, or bleeding. In some cases you will have help; in others you will be alone. You should always focus on life threats to airway, breathing, and circulation (the ABCs) before you begin the secondary assessment. In the cases just mentioned it is quite possible that you will never get to perform the secondary assessment because you will be too busy ensuring the patient has a clear airway, is breathing adequately, and is not bleeding to death.

These things are much more important than the secondary assessment. Said another way, it won't matter if you find the patient has a broken leg if he dies from lack of oxygen. An EMR must have a sense of calmness, focus, and priority in those crucial first minutes at the scene.

An EMT or paramedic will not be upset with you for not performing a secondary assessment. Incoming crews would much rather have a controlled scene and an alive patient rather than a detailed secondary assessment and a dead patient. It is that simple.

Remember the principles of Standard Precautions as you continue the assessment process. The precautions you take against disease initially may not be enough as you continue into the secondary assessment. If you identify bleeding not seen before or if the patient should suddenly vomit and require suction, additional precautions may be necessary. Keep this in mind during the secondary assessment.

Principles of Assessment

There are several methods used to perform an assessment. The methods you use to assess will depend on the patient's condition and the part of the body you suspect is injured or causing the illness.

The three general techniques of assessment are:

Observation—looking at the patient. This is very valuable to find injuries (for example, a broken leg may be deformed and visible) or to notice that the patient is clutching his chest or holding his abdomen indicating pain. Sometimes your observation may simply be that the patient looks "sick." All of these are valuable observations you will use in your assessment and care for the patient.

Auscultating—listening with your ears or with a stethoscope. You may hear a patient wheezing as you approach. You may use a stethoscope to determine if air is moving out of each lung adequately and equally.

Palpating—feeling with your hands. While this may seem to be the most effective because it is the most hands on, if you are good at observation many of the things you find during palpation may not be a surprise. Palpate easily at first, then apply more pressure if needed to fully assess an area. Deep palpation at first may cause unnecessary pain. Palpate areas where you know there is pain last. If you palpate there first, the pain you cause may distract the patient away from the areas you palpate next.

Any assessment you perform should be well thought out and organized. For example, a hands-on assessment is generally performed in a head-to-toe manner. Skipping around could lead to forgetting to assess a particular area.

In an example noted earlier, you may observe a patient's leg is obviously broken. The patient will likely be in pain and want you to treat the leg. Tell the patient that you can see his leg is injured and assure him that you will take care of it. Explain that you must check his whole body for injuries. The leg injury in this case is commonly referred to as a **distracting injury**. This means that it is the most obvious and painful—but it may not be the only injury. This obvious injury could distract you from finding more serious internal bleeding or head injury.

The education standards provide the mnemonic "DOTS" as a reminder of what to look for in the head-to-toe assessment. This stands for:

Deformity

Open injuries

Tenderness (or pain)

Swelling

Assessing Different Patients

The patient assessment process is the same for all patients. That is, each will receive the same major assessment points: scene size-up, primary assessment, secondary physical examination, history, and vitals. However, the order and priority you give to each examination will vary somewhat. This section will explain the assessment of four major types of patients: seriously ill or injured patients, nonseriously ill or injured patients, medical patients, and trauma patients. You will have various combinations of these patient types as you practice as an EMR in the field.

As you complete your primary assessment, you will have some idea of how serious your patient is. You should consider your patient as being serious—or potentially serious—if he appears to be very sick or if he has an altered mental status, severe pain, abnormal vital signs, or any problems with airway, breathing, or circulation. This significantly changes your secondary assessment priorities.

Although you may get to move into the secondary assessment, you should always look back at the primary assessment. The serious patients are more likely to need lifesaving care on a moment's notice. These patients may require ventilation or suctioning. The care performed in the primary assessment is always a priority initially and throughout the call. When your patient is very ill, you may not ever get to a secondary assessment. That is OK.

observation assessment findings found by direct visualization.

auscultating listening with your ears or with a stethoscope.

palpating assessment findings found by pressing on body areas.

distracting injury injury to one area that masks a more serious injury due to increased pain.

ASK YOURSELF

- What is the relationship between good communication skills and obtaining a patient's history?
- How would you identify the chief complaint?

Nonserious patients are those who do not seem to be seriously ill or injured. Consider a patient who fell and hurt his ankle or one who has the flu and wants transportation to the hospital because he is weak. You find that there are no life threats during the primary assessment. Both patients are responsive and answer your questions. The pace of the assessment may not be as urgent as with the serious patients mentioned earlier. You may not have to palpate the head if the only part injured is the ankle.

A word of caution about the patient who doesn't appear serious: Sometimes there are conditions or injuries that don't appear serious at first but become serious later. If in doubt, you should assign a high priority to the patient. It is better to consider the possibility early rather than be surprised later.

Indications a serious hidden condition exists include (but aren't limited to) the following:

- A significant mechanism of injury
- Altered mental status
- Pale, cool, and sweaty skin
- Chest pain or discomfort
- Difficulty breathing
- Severe pain anywhere
- Elevated pulse and respiratory rates

CASE STUDY

THE RESPONSE

You respond and observe a scene that does not appear to pose any dangers. There is one patient who is seated in a chair. He looks like he is having significant difficulty breathing and is pale and sweaty.

- Discussion: *Based on this initial information, do you think the patient is stable or unstable? What actions will you take based on what you see?*

✳ Stop, Review, Remember

Multiple Choice

Place a check next to the correct answer.

1. The primary assessment focuses on immediate life threats while the secondary assessment focuses on:

_____ a. patient history.

_____ b. investigation of complaints.

_____ c. determining type of assessment needed.

_____ d. all of the above.

2. The three principles of assessment are considered to be crucial to finding injuries or illnesses not readily identifiable. They are:

_____ a. auscultation, percussion, and palpation.

_____ b. auscultation, observation, and palpation.

_____ c. observation, palpation, and percussion.

_____ d. imaging, auscultation, and palpation.

3. A distracting injury is one that:

_____ a. focuses your attention thereby missing other assessment findings.

_____ b. is the only injury found in an assessment.

_____ c. always requires all your attention and resources.

_____ d. is found only in the extremities.

4. The trauma patient will usually benefit most from the assessment findings revealed in:

_____ a. surgical history-taking.

_____ b. past medical history-taking.

_____ c. head-to-toe exam.

_____ d. pain assessment.

Matching

Match the following descriptions with the appropriate term.

1. _____ A patient that presents with no immediate life threats

2. _____ A patient that presents with injuries as a result of outside forces

3. _____ A patient that presents with injuries or illnesses not readily identifiable by observation

4. _____ A patient that presents with injuries or illnesses that are immediate life threats

a. Seriously Ill Patient

b. Non-seriously Ill Patient

c. Medical patient

d. Trauma patient

Critical Thinking

Your patient was involved in a motor-vehicle collision where his car went off the road into some bushes. He has some bleeding from his head where he hit the overhead visor and is unconscious. You see no other injuries. He has a low respiratory rate and his heart rate is also slow.

1. Is this patient a seriously ill patient or non-seriously ill patient? Is he a medical patient or a trauma patient?

_____

_____

_____

2. Do his injuries seem consistent with how is he presenting? Would his small head lacerations cause him to be in shock?

_____

_____

_____

3. Is it possible that this patient was a medical patient first that became a trauma patient as a result of his illness?

_____

_____

_____

Medical Versus Trauma Assessment

Medical and trauma patients are different, and their assessments will vary somewhat. While most of the concepts are the same, the order and priorities are a little different. (Tables 12-1 and 12-2)

TABLE 12-1 Integrating the History and Physical Examination— Medical Patient

Patients usually present with complaints—not specific diseases—so your assessment will be based on the body region or system involved.

Cardiac and Respiratory Complaints (chest pain or discomfort, shortness of breath)

HISTORY QUESTIONS (USE SAMPLE/OPQRST)	RELATED PHYSICAL EXAMINATION
■ Obtain details of the pain using OPQRST. ■ If chest pain/discomfort, ask specifically about breathing difficulty. ■ If breathing difficulty, ask specifically about chest pain, discomfort, and palpitations.	■ Carefully assess breathing for adequacy. ■ Determine if breath sounds are present and equal on both sides of the chest. ■ Palpate the chest. ■ Look for other signs of cardiac and respiratory problems (e.g., swollen ankles indicating fluid buildup).

Altered Mental Status

HISTORY QUESTIONS (USE SAMPLE/OPQRST)	RELATED PHYSICAL EXAMINATION
■ Look to the medical history for clues: does the patient have a history of diabetes, seizures, stroke, or psychiatric crisis, or is evidence of drug or alcohol use present? ■ Ask family bystanders for information about the patient and what may have led up to the patient's illness.	■ Look for signs of alcohol or drug use (e.g., scan area around patient, breath odor, vomiting). ■ Perform specific exams as allowed by protocols (e.g., stroke scale, blood glucose). ■ Perform a general head-to-toe exam to look for injuries (e.g., head injury) that could cause the problem. You will need to rely on the physical exam if the patient is unable to answer questions.

Abdominal Pain (may include urinary and obstetrical/gynecological emergencies)

HISTORY QUESTIONS (USE SAMPLE/OPQRST)	RELATED PHYSICAL EXAMINATION
■ Ask the patient to describe the pain in his own words. ■ Have the patient describe the location of the pain (point to it if possible) and if it radiates anywhere. ■ Ask the patient about oral intake and bowel movements/urination. ■ Ask the patient if she is/could be pregnant.	■ Inspect the abdomen. ■ Palpate the abdomen. Palpate the areas of pain last.

General Medical Complaints (general weakness, malaise, nonspecific complaints)

HISTORY QUESTIONS (USE SAMPLE/OPQRST)	RELATED PHYSICAL EXAMINATION
■ Use the SAMPLE history as a general guide to determine if a more specific issue can be raised/discovered. ■ You will learn later in this text that nonspecific complaints, especially in women, the elderly, and diabetic patients, may actually be signs of heart attack. Don't simply dismiss it as nonserious when a patient feels something is wrong but can't tell you why.	■ Perform a general head-to-toe examination. ■ Examine any systems you believe may be affected.

TABLE 12-2 Integrating the History and Physical Examination— Trauma Patient

Remember: Consider mechanism of injury as you assess.

Head

PHYSICAL EXAM—AREAS TO EXAMINE "DOTS"	HISTORY—SPECIFIC QUESTIONS TO ASK
■ Visually inspect the head. ■ Palpate the skull and facial bones. ■ Look for discharge from the nose and ears. ■ Check the mouth for vomit, secretions, blood, and loose/dislodged teeth.	■ Did you hit your head? ■ Does your head hurt? ■ Did you pass out?

Neck (maintain cervical spine stabilization if indicated)

PHYSICAL EXAM—AREAS TO EXAMINE "DOTS"	HISTORY—SPECIFIC QUESTIONS TO ASK
■ Visually inspect the neck. ■ Examine the anterior (front), which contains the trachea. ■ Examine the posterior (back); palpate along the spine. ■ Look for bleeding from large vessels and soft tissue injuries.	■ Do you have any pain in your neck? (Never ask the patient to move his head to check for this.) ■ Does your neck feel stiff or abnormal in any way?

Chest

PHYSICAL EXAM—AREAS TO EXAMINE "DOTS"	HISTORY—SPECIFIC QUESTIONS TO ASK
■ Visually inspect the chest. ■ Palpate the anterior and lateral chest for deformity and to evaluate expansion (should be equal). ■ Ask the patient to take a deep breath. Determine if that causes pain. ■ Put slight pressure against the ribs as the patient takes another deep breath. Determine if this causes pain.	■ Does your chest hurt? If so, where? ■ Does the pain change when you take a breath? ■ Do you feel like you have trouble breathing?

Abdomen

PHYSICAL EXAM—AREAS TO EXAMINE "DOTS"	HISTORY—SPECIFIC QUESTIONS TO ASK
■ Visually inspect the abdomen—look for scars, distention, pregnancy, and open wounds. ■ Palpate the four quadrants of the abdomen gently. Palpate any areas in which the patient complains of pain last.	■ Do you have any pain or discomfort? (Note: Abdominal injuries can also be described as cramping, colicky, burning, and many sensations other than "pain.") ■ Can you describe the pain? ■ Have you vomited? ■ Are you pregnant?

Pelvis

PHYSICAL EXAM—AREAS TO EXAMINE "DOTS"	HISTORY—SPECIFIC QUESTIONS TO ASK
■ Visually inspect for deformity and open wounds (includes shortening/rotation of legs due to pelvic/hip injury). ■ Palpate pelvis for deformity and pain. Do not apply very firm pressure or try to "rock" pelvic bones.	■ Do you have any pain in your hips? (The term "hip" is used by patients to describe the region of the pelvis and hip joint.)

(continued)

TABLE 12-2 Integrating the History and Physical Examination—Trauma Patient, *continued*

Extremities	
PHYSICAL EXAM—AREAS TO EXAMINE "DOTS"	**HISTORY—SPECIFIC QUESTIONS TO ASK**
■ Visually inspect each extremity for deformity and open wounds. ■ Palpate each extremity to further examine for deformity, open wounds, and pain on palpation.	■ Do you have pain in your arms or legs? ■ Did you strike your arms or legs? ■ When you fell, did you try to catch yourself with your arm(s)?

Posterior (assess only if it does not injure the spine)	
PHYSICAL EXAM—AREAS TO EXAMINE "DOTS"	**HISTORY—SPECIFIC QUESTIONS TO ASK**
■ Visually inspect for deformity and other signs of injury. ■ Palpate the back (along the spine and soft tissues) for deformity and tenderness.	■ Does your back hurt? ■ What part of your back hurts? ■ Can you describe the pain? ■ Does your neck hurt? (Often back and neck injuries occur together.)

With a trauma patient the hands-on head-to-toe exam is usually the most beneficial for finding injuries. Trauma involves outside forces and frequently leaves anything from bruising to deformity—things you can see and often feel when you examine.

Medical patients have something wrong on the inside. You can't palpate a heart attack or a stroke, so your history provides a majority of the information. Since you can't see the pain, you need to have the patient give you detailed information about it. The SAMPLE history and OPQRST mnemonic will help you gather pertinent information. These were discussed in Chapter 11. (Scans 12-1 and 12-2)

This doesn't mean you will never take a history from a trauma patient or do a head-to-toe exam on a medical patient, just that you will focus your secondary assessment efforts on what gives the most and best information in the time you have. You will also integrate vital signs into your secondary examination.

One additional difference is that the trauma patient may have a suspected neck injury. In this case you or a member of your crew will have begun **manual stabilization** of the head and neck. This should be continued throughout the assessment process and until the patient has been fully immobilized on a backboard with a cervical spine immobilization collar in place.

Head-to-Toe Examination

The physical examination is traditionally done from head to toe. This section will provide detailed information on this examination.

First, observe the patient quickly from head to toe. Look for any obvious signs of injury such as deformity, blood soaking through clothing, or areas the patient is holding or complaining of pain. You may note that the patient winces when he breathes or is holding himself awkwardly, indicating pain or discomfort.

Observation may also reveal that one side of the body appears differently than the other. For example, one leg may look shorter and the foot is rotated differently than the other, or one side of the face appears uneven with the other. This **asymmetry** is an important sign of injury.

You may have to expose parts of the patient to perform the examination. Heavy clothing may hinder your ability to find injuries and perform a proper assessment.

manual stabilization
Using your hands to prevent movement of the head and neck.

asymmetry unevenness.

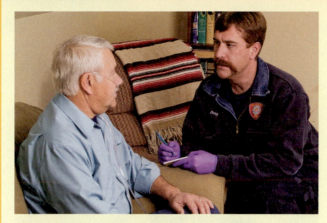

12-1a Obtain a history from the patient or bystanders. Take a history of the complaint.

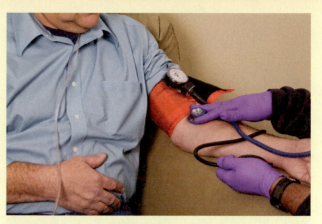

12-1b Vital signs: taking blood pressure.

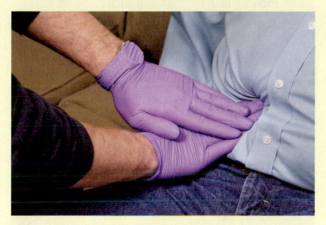

12-1c Perform an examination of specific complaint areas, (for example, palpate abdomen).

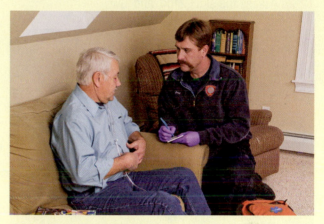

12-1d Obtain additional information about specific complaints, such as pain.

Items such as winter clothing and protective apparel worn in the workplace are particularly problematic.

There are several considerations when exposing a patient. Expose the patient in a way that protects the patient's modesty in public and minimizes unnecessary damage to clothing. In cold environments you will not fully expose your patient; instead you will expose briefly and then re-cover your patient.

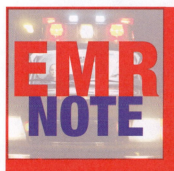

EMR NOTE

Be sure to learn the DOTS mnemonic as a reminder of things to look for in your exam:

Deformity
Open injury
Tenderness
Swelling

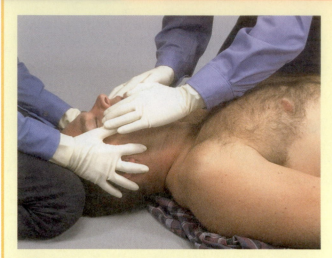

12-2a Assess the skull, face, and jaw.

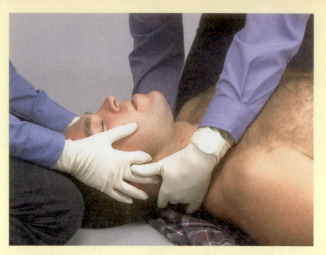

12-2b Examine both the front and back of the neck.

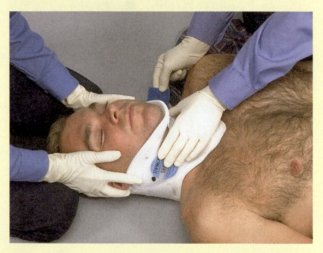

12-2c Apply a rigid cervical collar, if needed, and if you are trained and authorized to do so.

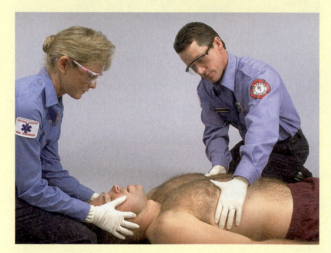

12-2d Examine the chest.

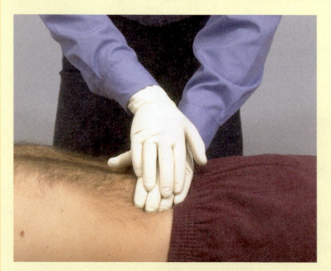

12-2e Palpate each quadrant of the abdomen.

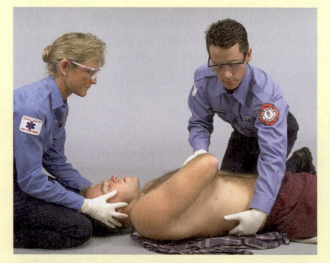

12-2f Examine the patient's back.

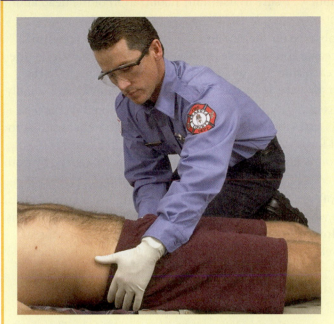

12-2g Examine the pelvis by applying gentle pressure.

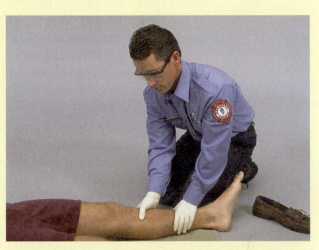

12-2h Observe and palpate each extremity.

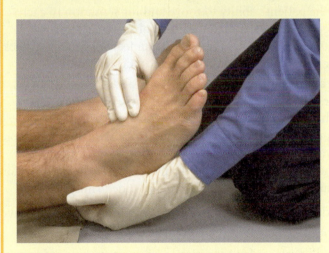

12-2i Also check the pulse in each extremity.

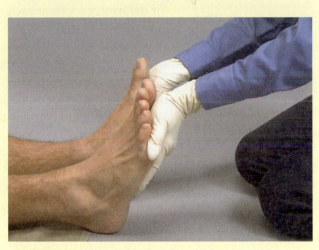

12-2j Check for sensation and the ability to move fingers and toes.

You will begin an assessment of the following areas:

Head—Assess for deformity of the entire head, including the skull and facial bones. Look for asymmetry of facial bones and discharge from the nose or ears. Check the mouth for secretions, vomit, injury, and bleeding that could affect the airway. Loose or damaged teeth may pose an airway hazard as well.

Neck—The neck holds several vital structures including the spine, the trachea, and the blood vessels that supply the brain. Injury to any of these can be fatal. Look for open wounds and deformity, palpate the spine at the back of the neck, and look for a **stoma**—a surgical opening created in the neck for the patient to breathe through.

stoma breathing hole in the neck directly into the trachea.

Observe for muscles that seem to protrude in the neck when the patient breathes. This is called accessory muscle use and indicates the patient is having difficulty breathing.

If you suspect a neck or spine injury, be sure to maintain stabilization of the head and neck throughout the assessment.

Chest—Look at the chest and observe for the rise and fall associated with breathing. The movement should be noticeable and adequate. It should also be symmetrical—the same amount of movement on each side. You or a fellow EMR may also listen to the chest with a stethoscope to hear air enter both sides of the chest adequately and equally.

Palpate the chest to feel for signs of injury, including deformity, and crepitus, the feeling created by broken bones (in this case ribs) rubbing together. Remember that trauma to the chest may be blunt (a direct force such as from a steering wheel in a crash) or penetrating (an open wound from a knife or gunshot). Look for injuries caused by both mechanisms of injury.

Abdomen—Observe for signs of pain, including the patient holding his abdomen. Your physical exam may reveal open wounds and in rare cases protruding abdominal organs. You may gently palpate the abdomen to see if this causes pain in any particular area. Your observations may also reveal scars from prior surgery or a suspicion that the patient may be pregnant.

Pelvis—Palpate the pelvis for pain and deformity. Palpate gently at first and apply pressure that increases slightly. Never palpate past the point that a patient feels pain.

Extremities—Observe all four extremities for deformity and open wounds. The extremities should be about the same length and symmetrical. Palpate each extremity for deformities. Check each for the patient's ability to move and for sensation in each extremity. Ask the patient to wiggle his fingers, then toes, and observe each for movement. Touch each extremity to determine if the patient can feel your touch. Check each extremity for pulses, capillary refill, and skin color to assess circulation.

laterally recumbent lying on one's side.

Posterior—The patient's back is actually the back of the chest and abdomen and can be the location or origin of the same serious injuries as the front of these important regions. You may not get to examine the back in some patients because moving them to do so would cause further injury. Only palpate the posterior if it will not cause further injury or if the patient is in a position that allows you to palpate the posterior without movement (such as **laterally recumbent**). Check the entire posterior from the neck to the buttocks for signs of injury (DOTS). Palpate along the spine to check for pain or deformity.

As you complete the secondary assessment, you will use the information you have found to:

- Determine what care you will perform for conditions or injuries uncovered in the assessment.
- Document your findings on appropriate reports (this may not be done at the exact time of assessment).
- Provide an accurate report of your findings to EMTs.

Some of the injuries you find in the secondary assessment will be treated right away. Life-threatening conditions are treated immediately. Stop the assessment process and treat the condition. An example might be finding bleeding you didn't see in the primary assessment, or noticing the patient's breathing has become shallow and inadequate when assessing the chest.

Certain factors can make your assessment more difficult or inaccurate. It is your responsibility as an EMR to rise above these issues to obtain the best and most accurate assessment possible. Some of these issues are:

- *Confusion and excitement at the scene*—Emergency scenes are often chaotic. You must focus and keep on track. Don't let the chaos control you. Remain calm.

- *Patients who are fearful or in denial*—Some patients don't want to admit they have pain because they are scared of hospitalization or in denial they are having a serious problem such as a heart attack. Observe your patient. Sometimes you will notice a patient is in pain (wincing, seeming uncomfortable) or minimizing symptoms. Provide a calm, reassuring presence and continue to assess the patient. Encourage him to communicate with you about his concerns as well as his condition.

- *Altered mental status*—Some patients will be unable to answer your questions. In this case you will depend more on your head-to-toe examination and information from family and bystanders.

- *Patients with disabilities*—You may find patients with **cognitive disabilities** and those with vision and hearing loss. Modify your exam to explain more of what you are doing as you assess. Use terms that the patient will understand and relate to. Do not talk down to the patient.

cognitive disabilities
impairment of thinking.

- *Heavy clothing*—Your physical assessment may be hindered by heavy clothing. This may occur in cold climates or in workplace settings where workers are required to wear heavy protective clothing. Your challenge will be assessing the patient while not aggravating injuries when removing the clothing. Sometimes the clothing can be removed, pushed aside for an exam, or in some cases cut from the patient.

- *Distracting injuries*—Patients generally only feel pain in one place. A patient with a broken bone or deep laceration may concentrate on only that one wound when there are other, more serious injuries. Be sure that you do not focus on the obvious and fail to find the more serious conditions if present.

ASK YOURSELF
- How would you obtain a patient history?

- *Difference among the ages*—Pediatric and geriatric patients will respond differently to conditions such as pain and may have physical differences and vital signs much different than an average adult.

✳ Stop, Review, Remember

Multiple Choice

Place a check next to the correct answer.

1. It is important when doing a head-to-toe exam to note any unequal responses between the two sides of the body as this can be a serious finding. This is referred to as:

   ____ a. asymmetry.

   ____ b. malformation.

   ____ c. improper equality.

   ____ d. proximate causation.

2. After assessing the head using the "DOTS" mnemonic, you should next observe the _____ using the same method.

   ____ a. chest

   ____ b. abdomen

   ____ c. neck

   ____ d. extremities

3. When observing the abdomen, it is important to note signs of previous surgery which will be most readily visible by:

   ____ a. auscultation for inappropriate bowel sounds.

   ____ b. observation of scars.

   ____ c. palpation of masses of scar tissue.

   ____ d. deep palpation of retroperitoneal tissues.

4. Patients who are unable to fully comprehend your questions or answer them appropriately must be given a thorough a(n):

   ____ a. head-to-toe exam.

   ____ b. abdominal exam.

   ____ c. chest exam.

   ____ d. head exam.

True/False

Mark whether each of the following statements is true (T) or false (F).

1. _____ All trauma patients should be completely exposed regardless of scene location and external conditions.

2. _____ Checking the mouth and airway is done during your assessment of the head.

3. _____ Life-threatening condition found only in the secondary assessment should be treated once the entire exam is complete.

4. _____ Age is a distracting condition that can alter your assessment findings.

Critical Thinking

You are assessing a patient who is suffering from chest pain. He is sweating and pale and says this is the worst pain that he has ever felt. It is in the center of his chest and radiates to his left arm and his jaw. He says he feels like he is having a heart attack again.

1. What body section is likely to reveal findings consistent with a heart attack?

_____

_____

_____

_____

2. What might you expect to observe/auscultate/palpate?

_____

_____

_____

_____

3. Will his injuries be readily identifiable by your assessment findings?

_____

_____

_____

_____

ASK YOURSELF

■ What is the importance of obtaining a baseline set of vital signs and comparing them to later sets of vital signs?

■ How would you explain the assessment of respirations, pulse, and blood pressure?

Vital Signs

Chapters 10 and 11 discussed how to accurately obtain vital signs. These include pulse; respiratory rate; skin color, temperature, and condition; and pupils. This section will help you apply these findings in your secondary assessment. You may also integrate pulse oximetry into your vital signs toolbox.

Remember that one set of vital signs is a baseline; two or more sets of vital signs show trends which are the most valuable when determining patient condition and stability. Depending on how close the ambulance is, you may only have time for one set of vital signs. In this case the ambulance crew can use yours as a baseline to compare their subsequent vital signs to.

If you have more time on the scene and the patient's condition allows (for example, you don't have more important priorities such as ventilating the patient) you should complete vital signs more frequently. They should be taken about every 5 minutes for unstable patients and at least every 15 minutes for patients who appear stable.

Any one part of the assessment process is valuable, but the true value comes when you consider the patient's complaint, the components of the primary and secondary assessments, mechanism of injury (in trauma patients), vital signs, and history together.

Table 12-3 provides examples of how you will correlate your findings in the secondary examination with the history and vital signs.

Reassessment

The secondary assessment isn't the end of the assessment process. You will continue to monitor the patient until the EMTs arrive and you turn the patient fully over to their care (Scan 12-3).

As mentioned already, assessment isn't a simple start-to-finish proposition. Patients' conditions often change during your care. Sometimes this is for the better; sometimes worse. The ongoing or **reassessment** process ensures you are prepared for all of the possible changes.

If you have completed your secondary assessment and treated all of the conditions you are able to and the EMTs still haven't arrived, continue reassessing the patient. Reassessments should be done every 5 minutes for the unstable patient (this means it is done almost continuously) and at least every 15 minutes for the stable patient, as follows:

1. Repeat the primary assessment. Carefully assess the ABCs and the patient's level of responsiveness.
   - *Level of responsiveness*—Changes in responsiveness are very indicative of the patient's condition. Patients who become more oriented are usually getting better. Those who show a decrease in responsiveness are usually getting worse and will require additional care.

ASK YOURSELF

- What are the differences in obtaining complete sets of vital signs from patients of various ages?
- How do you compare a patient's vital signs to the normal vital signs for a patient of his age?
- How do you relate abnormal skin colors and temperatures to their potential causes, including:
  - Pale skin
  - Cyanosis
  - Redness or flushed skin
  - Yellowish skin
  - Cool skin
  - Hot skin

reassessment strategic ongoing assessments of the patient's condition and your interventions until the arrival of EMS.

TABLE 12-3 Correlating Vital Signs to Patient Condition

CONDITION	VITAL SIGN CHANGES	PHYSICAL EXAM CORRELATIONS
Shock (e.g., internal injury from a car crash or violence)	■ Increasing pulse ■ Increasing respirations ■ Skin becomes cool, pale, and moist ■ Blood pressure drops (late sign)	■ Mechanism of injury indicating shock is possible ■ Increasing anxiety or restlessness ■ Physical exam showing chest, abdominal, or pelvis injury or multiple bone fractures
Chest pain or discomfort (responsive patient)	■ Abnormal pulse rate (may be high, low or irregular) ■ Elevated respiratory rate ■ Skin cool, pale, moist ■ Blood pressure may be elevated or low	■ Complains of chest pain, discomfort, or tightness ■ May deny chest pain but experiences difficulty breathing ■ May have a history of cardiac problems and take medications for this problem ■ May also have a history of high blood pressure, high cholesterol, or diabetes ■ Is the patient in the tripod position? Does he use accessory muscles to breathe or have other obvious signs of distress?
Serious closed head injury	■ Decreased pulse ■ Increased blood pressure ■ Abnormal respiratory patterns ■ Abnormal pupillary response	■ Mechanism of injury involving the head ■ May complain of a headache ■ Decreasing mental status

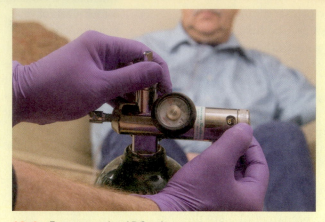

12-3a Reassess the ABCs. Assure you have oxygen in the cylinder and that it is reaching the patient.

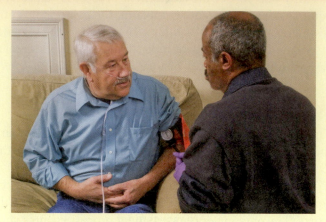

12-3b Reassess patient complaint(s).

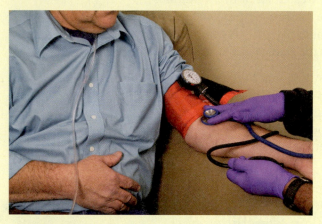

12-3c Reassess vital signs.

ASK YOURSELF

- What is the significance of finding that a patient has abnormally moist skin?
- How do you determine and interpret capillary refill time?

trending charting of upward or downward patterns in vital signs.

- *Airway*—Ensure that the airway remains open. This is especially important if the patient's mental status has deteriorated. Suction any blood, secretions, or vomit from the airway.
- *Breathing*—Assess the rate and depth of respirations. If either have slipped to an inadequate level, you must begin ventilating the patient. If you have administered oxygen, make sure the mask or cannula is still seated appropriately on the patient's face. Be sure the oxygen tank is at an adequate level and that the oxygen tubing is unobstructed and not kinked.
- *Circulation*—Check the patient's radial pulse (if responsive) or the carotid pulse (if unresponsive). Feel the patient's skin for temperature and condition. Note the patient's skin color.

2. Repeat vital signs. This allows **trending**, the ability to compare multiple sets of vital signs.
3. Check the patient's complaints. If a medical condition such as chest pain or difficulty breathing exists, determine if it is better or worse since the last time you checked. In trauma, check the level of pain. Also reassess for new

complaints that may have developed since the patient was in your care. For example, a patient with chest pain may now complain of difficulty breathing.

4. Check any interventions you have performed. Check your oxygen delivery devices, splints or bandages you have applied, and anything else you have done for your patient to ensure it is functioning properly and isn't causing harm.

If any of your interventions aren't functioning properly, adjust or reapply them. You may also need to change your intervention. For example, you may be administering oxygen by nasal cannula and the patient begins to deteriorate (he develops cool, moist, pale skin, and anxiety). You will switch to a mask or ventilate the patient if necessary.

CASE STUDY

TRANSITION

You approach the patient and he is as you suspected, in considerable distress and unstable. You update the ambulance immediately and begin caring for the patient's ABCs. The patient appears to be worsening before your eyes. His level of responsiveness has dropped considerably. You are concerned that his breathing may be inadequate and prepare to ventilate the patient.

- Discussion: *Will you be able to do a secondary assessment for this patient? Why or why not? How would your care change if two coworkers heard the call and stopped by to help?*

ASK YOURSELF

- What is the difference between blood pressure auscultation and palpation?

- What is the meaning of pulse oximetry values?

- How do you assess a patient's pupils?

- How do you relate the following findings to their potential causes?
  - Pupils that do not react to light
  - Dilated pupils
  - Constricted pupils
  - Unequal pupils

- How do you communicate concise, organized, pertinent patient histories and vital signs orally and in writing?

THE LAST WORD

Each part of the assessment process is important, from the foundational scene size-up to the lifesaving primary assessment, to the investigational secondary assessment, and finally the ongoing reassessment. Your patient assessment not only identifies things that may be wrong with the patient, but also directs the care you will need to perform until the EMTs arrive.

Chapter Review

Multiple Choice

Place a check next to the correct answer.

1. Blood pressure, pulse, and respiratory rate are part of:

   _____ a. primary assessment.

   _____ b. vital signs.

   _____ c. scene size-up.

   _____ d. general impression.

2. Patient conditions can often change as a result of the care you have given or not given. This is generally found by:

   _____ a. primary assessment.

   _____ b. reassessment.

   _____ c. vital signs.

   _____ d. secondary assessment.

3. Reassessment of a patient with chest pain during the ongoing assessment can reveal a change. Reassessing vital signs in the ongoing assessment creating a pattern is called:

    _____ a. trending.

    _____ b. vitalizing.

    _____ c. proximation.

    _____ d. signing.

4. Assessment findings found by direct visualization or exposure are referred to as:

    _____ a. palpating.

    _____ b. percussion.

    _____ c. observation.

    _____ d. auscultating.

5. A trauma patient found to have a suspected neck injury should have immediate _____ placed.

    _____ a. ongoing assessment

    _____ b. manual stabilization

    _____ c. long backboarding

    _____ d. direct pressure

6. An exam of the back or posterior should be comprehensive checking from the neck to the:

    _____ a. chest.

    _____ b. lower back.

    _____ c. buttocks.

    _____ d. feet.

7. Patients with disabilities will often not understand your assessment. These patients will need:

    _____ a. all tests explained to them to help them remain calm.

    _____ b. a less detailed exam.

    _____ c. more frequent physical exams.

    _____ d. less vital signs assessed.

8. Patients commonly only feel pain in one place and it may not be the most serious injury. This is more commonly referred to as:

    _____ a. trending.

    _____ b. distracting injury.

    _____ c. reassessment.

    _____ d. a broken leg.

True/False

Indicate whether each of the following is true (T) or false (F) on the line provided.

1. _____ A patient's airway needs to be reassessed constantly in the potentially unstable patient.

2. _____ Injuries not found during the primary assessment are not considered to be life threatening.

3. _____ A trauma patient will never receive a detailed medical history.

4. _____ The patient with a suspected spinal injury should be held in place via manual stabilization.

5. _____ The first set of vital signs obtained during patient contact are referred to as baseline vital signs.

6. _____ Obtaining at least two more sets of vital signs allows for trending.

7. _____ Proper palpation of an area always requires deep, constant pressure regardless of the amount of pain found.

8. _____ Exposing the chest of a nontrauma patient in cardiac arrest is not necessary for care of the patient.

Critical Thinking

The seriously ill patient requires an intense amount of care at varying levels. As such, a good foundation is necessary to create a starting point for care. Improper vital signs or assessment findings can greatly alter the care or services rendered from that point on by the care team. Listed on page 303 are some assessment findings or key terms. Describe the relevance of your findings as they would relate to the seriously ill patient.

1. Abnormal vital signs

_____

_____

_____

_____

2. Pain on palpation to the abdomen

_____

_____

_____

3. Unexplained pain to the head

_____

_____

_____

4. Unstable bones/joints in the pelvis

_____

_____

_____

Communication and Documentation

NAVIGATION GUIDE

The following items provide an overview to the purpose and content of this chapter. The Education Standard and Competency are from the National EMS Education Standards.

Education Standard Preparatory (Therapeutic Communication, EMS System Communication, Documentation)

Competency Uses simple knowledge of the EMS system, safety/well-being of the EMR, medical/legal issues at the scene of an emergency while awaiting a higher level of care. Practices principles of communicating with patients in a manner that achieves a positive relationship.

Knowledge Areas Therapeutic Communication
- Interviewing techniques
EMS System Communication
Communication needed to:
- Call for resources
- Transfer care of the patient
- Interact within the team structure
Documentation
- Recording patient findings

Objectives After reading this chapter, you should be able to:

1. Define key terms introduced in this chapter.
2. Explain the process of therapeutic communication.
3. Describe actions that will improve your communication with a patient in order to accomplish the goals of patient care.
4. Given a variety of scenarios, demonstrate effective therapeutic communications.
5. Discuss the role of body language in communications.
6. Use both open-ended and closed-ended questions to efficiently obtain pertinent information from patients.

7. Recognize pitfalls that can interfere with a successful patient interview.
8. Give a brief, organized, pertinent report to the EMS providers assuming care of the patient.
9. Use portable, mobile, or base station radios to communicate with emergency services personnel.
10. Describe the general rules of communicating by radio.
11. Discuss the special considerations in communicating with patients who are:
    a. Hearing impaired or deaf
    b. Visually impaired or blind
    c. Mentally impaired

NAVIGATION GUIDE (continued)

12. Explain the information that is recorded for each prehospital care report data element.
13. Describe the actions to be taken and documented when a patient refuses care and transportation.
14. Differentiate between subjective and objective patient information.
15. List examples of special reporting situations.

Key Terms Page references indicate first major use in this chapter. The Margin Glossary in this chapter provides definitions as you read.

Media Resources Please go to www.bradybooks.com to access mykit for this text. You will find quizzes, critical thinking scenarios, weblinks, animations, and videos related to this chapter—and much more. Look for online information on documentation and the PCR. You will also find a video clip on alternative methods of communicating with children.

INTRODUCTION

As an Emergency Medical Responder (EMR), communication and documentation will be an important part of your duties. While you may feel that studying care for patients suffering heart attacks and trauma is more important to prepare you as an EMR, communication and documentation will be a vital part of everything you do—including when you care for patients with heart attacks and trauma.

Imagine responding to a chaotic scene—or arriving to care for a patient who is panicking because of a badly broken leg. Your communication skills will be important for taking control, establishing a professional presence, and caring for your patient.

After you care for the patient, the ambulance will transport the patient to the hospital. How will the ambulance crew know what care you provided for the patient prior to their arrival? How will the hospital know what the patient's vital signs were very early in the call? The answer: your documentation.

CASE STUDY

THE CALL

You are dispatched to a holiday party for a patient who has passed out. You arrive to find the patient sitting on the carpet, leaning against the couch. She appears to be one of the youngest family members at the party, about 20 years old. There are 12 nervous family members standing over the patient as you arrive trying to decide what to do.

■ Discussion: *How should you approach this scene from a communication standpoint?*

ASK YOURSELF

■ How would you demonstrate effective therapeutic communications?

■ Can you define key terms introduced in this chapter?

■ What is the process of therapeutic communication?

therapeutic communication
conversing with a patient in a comforting and empathetic nature.

Communicating with Your Patient

While communication provides a flow of information back and forth between an EMR and a patient, there are many additional benefits to communication (Figure 13-1 ■).

Communication will provide answers to your questions and help you communicate with medical direction and arriving EMTs and paramedics. As part of your training, you have learned to take a patient history. Your communication also provides reassurance and a sense of order to a patient in crisis. Because of the many functions of communication, it is sometimes referred to as **therapeutic communication**.

The first step in any patient encounter should be to introduce yourself to the patient and any family members that are present. You learned in Chapter 3 that you are also required to obtain consent to perform patient care. This is performed after you introduce yourself to the patient.

You will even introduce yourself to critical patients and to family members of unresponsive patients. In these situations you will do so quickly so as not to waste time. But do not ignore this step. It is vital to develop trust and rapport with those on the scene. Something as simple as "My name is Dan. This is my partner, Sarah. We're Emergency Medical Responders and we are going to take care of your father today" provides a tremendous amount of comfort and even creates a foundation for those on scene to be confident in your abilities.

If you have ever been a patient, you know how important it is to feel comfortable with the people providing care.

ASK YOURSELF

■ What are some actions that will improve your communication with a patient in order to accomplish the goals of patient care?

Accurate and Efficient Communication

Communication should be more than polite. There are times you will need to obtain vital information quickly. This requires communication to be accurate and efficient as well as respectful.

You should talk with your patient in an area that allows for appropriate conversation. Avoid distractions (such as noise in a machine shop) and crowds (such as a large sports stadium). If the patient is stable and you don't believe he will be injured by movement, you may be able to either take the patient away from the situation or in some cases be able to reduce the noise. While the sports stadium won't quiet down for you, you may be able to ask to turn some machines in the shop off until the emergency scene has been cleared.

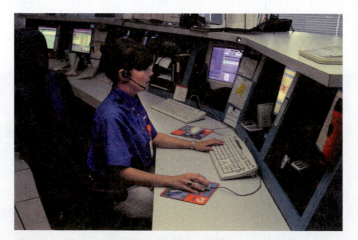

■ **Figure 13-1** A communication center.

You will need light to assess your patient. Adequate lighting also allows your patient to see you. This adds to a level of comfort. If you can't see your patient well, you may not be able to observe clinical signs such as when he winces in pain when he moves. You also need light to see subtle signs of respiratory distress.

Privacy is another major concern for patients. You will be asking about their medical conditions and medications as well as other details about their activities leading up to the emergency. If there are strangers, coworkers, or in some cases family members around, the patient may be uncomfortable telling you this information. It is important that you ensure your patient's privacy for his comfort and so that he will feel free to speak to you and tell you all relevant information.

When communicating with patients, you should create an environment as comfortable as possible given the emergency situation. One way you can do this is to position yourself appropriately in relation to the patient. You should take a position that puts you at the patient's eye level or slightly below.

Many times the patient will be sitting on the couch, lying on a bed, or even in a car that has crashed. In each of these situations, you can get to the patient's level by crouching or kneeling. If the patient is sitting on the ground or floor, squat down at his level when possible. The patient will be able to look directly at you. Standing above the patient can create an uncomfortable feeling or imply intimidation.

The exception to this rule is safety. If the patient appears potentially violent or is agitated, or if you have an uneasy feeling, maintain a greater distance and avoid placing yourself in a position (such as crouching) where it would be difficult to retreat from danger.

People have what has been referred to as a **personal space** around them. It is an area about 3 feet from the patient in all directions. Getting too close to a patient without his authorization to do so will make him uncomfortable.

Gaining access to personal space (which you will need to obtain vitals and provide care) isn't difficult. Introduce yourself, get down on the patient's level, and explain what you are going to do (such as check the pulse at the wrist). This is usually all that is required.

Some people will be a bit trickier. Those who have been assaulted, some patients experiencing a psychological emergency, children, and those with an altered mental status might take a little more time to get close to without causing an emotional outburst.

As you perform care, try to minimize interruptions. These may come from a family member trying to be helpful, a family pet who keeps trying to sit with the patient, or noise from phones or your portable radio. These distractions will keep the patient from adequately answering important questions and prevent you from listening in detail.

You should actively listen to your patients. Give them your full attention. This will result in hearing everything they say. If you listen actively you may notice that your patient seems hesitant to say something. You may also observe the patient deny pain when he looks like he is in pain.

If you pay careful attention, you will spot vital clinical clues that others who don't pay attention will miss. Listening is also a key way to indicate that what the patient is saying is important to you.

Many of the items already mentioned (such as noise, distraction, poor lighting) are considered **barriers to communication**. Equipment may also cause a barrier to communication.

You will also treat patients who have diminished sight or hearing. The patients will pose communication challenges to you as you provide the same high quality of care to them. Patients who are deaf or have difficulty hearing may need you to write down questions or use a sign language interpreter (often a family member) (Figure 13-2a ■). You will need to take a bit more time in your assessment and care. These patients will not see your hand movements or pointing, nor will they see you moving toward them with medical equipment. You must explain everything you are doing (Figure 13-2b ■).

personal space an area of approximately 3 feet around a patient where he feels comfortable.

barriers to communication distractions or physical objects that impede one's assessment and care.

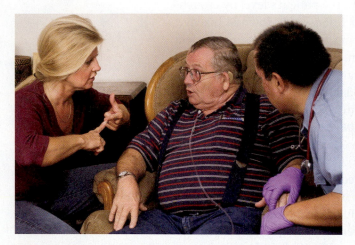

■ **Figure 13-2a** Deafness in patients is a communication challenge.

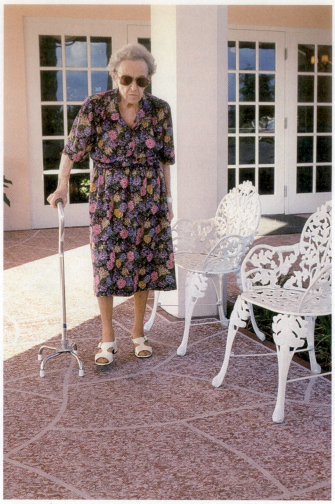

■ **Figure 13-2b** Blindness or any decrease in cognitive abilities is also a communication challenge.

ASK YOURSELF

■ What is the role of body language in communications?

The clipboard is one of these barriers. The way you interview a patient and take notes is important to the flow of information. Placing a large clipboard between you and the patient could be perceived as a barrier. Constantly writing notes while the patient is talking can cause the patient to stop talking while you catch up writing. Important information may be lost.

Balance your need to write down information with the need for uninterrupted conversation with your patient. Many EMS providers use a small pad to record information during the initial patient contact. That information is later transferred to a written or computerized run report. You must balance remembering accurate information with good patient interaction.

Medical equipment and procedures can also interfere with communication. Tasks such as taking a blood pressure are difficult to do while talking with a patient. Often both the conversation and the accuracy of the blood pressure suffer (Figure 13-3a ■).

Unless the patient is in serious condition (where it is acceptable to gain a history while performing other assessment and care steps to save vital time), pay close attention to the patient while talking. When taking vital signs or performing any other examinations, be sure to explain what you are doing to reduce anxiety (Figure 13-3b ■).

Finally, be aware of your body language as you speak with your patient. Face your patient and look directly at him while you communicate. Avoid crossing your arms, looking at your watch, or other actions that will make you appear disinterested (Figure 13-4 ■).

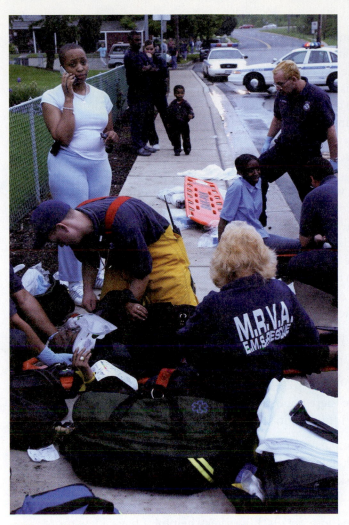

■ Figure 13-3a A chaotic scene may make it difficult to communicate with your patient and others. *(© Mark C. Ide)*

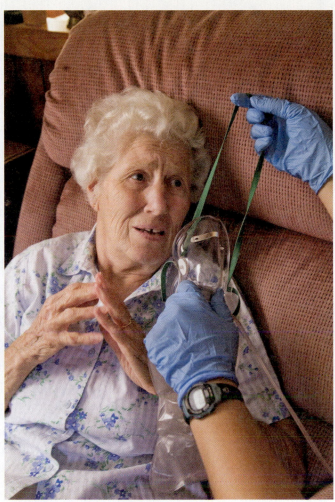

■ Figure 13-3b An anxious and scared patient may present a communication challenge.

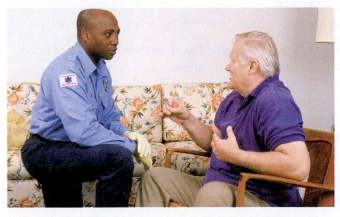

■ Figure 13-4 Use body language that shows you are open and interested in what the patient has to say. Be aware of your patient's body language as well.

Patient Interview Techniques

The prior sections have discussed ways to listen and make the patient feel comfortable. This section will center around techniques to get the most pertinent information from your patient. The way you ask questions can make a considerable difference in the quality and amount of information you receive.

ASK YOURSELF

■ What are some examples of both open-ended and closed-ended questions that will help you efficiently obtain pertinent information from patients?

■ What are the pitfalls that can interfere with a successful patient interview?

Start with general questions when you approach a patient. Even if you see a patient clutching his chest or holding an apparently broken arm, you will start with general questions—not questions about the patient's obvious complaints.

An **open-ended question** is one that can't be answered with a one-word answer such as yes or no. An example of an open-ended question is "How would you describe what is wrong?" or "How are you feeling?"

The opposite of an open-ended question is a **closed-ended question**. This may also be called a **direct question**. An example of a closed-ended question is "Does your chest hurt?" or "Did you fall?"

Never make assumptions when obtaining a history or examining a patient. It is always better to get a patient to explain what happened rather than to guess—or even worse, assume—what happened. The open-ended question is best for these early questions. There are times that patients can tell you something important that you might not have thought to ask if you give them a chance.

After you have begun with the more general open-ended questions, you may then ask pertinent, targeted questions. An example of how questions might progress with the patient with chest pain goes something like this:

You: Can you tell me why you called for an ambulance?

Patient: My chest hurts. Kind of feels heavy.

You: OK. Tell me more about the feeling in your chest.

Patient: It feels kind of like there is a band around my chest. It actually shoots up to my neck a bit now that I think of it.

The questions in this example resulted in the patient volunteering information that was clinically relevant and valuable. Getting the information in the patient's own words is important. Once you have asked open-ended questions, you may progress to more specific, closed-ended questions. They might continue like this:

You: Thanks for giving me those details. It was very helpful. I have a few more questions. Does it hurt or feel tight anywhere else?

Patient: No, it doesn't.

You: Do you have any difficulty breathing or any other problems?

In this exchange (which is designed to be an example and not a complete history) you see that there is a place to ask specific questions.

When you take the patient history, ask only one question at a time. Speak clearly and don't use medical terms, abbreviations, or mnemonics the patient may not be familiar with.

When you begin talking with a patient, he may ask you questions as well. It is a solid rule to answer the patient's questions honestly. If you don't know the answer, it is much better to say so rather than to make something up.

Other pitfalls to a successful patient interview include:

- Talking too much (not letting the patient talk).
- Interrupting the patient's answers to your questions.
- Appearing as if you are judging the patient or family members.
- Asking leading questions.
- Giving unwarranted or unauthorized advice.
- Providing false reassurance ("Everything is going to be OK"). Patients at some level are usually aware of the potential seriousness of a given situation. False reassurance indicates that you have no consideration of what the patient is going through or that you simply don't understand.

Stop, Review, Remember

Multiple Choice

Place a check next to the correct answer.

1. The type of communication utilized to help a patient and calmly reassure him is referred to as:

    _____ a. therapeutic communication.

    _____ b. open-ended communication.

    _____ c. closed-ended communication.

    _____ d. a barrier to communication.

2. You respond to a high school volleyball game for an injured player. Which is the most appropriate spot to discuss the female's medical history?

    _____ a. Gym volleyball court

    _____ b. Gym lobby

    _____ c. Back of the ambulance

    _____ d. Sidelines of the game

3. An effective part to communication is "getting on their level." When is it appropriate not to do this?

    _____ a. There is a difference greater than 2 feet in height.

    _____ b. Safety concerns exist.

    _____ c. You feel the patient won't appreciate the "personal touch."

    _____ d. Your patient is sitting on the floor.

4. When starting a patient interview, what type of question is best to ask?

    _____ a. Open-ended question

    _____ b. Closed-ended question

    _____ c. Therapeutic communication

    _____ d. Efficient communication

True/False

Mark whether each of the following statements is true (T) or false (F).

1. _____ Direct questions should be used to ask about specific problems or complaints.

2. _____ Effective communication is as important to patient care as complete knowledge of heart attack care.

3. _____ Lighting and noisy environments are characteristics not necessary to consider when interviewing a patient.

4. _____ As an EMR, you are able to use a note pad to take initial information on/from a patient for later transfer to the proper reporting instrument.

Critical Thinking

You are dispatched to the scene for a complaint of difficulty breathing. When you arrive, you find a person clutching his chest and appearing to be in respiratory distress. Your initial impression is that this patient needs immediate intervention to help life-threatening problems.

1. Is it still appropriate to ask open-ended questions during your initial interview of this patient to establish the problem, or do you have enough information to begin your care?

    _____

    _____

    _____

    _____

2. What types of closed-ended questions would be appropriate for this patient during your initial interview?

_____

_____

_____

_____

3. As this patient is most likely to be considered a critical patient, do you expect to have any barriers to care and what would they be?

_____

_____

_____

_____

ASK YOURSELF

■ How do you give a brief, organized, pertinent report to the EMS providers assuming care of the patient?

Communicating Patient Information to Other Providers

When you complete patient care, you will transfer the information you have gathered to the EMS provider taking over patient care. It is important that you transfer the information you have learned in an efficient manner. You will generally transfer the following information verbally:

- Patient condition—initially and currently
- Patient's age and sex
- Chief complaint
- Brief, pertinent history of what happened
- How you found the patient
- Relevant past medical and traumatic conditions
- Vital signs
- Pertinent physical exam findings
- Care given and the patient's response to that care

You will also introduce yourself, your patient, and your patient's family members to the incoming EMS crew.

At times you may need to communicate with other emergency services providers on the scene, including fire service and police personnel. These providers are often required to deal with scene hazards (violence or fire), as well as to provide assistance with patient care on scene.

Some scenes may be hectic. For example, in a major collision you may be responsible for initial patient care. The fire department may be dealing with a fuel spill and extrication of the patient who is trapped in the vehicle. The police will be looking for evidence and controlling traffic at the scene.

It is important to do your job with consideration for others at the scene. Everyone has a job to do and all intertwine. Remain calm and work together with the other emergency services personnel at the scene. In a large scene, the **incident command system** will be employed (see Chapter 28).

incident command system structure to allow for unified control of an incident.

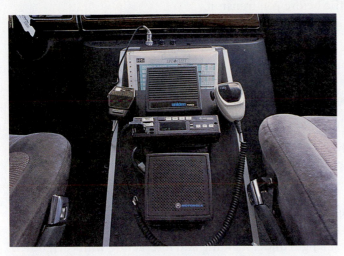

■ **Figure 13-5a**   An example of a vehicle mounted radio.

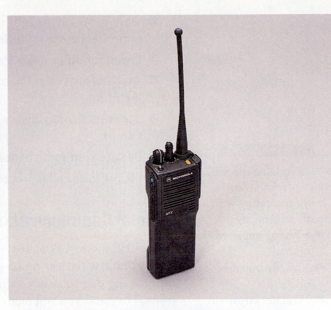

■ **Figure 13-5b**   An example of a hand-held portable radio.

Radio Communication

As an Emergency Medical Responder you may communicate with a dispatcher or other EMS providers by radio or phone. There are several types of radio devices. These include (Figures 13-5a and 13-5b ■):

Portable radios—two-way radios that can easily be carried on a belt and used from an emergency scene

Mobile radios—two-way radios mounted in a vehicle

Base station radios—radios found at fixed locations such as stations and hospitals

Cell phones may also be used in communication between the ambulance and the hospital and between the ambulance and dispatch (Figure 13-6 ■).

The following are general rules that all EMS providers should follow if they are required to use radios as part of their response:

- Speak slowly and clearly. Don't yell or speak very quickly. You will not be understood by others.

- Hold the radio or microphone about 4 inches from your mouth. Too close can result in garbling; too far can result in very low volume.

ASK YOURSELF

■ How do you use portable, mobile, or base station radios to communicate with emergency services personnel?

■ What are the general rules of communicating by radio?

portable radio   carried on one's person.

mobile radio   mounted in a vehicle.

base station radio mounted in a building.

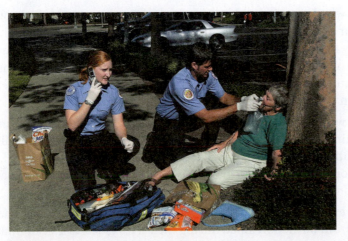

■ **Figure 13-6**   Cells phones may be used by EMRs.

- Only speak on the radio when necessary. Many others could be sharing the same radio frequencies at different emergency scenes.
- Listen for other radio traffic before you transmit.
- Avoid using patient names and other confidential (protected) information on the radio.
- Speak professionally. Avoid using other EMS providers' names, slang, jargon, or humor.
- Be sure your radio battery is charged and/or have a spare battery available.
- Follow local radio procedure and protocols.

Special Communication Situations

You will come across patients who have difficulty communicating. These patients may have trouble with hearing or sight, or they may have difficulties understanding or communicating due to issues such as Alzheimer disease, autism, and other possible conditions. They and you will face challenges understanding and interacting with each other.

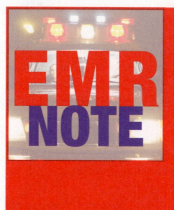

EMR NOTE

When you are called to a patient who has a challenge with hearing or sight, cognitive development issues, or other difficulties communicating, there are a few general rules to follow:

- Take your time. Determine the extent of the patient's difficulty either from the patient or a family member.
- Ask the patient or family member how it is best to communicate. You may be able to write your questions for a deaf person or have someone use sign language to translate.
- Do not assume the patient has reduced intelligence because of the reduced ability to communicate.
- Do not shout at the patient.

The following are guidelines for dealing with specific conditions:

- Patients who have impaired hearing or deafness may need to see your mouth to read your lips. Speak normally. Do not exaggerate your speech or shout. A friend or family member may know sign language and be able to relay your questions to the patient. You also might write down questions the patient can answer verbally or in writing. Patients with a hearing impairment may not speak clearly. This does not mean they have reduced intelligence.
- Patients who are blind are usually quite capable of getting around and functioning. However, an emergency can put the patient with visual impairment in a situation where assistance is needed. If your patient is blind, ask what help he needs. You may be asked to guide the patient and to explain any changes in the immediate surroundings.
- You will encounter many patients who have mental impairments that were present from birth, developed during their lives (such as a head injury), or are the result of aging (such as Alzheimer disease). There are many points to consider.

ASK YOURSELF

- What are the special considerations in communicating with patients who are:
  - Hearing impaired or deaf?
  - Visually impaired or blind?
  - Mentally impaired?

First, many patients have a level of function that will allow them to communicate with you and explain their condition. But some will not. You will need to rely on family members and other health care providers to tell you about the patient.

You should also differentiate altered mental status from the patient's communication difficulty. Explore how much of the patient's impairment is from an existing condition and how much is new or due to the present emergency. For example, a patient with Alzheimer disease could normally exhibit confused speech, but a stroke could make this worse. Family members may be able to report sudden or gradual changes in the patient that you would not be able to identify.

All patients deserve the best possible care delivered with compassion. Your efforts to communicate clearly will result in quality patient care and provide you with a sense of satisfaction that comes only with helping another.

CASE STUDY

THE RESPONSE

The patient seems alert and oriented. You introduce yourself, perform a primary assessment, and begin to ask the patient some history questions. Three or four family members are still lingering around trying to help the patient answer questions…yet the patient doesn't seem to want to answer any questions.

■ Discussion: *Why might the patient not want to answer questions? What can you do to fix this?*

✳ Stop, Review, Remember

Multiple Choice

Place a check next to the correct answer.

1. When turning over care of a patient to an EMS crew for transport, an effective report will introduce you, your patient, and:

    ____ a. his children.

    ____ b. his parents.

    ____ c. his siblings.

    ____ d. any of the above family members on the scene assisting with care.

2. Which of the following communication devices would be commonly carried by a rescue worker on an incident?

    ____ a. Portable radio

    ____ b. Mobile radio

    ____ c. Dictaphone

    ____ d. Base radio

3. Patients with hearing difficulties will often be able to communicate by seeing your ____ as you speak to them.

    ____ a. eyes

    ____ b. mouth and lips

    ____ c. tongue

    ____ d. facial contours

4. What type of medical condition may impair a person's ability to give you an appropriate response when asked what is wrong?

    ____ a. Hearing difficulty

    ____ b. Head/brain injury

    ____ c. Visual impairment

    ____ d. Tactile/sensation impairment

True/False

Mark whether each of the following statements is true (T) or false (F).

1. _____ A patient's medical history and the care you have provided should be given in a report to transfer care.

2. _____ The best way to communicate with a patient who doesn't answer your questions the first time is to yell because he probably can't hear you.

3. _____ A mobile radio would most commonly be found in a vehicle or piece of emergency apparatus.

4. _____ Blind patients are generally incapable of functioning on their own.

Critical Thinking

You are dispatched to an assisted living facility for a patient with an altered mental status. You arrive and find a male who is stumbling around his room. The nurse tells you she just came in to get him for lunch and found him like this.

1. In order to create a good plan to care for this patient, what is important to ask the nurse about his current mental status?

   _____

   _____

   _____

   _____

2. Since this is an assisted living facility, should you assume the patient will be blind or deaf or have Alzheimer disease?

   _____

   _____

   _____

   _____

3. In caring for this patient with an altered mental status, who is likely to give you most of your pertinent medical information and why?

   _____

   _____

   _____

   _____

Documentation

prehospital care report
paperwork for documenting your assessment and care of a patient.

As mentioned earlier in this chapter, you will likely be the first trained EMS provider on scene. Your observations, patient assessment, and patient care will be vital and must be documented so that others in the EMS system are aware of it.

This documentation is most commonly performed on the **prehospital care report** (Figure 13-7 ■). Commonly referred to as a PCR, this document is provided by your

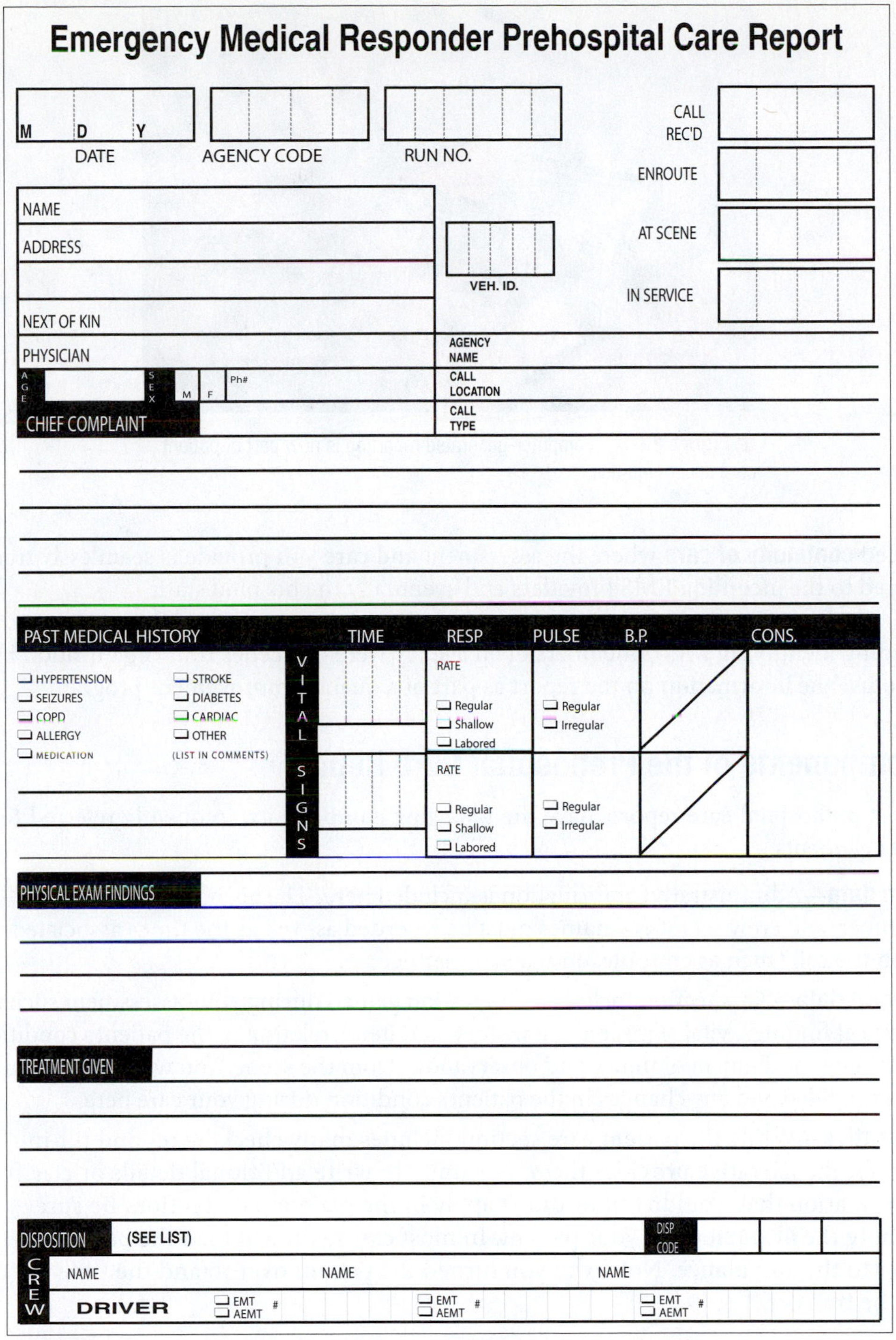
Emergency Medical Responder Prehospital Care Report

M D Y
DATE | AGENCY CODE | RUN NO.

CALL REC'D
ENROUTE
AT SCENE
IN SERVICE

NAME
ADDRESS
VEH. ID.
NEXT OF KIN
PHYSICIAN
AGENCY NAME
AGE | SEX M F | Ph#
CALL LOCATION
CHIEF COMPLAINT
CALL TYPE

PAST MEDICAL HISTORY
- HYPERTENSION
- SEIZURES
- COPD
- ALLERGY
- MEDICATION
- STROKE
- DIABETES
- CARDIAC
- OTHER (LIST IN COMMENTS)

VITAL SIGNS

TIME	RESP	PULSE	B.P.	CONS.
	RATE Regular Shallow Labored	Regular Irregular		
	RATE Regular Shallow Labored	Regular Irregular		

PHYSICAL EXAM FINDINGS

TREATMENT GIVEN

DISPOSITION (SEE LIST) | DISP CODE

CREW
NAME | NAME | NAME
DRIVER | EMT AEMT # | EMT AEMT # | EMT AEMT #

■ **Figure 13-7** An example of a prehospital care report for Emergency Medical Responders.

agency or regional or state EMS system for use in documenting your findings at the scene. Some systems use entirely computerized records (Figure 13-8 ■). You may input your data into a computer which will require the same information. The computer may transmit the material electronically or will allow a paper copy to print out.

The prehospital care report has several functions. The most common are for transfer of care from you as an EMR to other EMS providers in the field. This is part of a process

ASK YOURSELF

■ What information is recorded for each prehospital care report data element?

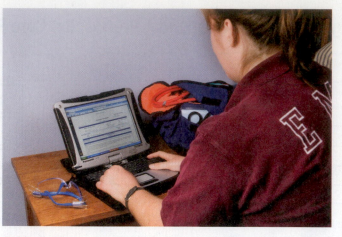

■ Figure 13-8 Computer-generated reporting is now part of patient care documentation.

called **continuity of care** where the assessment and care you provide is seamlessly transferred to the incoming EMS providers and eventually the hospital staff.

The prehospital care report also serves administrative purposes within an agency, including identifying which members of an agency were on scene. Your organization may also use the information on the report as part of a quality improvement program.

Components of the Prehospital Care Report

Most prehospital care reports have the following components, frequently referred to as data elements:

run data   administrative information such as agency and unit.

Run data—Administrative information is included here. The agency name, unit number, and crew members' names must be recorded as well as the times associated with the call (such as en route, on scene, in service).

patient data   clinical information concerning a patient.

Patient data—This section includes information gained during your assessment such as physical findings, vital signs, patient history, and items relating to the patient's condition including mechanism of injury and observations from the scene. You will note the care you provided and any changes in the patient's condition during your care here.

narrative   the details of a provider's care of a patient.

Narrative—While the patient care section includes many check boxes and fill-in spaces, the narrative provides the opportunity to write additional details or clarify information that wouldn't fit or didn't apply in the patient data section. Be sure to note the **disposition** of your patient. In most cases you will turn the patient over to the ambulance. Note who you turned the patient over to and the time of the transfer.

disposition   destination of a patient following your care.

Some patients may wish to refuse care and transportation. Most systems recommend having the ambulance continue to assist with assessment of the patient and to decide if the patient refusal is appropriate. In most cases, patients should be persuaded to accept your care and the care and transportation provided by personnel on the ambulance.

In the event of refusal of care, there are a series of facts that must be documented. Often this is performed on a specific refusal checklist. These items include that you:

- Advised the patient that further care and transportation is warranted.
- Advised the patient of the risks of refusing care and transportation. This usually includes worsening of the patient's condition up to and including death.
- Took steps to attempt to persuade the patient to accept care and transportation.

ASK YOURSELF

■ What are the actions to be taken and documented when a patient refuses care and transportation?

- Assured the patient was able to comprehend the consequences of not accepting transport.
- Advised the patient and his family that they could call back at any time.
- Encouraged the patient to seek care at a clinic, at a hospital, or with his family physician.
- Took steps to make sure someone could call again if the patient was stricken (for example, to have family members monitor him for a period of time).

Again, it is highly recommended that the EMTs or Paramedics on the ambulance continue to the scene and handle the patient refusal process when at all possible.

The prehospital care report is a legal document which may be subpoenaed for court proceedings in both civil and criminal cases. Your documentation must be relevant, accurate, and honest.

The term **objective** is often used to describe how you should document. Objective means you only document things that are factual or clearly observable such as vital signs, wounds, and mechanism of injury. Examples of objective statements include:

"The patient's blood pressure is 110/66."

"The patient fell 10 feet from a roof into a lawn."

"The patient complains of pain in his left lower leg."

There are times you will need to document information that you cannot personally observe, but is relevant to patient care. This is called **subjective** information. In cases where the patient tells you important clinical information, it must be documented. If your patient says she hasn't eaten for 3 days and you write "The patient hasn't eaten for 3 days" on your PCR, it appears as if it is something you know or could attest to. However, if you write "The patient reports not eating for 3 days," everyone knows how you received the information.

There may be something the patient says that is a legal issue or may be controversial. In this case document it in your narrative section by writing "The patient states . . ." and then write what the patient said and place it in quotes. Examples include:

The patient stated, "I was raped. And he left me for dead."

or

The patient stated, "I was abducted by aliens and then left on the highway."

It is always best to write clear, concise, honest prehospital care reports because, as legal records, they will be looked at again by someone else. It is a reflection of your work and the patient care you provided on scene. Sloppy and incomplete documentation implies that the care you gave was sloppy and incomplete.

In the unlikely event you are sued as a result of your action at the scene (you may be named in a lawsuit simply because you are one of many EMS providers at a scene), your documentation will be scrutinized as representative of the care you gave at the scene. In this case you will want to have neat, complete, and accurate documentation.

Special Reporting Situations

You learned about special reporting situations in Chapter 3. These include abuse and assault (including child, spousal, and elder abuse) as well as gunshot wounds, sexual assault, infectious disease, and other situations (Figure 13-9 ■).

As an EMR you will make the appropriate notifications as required by law. Follow the guidelines noted earlier for documentation of these situations. Since it is likely that your report will be viewed by others and may be introduced into court as evidence, you will want to make sure your report is thorough, objective, and accurate. Remember to avoid subjective opinions in your documentation.

objective factual documentation of events or conditions.

subjective impressions relayed from the patient.

ASK YOURSELF

- How do you differentiate between subjective and objective patient information?
- What are some examples of special reporting situations?

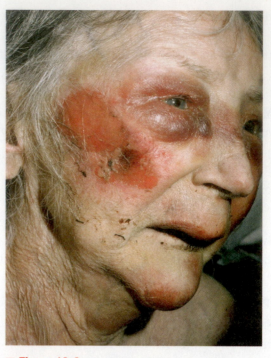

■ **Figure 13-9** You must report suspected elder abuse or any abuse.

THE LAST WORD

Whether for interpersonal, medical, or legal reasons, communication and documentation are vitally important for the Emergency Medical Responder.

When you are first at the scene your ability to take control of a challenging scene, gather vital information quickly, care for your patient, and transfer information to the EMTs will depend on your communication and documentation skills.

Multiple Choice

Place a check next to the correct answer.

1. Therapeutic communication can best be described as:
   - _____ a. a calming voice.
   - _____ b. an abrasive tone.
   - _____ c. a tone and wording that puts the patient at ease.
   - _____ d. a feeling felt only by the truly ill or injured.

2. When discussing a patient's medical history, you should seek a proper environment. What is the most appropriate location in an industrial facility?
   - _____ a. The break room
   - _____ b. A private office
   - _____ c. The production floor where the injury occurred
   - _____ d. The parking lot

3. Which of the following patients may create a challenge in establishing a rapport or relationship for providing care?
   - _____ a. A child just involved in a car accident
   - _____ b. An adult just involved in a car accident
   - _____ c. A teenager who hurt his elbow on the gym floor
   - _____ d. An adult with a terminal illness

4. What is a good distance to hold the microphone from one's mouth when attempting to communicate via radio?
   - _____ a. 1 inch
   - _____ b. 2 inches
   - _____ c. 4 inches
   - _____ d. 6 inches

5. All of the following techniques for dealing with a visually impaired patient are appropriate except:
   - _____ a. taking more time.
   - _____ b. explaining what you are doing.
   - _____ c. shouting.
   - _____ d. not talking down to the patient.

6. Continuity of care can be accomplished, most officially, in writing by completing a(n):
   - _____ a. notebook page.
   - _____ b. prehospital care report.
   - _____ c. event diary.
   - _____ d. assessment information sheet.

7. In addition to your normal assessment documentation, when documenting a refusal you must document:
   - _____ a. your notifying the patient to seek further aid should his symptoms worsen.
   - _____ b. your attempts to have the patient consent to your care.
   - _____ c. your explanation to the patient of the risks of his condition up to and including death.
   - _____ d. all of the above.

8. Which type of documentation should be avoided when detailing your assessment and interactions with a patient?
   - _____ a. Objective
   - _____ b. Subjective
   - _____ c. Written
   - _____ d. Verbal

True/False

Indicate whether each of the following is true (T) or false (F) on the line provided.

1. _____ Adequate lighting is an important aspect to patient communication.

2. _____ A family pet that continually tries to sit with the patient during your assessment can be viewed as a positive thing to keep the person on task with your questions.

3. _____ "Can you tell me about your chest pain?" is an appropriate opening question for a patient interview.

4. _____ It is important not to give false impressions to patients by saying "Everything will be OK."

5. _____ If you yell loud enough, even a deaf person can hear you.

6. _____ The EMR's subjective opinion of the living conditions surrounding an accident should be documented in the prehospital care report.

7. _____ Special reporting situations often involve crimes or cases that may end up in court and should be documented with extra thoroughness.

8. _____ A refusal of care will require a very small amount of documentation.

Critical Thinking

A person has been involved in a motor vehicle collision on the local interstate. He was the passenger in the vehicle and states that he is not injured. The driver ultimately requires helicopter transportation for his injuries to the trauma center.

1. Should this person be allowed to sign a refusal of care or be persuaded to go with the ambulance to the hospital?

   _____

   _____

   _____

2. Although this person is uninjured, if the other occupant requires air evacuation from the scene, would you say there is significant mechanism for injury? What would this tell you about the potential injuries this person may have?

   _____

   _____

   _____

3. Would it be better to take a more stern position with this patient versus a submissive and apologetic position and why?

   _____

   _____

   _____

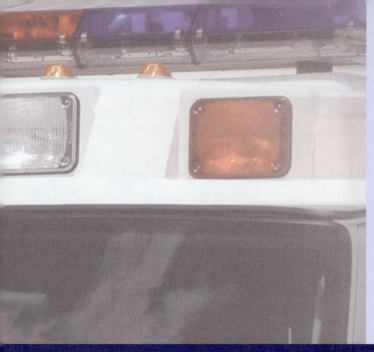

SECTION 3
Review and Practice Examination

Assess what you have learned in this section by checking the best answer for each multiple-choice question. When you are done, check your answers against the key provided in Appendix B.

1. Ducking behind a shrub to protect yourself from a violent individual at a scene is an example of:
   _____ a. concealment.
   _____ b. cover.
   _____ c. distraction.
   _____ d. retreat.

2. As you approach the scene of a reported motor vehicle collision, you can see that one of the vehicles involved is a tanker truck. Which of the following is the best course of action?
   _____ a. Approach the scene from the upwind side to avoid exposure to vapors.
   _____ b. Stop where you are and use binoculars to identify any placards on the truck or indications of a leak.
   _____ c. Approach the scene as long as the ambient temperature is less than 80°F.
   _____ d. Immediately notify dispatch that you are responding to a hazardous materials incident.

3. The best source of information for determining the safe distance from a particular type of hazardous material involved in a highway transportation incident is:
   _____ a. dispatch.
   _____ b. the fire department.

_____ c. the driver of the truck.
_____ d. the Emergency Response Guidebook.

4. You have responded to a call for a building that collapsed while under renovation. You can hear at least two people yelling for help from within the rubble. You should:
   _____ a. notify dispatch that you are on the scene and will be entering the structure to perform triage.
   _____ b. report this information to dispatch and ensure specialized rescue is en route.
   _____ c. put on self-contained breathing apparatus (SCBA) before entering the scene.
   _____ d. wait until other emergency personnel arrive on the scene before entering to search for and rescue survivors.

5. The EMR assesses mechanism of injury to determine:
   _____ a. who was at fault in a collision.
   _____ b. the type and severity of injuries to be suspected.
   _____ c. whether to take Standard Precautions.
   _____ d. whether EMS should continue to the scene.

6. The unrestrained vehicle occupant who takes a down-and-under pathway in a frontal impact would experience the most forceful impact to the:

    _____ a. upper extremities.
    _____ b. lower extremities.
    _____ c. lumbar spine.
    _____ d. head or face.

7. The piece of safety equipment that will work the best to prevent whiplash injuries is a(n):

    _____ a. lap belt and shoulder harness.
    _____ b. side-impact air bag.
    _____ c. front air bag.
    _____ d. headrest.

8. Your patient was the driver of a vehicle struck in the left side by another vehicle. Which of the following injuries should you most highly suspect?

    _____ a. Injury to the liver
    _____ b. Injury of the right hip
    _____ c. Head and neck injury
    _____ d. Whiplash injury

9. For an adult, you would consider the mechanism of injury to be significant if he fell from a distance of _____ feet or higher.

    _____ a. 3
    _____ b. 6
    _____ c. 9
    _____ d. 12

10. Which of the following best explains the purpose of the primary assessment?

    _____ a. Find and treat all patient problems.
    _____ b. Find and treat life-threatening problems.
    _____ c. Determine whether the scene is safe.
    _____ d. Get a complete medical history.

11. As you approach a patient who is sitting on the floor of his living room, you can see that he does not appear to be uncomfortable or in distress. Which of the following have you just completed?

    _____ a. Formed a general impression
    _____ b. The entire primary assessment
    _____ c. Assessed for disability
    _____ d. The scene size-up

12. Which of the following is the best example of a chief complaint?

    _____ a. A bystander tells you the patient was the driver of a vehicle that rolled over.
    _____ b. A patient's wife tells you he has a history of heart problems.
    _____ c. You can see that a patient has a severely deformed left lower leg.
    _____ d. A patient tells you that he is having a hard time catching his breath.

13. Which of the following situations should make you concerned that a patient is in serious, or potentially serious, condition?

    _____ a. You were called for a sick person who is vomiting into a basin as you enter the room.
    _____ b. You were called for an unknown problem and a patient tells you he has had lower back pain for 3 days.
    _____ c. You were called for difficulty breathing, but when you arrive, the patient seems combative.
    _____ d. You were called for a patient who tripped over a curb and has bleeding from a cut on his shin.

14. A 30-year-old male patient is awake and tells you his name is John. When you ask him what happened, he says he doesn't know. As you are evaluating him, he asks you several times if you can tell him what happened. How would you describe his level of consciousness?

    _____ a. Alert
    _____ b. Verbal
    _____ c. Pain
    _____ d. Unresponsive

15. You have approached a middle-aged male who does not answer you when you speak. After raising your voice, the patient still does not respond. You should next:

    _____ a. lightly slap the patient's cheeks.
    _____ b. gently shake the patient's shoulder.
    _____ c. apply pressure to the patient's thumbnail with the side of your pen.
    _____ d. document that the patient is unresponsive.

16. Your primary assessment of a patient has revealed that she is awake, alert, and speaking normally. Which of the following statements is true concerning additional assessment of this patient?
   _____ a. You should now check the patient's radial pulse.
   _____ b. The next step is to measure the patient's blood pressure.
   _____ c. No further assessment of circulation is needed.
   _____ d. You must determine whether the patient responds to painful stimuli.

17. Which of the following would you do to assess a patient for disability in the primary assessment?
   _____ a. Check the radial pulses.
   _____ b. Place your hands near the patient's hands and ask her to squeeze your fingers.
   _____ c. Hold up a finger and ask the patient to follow your finger with her eyes as you move it.
   _____ d. List five items, and ask the patient to remember them. Ask the patient to repeat the five items after several minutes.

18. When updating the incoming EMS units, which of the following should you include in your report?
   _____ a. The patient's age and name
   _____ b. A list of the patient's medications
   _____ c. The patient's marital status and ethnicity
   _____ d. The patient's level of consciousness

19. Which of the following is the most important factor in obtaining a patient's medical history?
   _____ a. Having good communication skills
   _____ b. Using proper medical terminology to ask questions
   _____ c. Making sure the patient gets to the point efficiently
   _____ d. Avoiding questions that may embarrass the patient

20. A patient tells you she called because she has chest pain, but she also feels nauseated. In this case, nausea is most accurately described as:
   _____ a. the patient's history.
   _____ b. a symptom.
   _____ c. a sign.
   _____ d. the chief complaint.

21. Which of the following statements is true regarding obtaining the patient's history?
   _____ a. It is not important to ask about medications if the patient's chief complaint is an injury.
   _____ b. Last oral intake is only important if the patient is nauseated or vomiting.
   _____ c. Food allergies are not the concern of the EMR, no matter what the patient's complaint.
   _____ d. Asking about the past medical history is important for all patients.

22. Which of the following statements is true concerning the EMR's role in obtaining vital signs?
   _____ a. Taking a blood pressure provides no useful information for the EMR, but is done to give information to incoming EMS units.
   _____ b. As long as a patient's vital signs are normal, the EMR does not need to repeat vital signs.
   _____ c. Both baseline and follow-up vital signs are important for all patients.
   _____ d. A blood pressure is only taken if the pulse is weak, irregular, too fast, or too slow.

23. Your patient is a 5-day-old infant. Which of the following respiratory rates should you consider abnormal in this patient?
   _____ a. 50
   _____ b. 40
   _____ c. 30
   _____ d. 20

24. When assessing an adult, you should expect the respiratory rate to be _____ per minute.
   _____ a. 25–50
   _____ b. 15–30
   _____ c. 12–20
   _____ d. 6–12

25. Your patient is a 7-year-old male who was struck by a car as he was riding his bicycle down the road. Which of the following would make you suspect that his perfusion is not adequate?
   _____ a. Capillary refill time less than 2 seconds
   _____ b. Pale, cool skin
   _____ c. Heart rate of 116
   _____ d. Blood pressure of 94/62

26. Upon trying to auscultate a patient's blood pressure, you were unable to hear distinct noises. Which of the following is the best course of action?

_____ a. Try palpating the blood pressure, instead.

_____ b. Record your best estimate of the blood pressure based on what you heard.

_____ c. Inflate the blood pressure cuff to the maximum pressure and try again, deflating the cuff very slowly.

_____ d. Treat the patient for shock.

27. Your patient is a 27-year-old female who was the driver of a vehicle involved in a minor collision. She is alert and complaining of pain in her left elbow. Her pulse is 78, respirations are 12, and blood pressure is 118/72. When you check her pupils, you do not see them constrict in response to your penlight. Which of the following makes the most sense?

_____ a. The patient has an injury to her brain.

_____ b. The patient is in shock.

_____ c. The patient is wearing contact lenses.

_____ d. There is too much light around you to assess the pupils.

28. Your patient is a 50-year-old male who was found unresponsive in his home. He does not respond to painful stimuli and has cool, pale, dry skin. His pulse is 60, respirations are 6, and blood pressure is 90/68. Upon checking his pupils, you find that they are very constricted and do not constrict further in response to your penlight. Which of the following is the most likely explanation for his constricted pupils?

_____ a. The patient has an injury to his brain.

_____ b. The patient is hypoxic.

_____ c. The patient has overdosed on a narcotic drug.

_____ d. Your penlight is not bright enough to cause the pupils to constrict further.

29. Your patient is a 19-year-old male with a history of asthma. He is mildly wheezing, but alert, and does not appear to be in significant respiratory distress. His pulse is 82, respirations are 20, and blood pressure is 124/74. When assessing his pulse oximetry reading, you get a reading of 72 percent with a pulse of 44. Which of the following is the most likely explanation?

_____ a. The patient is hypoxic.

_____ b. You are not getting an accurate pulse oximetry reading.

_____ c. Your initial vital sign assessment was inaccurate.

_____ d. The patient may have a high level of carbon monoxide.

30. Your patient is a 4-year-old child who has been vomiting for 2 days. He is pale, very drowsy, and slow to respond to you. He has a pulse of 140, respirations of 30, and blood pressure of 88/50. His pupils respond to light by constricting, and he has a capillary refill time of 4 seconds. Which of the following tells you the most about his perfusion status?

_____ a. The blood pressure

_____ b. His respiratory rate

_____ c. Capillary refill time

_____ d. The heart rate

31. After the primary assessment, which of the following will provide you with the most information about an alert patient with a medical complaint?

_____ a. A thorough medical history

_____ b. Pulse oximetry

_____ c. Palpating the abdomen

_____ d. A head-to-toe assessment

32. For which of the following patients should you apply manual stabilization of the head and neck as you begin the assessment?

_____ a. A 13-year-old male who was ejected from an all-terrain vehicle (ATV) into some tall grass

_____ b. A 50-year-old male who began having chest pain and difficulty breathing while shoveling snow from his driveway

_____ c. A 70-year-old female who says her knee "gave out" as she was walking across the lawn, causing her to fall to the other knee

_____ d. A 24-year-old female who was bitten on the forearm when she tried to break up a fight between her dog and another dog

33. An 80-year-old female stood up from her chair and felt a "snap" in her right hip, causing her to fall to the floor. On examination, the right leg is shorter than the left and the foot is turned outward. This is an example of:
_____ a. guarding.
_____ b. asymmetry.
_____ c. crepitus.
_____ d. deformity.

34. A 45-year-old female fell down a flight of 12 steps. Her chief complaint is pain in her right arm and shoulder. As you complete a head-to-toe exam, the patient takes in a sharp breath as you palpate her right thigh and states that she experienced pain when you touched the area. This finding is best described as:
_____ a. discomfort.
_____ b. deformity.
_____ c. guarding.
_____ d. tenderness.

35. A 60-year-old man fell about 10 feet from a ladder onto the lawn. He is complaining of pain in his right arm, which appears deformed and swollen. As you complete your examination, you note that there is bruising and tenderness over the right upper quadrant of the abdomen. Which of the following terms best describes the injury to the patient's arm?
_____ a. Secondary injury
_____ b. Distracting injury
_____ c. Collateral injury
_____ d. Priority injury

36. A 78-year-old female slipped on some ice and fell down six concrete steps. She is still on the ground when you arrive. She is complaining that she has pain in her ribs on the right side when she breathes and that it is getting harder to breathe. She is wearing a heavy coat and several layers of clothing. Responding EMS units are still about 10 minutes away. Which of the following is in the best interest of your patient?
_____ a. Cut away any clothing that is preventing you from assessing the area. The possibility of the patient getting colder is secondary to the need to assess the area.
_____ b. Keep the clothing intact to prevent the patient from catching a chill. The EMTs can assess the patient after they put her in the ambulance.
_____ c. Move the clothing aside, cutting as little as possible, so you can cover the patient up again after assessing the area. It is critical that you observe the area the patient is complaining about.
_____ d. If the patient can move, help her inside, where it is warm, so you can assess the area and prevent the patient from getting colder.

37. When assessing a patient's abdomen, you note that it is swollen. The correct way to refer to this when relaying your findings to the responding EMTs is to state that the patient's abdomen is:
_____ a. distended.
_____ b. bloated.
_____ c. distorted.
_____ d. guarded.

38. While you are palpating a patient's pelvis, the patient indicates to you that it is painful. You should:
_____ a. press more firmly to establish the extent of the injury.
_____ b. rock the pelvis gently from side to side.
_____ c. roll the patient onto his side and inspect the posterior aspect of the pelvis.
_____ d. make a note of the finding and move on to palpate the lower extremities.

39. You have responded to a call for a patient who fell from his roof onto his concrete driveway. When you arrive, the 51-year-old male patient is unresponsive and bleeding from a cut on the back of his head. You stabilize the cervical spine and open the patient's airway. You note that the patient's breathing is deep and rapid. A second EMR tells you that the patient's pulse is 52 per minute and his blood pressure is 188/104. Which of the following is indicated by these findings?
_____ a. Shock from internal bleeding
_____ b. Serious closed head injury
_____ c. Serious injury to the heart or lungs
_____ d. A medical problem not related to the fall

40. As you enter a residence on a call for an injured child, you note that the scene is noisy and chaotic. The television is very loud and the lights are dim. A small dog is barking excitedly. Which of the following will best allow you to establish control of the scene and gain the cooperation of those present?

_____ a. Turn off the television set as you walk past on your way to the patient.

_____ b. State, "Someone needs to get this dog out of here so I can do my job."

_____ c. Ask, "Could I have someone turn on some lights so I can take a look at the patient?"

_____ d. Immediately pick up the patient and take him into another room.

41. Your patient is a 23-year-old female who had a sudden onset of abdominal pain while at work. Her coworkers are anxiously gathered about as you arrive. The patient is alert, with good color and warm, dry skin. She seems a bit embarrassed and tells you she is feeling better and that she's sorry you had to respond for nothing. The responding EMS unit is 2 to 3 minutes away. Which of the following would be the best way to handle this situation?

_____ a. Ask the patient if you can take her vital signs, but wait to take the history.

_____ b. Obtain a SAMPLE history and OPQRST related to the chief complaint.

_____ c. Tell the coworkers that the patient is very sick and you need privacy to examine her.

_____ d. Tell the patient you understand she might feel uncomfortable, but it is important that she be truthful with you about the pain she is having.

42. Personal space, the distance from others in all directions that most people feel comfortable, is about _____ feet.

_____ a. 1

_____ b. 2

_____ c. 3

_____ d. 4

43. Your patient is a 33-year-old female who works at a gas station convenience store. She slipped on some wet tile and fell, injuring her arm. As you enter the store, you see the patient sitting on a chair, holding her left arm, which appears deformed, with her right. To obtain the most accurate and complete history, which of the following statements or questions should you start with?

_____ a. "It looks like you've got a really painful arm, there."

_____ b. "On a scale of 1 to 10, with 10 being the worst, how much pain are you having in your arm?"

_____ c. "Are you having any difficulty breathing?"

_____ d. "Hi, my name is Ben. What happened?"

44. The radio that you would take with you when you leave your vehicle and approach the patient is a _____ radio.

_____ a. base station

_____ b. mobile

_____ c. portable

_____ d. repeater

45. When speaking on the radio, you should hold the microphone:

_____ a. lightly touching your lips.

_____ b. about 1 inch from your lips.

_____ c. about 4 inches from your lips.

_____ d. about 12 inches from your lips.

46. You have been called to the home of a 72-year-old male who previously had a stroke, and today has a cough and fever. When the patient speaks, his speech is slurred and it is difficult to understand what he is saying. What should you do?

_____ a. Tell the patient you are having a hard time understanding and ask if he can write down what he wants to say.

_____ b. Speak louder and more clearly.

_____ c. Get the pertinent information from a family member.

_____ d. Skip the history to avoid frustrating the patient, but go ahead with the assessment.

47. When writing a patient care report, an example of patient data is:

_____ a. the location of the call.

_____ b. medications the patient is taking.

_____ c. to whom you turned over care of the patient.

_____ d. a written description of what you saw when you entered the scene.

48. Which of the following is an example of subjective information in your patient care report?

_____ a. "The patient was found lying on the floor on his left side."

_____ b. "Date of birth: 12/21/1961."

_____ c. "The patient rates his chest pain a 7 on a scale of 10."

_____ d. "The patient's skin was wet and cool to the touch."

49. You have responded to care for an elderly female who is bedridden and lives with her son and his family. Your examination reveals that the patient is very thin and has several deep bedsores on her buttocks. Which of the following reflects objective documentation of the facts?

_____ a. "The patient has four skin ulcers on her buttocks. There were no dressings on the wounds."

_____ b. "The patient had not been turned, resulting in the formation of bedsores."

_____ c. "The patient is not being given proper nutrition."

_____ d. "The patient receives inadequate care at home."

50. Which of the following is true concerning EMR prehospital care report documentation?

_____ a. It is not considered a legal document unless you provide emergency medical care.

_____ b. It can be subpoenaed in criminal, but not civil, court cases.

_____ c. The care with which it is written is assumed to be a reflection on the care you provided to the patient.

_____ d. The objective information can be used in court, but the subjective information cannot.

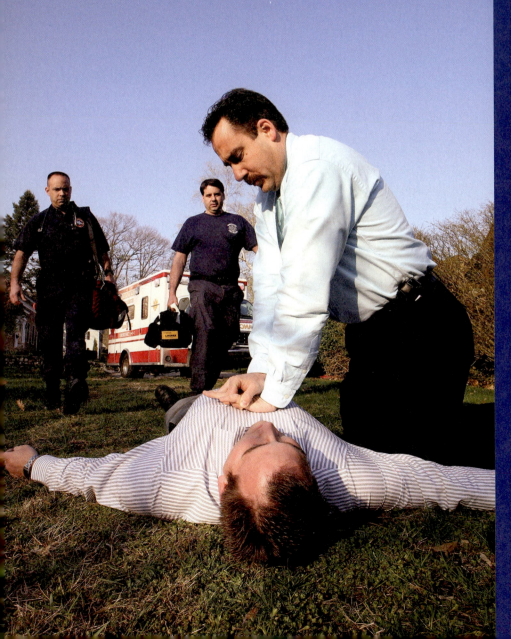

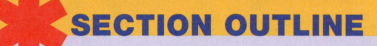

SECTION OUTLINE

In this section you will cover the following EMS Education Standard:

■ Medicine

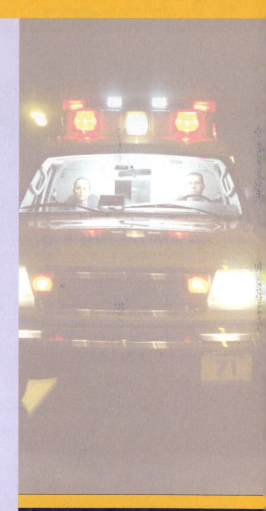

Cardiac and Respiratory Emergencies

NAVIGATION GUIDE

The following items provide an overview to the purpose and content of this chapter. The Education Standard and Competency are from the National EMS Education Standards.

Education Standard Medicine (Cardiovascular, Respiratory)

Competency Recognizes and manages life threats based on assessment findings of a patient with a medical emergency while awaiting additional emergency response.

Knowledge Areas Cardiovascular
Anatomy, signs, symptoms, and management of:
- Chest pain
- Cardiac arrest
Respiratory
Anatomy, signs, symptoms, and management of respiratory emergencies including those that affect the:
- Upper airway
- Lower airway

Objectives After reading this chapter, you should be able to:

1. Define new terms introduced in this chapter.
2. Describe how the cardiac and respiratory systems work together to bring oxygen to the cells and eliminate wastes.
3. Use assessment findings and patient complaints to recognize patients having cardiac and respiratory emergencies.
4. Formulate questions to obtain a relevant history from patients with cardiac and respiratory problems.
5. Recognize cardiac emergency patients who have both typical and atypical presentations.
6. Describe what happens in myocardial infarction and angina pectoris.
7. Describe what happens in asthma, chronic bronchitis, emphysema, congestive heart failure, and pneumonia.
8. Differentiate between patients with adequate breathing and patients with inadequate breathing.
9. Explain the importance of managing the airway, breathing, and circulation (ABCs), and administering oxygen to patients with cardiac and respiratory problems.
10. Demonstrate emergency care of patients with cardiac and respiratory problems.

NAVIGATION GUIDE (continued)

Key Terms Page references indicate first major use in this chapter. The Margin Glossary in this chapter provides definitions as you read.

Media Resources Please go to **www.bradybooks.com** to access mykit for this text. You will find quizzes, critical thinking scenarios, weblinks, animations, and videos related to this chapter—and much more. Look for online information on breath sounds, assessment tips, and asthma triggers as well as information about heart attacks and congenital heart defects. You will also find an animation on coronary artery disease and a video clip of AEDs.

INTRODUCTION

As an EMR you will see patients with cardiac and respiratory complaints frequently. Not only are these complaints frequent, they are also potentially serious. You learned about the resuscitation of cardiac patients using cardiopulmonary resuscitation (CPR) and a defibrillator in Chapter 8. This chapter will teach you to deal with patients with complaints such as heart attack, difficulty breathing, and other conditions that affect the cardiac and respiratory systems (See The Big Picture: Cardiac and Respiratory Emergencies).

ASK YOURSELF

- Can you define new terms introduced in this chapter?

- How do the cardiac and respiratory systems work together to bring oxygen to the cells and eliminate wastes?

CASE STUDY

THE CALL

You are called to the police station for a person in custody who the police report is having "some sort of attack." The dispatcher reports that the patient is conscious but agitated. You arrive to find three officers standing around the patient and holding him in a chair.

- Discussion: *What kind of attack do you think the patient had? Do his signs and symptoms point to a cardiac or respiratory condition?*

Although the systems are presented separately in this chapter, they are tightly interwoven. Many times what affects the cardiovascular system affects the respiratory system and vice versa.

The Big Picture
Cardiac and Respiratory Emergencies

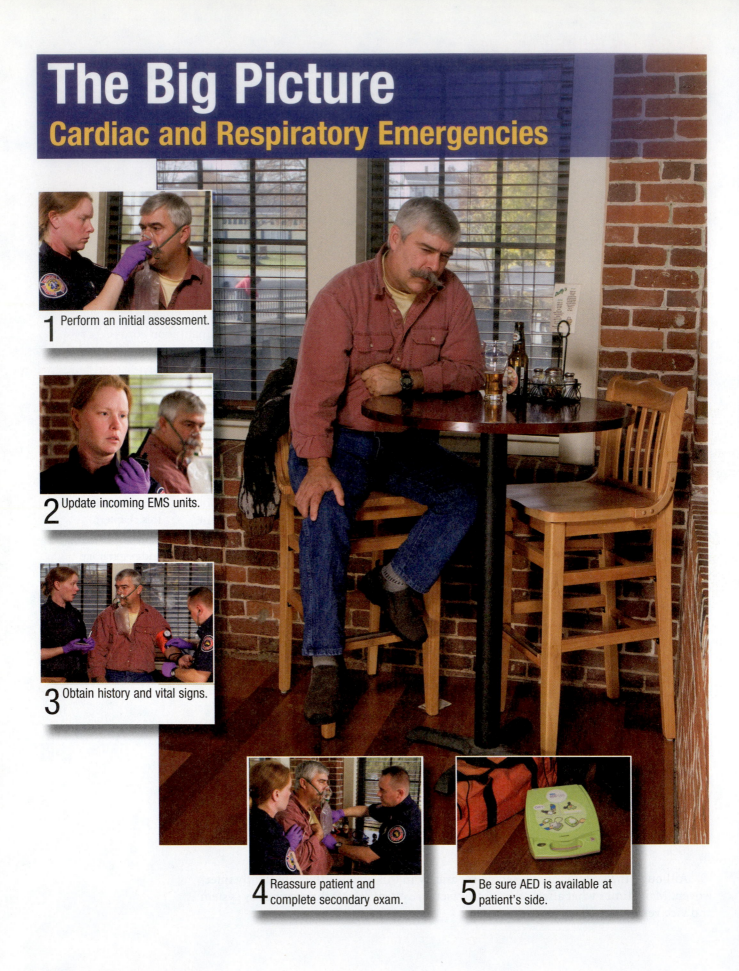

1 Perform an initial assessment.

2 Update incoming EMS units.

3 Obtain history and vital signs.

4 Reassure patient and complete secondary exam.

5 Be sure AED is available at patient's side.

Anatomy and Physiology: Respiratory System Review

The cardiac and respiratory systems work together to bring oxygen into the body, distribute the oxygen throughout the body via the bloodstream, and remove waste products from the cells for disposal. These systems are vital. Without either of the systems working properly, your patient will surely die (Figure 14-1 ■).

Air enters the mouth and nose during inspiration. It travels through the oropharynx and nasopharynx to the larynx, through the vocal cords, and into the lungs. The air passes from the trachea into increasingly smaller bronchi until it reaches the alveoli. It is in the alveoli that gas exchange takes place. Oxygen from the air is moved from the alveoli to red blood cells in the pulmonary capillaries while carbon dioxide from the blood cells is off-loaded and discarded through exhaled breaths.

The process of inhalation uses muscles. The intercostal muscles of the chest contract and move the ribs upward and outward. The diaphragm, itself a muscle, contracts and flattens. This causes air to rush into the chest. Exhalation is passive; that means it

ASK YOURSELF

■ How do you use assessment findings and patient complaints to recognize patients having cardiac and respiratory emergencies?

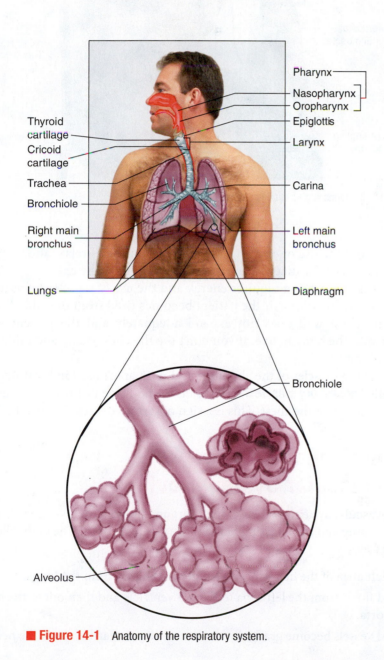

■ **Figure 14-1** Anatomy of the respiratory system.

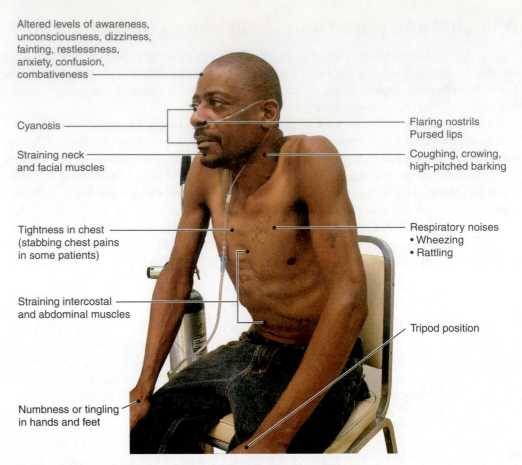

Altered levels of awareness, unconsciousness, dizziness, fainting, restlessness, anxiety, confusion, combativeness

Cyanosis

Straining neck and facial muscles

Flaring nostrils
Pursed lips

Coughing, crowing, high-pitched barking

Tightness in chest (stabbing chest pains in some patients)

Respiratory noises
• Wheezing
• Rattling

Straining intercostal and abdominal muscles

Tripod position

Numbness or tingling in hands and feet

■ **Figure 14-2** Signs and symptoms of respiratory distress.

ASK YOURSELF

■ How would you formulate questions to obtain a relevant history from patients with cardiac and respiratory problems?

accessory muscle use
abnormal use of the neck and intercostal muscles to assist in breathing.

happens without the use of energy. The intercostal muscles relax, allowing the ribs to fall back into place. The diaphragm rises. Air flows out of the chest.

The fact that breathing requires energy and the use of muscles helps us to understand inadequate breathing. If the patient becomes tired from the added work on the muscles, the chest wall does not expand adequately and the patient won't bring enough air into the body to live. If you don't see the chest rising and falling, air won't move in and out.

Normally the muscles of the abdomen and neck aren't used in breathing. If you see this, it is called **accessory muscle use**. It means the body is enlisting other muscles to help move air in and out of the chest. This is a sign of serious distress (Figure 14-2 ■).

Anatomy and Physiology: Cardiovascular System Review

The cardiovascular system consists of the heart and blood vessels. This system is responsible for pumping and transporting blood throughout the body. The path followed by the blood is as follows:

■ The left atria of the heart receive oxygenated blood from the lungs.

■ Blood flows from the left atria to the left ventricle and then out to the body via the aorta.

■ Blood vessels become gradually smaller as they get farther from the heart.

- Blood flows away from the heart in a system of arteries that turn into smaller arterioles and eventually capillaries.

- The exchange of oxygen and carbon dioxide occurs in the tissues of the body at the capillary level.

- From the capillaries, blood returns to the heart through venules and veins which gradually increase in size until they reach the inferior and superior vena cava, which return blood to the right side of the heart.

- From the right side of the heart (atria and ventricle), blood is pumped to the lungs where oxygen is obtained and carbon dioxide is excreted.

- The blood then returns back to the left side of the heart where the journey began.

The heart is a muscular organ that generally pumps about 80 times per minute. A significant volume of oxygen is required as fuel. This oxygenated blood supply is provided by the coronary arteries that encircle the heart.

Through this review of the respiratory and cardiac systems, we can begin to identify where problems may develop. Understanding the working of these systems will not only help you understand some of the common presentations but will also help you identify some conditions in the field, what treatment you will provide, and why it works. Consider the following problems:

- The smaller airways leading to the **alveoli** constrict, making it difficult to get air in and out. A common condition causing this is **asthma**. Air moving through these narrowed passageways makes a musical breath sound called **wheezing** that you can sometimes hear even without a **stethoscope**.

- Fluid builds up around the alveoli in the lungs because the heart doesn't pump efficiently. This makes the movement of oxygen to the capillaries difficult. Your patient will experience difficulty breathing. This is called **pulmonary edema** caused by **congestive heart failure**. Patients will more commonly call this "fluid in my lungs."

- One of the coronary arteries is blocked by a clot. This prevents blood (and needed oxygen) from getting to the heart muscle. The patient begins to feel pain, heaviness, and discomfort. The heart doesn't pump as efficiently and the patient may experience difficulty breathing. This is called a **myocardial infarction**, or heart attack. In severe cases the heart stops beating. This is called a **cardiac arrest** or "code."

Although you won't be diagnosing one condition from another, you have learned principles of anatomy and physiology that will help you understand why certain signs and symptoms are present in certain conditions (Figure 14-3 ■). This understanding will help you know what questions to ask the patient in the history and what parts of the body to assess.

Cardiac Emergencies

As noted in the preceding section, quite a few problems can happen with the cardiovascular system. It is important to note that you won't diagnose these conditions, and fortunately the treatments for all of the conditions you will learn are the same. Understanding the conditions will also help you when communicating with patients and other EMS providers who will likely use these terms (Figure 14-4 ■)

Cardiac conditions are generally caused by three basic problems: interruptions to the blood flow that supplies the heart muscle, problems with the heart's rhythm (electrical activity), and problems pumping. Many times these issues are interrelated.

alveoli small sacs at the end of the respiratory tree where gas exchange takes place.

asthma a respiratory condition that causes airway narrowing/constriction.

wheezing audible high-pitched breath sound heard when air passes through a constricted air opening.

stethoscope medical device used to auscultate or listen to noises not readily heard outside the body.

pulmonary edema fluid that builds up around the alveoli in the lungs when the heart does not pump efficiently.

congestive heart failure medical condition caused by backup of fluid in to the lungs from the heart's inability to properly pump.

myocardial infarction medical condition felt when a coronary artery becomes occluded or blocked.

cardiac arrest the heart stops beating.

ASK YOURSELF

- How do you recognize cardiac emergency patients who present with both typical and atypical presentations?

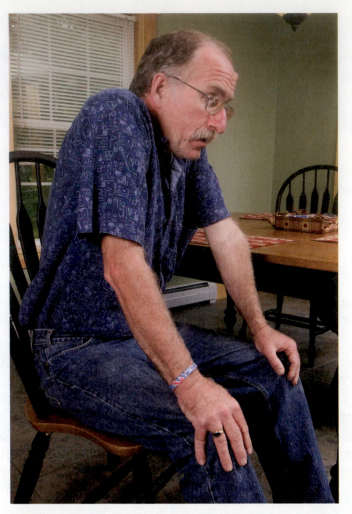

■ **Figure 14-3** Patient with respiratory distress.

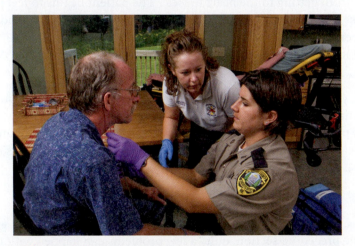

■ **Figure 14-4** Transfer of care to EMT.

ASK YOURSELF

■ How do you describe what happens in myocardial infarction and angina pectoris?

A myocardial infarction (also called acute myocardial infarction or MI) is when blood flow to one area of the heart is stopped by a clot in one of the coronary arteries. All blood flow to the section of the heart ceases. Since the heart is a muscular organ that needs oxygen to function, this is a very serious condition that, if not treated, results in death of heart muscle—and possibly death of the patient.

Angina pectoris is a condition where the heart is receiving reduced blood flow. This is usually from plaque that has built up in one or more coronary arteries. It could also be caused by a small clot that has lodged in one of the coronary arteries but has not occluded it completely. This reduced blood flow is enough to cause pain or discomfort but will not result in death of cardiac muscle.

Angina pectoris will be present when times of oxygen demand are high such as when a patient walks briskly or is under emotional stress. Rest will often cause the symptoms to subside or go away altogether.

You won't be able to differentiate a myocardial infarction from angina pectoris, and it isn't necessary to do so. Your care for anyone with chest pain or discomfort will be the same and is discussed later in the chapter.

The other problem you may encounter is the patient who is experiencing a heart rhythm disturbance. The most serious of these—ventricular fibrillation—was discussed in Chapter 8. Not all rhythm disturbances result in death or the heart stopping even temporarily. Many times the patient feels that his heart is beating irregularly or "skipping beats." This may be a sign of a serious condition, and the patient should be transported by the EMTs to the hospital.

Signs and Symptoms of Cardiac Emergencies

If five patients have a heart attack, each may have different signs and symptoms.

At one time, cardiac emergencies were thought to be primarily associated with chest pain or discomfort as the primary sign and symptom of heart attack. For many patients that simply isn't true. Consider the following patients' signs and symptoms:

- A 76-year-old female patient complains of being very weak.
- A 64-year-old male with diabetes complains of shortness of breath.
- An 87-year-old man who lives in a nursing home says he has some minor chest pain that changes when he takes a deep breath. He just isn't himself.
- A 54-year-old man was mowing the lawn when he became sweaty and pale. He complains of "a bit of indigestion."

You have probably guessed that all of these patients may be having a heart attack. Not all patients experience chest pain. Patients who are elderly or diabetics may not experience "classic" chest pain. Women who have heart attacks often experience other presenting symptoms including pain in the neck, back, and jaw; weakness or fatigue; and difficulty breathing.

Why is this important? You may be called to a residence for weakness. It may seem like a nonserious call. Your knowledge of the signs and symptoms of heart attack may help you identify that the weak female patient also looks uncomfortable. You ask her if she has any pain, and she tells you that her neck and between her shoulder blades feels funny. She may actually be having a heart attack.

As an EMR you won't be able to diagnose this for sure, but you can suspect and provide proper care. Be alert to the fact that the patient can worsen, requiring greater care including ventilation and CPR.

In some cases the only sign of heart attack will be **sudden cardiac death** without any warning signs or symptoms.

The following are signs and symptoms of cardiac emergency, including angina pectoris and myocardial infarction:

- Chest pain or discomfort (This may also be described as heaviness in the chest. The sensation may radiate to the neck, back, or jaw.)
- Difficulty breathing

sudden cardiac death phenomenon marked by cardiac arrest being the first cardiac symptom or arising soon after initial down time.

- Nausea
- Vomiting
- Weakness
- Dizziness or light-headedness
- Breaking into a sweat or developing cool, clammy skin
- A feeling of irregular or "skipped" heartbeats

Note that any one of the signs and symptoms or a combination of symptoms indicates a cardiac emergency. All signs and symptoms do not have to be present.

EMR Patient Assessment: The Cardiac Patient

Your cardiac assessment will have two components: a history and physical examination.

The patient history often contains some of the most vital information you will use to make decisions. It is also important to turn this information over to the ambulance personnel.

The signs and symptoms ("S" in the SAMPLE history) provide considerable information about the patient's condition. The mnemonic OPQRST is often used to remember the things you should ask about the symptoms of the patient with pain or discomfort:

Onset—What was the patient doing when the pain began? Was he active or at rest?

Provocation—Was the patient doing anything that made the pain begin or get worse? This may be exercise (which causes increased need for oxygen) or movement that makes the pain worse.

Quality—Ask the patient to describe the pain in his own words. This should elicit words that describe the pain (for example, heavy feeling or sharp pain) in greater detail. Simply saying the patient has pain without getting a description of the pain isn't a full assessment.

Region—Where is the pain exactly? Have the patient describe or point to the areas where pain is felt. There are other important "Rs" in addition to region. These include:

> **Radiation**—Does the pain radiate (begin at one point and seem to travel to another)?
>
> **Relief**—Does anything make it feel better (for example, stopping mowing the lawn)?

Severity—How bad is the pain? You may ask the patient to rate the pain on a 1–10 scale where 1 is very minor pain and 10 is the worst pain imaginable.

Time—How long has the patient had the pain?

The remainder of the SAMPLE history will also have value. Determine the patient's medications and prior medical conditions. If you determine your patient has had previous cardiac problems, ask if this feeling is anything like previous cardiac emergencies. Patients with hypertension, diabetes, and high cholesterol, and those who smoke are at a higher risk of cardiac problems.

The events component of the SAMPLE history is also valuable when done properly. Consider this part of getting the full patient history. You should determine if the patient was at rest or active when the pain came on. If the patient was active, determine if activity made the condition worse. Did stopping activity make the symptoms go away?

EMR Emergency Care: The Cardiac Emergency Patient

As mentioned earlier, you do not have to diagnose the exact problem to treat a suspected cardiac condition.

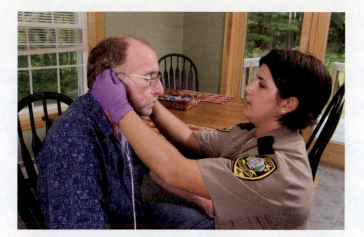

The most important decision you can make when treating a cardiac patient—or any patient—is to initially determine the patient's level of responsiveness and airway status. The care you provide and the order you provide it will be based on this determination. Consider the following two patients:

■ Your patient was said to have been complaining of "indigestion" before becoming unresponsive. You arrive to find him slumped over in a recliner. As you reach him, he vomits.

■ Your patient is sitting at the kitchen table. He is alert and oriented, telling you that he feels like he has some "pressure" in his chest and he feels uncomfortable. He appears to be breathing adequately.

Evaluation of the patient's level of responsiveness, airway and breathing are performed as part of the primary assessment and affect many things throughout the call. Applying this to the two patients just mentioned:

■ The patient who is unresponsive will be positioned supine on the floor, whereas the responsive patient will be placed in a position of comfort (usually sitting) (Figure 14-5 ■).

■ Your care of the unresponsive patient will focus on the ABCs, whereas you will have more time to do the history and examination on the responsive patient.

■ The unresponsive patient will require suction and will likely require ventilation with a pocket face mask or bag-valve mask. The responsive patient will receive oxygen by nasal cannula or nonrebreather mask.

The differences between these two patients are important to the EMR. Of course, the patient examples presented here are two ends of the spectrum. You will find many patients somewhere in between. You will also find patients who appear stable initially and then suddenly become unresponsive. It will be your responsibility to apply the following treatment steps to each patient based on the patient's overall status and individual needs.

To care for the patient with a suspected cardiac emergency (Scan 14-1):

1. Ensure the patient has adequate airway, breathing, and circulation as part of your primary assessment. Treat any problems you find immediately with suction, airway adjuncts, ventilation, CPR, and defibrillation if necessary.

2. Administer oxygen to the adequately breathing patient. Follow your local protocols as to the amount of oxygen and the delivery device. Some systems recommend the use of the nonrebreather mask delivering oxygen at 10–15

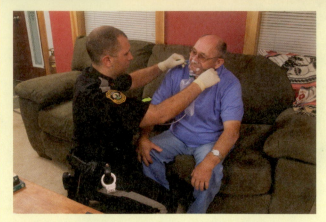

14-1a Administer oxygen and address life threats as necessary.

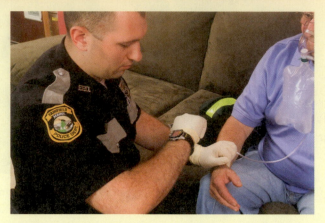

14-1b Perform a primary assessment.

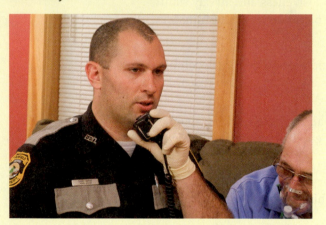

14-1c Update incoming EMS units.

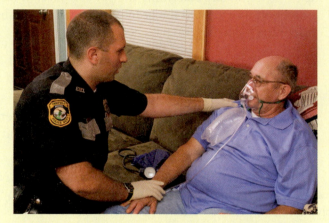

14-1d Assist the responsive patient to a position of comfort.

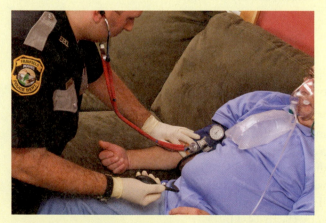

14-1e Perform a secondary exam, take vital signs, and monitor the patient until EMS arrives.

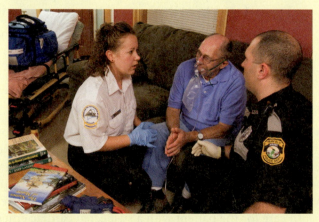

14-1f Transfer of care to incoming unit.

liters per minute (lpm). Others advise applying oxygen based on the patient's presentation and pulse oximetry readings. Recent science has found that too much oxygen may be harmful to patients experiencing a heart attack. In some cases no oxygen or minimal oxygen by nasal cannula may be recommended when the pulse oximetry reading is 95% or higher. Follow local protocols. Those who have lower oximetry readings, severe distress, or poor skin color would receive oxygen by nonrebreather mask at 10–15 lpm.

3. Update EMS units about the patient's complaint and status.
4. Obtain a patient history using SAMPLE and OPQRST.
5. Obtain vital signs.
6. Perform a physical examination concentrating on the cardiac and respiratory system, including palpating the chest and examining the body for fluid and edema.
7. Continue to monitor the patient until the ambulance arrives. The patient with chest pain, discomfort, or other suspected cardiac conditions should be considered unstable and monitored frequently with reassessment at least every 5 minutes:
   a. Look for changes in the patient's level of responsiveness.
   b. Look for changes in the patient's ABCs.
   c. Look for changes in the patient's complaint (better or worse?).
   d. Reassess vital signs.
   e. Ensure interventions (such as oxygen) are still working and effective.
8. Determine if the patient has taken any medications for his condition. The patient may have been instructed to take nitroglycerin or aspirin tablets in the event of chest pain.
9. Transfer care to incoming EMS units.

Note: Any time a patient becomes unresponsive and lifeless, use the C-A-B approach recommended by the American Heart Association.

✹ Stop, Review, Remember

Multiple Choice

Place a check next to the correct answer.

1. Air enters the body during inspiration by passing through the nose or mouth into the oropharynx or nasopharynx. After that, where does the inhaled air go in the respiratory system?
   _____ a. Pharynx
   _____ b. Larynx
   _____ c. Esophagus
   _____ d. Trachea

2. The abnormal use of the neck and intercostal muscles to facilitate respiration is referred to as:
   _____ a. accessory muscle usage.
   _____ b. paradoxical respirations.
   _____ c. "belly breathing."
   _____ d. tracheal breathing.

3. What part of the heart or associated vascular system is occluded or blocked when a myocardial infarction is occurring?
   _____ a. Aorta
   _____ b. Tricuspid valve
   _____ c. Ventricles
   _____ d. Coronary artery

4. When assessing a patient's pain, the "quality" should be asked by:
   _____ a. having the patient describe the pain in his own words.
   _____ b. having the patient pick from a list of usual responses.
   _____ c. asking the patient directly each type of quality it could be.
   _____ d. asking the patient's family what it thinks the quality would be based on the patient's behavior.

True/False

Mark whether each of the following statements is true (T) or false (F).

1. _____ The cardiac patient's mental status and airway are not as important as stopping the "heart attack" from spreading.

2. _____ A common way to describe the severity of the pain is to use a "1–10 scale."

3. _____ Sudden cardiac death is a phenomenon commonly seen by cardiac arrest being the first cardiac sign or symptom in a patient.

4. _____ Respiration and inspiration are terms that mean the same thing and can be used interchangeably.

Critical Thinking

Your patient is found in his residence on the toilet. His family found him slouched against the wall very disoriented and pale and sweaty. He has a "cardiac history" but the family can't tell you anymore than that.

1. What should your initial treatment of this patient be?

   _____

   _____

   _____

2. Is his altered mental status of more importance to you than establishing what may be going on with his heart?

   _____

   _____

   _____

   _____

3. How will your treatment vary if he is having a cardiac event or not?

   _____

   _____

   _____

   _____

Respiratory Emergencies

There are a wide variety of respiratory emergencies a patient may experience (Figure 14-3). Many times the condition you are called to treat is a worsening of an existing condition. This section will review the different types of respiratory emergencies as well as the assessment and care for these emergencies.

As with cardiac emergencies, you will not be required to diagnose exact conditions. Treatment for most respiratory emergencies is the same. There will also be some overlap between cardiac and respiratory emergencies since the systems are so closely related.

Common Respiratory Conditions

The most common respiratory conditions you will see in an emergency are asthma, chronic bronchitis, emphysema, congestive heart failure, and sometimes pneumonia. While there are many other diseases out there—enough to fill entire textbooks—these are the most common you will see.

You won't be required to tell the difference, but a basic knowledge of the diseases will allow you to understand patient presentations and converse with patients and other health care providers about the conditions.

Asthma is a disease that causes airway reactivity. That means there are triggers that cause the smaller airways to constrict. These triggers may be allergies, respiratory infections, or exercise, to name a few. People with asthma have what they refer to as an "attack." The airways will suddenly react and get smaller, which causes the patient to feel short of breath. You may hear wheezing with or without a stethoscope. The patient will be anxious. He may have an inhaler that sprays a medication into the airways that dilates, or opens, the airways.

Chronic bronchitis is a condition in which there is a long-term production of mucus in the lower airways. This is caused by inflammation that can result from smoking or exposure to industrial substances. Patients with chronic bronchitis often have a productive cough and chronic difficulty breathing. Calls for these patients usually occur when the inflammation and mucus production become worse, causing a worsening of breathing difficulties.

Emphysema can also be caused by smoking. Emphysema is a disease that results in the breakdown of the alveoli, reducing gas exchange between the lungs and the bloodstream. Patients will experience difficulty breathing and may be on oxygen all or most of the time.

Emphysema and chronic bronchitis are two diseases that are considered **chronic obstructive pulmonary disease (COPD)** (Figure 14-6 ■). Chronic means long term. Obstructive refers to the inability of air to move in and out and the reduced ability for exchange of gases. These conditions are frequently the cause of calls for difficulty breathing among older patients. The worsening of their conditions may be the result of a new respiratory infection aggravating the underlying disease.

Congestive heart failure is a problem with the heart that affects the lungs. The heart muscle weakens, either from tiring (for example, from overwork because of high blood pressure) or as a result of damage from a heart attack. Because the heart doesn't pump efficiently, blood backs up. When the left side of the heart fails, blood backs up into the lungs. This creates higher pressure in the pulmonary arteries, which results in fluid being

ASK YOURSELF

■ How do you describe what happens in asthma, chronic bronchitis, emphysema, congestive heart failure, and pneumonia?

chronic bronchitis medical condition marked by a long term accumulation of excess mucous in the lower airway.

emphysema respiratory disease often caused by smoking, resulting in a breakdown of the alveoli prohibiting gas exchange.

chronic obstructive pulmonary disease (COPD) term describing diseases which are long term in nature and cause an partial occlusion of the airway.

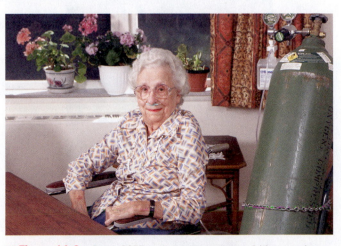

■ **Figure 14-6** Some COPD patients are on oxygen 24 hours a day.

forced from pulmonary capillaries into the space around the alveoli. In severe cases the fluid can seep into the alveoli. This significantly reduces the ability to exchange gases in the alveoli, resulting in hypoxia and respiratory distress.

When the left side of the heart fails, fluid accumulates in the lungs. When the right side of the heart fails, you may see accumulation of fluid in the body. Many times fluid accumulates in **dependent** places (such as the ankles) or the abdomen and flanks in bedridden patients. Patients may have fluid both in their lungs and in dependent parts of the body.

Pneumonia is an infection in the lungs. Although you might not get frequent calls for this, it can make patients quite sick. Patients with pneumonia often complain of chest congestion and cough. The cough may bring up thick sputum from the lungs. Patients may also have a fever, feel weak and achy, and even complain of pain in the chest.

dependent the lowest point in the body.

pneumonia infection of the lungs.

EMR Patient Assessment: Respiratory Complaints

As with cardiac patients, the most important determinations you can make with respiratory patients are in the primary assessment. The primary assessment is designed to identify and treat life threats. You must immediately determine if there are any airway problems (such as vomiting), if the patient is breathing adequately, and if the patient has a pulse. Your first priority is to address these life threats—with suction, oxygen, ventilation, CPR, or defibrillation, as appropriate.

You may observe the patient as soon as you enter the room and note difficulty breathing. How would you know a patient has difficulty breathing before you ask him? Look for these early and serious signs of distress:

- The patient has an altered mental status or is unresponsive.
- The patient is unable to speak more than a few words without catching his breath.
- There is minimal movement of the chest when the patient tries to breathe.
- The patient is working very hard to breathe. It looks difficult to breathe. The patient may use more muscles than usual to expand the chest. The patient may be sitting in the **tripod position** (Figure 14-7 ■).
- The patient has pale skin. The skin may also be cool and moist.

ASK YOURSELF

- How do you differentiate between patients with adequate breathing and patients with inadequate breathing?

tripod position sitting position used to assist the patient's respiration. This allows maximum chest capacity/maximum inspiration.

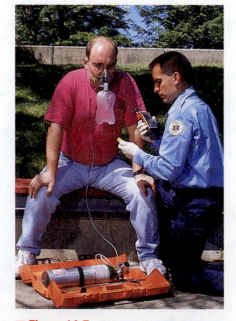

■ **Figure 14-7**   This man is seated in a tripod position, a sign of respiratory distress.

If you see any of the signs during your size-up and primary assessment, you should consider your patient to have a serious condition and carefully evaluate the ABCs.

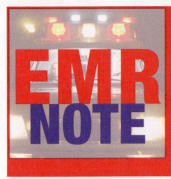

Adequate breathing involves *both* adequate rate of breathing *and* adequate depth of breathing. Monitor your patient throughout the call to make sure adequate breathing is present. If breathing becomes inadequate, you must ventilate the patient. Identifying inadequate breathing before the patient stops breathing is perhaps the most lifesaving action you can perform.

This history usually provides the most valuable information in the medical patient. This is where you will ask about the signs and symptoms as well as other items in the SAMPLE history. If you find the patient has a history of a respiratory or cardiac problem such as congestive heart failure or COPD, ask him if his current symptoms are similar to times in the past when he had that problem.

There are times when the patient can't accurately tell you his medical history. If you have time before the EMTs arrive and you have a drug reference, you can find out much about a patient's history from the medications he takes.

✳ Stop, Review, Remember

Multiple Choice

Place a check next to the correct answer.

1. The most common respiratory conditions you will see in an emergency are:

   _____ a. asthma, chronic bronchitis, emphysema, congestive heart failure, and sometimes pneumonia.

   _____ b. asthma, chronic bronchitis, emphysema, congestive heart failure, and collapsed lung.

   _____ c. asthma, chronic bronchitis, emphysema, congestive heart failure, and lung cancer.

   _____ d. asthma, chronic bronchitis, emphysema, congestive heart failure, and pneumothorax.

2. Which of the following is not an early sign of respiratory distress?

   _____ a. The patient has an altered mental status or is unresponsive.

   _____ b. The patient is able to speak more than a few words.

   _____ c. There is minimal movement of the chest when the patient tries to breathe.

   _____ d. The patient has pale skin. The skin may also be cool and moist.

3. The primary assessment is designed to identify:

   _____ a. life threats.

   _____ b. the patient's respiratory rate.

   _____ c. the need for suction or ventilation.

   _____ d. the condition from which the patient suffers.

True/False

Mark whether each of the following statements is true (T) or false (F).

1. _____ Pneumonia is an infection in the lungs.

2. _____ Emphysema and chronic bronchitis are two diseases that are considered asthma.

3. _____ Adequate breathing involves *both* adequate rate of breathing *and* adequate depth of breathing

Critical Thinking

1. Describe the early and serious signs of respiratory distress that you should note during primary assessment?

_____

_____

_____

_____

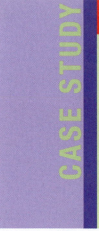

THE RESPONSE

The police cautiously move away from the patient. You observe that he appears to be a 25-year-old male who is breathing adequately but with difficulty. He is sitting with his hands on his knees. An unusual musical sound comes from the patient's chest when he exhales. He can't say many words without having to catch his breath.

■ Discussion: *Would you consider this patient to be serious or nonserious? What signs has he shown to lead you to that conclusion?*

ASK YOURSELF

■ What is the importance of managing the airway, breathing, and circulation, and administering oxygen to patients with cardiac and respiratory problems?

In most cases, the patient will tell you how he feels and what his signs and symptoms are. But there may be things he doesn't know to tell you. In many respiratory and cardiac patients, you may find additional important facts by asking the following questions:

■ Do you have trouble lying flat? Do you need a lot of pillows to sleep? (This may indicate a fluid problem in the lungs that worsens when the patient lies supine. Many patients actually sleep in a recliner when they develop congestive heart failure.)

■ Do you get winded or short of breath when you are active, such as walking up stairs? (Note: Don't ask a patient to do this as a test. It could cause harm.)

■ Have you gained weight in the past several days? (Fluid buildup causes a noticeable weight gain relatively quickly. Some patients will note that their clothes fit more snugly when they have congestive heart failure problems.)

■ Have you noticed any fluid accumulation in your body, such as swollen ankles?

■ Have you had a cough? Is the cough productive? Does the cough bring up any material from the bronchi or bronchioles? Does the sputum have any color to it? Look for other signs of illness, such as fever or chills.

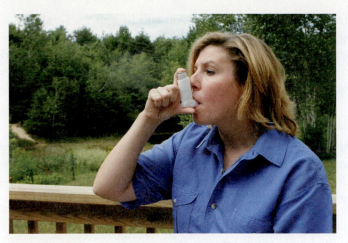

Figure 14-8 Inhalers are prescribed to patients who have breathing problems like asthma or COPD.

- Do you have any pain, heaviness, or discomfort in your chest, neck, jaws, arms, or back?
- Does it hurt when you breathe? When you take a deep breath? Describe and point to the pain.

Remember to monitor the patient throughout your time with him. As you talk with your patient, watch for signs of increasing anxiety or restlessness. This can indicate hypoxia. Any deterioration in mental status is a sign of the patient becoming increasingly unstable.

Complete a full set of vital signs. Respiratory and pulse rates that are above or below the normal limits (very fast or very slow) are a sign of a patient who is unstable.

Ensure the patient remains breathing adequately. Look for any physical signs of respiratory distress including accessory muscle use, jugular venous distention (neck veins bulging), poor skin color (pale, gray, or blue), or skin that is cool and moist. Note if the patient has any swelling of the ankles.

Determine if the patient has taken any medications for his breathing problems. Patients who have asthma and COPD often have prescribed inhalers (Figure 14-8 ■). If the patient has used an inhaler, determine how many times he used the device and if it made any difference in his respiratory distress. Be sure to note this to incoming EMS units in your handoff report.

You may have been taught to auscultate for breath sounds. This procedure is difficult for even experienced providers to perform and interpret. If you use your stethoscope to listen to the chest, the most important thing you can listen for is the sound of air moving in and out adequately and equally on both sides of the chest. If the sounds are significantly less on one side or the other, it could indicate a serious problem such as a **pneumothorax** (collapsed lung) or severe infection.

Listening for wheezing or signs of fluid in the lungs is more difficult. Fluid in the lungs may be a sign of congestive heart failure or other medical problems. The sounds you may hear, known as crackles (rales) and rhonchi, are the sound of air moving through this fluid in smaller airways. The sounds are very difficult to hear. Crackles are a fine popping sound that many describe as similar to the sound you hear when rubbing strands of hair together directly in front of your ear. Rhonchi are a coarser sound, more akin to bubbling or rattling.

Mentioned earlier, wheezing is a sound caused by air being forced through narrowed airways. This is often seen in asthma—although other conditions may present with wheezing as well. Wheezing is described as musical because of the various pitches of sound you may hear in one breath. You will hear this with and without a stethoscope.

ASK YOURSELF
- What are the emergency care steps of patients with cardiac and respiratory problems?

pneumothorax   a leak or tear in the lung causing air to fill in to the thoracic cavity.

To listen for abnormal lung sounds, you will listen to several areas of the patient's chest including the bases (lower lobes) of the lungs on the patient's back. Remember that these sounds are difficult to hear and interpret. Do not take valuable time doing this while you have other assessment or care tasks that are more important such as ensuring adequate breathing, administering oxygen, obtaining a history, and taking vital signs.

EMR Emergency Care: Respiratory Emergencies

Your care for the patient with a respiratory emergency will involve several components. Most importantly, you will monitor the patient's respiratory effort to ensure the patient is breathing adequately initially and throughout the call.

To care for the patient with difficulty breathing:

1. Position the patient for care. There are three ways you may position the patient depending on his condition:
   - If the patient is responsive and breathing adequately, you will place him in a position of comfort. This is up to the patient. In many cases the patient with respiratory distress will prefer to sit or slightly recline.
   - If the patient is breathing inadequately (the patient breathing inadequately isn't getting enough oxygen and will have an altered mental status ranging from severely anxious to unresponsive), you will position him for ventilation. If the patient tolerates it, lay the patient supine and use your bag-valve mask to ventilate him. If this makes the patient increasingly anxious, you may ventilate him in a sitting or semireclining position.
   - If the patient is not breathing, he will be placed in a supine position and ventilated.
2. Administer oxygen by nasal cannula, by nonrebreather mask, or through ventilation by pocket face mask or bag-valve mask.
3. Update incoming EMS units via phone or radio in reference to the patient's status and complaint.
4. Determine if the patient has taken any medications for his condition (such as a prescribed inhaler). Has this medication helped his condition?
5. Reassure the patient. Speak in a slow, calming tone. This has tremendous value to the patient with respiratory or cardiac conditions. Not only will it place the patient at ease, but it also has a positive medical effect. When the patient is calmer, the body requires less oxygen. The heart calms and slows. It then needs less oxygen to work. This can reduce chest pain and respiratory distress.

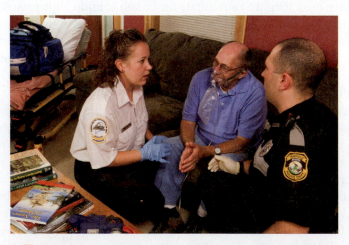

■ **Figure 14-9** Transfer of care from EMR to EMT, with the EMR providing a verbal report.

6. Monitor the patient carefully throughout the call.
7. Transfer care to the arriving EMS units (Figure 14-9 ■). Provide a thorough handoff report.

CASE STUDY

TRANSITION ✳

You have convinced the police that the patient's anxiety and behavior is at least partially due to the breathing condition. The patient tells you that he has asthma but his inhaler was in his car, which was towed by the police. You apply oxygen via nonrebreather mask and calm the patient while you complete a history, vitals, and physical exam. You provide the handoff report to the incoming Paramedics who assume care for the patient. He is transported to the hospital under police guard.

■ Discussion: *Sympathy played a role in the report to the police. Do you agree with this assessment?*

THE LAST WORD

Cardiac and respiratory complaints are common reasons people call for EMS. Not only are patients in need of your care for their medical condition, they are also in need of your calming and compassion. Many people you will encounter may believe they are about to die. There are few feelings more frightening than not being able to breathe.

This chapter is the first to cover specific types of emergencies. You have now seen how the primary assessment, history, vital signs, and secondary assessment apply to real patient conditions.

✳ *Chapter Review*

Multiple Choice

Place a check next to the correct answer.

1. What respiratory disease or condition is said to have "triggers" that cause airway reactivity and ultimately constrict the airways?

_____ a. Pneumonia

_____ b. Bronchitis

_____ c. Asthma

_____ d. Emphysema

2. Which disease, most often caused by smoking, results in a breakdown of the alveoli thereby not allowing gas exchange to take place?

_____ a. Pneumonia

_____ b. Bronchitis

_____ c. Asthma

_____ d. Emphysema

3. When asking a patient about secretion brought up from the bronchial tree, it is also important to note the _____ of the secretions.

_____ a. color

_____ b. size

_____ c. shape

_____ d. density

4. When auscultating breath sounds, you note that one side is particularly diminished to almost absect. What should you suspect is taking place?

_____ a. Congestive heart failure

_____ b. Coronary vascular accident

_____ c. Pneumothorax

_____ d. Myocardial infarction

5. When discussing the "OPQRST" mnemonic, which of the following is not one of the commonly used "R's?"

_____ a. Radiation

_____ b. Relief

_____ c. Region

_____ d. Recent history

6. A person who's first cardiac symptom is full cardiac arrest is said to be suffering from the phenomenon of

_____ a. congestive heart failure.

_____ b. sudden cardiac death.

_____ c. sudden pulmonary death.

_____ d. chronic obstructive pulmonary disease.

7. After blood passes through the left ventricle, where does it travel next in the circulatory system?

_____ a. The lungs

_____ b. The atria

_____ c. The aorta

_____ d. The brain

8. What cardiac condition can often present when the heart is under great oxygen demand but then subside entirely when that demand is ceased?

_____ a. Angina

_____ b. Myocardial infarction

_____ c. Heart attack

_____ d. Cerebral vascular accident

9. The cardiovascular system consists of the heart and the

_____ a. lungs.

_____ b. brain.

_____ c. blood vessels.

_____ d. abdominal organs.

10. The heart is a muscular organ. As such, it requires a great deal of _____ to act as fuel to make it beat.

_____ a. oxygen

_____ b. air

_____ c. blood

_____ d. plasma

True/False

Indicate whether each of the following is true (T) or false (F) on the line provided.

1. _____ The heart is a hollow organ.

2. _____ Oxygen is the principal gas taken in to the body during inspiration for the purpose of respiration at the alveolar level.

3. _____ Carbon dioxide is the primary gas exchanged during respiration.

4. _____ Patients who are having a hard time breathing will often be using accessory muscles to facilitate inspiration.

5. _____ Congestive heart failure is a cardiac condition and has nothing to do with the lungs.

Critical Thinking

Your patient is an elderly male who tells you that he has "CHF" or congestive heart failure. His chief complaint today is that his chest hurts and he feels like it is very hard for him to breathe. You hear what sounds like water bubbling every time he breathes. His blood pressure is high and he is visibly using accessory muscles to aid in breathing.

1. Is this person's problem primarily cardiac or respiratory in nature?

_____

_____

_____

2. Does it seem as though all his symptoms can be linked together? Why?

_____

_____

_____

3. What is your best course of action to help this patient?

_____

_____

_____

4. What important facts should you emphasize when turning the patient over to another emergency care provider?

_____

_____

_____

Altered Mental Status

✳ NAVIGATION GUIDE

The following items provide an overview to the purpose and content of this chapter. The Education Standard and Competency are from the National EMS Education Standards.

Education Standard Medicine (Neurology, Endocrine Disorders, Psychiatric, Toxicology)

Competency Recognizes and manages life threats based on assessment findings of a patient with a medical emergency while awaiting additional emergency response.

Knowledge Areas Neurology
Anatomy, presentations, and management of:
- Decreased level of responsiveness
- Seizure
- Stroke
Endocrine Disorders
Awareness that:
- Diabetic emergencies cause altered mental status
Psychiatric
Recognition of:
- Behaviors that pose a risk to the EMR, patient, or others
Toxicology
Recognition and management of:
- Carbon monoxide poisoning
- Nerve agent poisoning
- How and when to contact a poison control center

Objectives After reading this chapter, you should be able to:

1. Define key terms introduced in this chapter.
2. Describe the range of findings that indicate an altered mental status.

3. Give examples of conditions that can cause altered mental status, including underlying causes of:
   a. Seizures
   b. Behavioral emergencies

4. Given a scenario of a response to a patient with an altered mental status:
   a. Explain the special considerations for EMS personnel safety.
   b. Recognize scene findings that may be clues to the cause of a patient's altered mental status.
5. Given a description of a patient's response to stimuli, differentiate between patients who are alert, those who respond to verbal or painful stimuli, and those who are unresponsive.
6. Recognize common signs and symptoms of:
   a. Diabetic emergencies
   b. Stroke and transient ischemic attack
   c. Seizure
   d. Poisoning
   e. Behavioral emergencies
7. Given a scenario involving a patient with an altered mental status, demonstrate the appropriate assessment and care of the patient, including management of patients with:
   a. Diabetic emergencies
   b. Stroke
   c. Seizure
   d. Status epilepticus
   e. Poisoning, including drug and alcohol emergencies
   f. Behavioral emergencies
8. Give examples of specific questions that should be asked when obtaining the history of patients with:
   a. Diabetic emergencies
   b. Poisoning
   c. Behavioral emergencies, including assessment of suicide risk
9. Predict what will happen if a patient has either too little or too much insulin for the amount of glucose present in his blood.
10. Compare and contrast the characteristics of hyperglycemia (diabetic coma) and hypoglycemia.
11. Explain what happens when a patient has either an ischemic or a hemorrhagic stroke.
12. Demonstrate use of the Cincinnati Prehospital Stroke Scale.
13. Describe the phases of a generalized seizure.
14. Give examples of poisons that can enter the body by each of the four routes:
    a. Injection
    b. Ingestion
    c. Inhalation
    d. Absorption
15. Explain the importance of contacting poison control when managing a patient who has been poisoned.
16. Demonstrate techniques of calming patients with behavioral emergencies.

Key Terms Page references indicate first major use in this chapter. The Margin Glossary in this chapter provides definitions as you read.

altered mental status, p. 356

glucose, p. 358

insulin, p. 358

diabetes mellitus, p. 358

diabetes, p. 358

hyperglycemia, p. 358

hypoglycemia, p. 359

stroke, p. 364

transient ischemic attack (TIA), p. 364

seizure, p. 367

poison, p. 371

drug abuse, p. 377

overdose, p. 377

withdrawal, p. 377

carbon monoxide (CO), p. 379

behavior, p. 384

behavioral emergency, p. 384

Media Resources Please go to **www.bradybooks.com** to access mykit for this text. You will find quizzes, critical thinking scenarios, weblinks, animations, and videos related to this chapter—much more. Look for online information on strokes, stroke prevention, and diabetes.

INTRODUCTION

altered mental status
condition of decreased
alertness and responsiveness.

As an EMR, you will encounter medical patients who present with an **altered mental status**. This may be a result of a medical condition, such as diabetes, an infection, or stroke; temperature extremes; intentional actions, such as alcohol or substance abuse; or accidental poisonings.

Your responsibility will be to ensure your safety and your patient's safety, perform a patient assessment, and provide appropriate emergency medical care based on that assessment until EMS personnel arrive to continue care and transport.

CASE STUDY

THE CALL

It is a warm summer day, and you are assisting with a medical standby assignment at your community's annual softball tournament. The sun is shining, and there is a gentle breeze. The temperature is in the mid-80s with moderate humidity.

The third game of the day is well under way. The crowds are cheering their favorite teams, and people are frequenting the concession stands. All in all, this has been an uneventful day for medical response.

As the game progresses, you notice that one of the bystanders in the grandstand is yelling excessively and inappropriately. He is waving his arms about and trying to push away those trying to help. Some of the others nearby are starting to react to the unusual behavior, and your response is requested by tournament officials.

■ Discussion: *What is the first thing you must do as you approach the scene?*

ASK YOURSELF
■ Can you define the key terms?
■ What are the findings that indicate an altered mental status?
■ What are some examples of conditions that can cause altered mental status, including underlying causes of:
　■ Seizures?
　■ Behavioral emergencies?

Altered Mental Status

When we think about a person's mental status, we think about his alertness and orientation to his environment. A person is said to have a normal mental status when he is alert and oriented to person, place, time, and, some sources say, self. An altered mental status is a condition characterized by a decrease in the patient's alertness and responsiveness to the environment (Figure 15-1 ■). Altered mental status can occur rapidly or slowly. It can range from disorientation to combativeness to unresponsiveness. There are several reasons a person may experience an altered mental status, for example:

■ Hypoxia (decreased level of oxygen in the blood)
■ Diabetic emergencies
■ Stroke (loss of blood flow to part of the brain)
■ Seizures
■ Fever or infection
■ Poisoning or substance abuse (including drugs or alcohol)
■ Head injury or other trauma

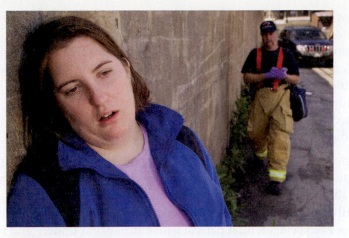

■ Figure 15-1 Patient with altered mental status.

- Psychiatric conditions
- Cardiac problems
- Respiratory problems
- Environmental exposures (excessive heat or cold)

This can seem overwhelming to the EMR, but your responsibility is to perform a patient assessment and provide appropriate emergency medical care based on that assessment until EMS personnel arrive to continue care and transport.

EMR Patient Assessment: Altered Mental Status

After ensuring scene safety and taking the appropriate Standard Precautions, proceed with your patient assessment. What is your general impression of the patient? What is the patient's mental status? Is he alert, responding to verbal stimuli, and responding to painful stimuli, or is he unresponsive to any stimuli? Is his airway open? Is he breathing? Is he breathing adequately? How is his circulation, skin color, and skin condition? Has EMS been requested to respond?

Attempt to obtain as accurate a history as possible. This may be obtained from the patient, the family, or bystanders and is a valuable asset in patient care. You may be the only provider able to get this information in a timely fashion. Perform an appropriate physical exam of the patient.

EMR Emergency Care: Altered Mental Status

If you suspect a patient has an altered mental status, you should immediately notify the responding EMS personnel and take appropriate Standard Precautions. Steps to providing care for this patient include:

1. Monitor and maintain the patient's airway, breathing, and circulation (ABCs). Be sure both breathing and circulation are adequate. If not adequate, take appropriate steps or correct.
2. Position the patient. If you do not suspect head or spine injury, place the patient in the recovery position. Be sure to monitor the patient's airway and breathing closely.
3. Administer oxygen. One of the most common causes of altered mental status is hypoxia. If the patient is breathing adequately, apply oxygen by nonrebreather mask or cannula, depending on the patient's condition and your protocols. If

ASK YOURSELF

- Given a scenario of a response to a patient with an altered mental status:
  - What are the special considerations for EMS personnel safety at an altered mental status scene?
  - How do you recognize scene findings that may be clues to the cause of a patient's altered mental status?

- Given a description of a patient's response to stimuli, how do you differentiate between patients who are alert, those who respond to verbal or painful stimuli, and those who are unresponsive?

the patient is not breathing adequately, assist with a pocket face mask or bag-valve-mask (BVM) device attached to an oxygen source.

4. Monitor the patient's mental status and vital signs frequently. This will help you see trends in the patient's condition. Is his condition getting better? Is his condition staying about the same? Is his condition getting worse?
5. Provide emotional support to the patient.
6. Be sure to notify the responding EMS personnel of any changes in the patient's condition.

Altered mental status can be a frightening experience for both the patient and the EMR. You should behave in a professional and empathetic manner and try not to act surprised by the abnormal physical findings you might encounter. In many cases the patient may be partially aware of his surroundings. A patient with a diabetic emergency may be very agitated or even belligerent. A patient with a stroke may understand what you're saying but not be able to respond verbally. A patient with a seizure may be incontinent (lose control of his bowels or bladder) which can be embarrassing. A patient who has taken an overdose may be aggressive. A patient with a behavioral problem may be violent.

The situation may also be very upsetting to the family. Attempt to reassure them that everything that can be done is being done and EMS will be arriving to transport the patient to the hospital for further care.

As an EMR, your role in the continuity of care is to ensure your personal safety, including appropriate Standard Precautions; assess the patient's condition in a systematic approach; provide care for both life-threatening and non-life-threatening conditions; and transfer care and information to the responding EMS personnel.

Through your efforts you can make a difference in the lives of those you serve.

Diabetic Emergencies

glucose a form of simple sugar that is the main source of fuel for the body's cells.

insulin hormone that allows glucose to enter the body's cells.

diabetes mellitus commonly referred to as diabetes, a condition that prevents individuals from producing enough insulin or from using insulin effectively.

diabetes common term for diabetes mellitus.

hyperglycemia high blood glucose.

Glucose, a form of simple sugar, is the main source of fuel for the body's cells. Glucose enters the body through what we eat and drink. It is carried to the cells by way of the bloodstream. Glucose is a large molecule and is unable to enter the body's cells by itself; it requires a helper. This helper is a hormone called **insulin**. Insulin is produced in the pancreas and allows glucose to enter the body's cells so it can be used for fuel (Figure 15-2 ■).

Like many body processes, glucose and insulin work in a delicate balancing act. Too much, or too little, glucose can cause problems. Too much, or too little, insulin can also cause problems.

Diabetes mellitus, commonly just referred to as **diabetes**, is a condition that prevents individuals from producing enough insulin (type 1 diabetes) or from not using insulin effectively (type 2 diabetes). Depending upon the extent of the diabetes, a patient may be managing his diabetes through a balanced diet, oral medications or, in more severe cases, insulin injections.

Generally there are two types of emergencies related to diabetes: hyperglycemia and hypoglycemia. Even though these two emergencies represent different ends of the glucose-insulin balancing act, the EMR management for each is the same. It will not be necessary for you to distinguish one condition from the other in order to care for your patient.

Many diabetic patients wear bracelets or necklaces that identify them as diabetics. When assessing any patient with altered mental status, make sure to check for the presence of such medical identification jewelry.

Hyperglycemia, or too high blood glucose, is the result of too much blood glucose and too little insulin. Common causes of hyperglycemia include the following:

- Infection
- Increased or prolonged stress

ASK YOURSELF

■ What are the common signs and symptoms of diabetic emergencies?

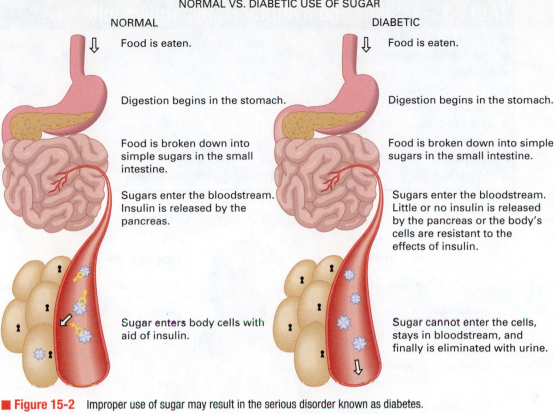

NORMAL VS. DIABETIC USE OF SUGAR

NORMAL	DIABETIC
⇩ Food is eaten.	⇩ Food is eaten.
Digestion begins in the stomach.	Digestion begins in the stomach.
Food is broken down into simple sugars in the small intestine.	Food is broken down into simple sugars in the small intestine.
Sugars enter the bloodstream. Insulin is released by the pancreas.	Sugars enter the bloodstream. Little or no insulin is released by the pancreas or the body's cells are resistant to the effects of insulin.
Sugar enters body cells with aid of insulin.	Sugar cannot enter the cells, stays in bloodstream, and finally is eliminated with urine.

■ **Figure 15-2** Improper use of sugar may result in the serious disorder known as diabetes.

- Failure of the patient to take his insulin or to take a sufficient amount of insulin
- Failure of the patient to take his oral diabetic medications or to take a sufficient amount of medication
- Eating too much food that contains or produces sugar

A hyperglycemic emergency is sometimes called a diabetic coma, even though the patient is not usually found in a coma.

EMR Patient Assessment: Hyperglycemia

Signs and symptoms for a patient with hyperglycemia are listed in Table 15-1 and shown in Figure 15-3 ■.

The onset of severe hyperglycemia is gradual, sometimes taking several days. Excessive hunger, thirst, and urination are usually some of the first signs. The patient often appears extremely ill and becomes sicker and weaker as the condition progresses. If the patient does not receive treatment, he may become unresponsive and possibly die. Improvement in the patient's condition is gradual, often occurring over 6 to 12 hours after insulin and intravenous (IV) fluids are administered.

EMR Patient Assessment: Hypoglycemia

Hypoglycemia, or too low blood glucose (sugar), is a result of too much insulin, too little glucose, or too much oral glucose control medication. This may be one of the more frequent diabetic emergency calls you will handle as an EMR. The onset of hypoglycemia is usually sudden, and the signs and symptoms are dramatic. Low blood glucose may occur in patients with diabetes, alcoholics, people who have ingested certain poisons, and people who are ill.

hypoglycemia low blood glucose.

TABLE 15-1 Signs and Symptoms: Hyperglycemia

- Altered mental status
- Sweet, fruity, or acetone-like breath
- Flushed, warm, dry skin
- Hunger and thirst
- Rapid weak pulse
- Intoxicated appearance, staggering, slurred speech
- Frequent urination
- Blurry vision
- Reports that the patient has not taken the prescribed diabetes medications

SIGNS AND SYMPTOMS OF A DIABETIC EMERGENCY

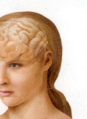

Hyperglycemia

Altered mental status

Sweet, fruity, or acetone-like breath

Hunger and thirst

Intoxicated appearance, staggering, slurred speech

Rapid, weak pulse

Frequent urination

Reports that patient has not been taking prescribed medications

Hypoglycemia

Rapid onset of altered mental status

Headache, hunger

Intoxicated appearance, staggering, slurred speech

Seizures

Cool, clammy skin

Rapid pulse rate

■ **Figure 15-3**   Signs and symptoms of a diabetic emergency.

Some additional common causes of hypoglycemia may include the following:

- Skipped meals, particularly for patients with diabetes
- Vomiting, especially with illness
- Strenuous exercise
- Physical stress from extreme heat or cold
- Emotional stress, such as weddings or funerals

The most recognized cause of low blood glucose is accidental overdose of insulin relative to inadequate ingestion of food.

Signs and symptoms for a patient with hypoglycemia are listed in Table 15-2.

TABLE 15-2 Signs and Symptoms: Hypoglycemia

- Rapid onset of altered mental status
- Intoxicated appearance, staggering, slurred speech
- Rapid pulse rate
- Cool, clammy skin
- Hunger and thirst
- Headache
- Seizures

When obtaining a history of a patient suffering a diabetic emergency, remember to ask him, "Have you eaten today?" "Did you take your medication today?" "Have you had any problems recently with your medication?" "Have you been sick or under stress lately?" Look for a medical identification tag during the physical exam. If the police are present, ask them to check the patient's wallet, too. If the patient is at home, you can check the refrigerator for diabetic medications such as insulin. You can also check around the house for needles and syringes or the presence of a discarded needle container.

EMR Emergency Care: Diabetic Emergency

You do not have to distinguish between hyperglycemia and hypoglycemia, but if you suspect a patient is having a diabetic emergency you should immediately notify the responding EMS personnel and take appropriate Standard Precautions. Steps to providing care for this patient include:

1. Monitor and maintain the patient's airway, breathing, and circulation.
2. Position the patient in a sitting position if responsive, or in a recovery position if unresponsive.
3. Administer high-flow oxygen.
4. Administer sugar, if allowed by your local protocol (Figures 15-4a and 15-4b ■). As mentioned earlier, you do not have to distinguish between hyperglycemia and hypoglycemia. Giving sugar will not harm the patient with hyperglycemia, but it could save the life of a patient with hypoglycemia. Before administering, be sure the patient is awake and is able to swallow. One of the following methods is suggested:
   a. Dissolve some sugar in a glass of water or juice and have the patient drink.

ASK YOURSELF

- Given a scenario involving a patient with an altered mental status, how do you demonstrate the appropriate assessment and care of the patient, including management of patients with diabetic emergencies?

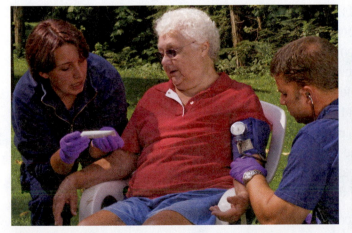

■ **Figure 15-4a**   EMRs assessing and treating a patient with a diabetic emergency.

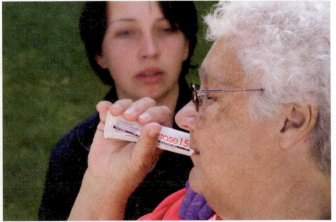

■ **Figure 15-4b**   A patient self-administering oral glucose.

b. Have the patient drink a beverage containing sugar. Do not use diet beverages as they do not contain sugar.

c. Use a commercially prepared glucose paste. The patient who is oriented and able to follow instructions may squeeze small amounts of paste into their mouth, swallow it and then squeeze in another small amount. Continue this until the tube is gone or until the patient develops a decreased mental status.

You may also squeeze a commercially prepared glucose paste onto a tongue depressor. Then, assist the patient in placing the tongue depressor between his cheek and gums. If the patient starts to gag or develops an altered mental status, remove the tongue depressor.

Never give a patient who cannot control his own airway anything to eat or drink. This might cause the patient to aspirate the substance into his lungs. Such aspiration might cause severe consequences, including death. When in doubt, contact medical direction for guidance.

5. Monitor the patient's mental status and vital signs frequently.

6. Provide emotional support to the patient.

7. Be sure to notify the responding EMS personnel that you administered sugar and what changes you noticed in the patient after administration.

CASE STUDY

THE RESPONSE

As you approach the grandstand, you take appropriate Standard Precautions and perform a scene size-up. There are several spectators gathered around a middle-aged male. The patient seems to be very agitated and is yelling at the other spectators. Some of the spectators are trying to calm him down. Within a few minutes, the patient is a little calmer and consents to your exam; however, he is still quite agitated. You contact the dispatch center and request an ambulance.

Your assessment reveals a 42-year-old male patient with a sudden onset of altered mental status. He is complaining of a headache and thirst. Bystanders state the patient was cheering the team when he suddenly started yelling at them and behaving erratically. The patient's initial vital signs are pulse of 142, respirations of 28, and blood pressure of 132/84. The patient's skin is cool and clammy. Upon examining the extremities, you notice a medical alert identification bracelet that indicates the patient is a diabetic.

You allow the patient to sit in a position of comfort while continuing to monitor his airway and breathing. You place the patient on oxygen at 15 lpm by nonrebreather mask. Following local protocol, you place glucose paste on a tongue depressor and place it between his gum and cheek.

Reassessment shows an improved mental status. Repeat vital signs are pulse of 92, respirations of 18, and blood pressure of 128/82.

■ Discussion: *Should you have tested the patient's glucose level before administering the glucose paste?*

Multiple Choice

Place a check next to the correct answer.

1. The main source of fuel for the body's cells is:

    ____ a. fructose.

    ____ b. sucrose.

    ____ c. maltose.

    ____ d. glucose.

2. All of the following are common causes of hyperglycemia EXCEPT:

    ____ a. infection.

    ____ b. increased stress.

    ____ c. not eating enough.

    ____ d. not taking enough insulin.

3. Your diabetic patient is complaining of a rapid onset of altered mental status. He has a rapid pulse and cool, clammy skin. Your patient is most likely suffering from:

    ____ a. hypoglycemia.

    ____ b. hyperglycemia.

    ____ c. hypothermia.

    ____ d. hyperthermia.

Emergency Medical Responder Practice

You respond to a family reunion for a diabetic patient with an altered mental status. The family says the patient has not felt well or acted like himself for a couple of days, but didn't want to miss the reunion. They also state he has been enjoying the variety of foods brought by relatives, but they are not sure when he last checked his blood sugar or took his insulin. When talking with the patient, you notice he has an unusual breath odor.

1. List four signs or symptoms you would expect to see with this patient.

    _____

    _____

    _____

    _____

2. Though it is not necessary that you distinguish between hypoglycemia and hyperglycemia to initiate emergency care, would you suspect this patient is suffering from hypoglycemia or hyperglycemia? Why?

    _____

    _____

    _____

    _____

3. What would the treatment for this patient include?

    _____

    _____

    _____

    _____

True/False

Mark whether each of the following statements is true (T) or false (F).

1. _____ A patient with a diabetic emergency might appear to be intoxicated.

2. _____ Insulin is the primary fuel for the body's cells.

3. _____ Hyperglycemia is the condition in which there is too little insulin and too much blood sugar.

4. _____ Hypoglycemia is too low blood sugar.

5. _____ Glucose is the hormone that helps the body's cells use insulin.

ASK YOURSELF

■ What are the common signs and symptoms of stroke and transient ischemic attack?

stroke a condition that interrupts the blood supply to the brain.

Stroke

Like the heart, the brain needs a steady supply of blood to deliver oxygen and nutrients and remove carbon dioxide and waste products. Any interruption in this blood supply will result in a stroke, previously called cerebrovascular accident (CVA). There are two types of stroke. One is caused by a blockage of the blood flow by a clot (ischemic stroke). The second type is caused when a blood vessel within the brain ruptures (hemorrhagic stroke). Ischemic strokes are much more common than hemorrhagic strokes.

Stroke is the third leading cause of death in the United States. It follows heart disease and cancer. To help emphasize the similarity between a stroke (interruption of blood supply to the brain) and a heart attack (interruption of blood supply to the heart), the American Stroke Association sometimes refers to a stroke as a "brain attack."

Though anyone can suffer from a stroke, it is more common in people over the age of 65. Additional risk factors include cardiac diseases, high blood pressure, diabetes, and smoking.

Some patients may experience signs and symptoms of a stroke that only last a short period of time. These temporary signs and symptoms may indicate a "mini-stroke" or **transient ischemic attack (TIA)**. TIAs are often a warning sign that an impending stroke will occur in the future. Patients who experience a TIA should not ignore the warning and should seek medical assistance.

transcient ischemic attack signs and symptoms of a stroke that only last a short period of time. These temporary signs and symptoms may indicate a "mini-stroke." TIAs are often a warning sign of an impending stroke.

There have been great strides in recent years to improve the outcomes of patients suffering a stroke. Programs such as the American Stroke Association's "Get with the Guidelines" and the Joint Commission's "Certificate of Distinction for Primary Stroke Centers" have helped to enhance patient care and ultimately the quality of life after a stroke.

EMR Patient Assessment: Stroke

The signs and symptoms you may see in a patient with a stroke (or TIA) include (Figure 15-5 ■):

- *Altered mental status.* This can range from a change in personality to seizures to unresponsiveness.
- *Inability to communicate.* The patient may either fail to speak normally or fail to understand what others say.
- *Impairment in one part (or side) of the body.* Use care when handling an extremity that appears paralyzed so as not to injure the patient (Figure 15-6 ■).

ASK YOURSELF

■ What happens when a patient has either an ischemic or a hemorrhagic stroke?

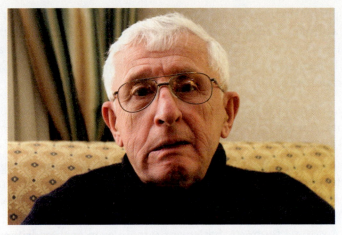

Figure 15-5 Facial asymmetry or facial droop is one sign of stroke.
© Daniel Limmer

Attempt to determine the exact time the patient started experiencing these signs and symptoms. This information may be obtained from the patient, family, or bystanders.

About half of all stroke patients have an increased blood pressure during a stroke. The combination of decreased mental status, increased blood pressure, slow pulse, and rapid or irregular breathing is a sign of a major stroke. You should also be prepared in case the patient experiences sudden convulsions.

ASK YOURSELF

■ Given a scenario involving a patient with an altered mental status, how do you demonstrate the appropriate assessment and care of the patient, including management of patients with stroke?

SIGNS AND SYMPTOMS OF STROKE

Altered mental status.

Change in personality.

Severe headache.

Pupils unequal in size.

Drooping eyelid and mouth on one side of face.

Loss of vision, dimness, or double vision.

Paralysis or weakness on one or both sides of the body.

Difficulty speaking or slurred speech.

Inability to speak.

Rapid or irregular breathing.

Elevated blood pressure.

Nausea or vomiting.

Slow, bounding pulse.

Sudden weakness or paralysis of face, arm, or leg.

Possible seizures.

Loss of bowel or bladder control.

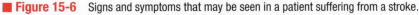

Figure 15-6 Signs and symptoms that may be seen in a patient suffering from a stroke.

There are specific prehospital tests that you can perform to help determine if the patient is having a stroke. One of the most common is the Cincinnati Prehospital Stroke Scale. This scale tests the nerves affected by a stroke. Be sure to report any abnormal findings to the EMTs responding to your scene. The Cincinnati Prehospital Stroke Scale has three major components:

■ *Facial droop* (Figure 15-7a ■). Ask the patient to smile while you note his facial movements. A normal finding is symmetry (equal movement on both sides). An abnormal finding is asymmetry, or drooping on one side and not the other.

■ *Arm drift* (Figure 15-7b ■). Ask the patient to hold both arms straight out in front of his body with the palms down. You may need to assist in supporting his arms. Then ask him to close his eyes and hold his arms in that position for about 30 seconds. Watch to see if one arm, and not the other, begins to fall or drift from position. A normal finding is both arms remain even or they drift evenly together. An abnormal finding is one arm drops or rises, while the other arm remains in position.

■ *Speech* (Figure 15-7c ■). Ask the patient to repeat a simple phrase aloud such as, "you can't teach an old dog new tricks." Listen for slurred speech while the patient talks. This will reveal a problem faster than yes or no answers. A normal finding is clear speech. An abnormal finding is slurred speech or the inability to accurately repeat a phrase. If the patient has had prior strokes ask a family member if there are changes from the patient's prior condition.

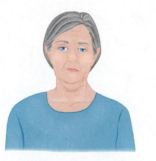

FACIAL DROOP

Normal Both sides of the face move equally.

Abnormal One side of the face does not move equally with the opposite side or it doesn't move at all.

■ **Figure 15-7a** Facial droop in a stroke patient.

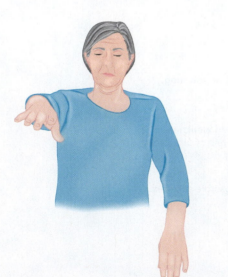

ARM DRIFT

Normal Both arms move equally or can be held steady.

Abnormal One arm drifts compared to the other.

■ **Figure 15-7b** Arm drift in a stroke patient.

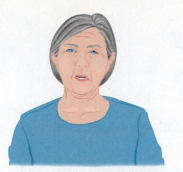

SPEECH

Normal   Patient uses correct words with no slurring.

Abnormal   Words are slurred, inappropriate, or the patient is unable to speak.

■ **Figure 15-7c**   Stroke patients often experience speech difficulties.

EMR Emergency Care: Stroke

If you suspect a patient is having a stroke, you should immediately notify the responding EMS personnel and take appropriate Standard Precautions. Steps to providing care for this patient include:

1. Monitor and maintain the patient's airway, breathing, and circulation.
2. Position the patient. If tolerated, the patient's head should be kept as flat as possible to maximize blood to the brain.
3. Administer oxygen if the pulse oximetry reading is below 95% or as directed by local protocols. Current science indicates it is possible to administer too much oxygen to a stroke patient. If you don't have a pulse oximeter or if the patient appears hypoxic, administer oxygen per protocol.
4. Monitor the patient's mental status and vital signs frequently.
5. Provide emotional support to the patient.
6. Never give a patient with suspected stroke anything to eat or drink. The airway may be compromised by the paralysis. Also, food or drink may cause complications if surgery is needed.
7. Be sure to notify the responding EMS personnel that you suspect a stroke. It is important to note the exact time the patient started experiencing signs and symptoms.

The loss of mental or motor function may be extremely frightening for your stroke patient. Continue to communicate with the patient, even if he is having difficulty responding to you. Do not make any statements about long-term disability.

Seizure

A **seizure** is a sudden change in behavior or movement caused by irregular electrical activity in the brain. It can last from a few seconds to several minutes. Symptoms can range from a twitch of a part of the body to the entire body muscle contractions. Having a seizure is strenuous on the body, and many patients are very sleepy afterward. Though not usually life threatening, they can indicate a serious underlying problem. Common causes of seizures include the following:

■ Chronic medical conditions
■ Epilepsy
■ Hypoglycemia
■ Poisoning
■ Substance abuse
■ Stroke
■ Fever (most commonly in children)

seizure   a sudden change in behavior or movement caused by irregular electrical activity in the brain.

ASK YOURSELF

■ What are the common signs and symptoms of seizure?

ASK YOURSELF

■ Given a scenario involving a patient with an altered mental status, how do you demonstrate the appropriate assessment and care of the patient, including management of patients with seizure?

■ Infection

■ Head injury

■ Brain tumors

■ Hypoxia

■ Complications of pregnancy

EMR Patient Assessment: Seizure

Most commonly you will be called to the scene for a patient having a generalized tonic-clonic seizure (formerly called a grand mal seizure). This type of seizure affects the entire body. There are four phases to this type of seizure:

■ *Aura phase.* The patient becomes aware that a seizure is going to happen. He may describe the aura as an unusual smell or visual image. This usually occurs in the moments prior to the seizure. Not all patients have auras prior to a seizure.

■ *Tonic phase.* The patient becomes unresponsive and collapses to the ground. Then, all the muscles of the body contract. This can force a scream out of the patient. This can also force sputum, which may look like foam, out of the mouth. During this phase, some patients may stop breathing briefly.

■ *Clonic phase.* The patient's muscles alternate between contraction and relaxation. The patient may become incontinent (unable to control his bladder or bowels). Because the patient may bite his cheek, there may be blood in the mouth.

■ *Postictal phase.* The patient gradually regains responsiveness. At first, the patient is confused and even combative. Gradually, the patient becomes aware of his surroundings.

ASK YOURSELF

■ Given a scenario involving a patient with an altered mental status, how do you demonstrate the appropriate assessment and care of the patient, including management of patients with status epilepticus?

EMR Emergency Care: Seizure

If you suspect a patient is having a seizure, you should immediately notify the responding EMS personnel and take appropriate Standard Precautions. Steps to providing care for this patient include (Figures 15-8a and 15-8b ■):

1. Remain calm and wait for the seizure to end. This will usually only be a few minutes.

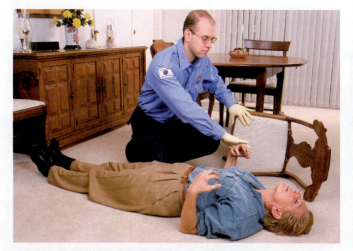

■ **Figure 15-8a**   Move objects away from the seizure patient to help prevent injury.

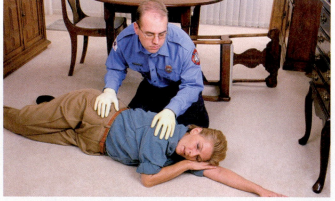

■ **Figure 15-8b**   When the seizure stops, position the patient to allow drainage of saliva and vomit.

2. Prevent any further injury. Move objects away from the patient. If you cannot move the objects, place some type of padding, such as a blanket or coat, between the patient and the object. Place some padding beneath the patient's head to help avoid injury.
3. Remove the patient's eyeglasses, if he is wearing a pair.
4. Do not force anything into the patient's mouth. During the seizure, the object may break and cause an airway obstruction.
5. Do not try to restrain the patient. The muscle contractions during a seizure may be extensive. If the patient is being held down, an injury may result.

Steps to providing care for a patient who is no longer seizing include:

1. Monitor and maintain the patient's airway, breathing, and circulation.
2. Place the patient in the recovery position.
3. Administer high-flow oxygen.
4. Provide emotional support to the patient and family.
5. Be sure to notify the responding EMS personnel that you suspect a seizure. Describe the seizure in as much detail as possible: How long did it last? Was only part of the body seizing or was the whole body involved? Has the patient had previous seizures? Was there any previous head injury, no matter how minor?

Some patients may experience a continuous seizure or two or more seizures in a row without a period of responsiveness between them. This indicates a true medical emergency called **status epilepticus**, and can be fatal. Complications of status epilepticus include aspiration, hypoxia, hyperthermia (elevated body temperature), and heart problems. If you suspect status epilepticus:

1. Notify responding EMS personnel immediately. Transportation should not be delayed.
2. Monitor and maintain the patient's airway, breathing, and circulation.
3. Position the patient.
4. Administer high-flow oxygen.
5. Provide emotional support to the patient.
6. Be sure to notify the responding EMS personnel that you suspect status epilepticus.

ASK YOURSELF
■ What are the phases of a generalized seizure? Provide a description of each phase.

status epilepticus a continous seizure or two or more seizures in a row without a period of responsiveness.

✳ Stop, Review, Remember

Multiple Choice

Place a check next to the correct answer.

1. An interruption of the blood supply to the brain is called a(n):

_____ a. seizure.

_____ b. diabetic emergency.

_____ c. stroke.

_____ d. aneurysm.

2. Strokes are the:

_____ a. leading cause of death in the United States.

_____ b. second leading cause of death in the United States.

_____ c. third leading cause of death in the United States.

_____ d. fourth leading cause of death in the United States.

3. A sudden change in behavior or movement caused by irregular electrical activity in the brain is called a(n):

_____ a. seizure.

_____ b. diabetic emergency.

_____ c. stroke.

_____ d. aneurysm.

4. The condition in which a patient has a continuous seizure or two or more seizures in a row without a period of responsiveness between them is status:

_____ a. asthmaticus.

_____ b. epilepticus.

_____ c. glycemious.

_____ d. myocardicus.

Emergency Medical Responder Practice

You are treating a patient complaining of weakness on her right side and difficulty speaking. She has right-sided facial droop, and she is unable to keep her right arm elevated.

1. What emergency situation do you suspect your patient is experiencing?

_____

_____

_____

2. What emergency care should you provide this patient?

_____

_____

_____

You respond to a local office building for a patient having a seizure. When you arrive, you are led to a conference room where you find the patient lying on the floor still having a seizure.

3. What emergency care would you provide for this patient?

_____

_____

_____

4. The seizure ends. Now what emergency care should you provide?

_____

_____

_____

List

1. List the three components of the Cincinnati Prehospital Stroke Scale. Describe how to check each and what normal and abnormal signs are.

_____

_____

_____

2. The most common type of seizure you will encounter is a generalized tonic-clonic seizure. List and describe the four phases of a generalized tonic-clonic seizure.

_____

_____

_____

Poisoning

A **poison** is any substance that can harm the body. Poisoning can occur in a variety of settings; however, many occur in the home (Figure 15-9 ■). Poisons enter the body through one of four routes:

- *Injection.* These poisons enter the body through a puncture or break in the skin (Figure 15-10a ■). Sources include bites and stings of insects and other animals or the injection of drugs or chemicals through hypodermic needles.

- *Ingestion.* These poisons enter the body through the mouth into the digestive tract. Each year in the United States there are over 8 million reported cases of ingested poisons. Of these, aspirin and alcohol are among the top agents. Sources may include biological weapons like nerve agents, medications, cleaning chemicals, lead paint, and tainted foods.

- *Inhalation.* These poisons enter the body through the respiratory tract in the form of a gas or a fine mist. (Figure 15-10b ■). A common type of poisonous gas is carbon monoxide. Carbon monoxide (CO) is a result of incomplete combustion. Smoke is a visual sign of incomplete combustion. CO is odorless and many poisonings occur without the presence of identifiable smoke. Another poisonous gas that may be given off during a fire is cyanide. Cyanide results from the burning of certain types of plastics. Other sources of poisonous gases include nerve agents, wastewater treatment plants and manufacturing facilities that may give off carbon dioxide (CO_2), water treatment plants and swimming pools that may give off chlorine gas, and transportation accidents that may give off a variety of gases if the cargo is damaged.

poison any substance that can be harmful to the body.

ASK YOURSELF

- What are the common signs and symptoms of poisoning?

ASK YOURSELF

- Given a scenario involving a patient with an altered mental status, how do you demonstrate the appropriate assessment and care of the patient, including management of patients with poisoning, including drug and alcohol emergencies?

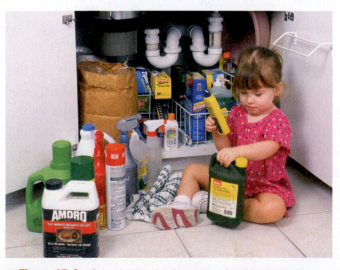

■ **Figure 15-9** Poisoning is a leading cause of accidental death among children.

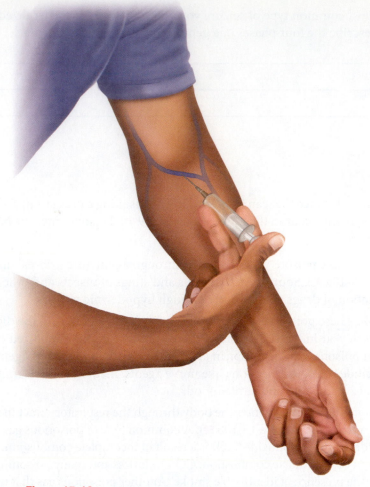

■ **Figure 15-10a**   Intravenous drug use is an example of injected poison.

■ *Absorption.* These poisons enter the body through the intact skin (Figure 15-10c ■). Sources include contact with poisonous plants such as poison ivy, poison sumac, and poison oak, or chemicals such as nerve agents, herbicides, pesticides, cleaning products, and industrial chemicals.

There are a variety of reasons a patient may be poisoned. The following are just a few examples:

■ A small child is curious to see what a particular product tastes like.

■ A teenager is so overwhelmed by the physical and emotional changes of life that he attempts to take his own life with drugs or volatile chemicals.

■ A college student on a hike accidentally walks through a patch of poison ivy.

■ A young adult industrial worker is exposed to a chemical during an industrial accident.

■ A middle-aged person has been under excessive stress, so he turns to alcohol or drugs to make things "better."

■ An elderly person forgets he took his daily medications, and takes them again.

Our daily lives brings us in frequent contact with a variety of natural and manufactured substances that, if used properly, can help improve our quality of life but, if used improperly, can have a negative impact on our health, or even our lives.

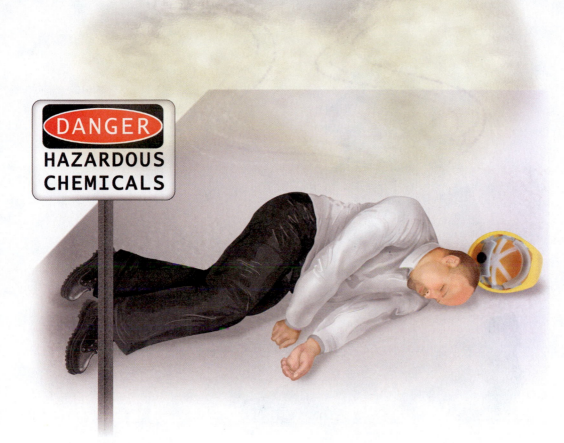

■ **Figure 15-10b**   Inhaled poison.

Your primary responsibility is your personal safety. While your zeal to help those in need is admirable, you will not help the situation if you are hurt, or even killed. Be sure to perform an appropriate scene size-up, including identifying potential hazards. As with any patient, use appropriate Standard Precautions. In addition, you may need specialized equipment and training to enter certain hazardous environments.

Stop and think about the route of exposure and how this may impact your treatment. If the poison was inhaled, you will want to remove the patient as quickly as possible to fresh air. If you use your bag-valve-mask device on room air to assist ventilations without moving the patient to fresh air, you are only pushing more poisons into the respiratory tract. If the poison was ingested, residue may be on the patient's lips, making mouth-to-mouth ventilations more hazardous. If the poison was absorbed, residue might be on the patient's clothing or skin. Improper handling of this substance may spread the contamination. If needles were used to inject the substance, there may be exposed needles lying around that could injure you or your team.

EMR Patient Assessment: Poisons

Altered mental status is one of the most common signs of poisoning. Each route of exposure will present with different signs and symptoms which will be discussed later in this chapter.

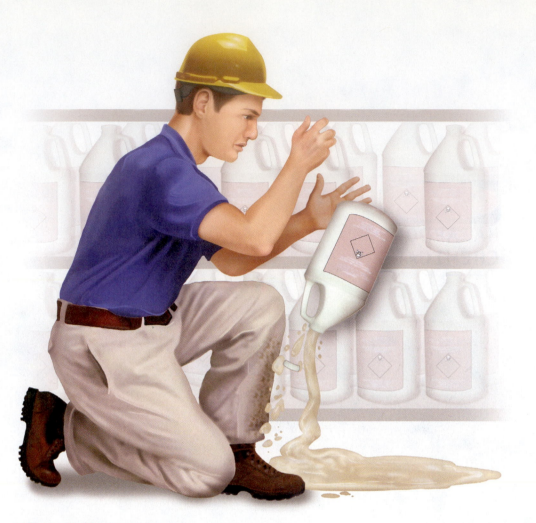

■ **Figure 15-10c** Absorbed poison.

In obtaining a history of the present situation, try to answer the following questions:

■ What was the substance involved?
■ How much of the substance was involved?
■ When did the poisoning occur?
■ What is the patient's approximate weight?
■ What has the patient or others done to relieve the signs and symptoms?

EMR Emergency Care: Poisons

If you suspect a patient has been exposed to a poison, you should immediately notify the responding EMS personnel and take appropriate Standard Precautions. Steps to providing care for this patient include (Scan 15-1):

1. Monitor and maintain the patient's airway, breathing, and circulation.
2. Position the patient.
3. Administer high-flow oxygen.
4. Identify the substances involved, if possible. Look for any bottles or containers that might have contained the substance. They may include information helpful in the continued patient care. In an industrial setting, try to obtain a material safety data sheet (MSDS) for the substance involved.

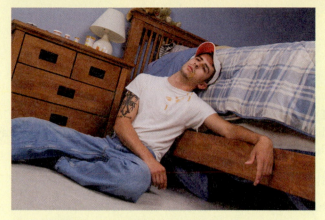

15-1a Perform a scene size-up. Assure scene safety. Be alert for substances involved in the poisoning.

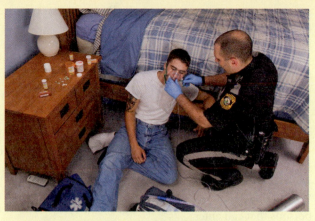

15-1b Perform the primary assessment while monitoring the airway. Watch for vomiting.

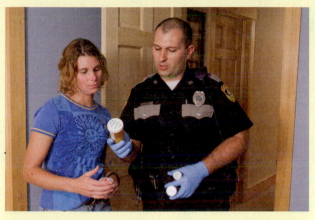

15-1c Attempt to identify the substances involved. Ask family or friends.

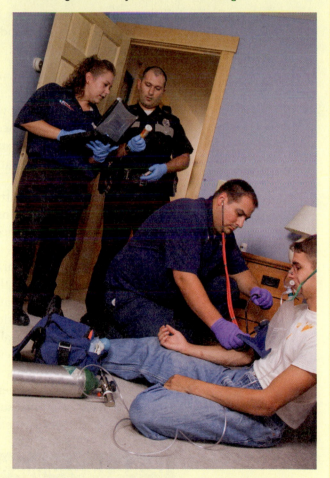

15-1e Follow the poison control or medical direction instructions and transition the patient to an EMT with proper documentation.

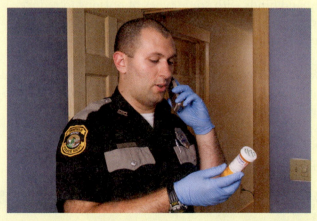

15-1d Contact medical direction or poison control, per protocol.

ASK YOURSELF

■ What is the importance of contacting poison control when managing a patient who has been poisoned?

5. Contact poison control (1-800-222-1222) or medical direction. They can provide additional information on the substance. Follow your local protocol.
6. Provide emotional support to the patient.
7. Be sure to notify the responding EMS personnel of the substance involved.

Specific Types of Poisons

Ingested Poisons

Be alert for clues to the poison. Do you see any empty or spilled bottles or containers? Do you see any overturned plants? Is there any drug paraphernalia lying around? These may be clues to help identify both what was ingested and how much.

ASK YOURSELF

■ What are some poisons that can enter the body by injection?

EMR Patient Assessment: Ingested Poisons

The signs and symptoms of an ingested poison are listed in Table 15-3.

EMR Emergency Care: Ingested Poisons

If you suspect a patient has ingested a poison, you should immediately notify the responding EMS personnel and take appropriate Standard Precautions. Steps to providing care for this patient include:

1. Monitor and maintain the patient's airway, breathing, and circulation.
2. Position the patient.
3. Administer high-flow oxygen.
4. Identify the substances involved. Look for any bottles or containers that might have contained the substance. They may include information helpful in the continued patient care. In an industrial setting, try to obtain the MSDS for the substance involved.
5. Contact poison control (1-800-222-1222) or medical direction. They can provide additional information on the substance. Follow your local protocol.
   a. Your local protocols may permit the administration of activated charcoal for certain types of poisons. Activated charcoal is a finely ground charcoal that is very absorbent and binds with some types of poisons to reduce absorption into the digestive system. Administration may increase the nausea and vomiting. Closely monitor the patient's airway and be prepared to suction.
   b. If the patient swallows an acid, corrosive, or petroleum product, your local protocols may permit the administration of water or milk to help dilute the poison. Administration may increase the nausea and vomiting. Closely monitor the patient's airway and be prepared to suction.
6. Provide emotional support to the patient.
7. Be sure to notify the responding EMS personnel of the substance involved.

TABLE 15-3 Signs and Symptoms: Ingested Poisons	
■ Altered mental status	■ Nausea and vomiting
■ History of ingesting the poison	■ Diarrhea
■ Odd breath odors	■ Burns around the mouth
■ Excessive salivation	■ Dilated or constricted pupils
■ Tearing or sweating	■ Vision problems
■ Abdominal pain	■ Seizures

Another area that can be considered an ingested poison is the misuse of drugs and alcohol. **Drug abuse** is the self-administration of one or more drugs in a way that differs from the approved medical or social practice. An **overdose** is an emergency that involves poisoning by drugs or alcohol. The term **withdrawal** refers to the effects on the body that occur after a period of abstinence from the drug or alcohol to which the body has become accustomed.

A drug overdose may be the result of long-term drug abuse, miscalculation, confusion, use of more than one drug, or a suicide attempt. No one is exempt from potential drug or alcohol abuse (Figure 15-11 ■).

While there are drugs that have been around for some time, new drugs do appear periodically. One of these is **bath salts**. A stimulant, bath salts may be ingested, snorted or injected. Of particular concern is that the drug has been available on the Internet as well as in convenience stores and head shops. Many states have taken action to make bath salts illegal. There are no legitimate uses of bath salts.

Since bath salts are a stimulant, you could expect to see increased heart rate and respirations, insomnia, agitation, chest pain, nausea and vomiting. More severe symptoms include worsening altered mental status, seizures, delusions and impaired perception of reality

Bath salts are packaged as a fine white, off-white or slightly yellowed powder. It may simply be called "bath salts" or by street names such as Snow Leopard, Ivory Wave, Bliss, Vanilla Sky, White Lightening and others.

Care for patients who have ingested bath salts is the same as for other drug emergencies covered in this chapter.

Many of these drugs can cause changes in the respiratory, circulatory, and central nervous systems. Some are stimulants like bath salts, which increase the body's processes; some are depressants, which decrease the body's processes. Others may cause a variety of sensory- or behavior-altering effects. In addition, several major medical problems can result from a drug or alcohol overdose or from sudden withdrawal. Among these are respiratory problems, internal injuries, seizures, hypothermia, hyperthermia, and even cardiac arrest.

drug abuse the self-administration of one or more drugs in a way that differs from the approved medical or social practice.

overdose an emergency that involves poisoning by drugs or alcohol.

withdrawal the effects on the body that occur after a period of abstinence from the drug or alcohol to which the body has become accustomed.

bath salts a stimulant drug found in powder form. It can be purchased in some stores and on the internet.

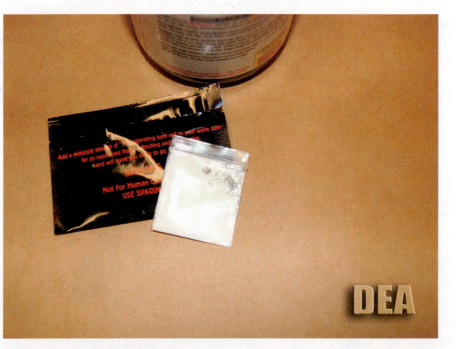

■ **Figure 15-11**   Bath salts. (© DEA)

EMR Patient Assessment: Drug or Alcohol Emergency

Signs and symptoms you may see in a drug or alcohol emergency are listed in Table 15-4 and shown in Figure 15-12 ■.

EMR Emergency Care: Drug or Alcohol Emergency

If you suspect a patient is experiencing a drug or alcohol emergency, you should immediately notify the responding EMS personnel and take appropriate Standard Precautions. Steps to providing care for this patient include:

1. Monitor and maintain the patient's airway, breathing, and circulation.
2. Position the patient.
3. Administer high-flow oxygen.
4. Monitor the patient's mental status and vital signs frequently.
5. Maintain the patient's body temperature.

TABLE 15-4 Signs and Symptoms: Drug or Alcohol Emergency

- Altered mental status or unresponsiveness
- Respiratory difficulties
- Abnormal or irregular pulse rate
- Nausea and vomiting
- Seizures
- Odor of alcohol on the breath
- Swaying and unsteadiness
- Slurred speech
- Flushed face
- Violent, destructive, or erratic behavior
- Self-injury, usually without realizing it

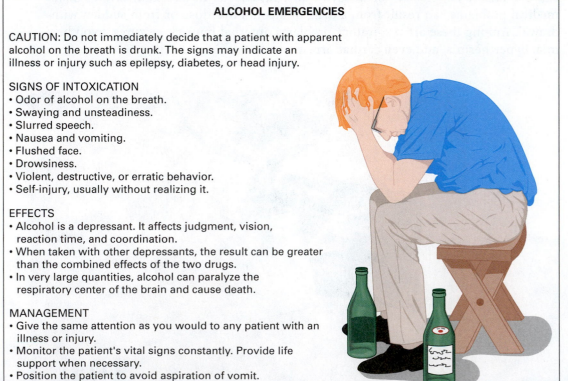

ALCOHOL EMERGENCIES

CAUTION: Do not immediately decide that a patient with apparent alcohol on the breath is drunk. The signs may indicate an illness or injury such as epilepsy, diabetes, or head injury.

SIGNS OF INTOXICATION
• Odor of alcohol on the breath.
• Swaying and unsteadiness.
• Slurred speech.
• Nausea and vomiting.
• Flushed face.
• Drowsiness.
• Violent, destructive, or erratic behavior.
• Self-injury, usually without realizing it.

EFFECTS
• Alcohol is a depressant. It affects judgment, vision, reaction time, and coordination.
• When taken with other depressants, the result can be greater than the combined effects of the two drugs.
• In very large quantities, alcohol can paralyze the respiratory center of the brain and cause death.

MANAGEMENT
• Give the same attention as you would to any patient with an illness or injury.
• Monitor the patient's vital signs constantly. Provide life support when necessary.
• Position the patient to avoid aspiration of vomit.
• Protect the patient from hurting him- or herself.

■ **Figure 15-12** Emergency care for a patient with an alcoholic emergency includes EMR safety, airway management, and treatment for life-threatening conditions.

6. Take measures to prevent shock.
7. Provide emotional support to the patient.
8. Be sure to notify the responding EMS personnel of any changes in the patient's condition.

Inhaled Poisons

Many poisonous gases are odorless, colorless, and tasteless (Figure 15-13 ■). Just because you cannot smell, see, or taste anything does not mean you are not in danger from exposure to a poisonous gas. You will have to rely upon a careful size-up of the scene and any dangers that may be present. Remember, your first priority is your own safety.

As inhaled poisons affect the respiratory system, you must pay special attention to the patient's airway.

EMR Patient Assessment: Inhaled Poisons

The signs and symptoms of an inhaled poison are listed in Table 15-5.

Carbon monoxide (CO) is a poisonous gas that can be especially lethal. The most common sources of CO include kerosene heaters, gas water heaters, car exhaust, and smoke inhalation. Some response agencies are equipped with CO oximeters to detect the level of CO in the patient's bloodstream (Figure 15-14a ■).

ASK YOURSELF

■ What are some poisons that can enter the body by inhalation?

■ What are some specific questions that should be asked when obtaining the history of patients with poisoning?

carbon monoxide (CO)
an odorless, colorless, tasteless poisonous gas that can be especially lethal.

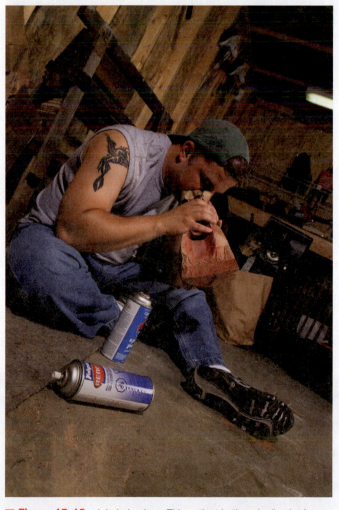

■ **Figure 15-13** Inhaled poison. This patient is "bagging" paint fumes to obtain a "high."

TABLE 15-5 Signs and Symptoms: Inhaled Poisons

- Soot, burns, or singed hair around the mouth or nose
- Breathing difficulty
- Altered mental status
- Chest pain
- Cough, hoarseness, or burning sensation in the throat
- Cyanosis
- Dizziness, headache
- Seizures, unresponsiveness (usually a late sign)

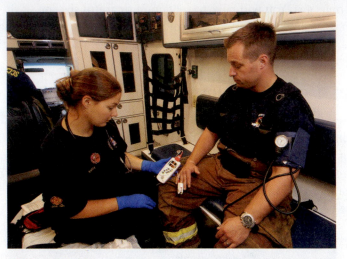

■ **Figure 15-14a** CO oximeters are used to detect the level of CO in the patient's bloodstream.

ASK YOURSELF

- What are some poisons that can enter the body by inhalation?

If you respond to a scene where several individuals are complaining about the same signs and symptoms, you should consider potential carbon monoxide poisoning. CO will also affect pets, so be alert if the family dog, cat, or other pet also appears sick.

EMR Patient Assessment: Carbon Monoxide Poisoning

The signs and symptoms of carbon monoxide poisoning are listed in Table 15-6.

EMR Emergency Care: Carbon Monoxide Poisoning

If you suspect a patient has carbon monoxide poisoning, you should immediately notify the responding EMS personnel and take appropriate Standard Precautions. Steps to providing care for this patient include:

1. Do not enter the scene unless properly equipped and trained.
2. When safe to do so, quickly remove the patient from the source of the poison.

TABLE 15-6 Signs and Symptoms: Carbon Monoxide Poisoning

- Throbbing headache and agitation
- Nausea, vomiting
- Confusion, poor judgment
- Diminished vision, blindness
- Breathing difficulty with rapid pulse
- Dizziness, fainting, unresponsiveness
- Seizures
- Paleness
- Cherry-red color to skin (very late sign)

3. Monitor and maintain the patient's airway, breathing, and circulation.
4. Position the patient.
5. Administer high-flow oxygen.
6. Monitor the patient's mental status and vital signs frequently.
7. Provide emotional support to the patient.
8. Be sure to notify the responding EMS personnel of any changes in the patient's condition.

All patients exposed to carbon monoxide need medical evaluation. In severe cases, the patient may be transported to a hospital with specialized equipment, such as a hyperbaric chamber, for further treatment.

ASK YOURSELF

■ What are some specific questions that should be asked when obtaining the history of patients with poisoning?

■ What are some poisons that can enter the body by absorption?

Absorbed Poisons

Exposure to an absorbed poison is probably the easiest to identify. Look for any spilled containers that contained liquid or powder substances. Size-up the scene for the presence of poisonous plants. Oil-based poisons, including petroleum products and plant extracts, can easily spread from person to person. Be sure to use appropriate Standard Precautions when assessing and caring for your patient. If the poison involved hazardous materials, follow your local protocol for the proper hazmat response team.

EMR Patient Assessment: Absorbed Poisons

The signs and symptoms of exposure to an absorbed poison are listed in Table 15-7.

EMR Emergency Care: Absorbed Poisons

If you suspect a patient has been exposed to an absorbed poison, you should immediately notify the responding EMS personnel and take appropriate Standard Precautions. Steps to providing care for this patient include:

1. Do not enter the scene unless properly equipped and trained.
2. When safe to do so, quickly remove the patient from the source of the poison.
3. Monitor and maintain the patient's airway, breathing, and circulation.
4. Position the patient.
5. Administer high-flow oxygen.
6. Carefully remove the contaminated clothing.
7. Carefully remove the excess poison (Figure 15-14b ■):
   a. If the poison is dry, brush it off.
   b. If the poison is wet, blot it off.
8. After removing as much poison as possible, flood the area with copious amounts of water. Attempt to contain the runoff.
9. Monitor the patient's mental status and vital signs frequently.
10. Provide emotional support to the patient.
11. Notify the responding EMS personnel of any changes in the patient's condition.

TABLE 15-7 Signs and Symptoms: Absorbed Poisons	
■ Liquid or powder on the skin	■ Excessive salivation and tearing
■ Burns	■ Redness, rash, blisters
■ Itching, irritation	

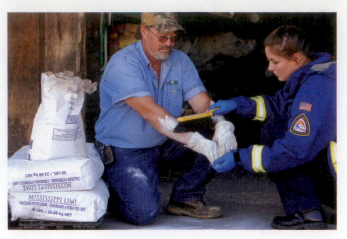

■ **Figure 15-14b** Absorbed poison. If the poison is dry, brush it off the skin.

ASK YOURSELF

■ What are some specific questions that should be asked when obtaining the history of patients with poisoning?

■ What are some poisons that can enter the body by injection?

Injected Poisons

An injected poison may be a drug that enters the body by way of a hypodermic needle. The signs, symptoms, and emergency care for this type of injected poison were discussed earlier in this chapter under "Ingested Poisons."

An injected poison may also be the result of bites and stings from insects, spiders, snakes, and marine animals. The venom from these creatures can cause a mild allergic reaction, a severe allergic reaction known as anaphylaxis, or in extreme cases even death.

✳ Stop, Review, Remember

Multiple Choice

Place a check next to the correct answer.

1. _____ _____ is very absorbent and binds with some types of poisons to reduce absorption into the digestive system.

    ____ a. Instant glucose

    ____ b. Activated charcoal

    ____ c. Ipecac syrup

    ____ d. Activated glucose

2. An emergency that involves poisoning by drugs or alcohol is called a(n):

    ____ a. drug abuse.

    ____ b. withdrawal.

    ____ c. delirium tremens.

    ____ d. overdose.

3. Which of the following patients presents a history of an absorbed poison?

    ____ a. A 48-year-old farmer who spilled powdered herbicide on his arms

    ____ b. A 16-year-old who swallowed some illegal mushrooms

    ____ c. A 32-year-old who works on his motorcycle in a closed garage

    ____ d. An 8-year-old who was stung by a bee on the school playground

Emergency Medical Responder Practice

1. A 2-year-old toddler has gotten into a cabinet containing household cleaners. What emergency care should you provide this patient?

_____

_____

_____

_____

2. You are assessing a patient who was working on a lawn mower in his garage when he was overcome by exhaust fumes. What signs and symptoms would you expect to see?

_____

_____

_____

_____

3. What emergency care would you provide for the patient in question 2?

_____

_____

_____

_____

Matching

Match the following routes of poisoning with the appropriate description.

1. _____ Enter the body through the respiratory tract

2. _____ Enter the body through a puncture or break in the skin

3. _____ Enter the body through the mouth into the digestive tract

4. _____ Enter the body through the intact skin

a. Injection
b. Ingestion
c. Inhalation
d. Absorption

Critical Thinking

1. When assessing a patient who has been poisoned, what questions should you ask?

_____

_____

_____

_____

Behavioral Emergencies

behavior the manner in which we act.

behavioral emergency any situation in which a patient's behavior is unacceptable or intolerable to the patient, the family, or the community.

Behavior is simply the manner in which we act. A **behavioral emergency** is any situation in which a patient's behavior is unacceptable or intolerable to the patient, the family, or the community. The following factors may influence a patient's behavior:

- Situational stresses
- Medical illnesses
- History
- Psychiatric problems
- Alcohol or drugs
- Patient not taking his psychiatric medication

You must consider all patients who exhibit abnormal behavior to be suffering from a physical condition until proven otherwise. Such conditions may include the following:

- Low blood glucose
- Lack of oxygen
- Shock
- Head trauma
- Mind-altering substances
- Psychiatric conditions
- Excessive cold; excessive heat
- Brain infection
- Seizure disorders
- Poisoning or overdose
- Withdrawal from drugs or alcohol

Patients with behavioral emergencies may appear agitated and display bizarre thinking, such as hallucinations or paranoia. They may be a danger to themselves as a result of self-destructive behavior or even a suicide attempt. They may be a danger to others, including the EMR, as a result of threatening behavior, violence, or even the use of weapons.

Remember, your personal safety is your primary concern. Be alert for any rapid change in the patient's mannerisms or behavior. Is the patient showing an aggressive stance, such as holding a weapon, clenching his fists, making aggressive gestures, or displaying others signs of violence?

EMR Patient Assessment: Behavioral Emergency

The signs and symptoms of a behavioral emergency are listed in Table 15-8.

ASK YOURSELF

- What are the common signs and symptoms of behavioral emergencies?
- Given a scenario involving a patient with an altered mental status, how do you demonstrate the appropriate assessment and care of the patient, including management of patients with behavioral emergencies?

TABLE 15-8 Signs and Symptoms: Behavioral Emergency

- Altered mental status
- Poor appearance or hygiene
- Altered speech
- Agitated stance or gait
- Variations in mood, thought processes, perception, judgment, memory, or attention
- Violent or aggressive behavior
- Patient hearing voices that are not really there (auditory hallucinations)

Assessment for Suicide Risk

Occasionally you may encounter a patient who is at risk for attempting or committing suicide. To help assess the risk, ask the following questions:

- Does the patient have any weapons on self or in a purse? Ask police to check.
- Has the patient been depressed?
- Has the patient had a recent major life event, such as divorce, loss of a loved one or close friend, loss of a job or other similar event, or diagnosis of a terminal illness?
- Has the patient said or done anything that would indicate the possible risk of suicide or violence against self or others?
- How does the patient feel?
- Is the patient thinking about hurting or killing self or anyone else?
- Is the patient a threat to self or others?
- Is there a medical problem?
- Is there trauma involved?
- Is the patient being treated for any behavioral problems?

ASK YOURSELF

- What are some specific questions that should be asked when obtaining the history of patients with behavioral emergencies, including assessment of suicide risk?

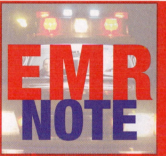

EMR NOTE

According to the National Institute of Mental Health's 2004 statistics, suicide was the third leading cause of death in persons ages 10–24.

In children ages 10–14, the suicide death rate was 1.3 per 100,000.

In adolescents ages 15–19, the suicide death rate was 8.2 per 100,000.

In young adults ages 20–24, the suicide death rate was 12.5 per 100,000.

In people age 65 and older, the suicide death rate was 14.3 per 100,000.

The national average was 10.9 suicide deaths per 100,000 in the general population.

Methods to Calm Behavioral Emergency Patients

A behavioral emergency can be a trying experience for both the EMR and the patient. In addition to identifying and correcting any life-threatening problems, your efforts should be focused on keeping the patient calm (Figure 15-15 ■). The following are a few methods to assist in calming the patient:

- Protect the patient and yourself.
- Acknowledge that the person seems upset.
- Restate that you are there to help.
- Inform the patient about what you are doing.
- Ask questions in a calm, reassuring voice.
- Maintain a comfortable distance.
- Encourage the patient to state what is troubling him.
- Do not make quick moves.

ASK YOURSELF

- How would you demonstrate with a fellow student the techniques of calming patients with behavioral emergencies?

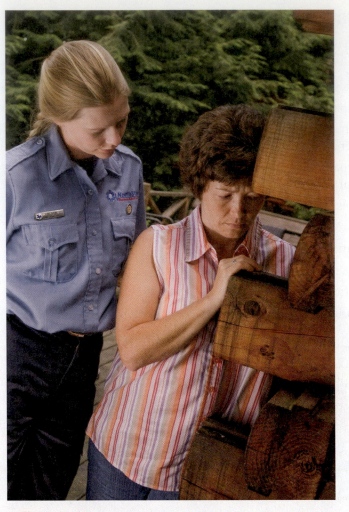

■ **Figure 15-15** Emergency care for a patient with a behavioral emergency includes EMR safety, treatment for life-threatening conditions, and trying to keep the patient calm.

- Respond honestly to the patient's questions.
- Do not threaten, challenge, or argue with disturbed patients.
- Tell the truth; do not lie to the patient.
- Do not "play along" with visual or auditory disturbances of the patient.
- Involve trusted family members or friends.
- Be prepared to stay at the scene for a long time. Always remain with the patient until you transfer care.
- Avoid unnecessary physical contact.
- Use good eye contact.
- Avoid threatening postures.
- Always try to talk the patient into cooperation.
- Do not belittle or threaten patients.
- Be calm and patient in your attitude.
- Reassure the patient.
- Lower distressing stimuli, if possible.

- Avoid restraints unless necessary.
- Treat the patient with respect.
- Call additional help if needed.

EMR Emergency Care: Behavioral Emergency

If you suspect a patient has a behavioral emergency, you should immediately notify the responding EMS personnel and take appropriate Standard Precautions. Steps to providing care for this patient include:

1. Do not enter the scene unless safe to do so.
2. Attempt to establish a rapport with the patient.
3. Acknowledge that you are listening to the patient.
4. Avoid threatening actions, statements, or questions.
5. Attempt to calm the patient.
6. Do not leave the patient alone, unless the situation becomes unsafe.
7. Consider the need for law enforcement.
8. Assist other EMS responders with restraint if necessary.
9. Monitor the patient's mental status and vital signs frequently, if the patient permits.
10. Treat any injuries, if the patient permits.
11. Provide emotional support to the patient.
12. Be sure to notify the responding EMS personnel of any changes in the patient's condition.

THE LAST WORD

There are several situations that can cause a patient to have an altered mental status. Some may be medical in nature: hypoglycemia, too low blood glucose; hyperglycemia, too high blood glucose; stroke; and seizure. Others may be environmental in nature: poisonings, whether through ingestion, inhalation, absorption, or injection; drug overdose; and alcohol abuse. And still others may be psychological, such as behavioral emergencies.

Your role as an EMR is to support the patient's airway, breathing, and circulation in a professional and caring manner.

Chapter Review

Multiple Choice

Place a check next to the correct answer.

1. Your patient is an 18-year-old female who has had a sudden onset of altered mental status. Her airway is patent and her breathing is adequate. She has a rapid pulse; cool, clammy skin; and a headache. There is no reason to suspect a head or spine injury. She has no history of medical problems. You should:

   _____ a. treat her for low blood sugar and administer glucose.

   _____ b. monitor her ABCs closely and administer oxygen.

   _____ c. manually stabilize her head and neck.

   _____ d. administer activated charcoal.

2. The term *hypoglycemia* refers to:

   _____ a. high blood pressure.

   _____ b. low blood sugar.

   _____ c. seizures.

   _____ d. stroke.

3. Patients with altered mental status who have a history of diabetes should receive oral glucose or sugar solution if they are:

   _____ a. awake and not able to control their own airway.

   _____ b. awake and able to control their own airway.

   _____ c. unresponsive and not able to swallow.

   _____ d. unresponsive but able to swallow.

4. Your patient has been found unconscious, with no suspected trauma. His wife tells you that he has diabetes. Which of the following should you do first?

   _____ a. Assist in administering oral glucose.

   _____ b. Ensure an open airway and adequate breathing.

   _____ c. Get permission to administer an antidote.

   _____ d. Question bystanders about a possible overdose.

5. Which of the following statements about stroke is false?

   _____ a. Stroke patients may have weakness on one side of the body.

   _____ b. Prompt identification and treatment of stroke is critical.

   _____ c. Patients rarely delay seeking medical care for stroke.

   _____ d. Stroke is sometimes referred to as a "brain attack."

6. Emergency Medical Responder care for the seizing patient includes all of the following except:

   _____ a. placing padding under the patient's head.

   _____ b. moving dangerous items away from the patient.

   _____ c. monitoring the patient's airway and breathing.

   _____ d. placing something in the mouth to prevent injury.

7. All of the following are common causes of seizures except:

   _____ a. stroke.

   _____ b. allergic reaction.

   _____ c. alcohol poisoning.

   _____ d. complications of pregnancy.

8. Emergency medical care for a patient who has absorbed a poisonous chemical powder through his skin includes:

   _____ a. brushing off the poison and flushing the skin with water.

   _____ b. administering activated charcoal to absorb the poison.

   _____ c. leaving the patient's clothes on to absorb the poison.

   _____ d. neutralizing the poison with an alkaline agent.

9. Your adult patient tells you that he has ingested an unknown number of pills he bought illegally. You should ask all of the following questions except:

_____ a. What kind of pills and how many did you take?

_____ b. Has anyone tried to treat you with anything?

_____ c. Who sold the pills to you? What is his name?

_____ d. What time was it when you took the pills?

10. Which of the following is a good way to calm a behavioral emergency patient?

_____ a. Lie if it seems like the truth will upset him.

_____ b. Talk about anything except the current problem.

_____ c. Use a calm, reassuring tone when you speak to him.

_____ d. Pat him on the back, touch his elbow, and stay close.

Matching

Match the following descriptions with the appropriate term.

1. _____ An emergency that involves poisoning by drugs or alcohol
2. _____ An odorless, colorless, tasteless poisonous gas that can be especially lethal
3. _____ Low blood glucose
4. _____ The effects on the body that occur after a period of abstinence from the drug or alcohol to which the body has become accustomed
5. _____ Any situation in which a patient's behavior is unacceptable or intolerable to the patient, the family, or the community
6. _____ Commonly known as a stroke, a condition that interrupts the blood supply to the brain
7. _____ High blood glucose
8. _____ The self-administration of one or more drugs in a way that differs from the approved medical or social practice
9. _____ Commonly referred to as diabetes, a condition that prevents individuals from producing enough insulin or from not using insulin effectively
10. _____ Hormone that allows glucose to enter the body's cells
11. _____ Any substance that can be harmful to the body
12. _____ Condition of decreased alertness and responsiveness
13. _____ Common term for diabetes mellitus
14. _____ The manner in which we act
15. _____ A condition that interrupts the blood flow to the brain
16. _____ A form of simple sugar that is the main source of fuel for the body's cells
17. _____ A sudden change in behavior or movement caused by irregular electrical activity in the brain

a. Altered mental status
b. Glucose
c. Insulin
d. Diabetes mellitus
e. Diabetes
f. Hyperglycemia
g. Hypoglycemia
h. Cerebrovascular accident (CVA)
i. Stroke
j. Seizure
k. Poison
l. Drug abuse
m. Overdose
n. Withdrawal
o. Carbon monoxide (CO)
p. Behavior
q. Behavioral emergency

Emergency Medical Responder Practice

You are called to an unconscious patient. When you arrive on scene, you find a male patient, about 45 years old, who is lying on the ground. He does not respond to your voice but moans when you pinch the webbing between his thumb and index finger. His wife says she found him that way a short time ago. She also tells you that he is a diabetic and has been since childhood. He takes insulin but lately has been having trouble keeping his blood sugar at normal levels.

1. What initial assessment steps would you take for this patient?

_____

_____

_____

_____

2. Would you consider giving glucose to the patient? Explain your answer.

_____

_____

_____

_____

3. In your update to the incoming ambulance, would you describe this patient as unstable (in serious condition)? Explain your answer.

_____

_____

_____

_____

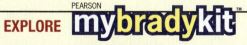

EXPLORE **PEARSON** **mybradykit**™

Please go to **www.bradybooks.com** to access mykit for this text. You will find quizzes, critical thinking scenarios, weblinks, animations, and videos related to this chapter— and much more. Look for online information on strokes and stroke prevention and diabetes.

Register your access code from the front of your book by going to **www.bradybooks.com** and selecting the mykit links.

Medical Emergencies

✳ NAVIGATION GUIDE

The following items provide an overview to the purpose and content of this chapter. The Education Standard and Competency are from the National EMS Education Standards.

Education Standard Medicine (Medical Overview, Abdominal and Gastrointestinal Disorders, Immunology, Genitourinary/Renal)

Competency Recognizes and manages life threats based on assessment findings of a patient with a medical emergency while awaiting additional emergency response.

Knowledge Areas Medical Overview
Assessment and management of a:
- Medical complaint
Abdominal and Gastrointestinal Disorders
Anatomy, presentations, and management of shock associated with abdominal emergencies
- Gastrointestinal bleeding
Immunology
Recognition and management of shock and difficulty breathing related to:
- Anaphylactic reactions
Genitourinary/Renal
- Blood pressure assessment in hemodialysis patients

Objectives After reading this chapter, you should be able to:

1. Define key terminology introduced in this chapter.
2. Describe the EMR's responsibility in caring for patients with a medical emergency while awaiting EMS response.
3. Given a scenario in which a patient has a general medical complaint, demonstrate assessment and management of the patient.
4. List special considerations in the assessment of patients with a hemodialysis access site (shunt or fistula).

5. Describe the basic pathophysiology and presentation of patients with:
   a. Anaphylaxis and allergic reactions
   b. Abdominal complaints and emergencies
   c. Emergency complications of hemodialysis
6. Anticipate the effects on the patient of administration of an epinephrine auto-injector.
7. If allowed by local protocol, demonstrate the administration of epinephrine by auto-injector.

NAVIGATION GUIDE (continued)

Key Terms Page references indicate first major use in this chapter. The Margin Glossary in this chapter provides definitions as you read.

allergen, p. 394	*anaphylaxis, p. 394*	*fetal position, p. 400*
antibodies, p. 394	*anaphylactic shock, p. 394*	*distended, p. 400*
allergic reaction, p. 394	*acute abdomen, p. 399*	*hemodialysis, p. 403*

Media Resources Please go to **www.bradybooks.com** to access mykit for this text. You will find quizzes, critical thinking scenarios, weblinks, animations, and videos related to this chapter—and much more. Look for online information on anaphylaxis and kidney dialysis.

ASK YOURSELF

- Can you define the key terms introduced in this chapter?

INTRODUCTION

A medical emergency is any situation not caused by trauma. During your career as an Emergency Medical Responder (EMR), you will deal with a variety of medical patients. Some of these patients will have very specific complaints, while others are more vague. In this chapter we will discuss some of the more common medical emergencies not previously covered in this text.

Remember that your responsibility as an EMR is to ensure safety, perform a patient assessment, and provide appropriate emergency medical care based on that assessment until EMS personnel arrive to continue care and transport.

CASE STUDY

THE CALL

It is the first day of fall and the forecast is for sunny skies, mild temperatures, and a gentle breeze. Several of you are doing some work around the station when 911 dispatches you to a private residence for a male patient who hasn't been feeling well and who is not responding appropriately.

As you approach the residence, you perform a scene size-up and determine it is safe to proceed. You and your partner have donned the appropriate Standard Precautions. You grab your gear and proceed toward the house.

You find the patient in the living room sitting on the couch. Family members are on both sides of the patient talking with him.

■ Discussion: *How did you determine the scene is safe?*

General Medical Complaints

One of the more challenging patients you will encounter is the patient with a general medical complaint. Unlike the medical patient who says, "My chest hurts" (leading you to suspect a cardiac problem as discussed in Chapter 14) or the patient who presents with signs and symptoms of a stroke (as discussed in Chapter 15), the patient whose only com-

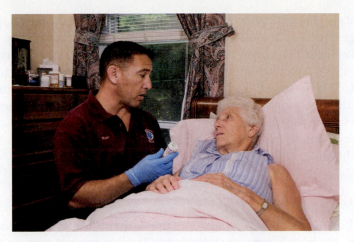

■ **Figure 16-1** EMR obtaining a history from the patient.

plaint is "I just don't feel well" presents a challenge not only to the EMR but to all the patient care personnel who follow in the continuum of care. An appropriate assessment of your patient will help guide your emergency care.

Given such vague complaints, the patient may be extremely frightened and concerned for his overall health. You should remain calm and treat the patient in a professional manner. You may also have family members present who are very concerned. Be truthful and empathetic with your patient and the family. You might say that though you do not know exactly what the problem is, you're doing all that is possible. Let them know you have arranged for transport to the hospital for further evaluation and treatment as needed.

EMR Patient Assessment: General Medical Complaints

After ensuring scene safety and taking the appropriate Standard Precautions, proceed with your patient assessment. Remember what you learned in the Assessment chapters? What is your general impression of the patient? What is the patient's mental status? Is he alert, responding to verbal stimuli, and responding to painful stimuli, or is he unresponsive to any stimuli? Is his airway open? Is he breathing? Is he breathing adequately? How is the circulation, skin color, and skin condition? Has EMS been requested to respond?

Attempt to obtain as accurate a history as possible (Figure 16-1 ■). This may be obtained from the patient, the family, or bystanders and may be a valuable asset in patient care. You may be the only provider able to get this information in a timely fashion. Perform an appropriate physical exam of the patient.

EMR Emergency Care: General Medical Complaints

If a patient has a general medical complaint for which you are unable to determine a more specific complaint or if you are unable to obtain a pertinent history, you should update the responding EMS personnel and take appropriate Standard Precautions. Steps to providing care for this patient include:

1. Monitor and maintain the patient's airway, breathing, and circulation. Be sure both breathing and circulation are adequate. If not adequate, take immediate steps to correct these life-threatening conditions.
2. Position the patient. If the patient is conscious and there are no suspected spine injuries, allow the patient to get in a position of comfort.
3. Administer oxygen. If the patient is breathing adequately, apply high-flow oxygen by nonrebreather mask to patients who appear to be in distress or have an altered

ASK YOURSELF

■ What are your responsibilities as an EMR in caring for patients with a medical emergency while awaiting EMS response?

ASK YOURSELF

■ How would you demonstrate assessment and management of the patient with a general medical complaint?

- How would you describe to a fellow student the basic pathophysiology and presentation of patients with:
  - Anaphylaxis and allergic reactions?
  - Abdominal complaints and emergencies?
  - Emergency complications of hemodialysis?

allergen any substance that causes an abnormal immune response or hypersensitivity.

antibodies protein molecules produced by B cells as a primary immune defense.

allergic reaction an exaggerated immune response.

anaphylaxis a severe, potentially life-threatening allergic reaction.

anaphylactic shock another term for anaphylaxis.

mental status. Patients who appear oriented and in less distress may receive oxygen by nasal cannula. If the patient is not breathing adequately, assist with a pocket face mask or bag-valve-mask (BVM) device attached to an oxygen source.

4. Monitor the patient's mental status and vital signs frequently. This will help you see trends in the patient's condition. Is his condition getting better? Is his condition staying about the same? Is his condition getting worse?
5. Provide emotional support to the patient.
6. Be sure to notify the responding EMS personnel of any changes in the patient's condition.

Anaphylaxis

The human body is constantly being bombarded by substances in the environment. For the most part, the body's immune system works well to prevent these invaders from doing harm. Simply put, the immune system classifies everything it comes in contact with as "self" or "nonself." Those substances classified as self are allowed to go about their business. Those substances classified as nonself are dealt with on either a nonspecific level or a specific level. In most cases, the person does not even realize that the immune system is dealing with a substance.

An **allergen** is any substance that causes an abnormal immune response or hypersensitivity. When first exposed to an allergen, a person will not have an allergic reaction. This is because the immune system has not learned to recognize the allergen. Once exposed to an allergen, the immune system will develop **antibodies**. These antibodies are specific to the particular allergen. The second time a person is exposed to the same allergen, the antibodies will attack the allergen, releasing various chemicals that cause the blood vessels to dilate and bronchioles to constrict. You have probably heard commercials for allergy medications that work to control histamine and leukotrienes. These are chemicals released as part of the immune system's response to an allergen.

Some patients will only experience a mild **allergic reaction**, an exaggerated immune response. Signs and symptoms may include watery eyes, runny nose, localized redness, itching, or hives (Figure 16-2 ■).

Still other patients will experience a severe, potentially life-threatening allergic reaction called **anaphylaxis** (also called **anaphylactic shock**). Anaphylaxis may occur within seconds or minutes after exposure. The patient may go into shock, thus decreasing perfusion. The blood pressure may drop suddenly, decreasing circulation. And the airway passages may narrow, constricting normal breathing (Table 16-1).

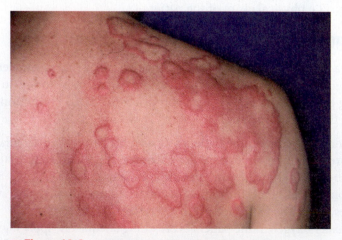

■ **Figure 16-2**   A patient with hives. (© *ISM/Phototake*)

The following are common causes of an allergic reaction or anaphylaxis:

- *Insects.* Stings from bees, yellow jackets, wasps, and hornets can lead to reactions that are often rapid and severe.
- *Foods.* Nuts, dairy products, and seafood are common examples. Most food reactions have a slower onset than those caused by stings because they are ingested. The exception to this is peanuts. A reaction to peanuts is usually quite rapid and severe.
- *Plants.* Examples are poison ivy, poison oak, and poison sumac. Reactions result from exposure to plant pollen and oils. These are usually localized reactions.
- *Medications.* Antibiotics such as penicillin are a common cause of allergic reaction or anaphylaxis.
- *Others.* Latex, dust, chemicals, soaps, makeup, and many other substances can also cause allergic or anaphylactic reactions.

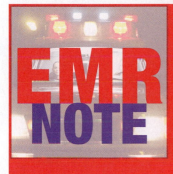

When the signs and symptoms of a patient's allergic reaction include either respiratory distress or suspected shock (hypoperfusion), assume that it is anaphylaxis.

EMR Patient Assessment: Anaphylaxis

The signs and symptoms you may see in a patient with anaphylaxis are listed in Table 16-1.

EMR Emergency Care: Anaphylaxis

If you suspect a patient has anaphylaxis, you should immediately notify the responding EMS personnel and take appropriate Standard Precautions. Follow these steps to provide care for this patient:

1. Monitor and maintain the patient's airway, breathing, and circulation.
2. Place the patient in a position of comfort.

TABLE 16-1 Signs and Symptoms: Anaphylaxis

Respiratory	Nervous
Severe respiratory distress	Altered mental status
Wheezing	Gastrointestinal
Cardiovascular	Nausea, vomiting
Rapid pulse	
Low blood pressure	
Skin	
Pale, red, cyanotic	
Hives (Figure 16-2)	
Itching	
Swelling around eyes, mouth, tongue	

3. Administer high-flow oxygen. Ventilate the patient if necessary.
4. Remove the allergen, if possible.
5. Ask if the patient has used or has his epinephrine auto-injector.
6. Monitor the patient's mental status and vital signs frequently.
7. Provide emotional support to the patient.
8. Be sure to notify the responding EMS personnel of any changes in the patient's condition.

Patients with a previous history of a severe allergic reaction or anaphylaxis may be carrying an epinephrine auto-injector (EpiPen). When used, this device injects a medication called epinephrine into the patient's muscle (usually the leg). Epinephrine is a hormone produced by the body. As a medication, it constricts blood vessels and dilates respiratory passages. This medication works quickly to help relieve the life-threatening signs and symptoms of anaphylaxis.

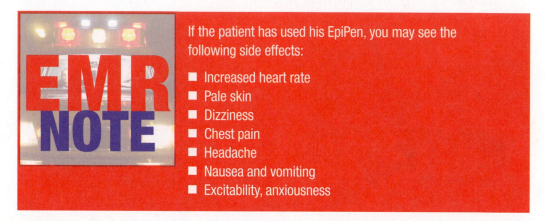

EMR NOTE

If the patient has used his EpiPen, you may see the following side effects:

- Increased heart rate
- Pale skin
- Dizziness
- Chest pain
- Headache
- Nausea and vomiting
- Excitability, anxiousness

ASK YOURSELF

- How would you explain or anticipate the effects of administration of an epinephrine auto-injector on a patient?

- With your instructor's guidance, how would you demonstrate the administration of epinephrine by auto-injector?

In most cases, the patient will have already administered his epinephrine auto-injector prior to your arrival. Be careful if you handle the auto-injector as the needle may be exposed. If signs and symptoms of a severe anaphylactic reaction have not improved within 10 minutes, a second dose of epinephrine may be needed. Patients should consider carrying a second EpiPen auto-injector. To help meet the possible need for a second dose of epinephrine, the Twinject auto-injector is available. This is a single device that contains two doses of epinephrine.

Local protocols may permit the Emergency Medical Responder to either assist a patient in using his EpiPen auto-injector or to use one that the EMR is carrying in the response kit. The steps in using an EpiPen auto-injector are summarized in Scan 16-1 and listed as follows:

1. Unscrew the yellow or green cap off the EpiPen (adult dose unit) or EpiPen Jr. (pediatric dose unit) carrying tube and remove the EpiPen or EpiPen Jr. auto-injector from its storage tube.
2. Grasp the unit with the black tip pointing downward.
3. Form a fist around the unit (black tip down).
4. With your other hand, pull off the gray safety release (cap).
5. Hold the black tip near the outer thigh.
6. Push firmly into the outer thigh until it clicks so that the unit is perpendicular (at a 90° angle) to the thigh. The auto-injector is designed to work through clothing.
7. Hold firmly against the thigh for approximately 10 seconds. The injection is now complete. The window on the auto-injector will show red.
8. Remove the unit from the thigh and massage the injection area for 10 seconds.

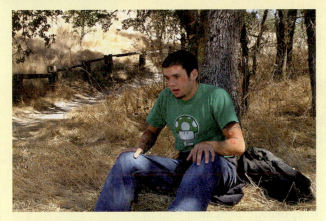

16-1a Recognize the anaphylactic shock patient and perform primary assessment. Administer oxygen by nonrebreather mask.

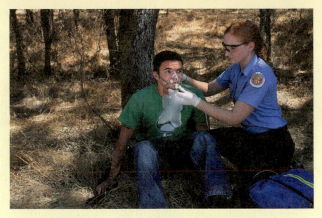

16-1b Administer oxygen. Assist with ventilations if necessary.

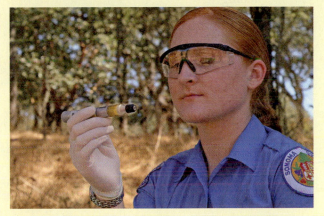

16-1c If permitted by medical direction, check the EpiPen epinephrine auto-injector to ensure it is prescribed for the patient. Check the expiration date and clarity of the drug. Remove the safety cap from the EpiPen.

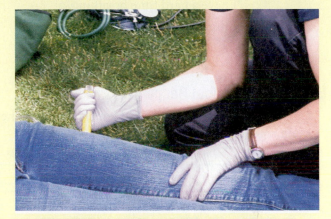

16-1d Place the tip of the auto-injector on the lateral aspect of the thigh, midway between the hip and knee. Push the injector firmly against the thigh until it activates. Hold it in place until the medication is injected.

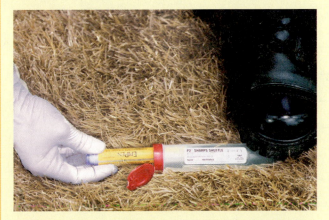

16-1e Properly dispose of the auto-injector. Record the time of the epinephrine injection.

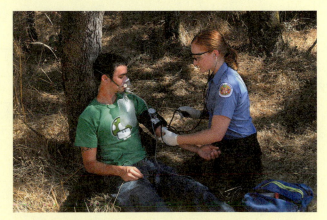

16-1f Check vital signs upon reassessment.

9. Carefully place the used auto-injector (without bending the needle), needle end first, into the storage tube of the carrying case that provides built-in needle protection after use. Then screw the cap of the storage tube back on completely and give it to the responding EMT personnel.

Be sure to follow your local protocols on the use of this device.

✳ Stop, Review, Remember

Multiple Choice

Place a check next to the correct answer.

1. Which of the following is an example of a general medical complaint?

   _____ a. "My chest hurts."

   _____ b. "I feel weak."

   _____ c. "I have a hard time breathing."

   _____ d. "I think I broke my ankle."

2. Which of the following patients may be in anaphylactic shock?

   _____ a. Patient with a running nose

   _____ b. Patient with localized redness and itching

   _____ c. Patient with hives and trouble breathing

   _____ d. Patient with itching and hives

Emergency Medical Responder Practice

1. You are treating a 43-year-old female who says she is weak and doesn't feel well. What would emergency care for this patient include?

   _____

   _____

   _____

   _____

You and your partner are called to a local park for a child stung by a bee. You find the patient sitting at a picnic table having trouble catching her breath.

2. List four signs or symptoms you might expect to see.

   _____

   _____

   _____

   _____

3. What would treatment for this child include?

   _____

   _____

   _____

   _____

Abdominal Emergencies

When a patient experiences a sudden onset of severe abdominal pain, the condition is termed an **acute abdomen**. As you learned in Chapter 5, "Anatomy and Physiology," the abdominal cavity contains several organs and major blood vessels. Abdominal emergencies may result from a variety of sources including digestive tract organs (such as the esophagus, stomach, and intestines), accessory organs (such as the spleen, liver, pancreas, and gallbladder), urinary tract organs (such as the kidneys and urinary bladder), or reproductive organs (Figure 16-3 ■).

acute abdomen a sudden onset of severe abdominal pain.

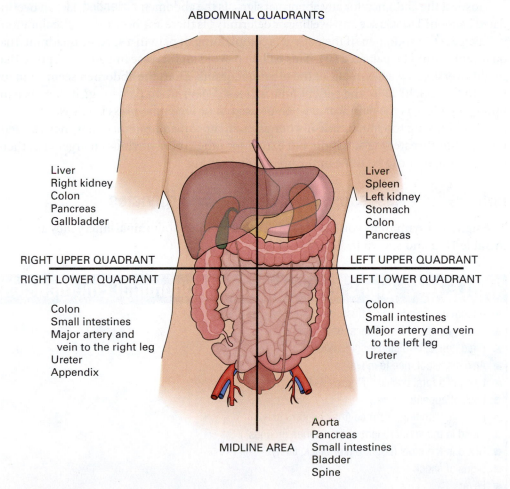

ABDOMINAL QUADRANTS

Liver
Right kidney
Colon
Pancreas
Gallbladder

Liver
Spleen
Left kidney
Stomach
Colon
Pancreas

RIGHT UPPER QUADRANT

LEFT UPPER QUADRANT

RIGHT LOWER QUADRANT

LEFT LOWER QUADRANT

Colon
Small intestines
Major artery and
 vein to the right leg
Ureter
Appendix

Colon
Small intestines
Major artery and vein
 to the left leg
Ureter

MIDLINE AREA

Aorta
Pancreas
Small intestines
Bladder
Spine

■ **Figure 16-3** The abdominal quadrants.

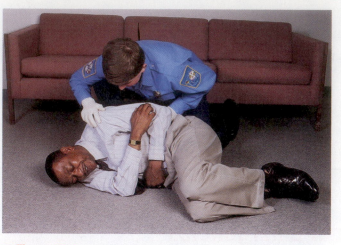

■ **Figure 16-4** A patient in the fetal position, guarding his abdomen.

You may find the patient lying on his side with his legs drawn up and his arms across his abdomen. This position is called the **fetal position** (Figure 16-4 ■). It helps reduce tension on the abdominal muscles, thus reducing pain.

Gather as much history as possible from the patient, family, or bystanders. What was the patient doing when the pain started? When did the pain start? What does the pain feel like? When did the patient last eat? What did the patient last eat? Has the patient had similar pain before?

Inspect the abdomen for any abnormal signs. Is the abdomen **distended**, like an overinflated balloon? Do you see any swelling or deformity? Is there any bruising or discoloration?

Palpate the abdomen. If the patient is complaining of pain in a specific quadrant, that quadrant should be palpated last. This will help avoid an increase in pain perception that might overshadow assessment of the other quadrants. Does the abdomen seem rigid, or hard to the touch? Does the patient note increased pain when palpating? If there is pain upon palpation, is the pain worse when pressed in or when the press is released?

Avoid taking too much time in your assessment. An abdominal emergency can represent a life-threatening situation, but except for other more obvious emergencies, there may be little that can be done in the prehospital setting.

EMR Patient Assessment: Abdominal Emergencies

The signs and symptoms you may see in a patient with an abdominal emergency are listed in Table 16-2 and shown in Figure 16-5 ■.

TABLE 16-2 Signs and Symptoms: Abdominal Emergencies
■ Abdominal pain (local, diffuse, or crampy)
■ Abdominal tenderness, local or diffuse
■ Rigid, tense, or distended abdomen
■ Anxiety, reluctance to move
■ Lying in a fetal position (Figure 16-4)
■ Loss of appetite
■ Nausea, vomiting, diarrhea (may be extensive)
■ Blood in the vomit (bright red or "coffee grounds")
■ Blood in the stool (bright red or black, tarry)
■ Signs of shock
■ Fever

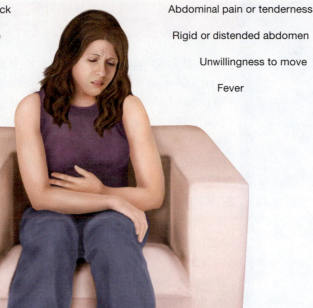

Signs of shock

Loss of appetite

Nausea, vomiting, diarrhea

Blood in vomit (bright
red or coffee grounds)

Blood in stool (bright
red or tarry black)

Abdominal pain or tenderness

Rigid or distended abdomen

Unwillingness to move

Fever

■ **Figure 16-5** Signs and symptoms of an abdominal emergency.

If vomiting or diarrhea is excessive, your patient may be in shock. This is especially true with pediatric patients. Abdominal pain in the elderly patient may also be a sign of possible heart attack.

Some patients may be experiencing internal gastrointestinal bleeding. This may be a result of esophageal damage, ulcers, intestinal damage or conditions, or a variety of conditions that may cause the digestive tract to bleed. These patients may appear to be in shock even though there are no external signs of bleeding. They may have bright red or "coffee grounds" emesis. They might also have stools that are dark red or black in color and tarry in texture (Table 16-2).

EMR Emergency Care: Abdominal Emergencies

If you suspect a patient has an abdominal emergency, you should immediately notify the responding EMS personnel and take appropriate Standard Precautions. Steps to providing care for this patient include the following:

1. Monitor and maintain the patient's airway, breathing, and circulation.
2. Place the patient in a position of comfort.
3. Administer high-flow oxygen.
4. Monitor the patient's mental status and vital signs frequently.
5. Provide emotional support to the patient.
6. Be sure to notify the responding EMS personnel of any changes in the patient's condition.

THE RESPONSE

The first thing you notice when you look at the patient is his color. He is very pale, almost ghostly white. There is no sparkle in his eyes and he generally looks sick. He does answer questions but somewhat slowly. The airway appears clear and breathing appears slightly fast. His pulse is rapid, but it is hard to palpate because it is very weak. The patient's initial vital signs are pulse of 146 and very weak, respirations of 28 and nonlabored, and blood pressure of 88/40.

The patient states he is "very weak" and just "doesn't feel well." He is sitting up and is comfortable in that position. The family states he has no allergies and takes medication for high blood pressure, which he last took this morning as prescribed. The patient ate some toast about 2 hours ago, but hasn't had much of an appetite lately. This is the first time this has happened to him. The patient says he has not been feeling his usual self for a couple of weeks, but today he suddenly feels much worse.

You place the patient on oxygen at 15 lpm by nonrebreather mask and begin your physical exam. There is nothing remarkable about the exam except some generalized tenderness as you palpate the abdomen. You ask the patient if he has had any unusual bowel movements since he has been sick. He says he has had several black stools over the past couple of weeks.

Reassessment shows little change in the patient's condition. Repeat vital signs are pulse of 132 and still very weak, respirations of 26 and nonlabored, and blood pressure of 90/42.

■ Discussion: *What decision regarding transport would you recommend and why?*

✳ Stop, Review, Remember

Multiple Choice

Place a check next to the correct answer.

1. A patient with a sudden onset of abdominal pain is said to have a(n):

   _____ a. acute abdomen.

   _____ b. distended abdomen.

   _____ c. rigid abdomen.

   _____ d. tender abdomen.

2. When palpating the abdomen, palpate the quadrant with the pain:

   _____ a. first.

   _____ b. second.

   _____ c. third.

   _____ d. fourth.

Renal Emergencies

You may be called to treat a patient who has a history of kidney (renal) failure. Many of these patients undergo **hemodialysis**, commonly called dialysis, on a regular basis. During hemodialysis, the patient's blood passes through a dialysis machine which filters out excess water and waste products. The dialysis machine is connected to the patient through a fistula, a shunt, or another type of access port.

EMR Emergency Assessment: Dialysis Patients

Dialysis patients may suffer from any of the medical or traumatic emergencies as your other patients. When assessing a dialysis patient, *do not* attempt to obtain a blood pressure in the arm with the fistula or shunt. By doing so you may alter the pressure and flow in that extremity's vascular system and damage the fistula or shunt.

Life-threatening emergencies associated with dialysis patients include:

- Low blood pressure
- Nausea and vomiting
- Irregular pulse
- Cardiac arrest

hemodialysis treatment where a patient's blood passes through a dialysis machine which filters out excess water and waste products; commonly called dialysis.

ASK YOURSELF

- What are the special considerations in the assessment of patients with a hemodialysis access site (shunt or fistula)?

- Bleeding from the access site
- Difficulty breathing (possibly from a missed dialysis treatment)

EMR Emergency Care: Dialysis Patients

You should treat a dialysis patient with a medical or traumatic emergency like you would any other patient in a similar situation:

1. Monitor and maintain the patient's airway, breathing, and circulation.
2. Stop bleeding from the shunt, if present.
3. Position the patient lying flat if he shows signs of shock. Position the patient sitting upright if he is having difficulty breathing.
4. *Do not* obtain a blood pressure in the arm with the fistula or shunt.
5. Reassure the patient.
6. Notify responding EMS personnel of any changes in condition.

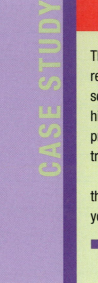

CASE STUDY

TRANSITION

The EMTs arrive, and you transfer patient care to them. Your verbal report includes information on the condition in which you found the scene and patient. You inform the EMTs of your assessment and history, being sure to mention the black stools and the treatment you provided. You note that the patient has not really improved much after treatment.

You assist the EMTs in loading the patient into the ambulance. You then proceed to restock your supplies and document the response in your written report.

- Discussion: *While your job is not to diagnose an illness, what was the indication that the patient may have a serious illness? Why?*

THE LAST WORD

In addition to medical patients with specific complaints, such as chest pain or shortness of breath, you will encounter medical patients with vague complaints, such as "I don't feel well."

These patients may present a challenge to the Emergency Medical Responder. You can significantly improve the comfort and condition of the patient by being professional; performing an appropriate assessment and physical exam; supporting the airway, breathing, and circulation; and gathering information for the responding EMS personnel.

Patients experiencing a mild allergic reaction or slight abdominal discomfort may only need general supportive care, while those experiencing an anaphylactic reaction or severe internal abdominal bleeding may be in need of rapid, life-supporting care.

Your role as an Emergency Medical Responder is a vital link in your patient's continuity of care and may make the difference in the patient's quality of life.

Multiple Choice

Place a check next to the correct answer.

1. Which of the following patients would be categorized as having a general medical complaint?

   a. _____ A 66-year-old patient who feels sick

   b. _____ An 8-year-old having an asthma attack

   c. _____ A 23-year-old patient who has been in a motorcycle crash

   d. _____ A 43-year-old with chest discomfort

2. When assessing a patient with a medical complaint, the best way to determine the problem is to:

   a. _____ identify the medications the patient is taking.

   b. _____ perform a thorough physical exam and obtain a history.

   c. _____ assess the mechanism of injury.

   d. _____ determine the chief complaint.

3. When first exposed to an allergen, a person will not have an allergic reaction because _____ have not been developed.

   a. _____ antibodies

   b. _____ antigens

   c. _____ antihistamines

   d. _____ antidotes

4. Your patient has a particularly painful insect sting on his upper right arm. He also tells you that his face feels tingly and his eyes are getting watery and itchy. Upon hearing this, you determine that you should be prepared for:

   a. _____ stroke or seizures.

   b. _____ other imaginary symptoms.

   c. _____ respiratory difficulties.

   d. _____ drug or alcohol poisoning.

5. When using an EpiPen, you should hold the injector firmly against the thigh for:

   a. _____ 2 seconds.

   b. _____ 5 seconds.

   c. _____ 10 seconds.

   d. _____ 20 seconds.

6. The appendix is located in the:

   a. _____ right upper quadrant.

   b. _____ right lower quadrant.

   c. _____ left upper quadrant.

   d. _____ left lower quadrant.

7. Which of the following patients is suffering from an acute abdomen?

   a. _____ A 71-year-old female with respiratory distress complaining of nausea

   b. _____ A 37-year-old male with a history of drug abuse and liver disease

   c. _____ A 62-year-old male with no medical history and a sudden pain in the lower abdomen

   d. _____ A 17-year-old pregnant female whose delivery date is next month

8. A patient with gastrointestinal bleeding may present with all of the following except:

   a. _____ increased appetite.

   b. _____ "coffee grounds" vomit.

   c. _____ black, tarry stools.

   d. _____ signs of shock.

9. The treatment that removes excessive water and wastes from the blood is called:

   a. _____ hyperdialysis.

   b. _____ hypodialysis.

   c. _____ hemodialysis.

   d. _____ heptodialysis.

10. When obtaining a blood pressure in a dialysis patient, you should only obtain the blood pressure in the:

a. _____ left arm.

b. _____ right arm.

c. _____ arm without the fistula or shunt.

d. _____ arm with the fistula or shunt.

Matching

Match the following descriptions with the appropriate term.

1. _____ Another term for anaphylaxis
2. _____ Presence of excessive air, usually in the abdominal cavity
3. _____ Treatment that filters out excess water and waste from the blood
4. _____ Lying on one's side with legs drawn up and arms across the abdomen
5. _____ Exaggerated immune response
6. _____ Any substance that causes an abnormal immune response or hypersensitivity
7. _____ Severe, potentially life-threatening allergic reaction
8. _____ Sudden onset of abdominal pain

a. Allergen
b. Allergic reaction
c. Anaphylaxis
d. Anaphylactic shock
e. Acute abdomen
f. Fetal position
g. Distended
h. Hemodialysis

Emergency Medical Responder Practice

You and your partner have been called to the scene for a 58-year-old man who "doesn't feel well." All this tells you is that you should probably expect a medical rather than a trauma patient, but even that isn't a sure thing.

1. What is the first thing you should do when you arrive on the scene?

_____

_____

_____

_____

You and your partner are met at the door of the house by a woman. "I'm Mrs. Kennedy," she says. "My husband, Patrick, is in the bedroom." You find Patrick in bed, lying on his side, holding his stomach and moaning.

2. What signs and symptoms would you expect to see in this patient?

_____

_____

_____

_____

3. After completing your assessment, you determine your patient is suffering from acute abdominal pain. What treatment would you provide this patient?

_____

_____

_____

_____

PEARSON
EXPLORE **mybradykit**™

Please go to **www.bradybooks.com** to access mykit for this text. You will find quizzes, critical thinking scenarios, weblinks, animations, and videos related to this chapter— and much more. Look for online information on anaphylaxis and kidney dialysis.

Register your access code from the front of your book by going to **www.bradybooks.com** and selecting the mykit links.

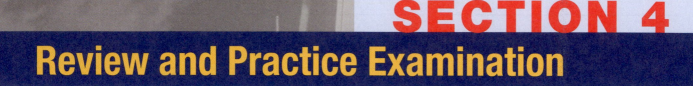

Review and Practice Examination

Assess what you have learned in this section by checking the best answer for each multiple-choice question. When you are done, check your answers against the key provided in Appendix B.

1. Oxygenated blood leaving the lungs returns to the _____ of the heart.
   a. _____ right atrium
   b. _____ left atrium
   c. _____ right ventricle
   d. _____ left ventricle

2. The exchange of oxygen and carbon dioxide between the blood and the cells of the body occurs at the level of the:
   a. _____ aorta.
   b. _____ arteries.
   c. _____ capillaries.
   d. _____ venules.

3. The heart muscle receives oxygenated blood from the _____ arteries.
   a. _____ coronary
   b. _____ cerebral
   c. _____ pulmonary
   d. _____ systemic

4. Wheezing in asthma is caused by:
   a. _____ fluid in the alveoli.
   b. _____ infection of the larynx.
   c. _____ constriction of the small airways.
   d. _____ inflammation of the oropharynx.

5. Chest pain, heaviness, or discomfort due to a myocardial infarction is due to:
   a. _____ inflammation of the lung tissue.
   b. _____ lack of oxygen to the heart muscle.
   c. _____ a spasm of the heart muscle.
   d. _____ fluid in the alveoli.

6. A reduction in blood flow to the heart muscle, causing pain but not death of heart muscle, is known as:
   a. _____ angina pectoris.
   b. _____ congestive heart failure.
   c. _____ myocardial infarction.
   d. _____ ventricular fibrillation.

7. A patient experiences pain in the chest while doing yard work, but the pain goes away after a few minutes of rest. This pattern is most typical with:
   a. _____ myocardial infarction.
   b. _____ heart attack.
   c. _____ congestive heart failure.
   d. _____ angina pectoris.

8. Which of the following is most likely to be experienced by the patient in ventricular fibrillation?
   a. _____ Palpitations
   b. _____ Cardiac arrest
   c. _____ Shortness of breath
   d. _____ Nausea

9. A patient states that he has pain in his chest that feels like it "goes through to my back." Which of the following is the most accurate description of the patient's complaint?
   a. _____ Onset of pain is in the chest.
   b. _____ Chest pain radiates to the back.
   c. _____ Provocation of chest pain is to the back.
   d. _____ Pain is radiating in quality.

10. A 50-year-old female is complaining of difficulty breathing and pain in her left shoulder, along with some "heartburn." She is alert and seems anxious. Which of the following should you do first?
    a. _____ Administer oxygen
    b. _____ Have the patient lie down.
    c. _____ Apply the AED pads.
    d. _____ Obtain a SAMPLE history.

11. A 60-year-old male is lying on the kitchen floor. His wife reports he collapsed while sitting at the table and fell to the floor. He does not respond to painful stimuli, his skin is cool and dry, he is breathing shallowly 8 times per minute, and he has a carotid pulse of 44 per minute. Of the following, which should you do first?
    a. _____ Obtain a blood pressure.
    b. _____ Apply the AED pads.
    c. _____ Perform a head-to-toe exam.
    d. _____ Assist breathing with a bag-valve mask.

12. A 55-year-old male complains of a sudden onset of severe, "crushing" chest pain while working in his home office. He is pale and cool, and has diaphoretic skin. His radial pulse is 74 per minute, and respirations are 20. Which of the following will benefit the patient the most at this time?
    a. _____ Asking if he has a family history of heart disease
    b. _____ Administering oxygen by nonrebreather mask
    c. _____ Determining the OPQRST of the pain
    d. _____ Locate the patient's nitroglycerin

13. A 70-year-old male patient has a history of a previous heart attack. His physician has instructed him that if he experiences chest pain and believes he is having another heart attack, he should call 911 and take two medications. These two medications are most likely:
    a. _____ albuterol and aspirin.
    b. _____ nitroglycerin and albuterol.
    c. _____ nitroglycerin and aspirin.
    d. _____ epinephrine and nitroglycerin.

14. A patient who has smoked for many years has ongoing inflammation of the lower airways, along with increased mucus production, difficulty breathing, and a productive cough. He has periods when his symptoms are better, but he calls 911 when he has episodes in which his breathing becomes worse. This description is most consistent with:
    a. _____ asthma.
    b. _____ chronic bronchitis.
    c. _____ emphysema.
    d. _____ pneumonia.

15. When the left side of the heart cannot keep up with the amount of blood returned to it, causing blood to back up into the lungs, this is called:
    a. _____ pneumonia.
    b. _____ chronic bronchitis.
    c. _____ emphysema.
    d. _____ congestive heart failure.

16. You are on the scene with a 16-year-old male who has a history of asthma. He does not have his inhaler with him. He began wheezing and having difficulty breathing during gym class at school. You have applied a nonrebreather mask with 15 liters per minute of oxygen. The patient's wheezing has decreased, and the chest wall is moving much less than when you first arrived. Initially, the patient was "fighting" you as you tried to assess him and provide oxygen. He now seems very tired and sleepy. Of the following, which should you do first?
    a. _____ Ensure an open airway and assist ventilations with a bag-valve mask.
    b. _____ Switch to a nasal cannula now that the patient is calmer.
    c. _____ Advise the incoming EMS crew that the patient's condition has improved.
    d. _____ Call the parents for permission to perform further assessment and treatment.

17. You are called to a residence for difficulty breathing at 3:00 a.m. You find a 79-year-old female sitting in a recliner with several pillows behind her head. Her respiratory rate is 24 per minute, her radial pulse is 88, and her skin is cool and moist. Which of the following pieces of information would lead you to believe that the patient has congestive heart failure?
    a. _____ She complains of fever and chills.
    b. _____ She always sleeps in the recliner.
    c. _____ She takes an aspirin every day.
    d. _____ She uses an inhaler for her difficulty breathing.

18. When auscultating a patient's lungs you hear coarse, bubbling, rattling sounds. These sounds are best described as:
    a. _____ crackles (rales).
    b. _____ wheezes.
    c. _____ rhonchi.
    d. _____ stridor.

19. You are caring for an alert patient who is complaining of difficulty breathing. The most important thing you can do is:
    a. _____ determine why the patient is having difficulty breathing.
    b. _____ identify any abnormal breath sounds.
    c. _____ obtain a pulse oximetry reading.
    d. _____ administer oxygen.

20. Which of the following is the most important reason to calm and reassure the patient who is anxious due to difficulty breathing?
    a. _____ The body requires more oxygen during states of anxiety.
    b. _____ It is difficult to get a good history from an anxious patient.
    c. _____ When the patient is anxious, it makes everyone else anxious.
    d. _____ Vital signs will not be accurate if the patient is anxious.

21. What is the most important thing to realize when you discover that a patient does not have breath sounds on one side of the chest?
    a. _____ It could be a pneumothorax.
    b. _____ It could be pneumonia.
    c. _____ There is nothing you can do about this finding.
    d. _____ The patient is not adequately oxygenated.

22. Which of the following best describes the responsibility of the EMR in assessing and managing the patient who is unresponsive?
    a. _____ Determining if the patient is having a stroke
    b. _____ Maintaining the patient's airway, breathing, and circulation
    c. _____ Preventing seizures
    d. _____ Administering oral glucose paste between the cheek and gums

23. The main source of fuel for the body's cells is:
    a. _____ glucose.
    b. _____ oxygen.
    c. _____ sodium.
    d. _____ insulin.

24. Your patient is a 57-year-old male found sitting at the bus station. He opens his eyes when you speak to him, but gives confused answers. The bus station manager called 911 because he believes the patient is drunk. Which of the following would concern you the most if found during your assessment?
    a. _____ A pulse of 64
    b. _____ Respirations of 20
    c. _____ Warm skin
    d. _____ A fruity odor to his breath

25. Which of the following best describes the role of insulin in the body?
    a. _____ It raises the blood glucose level.
    b. _____ It is the primary source of fuel for the body's cells.
    c. _____ It is a helper that allows glucose to enter the body's cells.
    d. _____ It stimulates the pancreas to release glucose into the blood.

26. You have responded to a residence where a woman states that her husband has been urinating frequently and drinking an excessive amount of water. He has been increasingly confused and sleepy over the past 3 days. She tells you she is sure that her husband has a kidney infection, but she cannot get him to see a doctor. She states he does not have any known medical history and does not take medications. Your assessment reveals a 65-year-old male who is moderately obese and who responds to painful stimuli by weakly trying to push your hand away. His skin is flushed, warm, and dry. Vital signs are pulse 100, respirations 24, and blood pressure 102/62. The patient's condition is most consistent with:

a. _____ stroke.
b. _____ hypoglycemia.
c. _____ seizure.
d. _____ hyperglycemia.

27. A 25-year-old male with a history of diabetes began acting confused just before lunchtime. The patient is awake, but unable to answer your questions intelligibly. He keeps trying to walk away from you. He is sweating profusely, has a pulse of 96, and has respirations of 18, but he will not cooperate with allowing you to take a blood pressure. Which of the following is the best course of action?
    a. _____ Add some sugar to a glass of juice and encourage the patient to drink it.
    b. _____ Get the patient to lie on his left side until EMS arrives.
    c. _____ Avoid giving sugar to prevent a dangerously high blood glucose level.
    d. _____ Contact law enforcement to ensure your safety before taking any additional action.

28. To which of the following is a stroke most similar in the way it causes damage to the body?
    a. _____ Seizure
    b. _____ Hypoglycemia
    c. _____ Heart attack
    d. _____ Diabetes

29. Which of the following statements regarding stroke is most accurate?
    a. _____ The signs and symptoms last only a few minutes but should not be ignored.
    b. _____ There are treatments available that can reverse the signs and symptoms of stroke in some patients if they are treated early enough.
    c. _____ Talking to a patient who is having difficulty speaking will confuse and agitate him.
    d. _____ Patients having signs and symptoms of stroke require treatment by placing a glucose gel between the cheek and gums.

30. The three components assessed using the Cincinnati Prehospital Stroke Scale are:
    a. _____ pupil reaction, equality of grip strength, and ability to speak.
    b. _____ ability to speak, arm drift, and facial droop.

c. _____ memory, facial droop, and pupil reaction.
d. _____ arm drift, facial droop, and blood pressure.

31. Your patient is a 50-year-old female who experienced a sudden weakness of her left arm, slightly slurred speech, and weakness of the right side of her face. She is alert and oriented, though a bit difficult to understand. Her blood pressure is 144/88, pulse is 88, and respirations are 16. Which of the following makes the most sense?
    a. _____ This is most consistent with hypoglycemia, and the patient needs oral glucose.
    b. _____ This is most consistent with a seizure, and the patient needs high-flow oxygen.
    c. _____ The patient is most likely having a stroke and needs oxygen.
    d. _____ The patient most likely took an overdose of medications and you should contact poison control immediately.

32. A prolonged seizure or two or more seizures that occur without a period of responsiveness in between is called:
    a. _____ tonic-clonic seizure.
    b. _____ epilepsy.
    c. _____ transient ischemic attack.
    d. _____ status epilepticus.

33. A 3-year-old male has drunk some lamp oil from a decorative oil lamp. This is an example of poisoning by:
    a. _____ inhalation.
    b. _____ ingestion.
    c. _____ injection.
    d. _____ absorption.

34. You have received a call for a possible poisoning by inhalation resulting from a young man mixing ammonia and bleach together, producing vapors that caused difficulty breathing. The most critical action you can take for this patient is to:
    a. _____ carefully survey the scene for indications of danger.
    b. _____ protect the patient's airway, and ensure breathing and circulation.
    c. _____ call poison control.
    d. _____ find out how much of each substance was used in the mixture.

35. A substance that causes a hypersensitivity response when the body is exposed to it is known as a(n):
    a. _____ antibody.
    b. _____ allergen.
    c. _____ histamine.
    d. _____ leukotriene.

36. The signs and symptoms of an allergic reaction are caused by:
    a. _____ the substance to which the patient is allergic.
    b. _____ epinephrine.
    c. _____ antihistamines.
    d. _____ leukotrienes and histamine.

37. Your patient is a 26-year-old female complaining of "breaking out in hives." She believes she may be allergic to an antibiotic prescribed to her for a urinary tract infection. She is awake and alert, with warm, moist skin and good color. She has hives on her face, arms, and chest. She is having no respiratory difficulty. She has a respiratory rate of 16, pulse of 88, and blood pressure of 116/78. Which of the following is the most likely cause of the patient's chief complaint and presentation?
    a. _____ The patient is experiencing a mild allergic reaction, possibly to the antibiotic she is taking.
    b. _____ The urinary tract infection has spread, becoming a generalized infection.
    c. _____ The patient is experiencing anaphylactic shock, probably due to the antibiotic she is taking.
    d. _____ The patient has taken an overdose of the antibiotic, causing a toxic reaction.

38. A bee stung a 10-year-old male. By the time you arrive, the patient is having difficulty breathing, and is pale, cool, and diaphoretic. He is awake and anxious, with a weak radial pulse of 130, respirations of 24 with obvious wheezing, and a blood pressure of 92/64. Which of the following should have the lowest priority in further assessment and management of this patient?
    a. _____ Obtain a pulse oximetry reading.
    b. _____ Find out if the patient has an epinephrine auto-injector.
    c. _____ Apply oxygen by nonrebreather mask.
    d. _____ Inspect the site of the sting to see if the stinger is still present.

39. A patient informs you that she used an epinephrine auto-injector following the onset of signs and symptoms of anaphylaxis due to ingesting sesame seeds. If the epinephrine is having an effect, which of the following would you expect to find in your assessment?
    a. _____ Pale skin, chest pain, anxiousness
    b. _____ Low blood pressure, confusion, wheezing
    c. _____ Stomach cramps, vomiting, hives
    d. _____ Swelling of the tongue and lips, drowsiness, pale skin

40. Your patient is a 5-year-old male with a history of food allergies. After eating a treat at a birthday party, the patient began having difficulty breathing and complaining of stomach cramps. The patient vomited, and now appears pale and diaphoretic. The child does not have an epinephrine auto-injector. Which of the following has the highest priority in your assessment and treatment of this patient?
    a. _____ Finding out to what foods the child has an allergy
    b. _____ Maintaining the airway and applying high-flow oxygen
    c. _____ Getting a full set of vital signs
    d. _____ Contacting the mother to get permission to treat the patient

41. A 40-year-old male with a history of bee sting anaphylaxis used his epinephrine auto-injector about 15 minutes ago while awaiting your arrival. He initially experienced some relief of his difficulty breathing and feeling of weakness. On your arrival, he states he is having more trouble breathing and is feeling more light-headed. Which of the following should you do?
    a. _____ Assume that the patient's auto-injector was expired and ineffective.
    b. _____ Ask the patient if he is sure he was stung by a bee, since the epinephrine does not seem to be working.
    c. _____ Irrigate the site of the sting with water to remove any venom on the skin.
    d. _____ Ask if the patient has a second dose of epinephrine and assist him with its use.

42. After inserting an EpiPen into the thigh, the next step is to:
    a. _____ pull off the gray safety release cap.
    b. _____ unscrew the green or yellow cap from the storage tube.
    c. _____ hold the unit firmly against the thigh for 10 seconds.
    d. _____ remove the unit from the thigh and massage the injection area for 10 seconds.

43. Usually, the patient with acute abdominal pain will feel most comfortable if positioned:
    a. _____ prone.
    b. _____ on his side with his legs drawn up.
    c. _____ supine.
    d. _____ sitting straight up.

44. A 50-year-old woman is complaining of right upper quadrant pain, pain in her right shoulder, nausea, and vomiting. She states the symptoms began about 30 minutes after she ate dinner. She is awake and alert, but appears uncomfortable and continues vomiting. Which of the following is the most important part of your assessment and management?
    a. _____ Place the patient on her left side.
    b. _____ Find out what she ate.
    c. _____ Ask if she has an epinephrine auto-injector.
    d. _____ Palpate the abdomen.

45. Your patient is a 79-year-old male who had a sudden onset of bright red bleeding from the rectum. On your arrival you can see that there is a significant amount of blood in and around the toilet, and on the patient. The patient is pale and diaphoretic, and is having difficulty paying attention to you as you ask questions. Which of the following must you do first?
    a. _____ Obtain a complete set of vital signs.
    b. _____ Lay the patient flat and apply oxygen by nonrebreather mask.
    c. _____ Estimate as accurately as possible the amount of blood that has been lost.
    d. _____ Ask the patient if anything like this has happened to him in the past.

46. You have provided initial care to a 16-year-old male complaining of lower right quadrant abdominal pain and nausea that began about 4 hours ago. You have placed him on oxygen and determined that his initial vital signs are blood pressure 122/78, pulse 88, and respirations 20.

The patient has had no pertinent past illnesses or surgeries, takes no medications, has no allergies, and last ate 6 hours ago. EMS is 10 minutes away. What should you do while awaiting the arrival of EMS?
    a. _____ Give small sips of water to prevent dehydration.
    b. _____ Reexamine the abdomen.
    c. _____ Retake the vital signs to detect any trends.
    d. _____ Retake the history to see if the patient adds information.

47. Your patient is a 70-year-old female complaining of abdominal pain accompanied by vomiting. She says the material she vomited "looked like coffee." Which of the following should concern you the most about this patient?
    a. _____ Blood pressure is 128/84.
    b. _____ Heart rate is 124.
    c. _____ Pulse oximetry is 97 percent on room air.
    d. _____ Last oral intake was a piece of toast and tea last night.

48. Your patient, a 35-year-old female, is complaining of severe abdominal pain in the left lower quadrant. When palpating the abdomen, at which point is the left lower quadrant palpated?
    a. _____ First
    b. _____ Second
    c. _____ Third
    d. _____ Fourth

49. When a patient receives dialysis, this means he is suffering from:
    a. _____ kidney failure.
    b. _____ diabetes.
    c. _____ cancer.
    d. _____ liver failure.

50. A 60-year-old female received dialysis earlier in the day and is now having bleeding from the shunt in her right forearm. She is alert, with warm, dry skin. Which of the following is most important in the treatment of this patient?
    a. _____ Determine the blood pressure in the right upper extremity.
    b. _____ Administer high-flow oxygen by nonrebreather mask.
    c. _____ Apply direct pressure over the site of bleeding.
    d. _____ Apply a tourniquet above the site of bleeding.

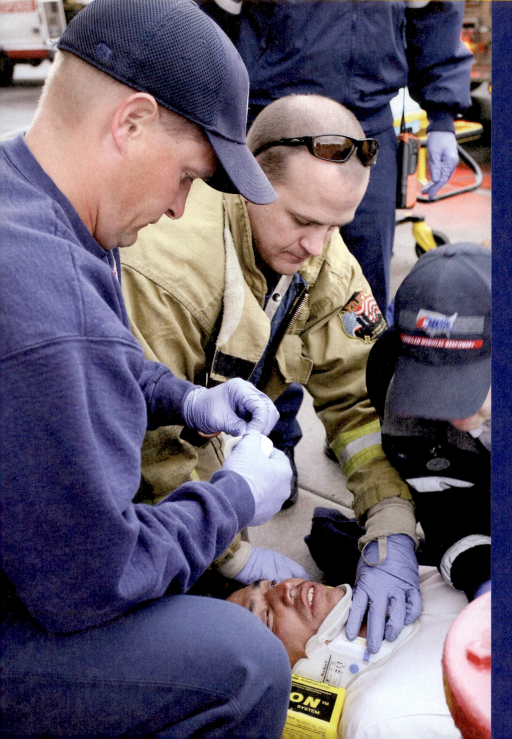

SECTION 5
Trauma

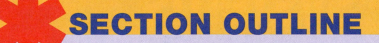

SECTION OUTLINE

In this section, you will cover the following EMS Education Standards:

- **Shock and Resuscitation**
- **Trauma**

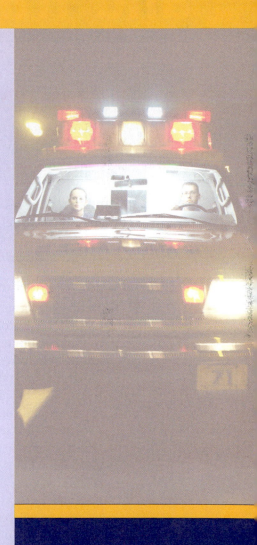

Overview of Trauma and Trauma Systems

NAVIGATION GUIDE

The following items provide an overview to the purpose and content of this chapter. The Education Standard and Competency are from the National EMS Education Standards.

Education Standard Trauma (Trauma Overview)

Competency Uses simple knowledge to recognize and manage life threats based on assessment findings for an acutely injured patient while awaiting additional emergency medical response. This level of provider does not transport patients but should be able to identify and categorize trauma patients and activate the appropriate trauma system response.

Objectives After reading this chapter, you should be able to:

1. Define key terms introduced in this chapter.
2. Outline key historical events that contributed to the development of EMS systems as we know them today.
3. Describe how trauma centers contribute to the survival of trauma patients.
4. Compare and contrast assessment of trauma patients with assessment of medical patients.
5. Given a scenario of a trauma call, perform each of the following components of the scene size-up:
   a. Scene safety
   b. Standard Precautions
   c. Mechanism of injury
   d. Number of patients
   e. Resource determination
6. Given a scenario of a trauma call, perform a primary assessment.
7. Identify trauma patients for whom cervical spine stabilization is needed during airway maneuvers.
8. Describe how the head-to-toe exam of a trauma patient will vary according to the patient's condition and mechanism of injury.
9. Inspect and palpate each of the following body areas to assess for indications of injury:
   a. Head
   b. Neck
   c. Chest
   d. Abdomen
   e. Pelvis
   f. Extremities
   g. Back
10. Determine a patient's level of responsiveness according to the Glasgow Coma Scale score.
11. Discuss the importance of each of the following concepts in the care of trauma patients:
    a. Priority of the ABCs
    b. Avoiding unnecessary movement
    c. Keeping the scene time short
    d. Determining patient criticality

NAVIGATION GUIDE (continued)

Media Resources Please go to www.bradybooks.com to access mykit for this text. You will find quizzes, critical thinking scenarios, weblinks, animations, and videos related to this chapter—and much more. Look for online information on gun violence and trauma scenarios. You will also find an animation on types of injuries and the mechanisms of injuries in motor vehicle collisions.

INTRODUCTION

ASK YOURSELF
- Can you define key terms introduced in this chapter?
- What key historical events contributed to the development of EMS systems as we know them today?

This chapter is designed to introduce you to trauma and caring for trauma patients. A trauma patient is one who is injured—as opposed to ill. A force of some sort has caused a physical injury. It may be a patient who has fallen, one who was involved in a car crash, or perhaps a patient who was assaulted. All of these and more are traumatic injuries.

The role of the Emergency Medical Responder (EMR)—and the entire EMS system—has changed dramatically in its response to patients who have experienced trauma (See The Big Picture: Trauma and Trauma Systems).

CASE STUDY

THE CALL

You are called to a motor vehicle collision in the business district. You are waved over by several bystanders and find a man lying in the road. You ensure safety from oncoming traffic and approach. A bystander excitedly tells you that she witnessed the patient get hit by the car and "thrown through the air." You see a dented bumper and hood of a car nearby.

- Discussion: *What has the mechanism of injury told you about how serious the patient's condition may be? What injuries might you expect to see in the patient?*

The History of Trauma Care

In 1966 patients were often transported to the hospital by local funeral homes who operated ambulances with providers who only had basic first aid cards. People dying on the highways spurred an interest in EMS—and treating trauma patients. It was out of the desire to care for trauma patients on the highway that our EMS system as we know it today was born.

As we were planning our national EMS system, the country was at war. During wartime we sadly lose many to trauma—but medicine also advances significantly in trauma care. Mobile army surgical hospital (MASH) units were introduced in the Korean war. Helicopters were also used there to rapidly evacuate casualties from the front lines and deliver them to the MASH units.

While we were making great strides to save the lives of soldiers on the battlefield, we were losing lives on the highways. The paper *Accidental Death and Disability: The Neglected Disease of Modern Society*, which was published by the National Academy of Sciences,

The Big Picture
Trauma and Trauma Systems

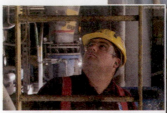
1 Scene size-up. Observe mechanism of injury.

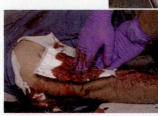
2 Perform initial assessment (bleeding control, oxygen, pulse check).

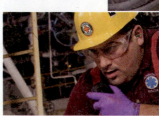
3 Update EMS. Determine criticality.

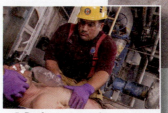
4 Perform secondary exam. Head to toe.

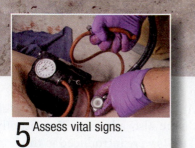
5 Assess vital signs.

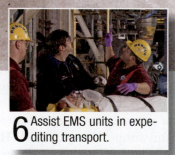
6 Assist EMS units in expediting transport.

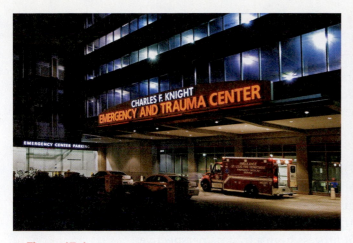

■ **Figure 17-1** Trauma center. (© Ray Kemp/911 Imaging)

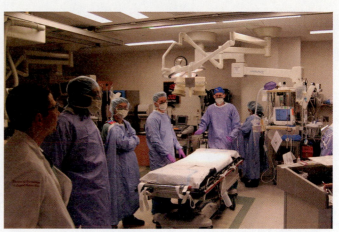

■ **Figure 17-2** The trauma room is available for large trauma cases and codes. (© Edward T. Dickinson, MD)

noted that soldiers could be injured on the battlefield and receive better care than if they were injured crossing the street back at home.

The EMS system as we know it started at this point.

Trauma Centers

Hospitals that meet strict criteria set by the American College of Surgeons or state authorities may be designated as **trauma centers** (Figure 17-1 ■). This designation is a very high standard and requires hospitals to have certain capabilities 24 hours per day. This includes trauma surgeons as well as specialty surgeons, full surgical capabilities, and diagnostic equipment available in the hospital at all times (Figure 17-2 ■).

Serious trauma patients should be transported to trauma centers for the best chance of survival when possible. Not all geographical areas have a trauma center. Your assessment at the scene may cause you to activate a helicopter to transport a patient to the trauma center (Figure 17-3 ■).

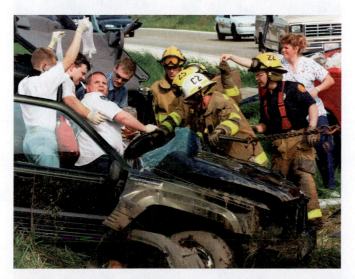

■ **Figure 17-3** The patient is attended by EMRs while rescuers work to release him from the vehicle. (© Jacksonville Journal Courier/The Image Works)

ASK YOURSELF

- How would you compare and contrast the assessment of trauma patients with the assessment of medical patients?
- Given a scenario of a trauma call, how would you perform each of the following components of the scene size-up?
  - Scene safety
  - Standard Precautions
  - Mechanism of injury
  - Number of patients
  - Resource determination

EMR Assessment and Care: Identification and Categorization of Trauma Patients

You have spent some time in the last several chapters learning about assessment and care of medical emergencies. Medical emergencies and trauma emergencies are very different. These differences span the full gamut from assessment to care.

Trauma Assessment

Trauma assessment is a largely hands-on process. The majority of your findings will come from a physical examination of the patient. You can see or feel most traumatic injuries—or determine the force that caused them. This isn't so for medical emergencies.

With the understanding that trauma is a physical process, let's review the components of the patient assessment process from a trauma perspective.

Scene Size-Up

There are five decisions in the scene size-up. Each has an important place in the assessment of all patients but many of these decisions have strong relevance to the trauma call.

- *Scene safety.* The trauma call may be a result of violence, motor vehicle collisions, machinery, falls, or other causes. The point to remember in the scene size-up is

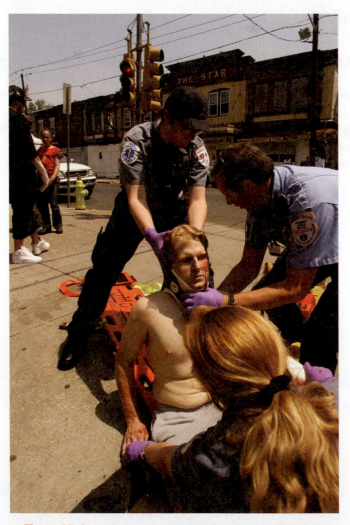

■ **Figure 17-4**   EMRs assist a minor trauma patient. *(© Mark C. Ide)*

that you could be a victim of the same trauma as your patient. Scene safety is always your primary concern while approaching—and at the scene.

- *Standard Precautions*. When patients have open wounds, there will be blood. You must take Standard Precautions. Gloves aren't always enough. Remember to protect your face when the blood or other fluids may spray. For very severe bleeding you will also protect your clothes with a gown.

- *Mechanism of injury and determining criticality*. As you approach the scene you will look for a mechanism of injury. This is the force that caused the patient's trauma. It may be the damage from a motor vehicle crash, the distance a patient fell from, or what the patient was struck with. The mechanism of injury gives you an idea of how serious or critically injured the patient may be. Alone it is not a guarantee of injury, but it helps you develop an **index of suspicion** (Figure 17-4 ■).

- *Number of patients*. You are much more likely to have more than one patient in a trauma emergency than you are with a medical emergency. Violence and motor vehicle crashes are examples of incidents that can result in multiple patients.

- *Resource determination*. Trauma may require the power company for downed wires, fire units for extrication, and additional EMRs and ambulances for multiple patients. (Figure 17-5 ■)

index of suspicion a general idea of how bad a person's injuries may be based upon the mechanism of injury.

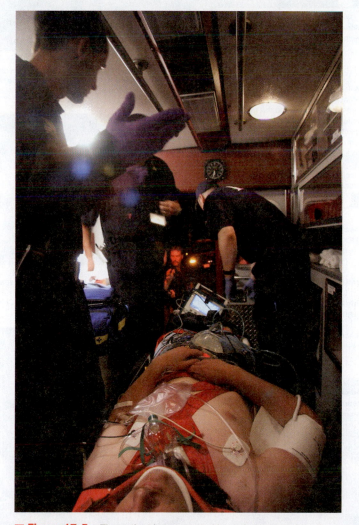

■ **Figure 17-5** The patient is transported by ambulance to the hospital. *(© Mark C. Ide)*

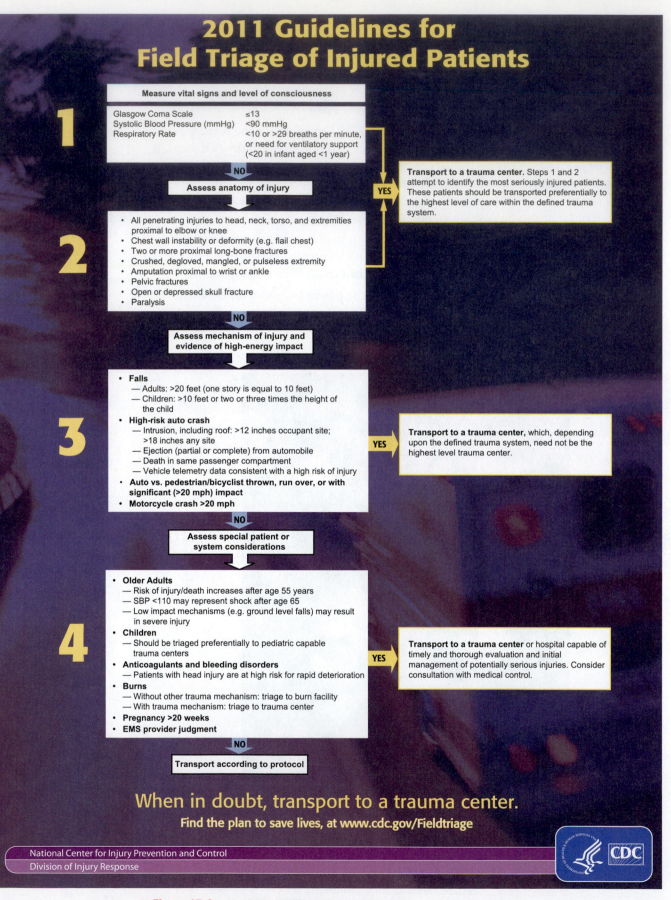

2011 Guidelines for Field Triage of Injured Patients

1 Measure vital signs and level of consciousness

Glasgow Coma Scale	≤13
Systolic Blood Pressure (mmHg)	<90 mmHg
Respiratory Rate	<10 or >29 breaths per minute, or need for ventilatory support (<20 in infant aged <1 year)

NO ↓

Assess anatomy of injury

YES → **Transport to a trauma center.** Steps 1 and 2 attempt to identify the most seriously injured patients. These patients should be transported preferentially to the highest level of care within the defined trauma system.

2
- All penetrating injuries to head, neck, torso, and extremities proximal to elbow or knee
- Chest wall instability or deformity (e.g. flail chest)
- Two or more proximal long-bone fractures
- Crushed, degloved, mangled, or pulseless extremity
- Amputation proximal to wrist or ankle
- Pelvic fractures
- Open or depressed skull fracture
- Paralysis

NO ↓

Assess mechanism of injury and evidence of high-energy impact

3
- **Falls**
  — Adults: >20 feet (one story is equal to 10 feet)
  — Children: >10 feet or two or three times the height of the child
- **High-risk auto crash**
  — Intrusion, including roof: >12 inches occupant site; >18 inches any site
  — Ejection (partial or complete) from automobile
  — Death in same passenger compartment
  — Vehicle telemetry data consistent with a high risk of injury
- **Auto vs. pedestrian/bicyclist thrown, run over, or with significant (>20 mph) impact**
- **Motorcycle crash >20 mph**

YES → **Transport to a trauma center,** which, depending upon the defined trauma system, need not be the highest level trauma center.

NO ↓

Assess special patient or system considerations

4
- **Older Adults**
  — Risk of injury/death increases after age 55 years
  — SBP <110 may represent shock after age 65
  — Low impact mechanisms (e.g. ground level falls) may result in severe injury
- **Children**
  — Should be triaged preferentially to pediatric capable trauma centers
- **Anticoagulants and bleeding disorders**
  — Patients with head injury are at high risk for rapid deterioration
- **Burns**
  — Without other trauma mechanism: triage to burn facility
  — With trauma mechanism: triage to trauma center
- **Pregnancy >20 weeks**
- **EMS provider judgment**

YES → **Transport to a trauma center** or hospital capable of timely and thorough evaluation and initial management of potentially serious injuries. Consider consultation with medical control.

NO ↓

Transport according to protocol

When in doubt, transport to a trauma center.
Find the plan to save lives, at www.cdc.gov/Fieldtriage

National Center for Injury Prevention and Control
Division of Injury Response

CDC

■ **Figure 17-6** The CDC's Field Triage Decision Scheme.

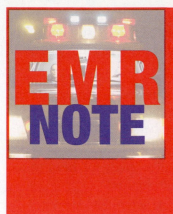

Remember that the scene size-up sets the foundation for the efficiency and success for the remainder of the call. If you don't address the issues properly during the size-up, you will experience them with greater severity later in the call.

For example, if you come upon a scene with multiple patients and you don't tell dispatch and request additional resources, by the time ambulances arrive—even minutes later—you have lost valuable time for the patients who must now wait for care.

Experienced EMS providers have learned that if you begin patient care before completing the scene size-up, you will lose track of time and forget to call for the help you need. It can't be said enough: Never begin patient care until the size-up is completed. It is an investment for you and your patient.

Primary Assessment

The primary assessment contains the same steps for a medical patient as it does for a trauma patient. Each trauma patient will be evaluated and treated immediately for any problems observed with airway, breathing, and circulation (the ABCs). For the trauma patient there may be a need for cervical spine stabilization during airway maneuvers. Check the ABCs as follows:

- *Airway.* Open the airway and make sure it remains open. Suction if necessary and insert an oral airway. Trauma patients may have blood, teeth, and tissue in the airway which must be removed by suctioning and finger sweeps. Take and maintain c-spine stabilization if indicated by mechanism or patient complaint.

- *Breathing.* Ensure the patient is breathing and breathing adequately. Administer oxygen or ventilate the patient. Chest injuries may make breathing difficult and inadequate. Conditions such as head injuries can cause breathing irregularities. Low blood volume and shock can increase a patient's need for oxygen. If you must ventilate the patient, remember that you will also maintain stabilization of the head as long as ventilations can be effectively delivered. Seal any open chest wounds.

- *Circulation.* The check for bleeding is very important in the trauma patient. Bleeding is not always obvious. Blood may soak into carpets or clothing and be hidden. The circulation check can also help you identify shock early in the call. You will learn that shock presents with a rapid pulse and cool, clammy skin. A quick check of the radial pulse can identify a rapid pulse as well as cool, clammy skin. The absence of a radial pulse is an indication of very low blood pressure indicating shock.

ASK YOURSELF

- Given a scenario of a trauma call, how would you perform a primary assessment?
- How would you identify trauma patients for whom cervical spine stabilization is needed during airway maneuvers?
- What is the importance of each of the following concepts in the care of trauma patients?
  - Priority of the ABCs
  - Avoiding unnecessary movement
  - Keeping the scene time short
  - Determining patient criticality

- How will the head-to-toe exam of a trauma patient vary according to the patient's condition and mechanism of injury?
- How do you inspect and palpate each of the following body areas to assess for indications of injury?
  - Head
  - Neck
  - Chest
  - Abdomen
  - Pelvis
  - Extremities
  - Back

Head-to-Toe Exam

The head-to-toe exam is done to identify injuries the patient may have sustained. The exam you perform will depend on a number of issues. In some cases you may not get to do the exam at all. For example:

- If a patient is in serious condition and requires airway care and/or ventilation, and you are alone or possibly with one other EMR, you may be too busy with the airway to provide additional care or assessment. Remember one EMR will be stabilizing the c-spine while the other provides airway care.

- Patients who have a significant mechanism of injury will receive a full head-to-toe exam. This will usually be done quickly to look for major injuries.

- Patients who have minor or isolated injuries (for example, a twisted ankle) will receive an exam of the injured area only. Be sure to look for more than one injury. Sometimes the pain of one injury will mask another injury.

The head-to-toe exam involves inspecting (looking at) and palpating (feeling) the following areas:

- Head
- Neck
- Chest
- Abdomen
- Pelvis
- Extremities

The patient's back (posterior) will also be assessed, but you should not move the patient and aggravate any spinal injuries to do so. The back can be assessed when the patient is rolled onto a backboard.

Look for signs of injury including deformity, open wounds, tenderness upon palpation, and swelling. The mnemonic DOTS can be used to remember what to look for.

Although the next chapters will teach you to deal with many different types of traumatic injuries, the principles of assessment will apply regardless of the type of traumatic injury.

Depending on where you will practice as an EMR, the EMTs may be on scene by this point. If this is the case, you will assist them with patient care and preparation for transport. If you have completed your assessment and the EMTs haven't yet arrived, you will perform ongoing assessments paying special attention to the ABCs and spinal stabilization.

Stop, Review, Remember

Multiple Choice

Place a check next to the correct answer.

1. Hospitals that maintain high standards set forth by the American College of Surgeons, which includes having certain services available 24 hours a day, are said to be:

   ____ a. surgery centers.

   ____ b. trauma centers.

   ____ c. emergency departments.

   ____ d. stroke centers.

2. In a trauma assessment, the majority of your relevant information will come from:

   ____ a. the patient's medical history.

   ____ b. the patient's story of his symptoms.

   ____ c. your physical assessment.

   ____ d. your medical equipment.

3. Providers who are treating a trauma patient with arterial bleeding must be sure to use all protective equipment including gloves and:

_____ a. goggles, mask, and gown.

_____ b. protective boots.

_____ c. X-ray proof vest.

_____ d. gloves alone.

4. A patient who is in shock will often present with a _____ pulse and cool, clammy skin.

_____ a. weak

_____ b. slow

_____ c. rapid

_____ d. strong

True/False

Mark whether each of the following statements is true (T) or false (F).

1. _____ Serious trauma patients should be transported to a trauma center for the best chance of survival.

2. _____ It is not possible to see or feel most traumatic injuries.

3. _____ A significant mechanism of injury guarantees significant physical injury.

4. _____ If a patient requires airway care, the EMR may not be able to perform a full physical assessment.

Critical Thinking

Your trauma patient was involved in a motor vehicle collision and has a compromised airway. He is not responsive and is still in the vehicle.

1. What is your primary responsibility as an EMR? Why?

_____

_____

_____

_____

2. If you are the sole provider, what should you accomplish before anyone else arrives?

_____

_____

_____

_____

3. Does your primary assessment change if this patient was deemed to have a medical problem that preceded the accident?

_____

_____

_____

_____

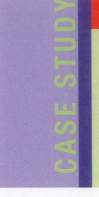

CASE STUDY

You arrive at the patient's side and find the patient's eyes closed. She is bleeding from a wound on her forehead and has an obviously deformed right leg.

- Discussion: *What are your priorities here? What priority would you assign this patient? What would you radio to incoming EMS units?*

Glasgow Coma Scale

Glasgow Coma Scale
assessment tool used to determine a person's level of consciousness based upon certain factors.

You may be taught to use the **Glasgow Coma Scale**. This scale helps EMS providers determine patient severity. It is also used in many EMS systems as one indicator in triage decisions (for example, patients with a Glasgow Coma Scale score of less than 14 should be transported to a trauma center, or a helicopter should be requested when appropriate). Another benfit to using the coma score is that there will be a record of the patient's status early in the call which can be compared later to determine trends in the patient's condition.

The Glasgow Coma Scale has three components (Table 17-1). They are as follows:

ASK YOURSELF

- How do you determine a patient's level of responsiveness according to the Glasgow Coma Scale score?

- *Eye opening.* Look to see if the patient's eyes open spontaneously (4 points). If they do not open spontaneously, see if they will open when the patient is asked to open them or when you talk to him (3 points). If the eyes aren't open after verbal stimulation, attempt a trapezius pinch as painful stimulus (2 points). If the eyes don't open in response to this, assign 1 point.

TABLE 17-1 Glasgow Coma Scale Score

Eye Opening

4—Spontaneous eye opening
3—Eyes open to speech
2—Eyes open to pain
1—No eye opening

Verbal Response

5—Alert and oriented
4—Confused, yet coherent, speech
3—Inappropriate words and jumbled phrases consisting of words
2—Incomprehensible sounds
1—No sounds

Motor Response

6—Obeys commands fully
5—Localizes to noxious stimuli
4—Withdraws from noxious stimuli
3—Abnormal flexion (decorticate posturing)
2—Extensor response (decerebrate posturing)
1—No response

- *Verbal response*. Evaluate the patient's verbal response as follows: alert and oriented (5 points), confused but coherent (4 points), words that are jumbled with no context (3 points), incomprehensible sounds (2 points), and no sounds (1 point).

- *Motor response*. The motor response is a scale of 6 points. If the patient can follow commands, assign a score of 6 points. If you apply a painful stimulus and the patient reaches toward that stimulus, assign 5 points. If the patient withdraws from the stimulus, assign 4 points. If the patient experiences decorticate posturing (elbows flexed toward torso), assign 3 points. If the patient experiences decerebrate posturing (arms extended away from torso), assign 2 points. If there is no response, assign 1 point.

The final score is determined by adding the values of the three sections. The maximum score is 15 and the minimum score is 3. Patients who are accurately scored at less than 12 are generally considered to be at risk for a serious injury, while a score of 8 or below is critical with the patient considered to be in a coma.

It is important to note that this score is not a priority. The primary assessment should always come first. Lifesaving care should never be withheld to determine a Glasgow Coma Scale score. This material is presented in the event it is used in your system as part of a priority determination or a criterion for request of a medical helicopter.

After you have completed the primary assessment and identified and treated any life threats, you will move on to a full physical exam to identify specific injuries. This is often called the secondary trauma assessment and will be covered in the next chapter.

CASE STUDY

TRANSITION

You provide manual stabilization while your partner applies oxygen. The patient opens her eyes and mumbles incoherent sounds. The patient has a rapid radial pulse and cool moist skin. EMS arrives relatively quickly and you tell them this is all you have found out thus far.

- Discussion: *What can you do to help the EMS providers? Is it an issue that you only got to stabilize the patient's spine and begin the ABCs before EMS arrived?*

THE LAST WORD

In addition to reviewing some trauma history and concepts, one of the most important parts of this chapter is *putting it all together* in your care of trauma patients.

The next chapters will teach you about many types of traumatic injuries and conditions such as bleeding, shock, internal injuries, spine injury, and musculoskeletal trauma. The following components are fundamental to trauma assessment and apply to all of these patients:

- The ABCs *always* take priority over all else. Once you are on a safe scene, the ABCs are the most important priority. On some serious calls, you may find a facial wound that is bleeding into the mouth. If the patient is unresponsive, that wound is fatal because it will cause blood to flow into the airway. If the first and only thing you get to do is keep the airway clear until the EMTs arrive, you will have done an excellent job.

- Moving the patient may cause injury. Patients who have experienced trauma may have spinal injury. In this case, moving the patient can worsen the injury up to and including paralysis. While you should avoid *unnecessary* movement, you may need to move the patient who is in danger or who requires positioning for airway care. In short, the risk of death outweighs the risk of paralysis.

- Time is of the essence. It has been proven that for a trauma patient to survive, he needs transport to a facility where surgeons are available to operate to correct life-threatening internal injuries. Emergency Medical Responders can help in this regard by identifying critical patients early and advising incoming units, ensuring the ABCs are assessed and treated, and preparing the scene for incoming units. You may be asked to stay and help with log rolling and backboarding the patient. This will be taught in Chapter 21, "Injuries to the Head and Spine."

- Determine criticality. In order to notify incoming EMS units of critical patients, you must be able to identify those who are critical—and those who may be critical. This will be done based on the mechanism of injury, your assessment findings, and the patient's vital signs.

Chapter Review

Multiple Choice

Place a check next to the correct answer.

1. Which of the following scales is used to determine a patient's severity and sometimes as a triage factor?

_____ a. Glasgow Coma Scale

_____ b. Advanced Trauma Scale

_____ c. START Triage Scoring

_____ d. Apgar Scoring

2. Which of the following is not included in the Glasgow Coma Scale score?

_____ a. Eye opening

_____ b. Verbal response

_____ c. Motor response

_____ d. Auditory response

3. What is the most important thing to accomplish once the scene is safe in a patient with traumatic injuries?

_____ a. OPQRST

_____ b. Apgar

_____ c. ABC

_____ d. DCAP BTLS

4. One way for an EMR to assist ensuring the trauma patient is transported to the proper facility is to:

_____ a. identify the critically injured patient.

_____ b. provide all care possible for the patient.

_____ c. transport the patient in a personal vehicle.

_____ d. stop bleeding before the person has a unctioning airway.

5. What is a proper time to assess the posterior of the patient with a suspected spinal injury?

_____ a. As soon as patient contact is established

_____ b. When rolling the patient to place on a backboard

_____ c. After assessing the head and neck

_____ d. Once bleeding is controlled

6. When ventilating the trauma patient, it is also important to ensure:

_____ a. he is secured to a long backboard.

_____ b. he has been given a full trauma assessment.

_____ c. the cervical spine is stabilized.

_____ d. all bleeding is controlled.

7. The trauma patient is more likely to require _____ transport from rural areas without trauma center capabilities.

_____ a. boat

_____ b. helicopter

_____ c. fixed-wing airplane

_____ d. four-wheel drive

True/False

Indicate whether each of the following is true (T) or false (F) on the line provided.

1. _____ It may be necessary to move a trauma patient for the purpose of airway control or to protect him from danger.

2. _____ EMS providers who begin care prior to ensuring proper units are en route often lose track of time and forget to call for additional resources.

3. _____ The ABCs can be bypassed to provide care for a patient with other traumatic injuries.

4. _____ Medical patients often require additional resources such as the power company or public works department.

5. _____ If you have completed your primary assessment and the EMTs haven't arrived yet, you may be required to complete ongoing assessments.

6. _____ Trauma patients with serious physical injuries should be given a rapid head-to-toe exam to identify other injuries.

7. _____ Scene safety is not of paramount concern in a trauma-related call.

Critical Thinking

Your patient fell from a ladder while trying to clean his gutters. His ladder had become entangled in power lines which have now fallen with him to the ground. He appears to be breathing and has an obvious open fracture to his upper left leg.

1. What is the EMR's primary concern when approaching this call? Why?

_____

_____

_____

_____

2. Once that issue has been dealt with, what should the EMR assess next?

_____

_____

_____

_____

3. Does this patient appear to be a critical trauma patient requiring transport to a trauma center? Why?

_____

_____

_____

_____

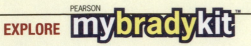

Bleeding and Shock

NAVIGATION GUIDE

The following items provide an overview to the purpose and content of this chapter. The Education Standard and Competencies are from the National EMS Education Standards.

Education Standard Trauma (Bleeding); Shock and Resuscitation

Competencies Uses assessment information to recognize shock, respiratory failure or arrest, and cardiac arrest based on assessment findings, and manages the emergency while awaiting additional emergency response.

Uses simple knowledge to recognize and manage life threats based on assessment findings for an acutely injured patient while awaiting additional emergency medical response.

Knowledge Area Bleeding
- Recognition and management of

Objectives After reading this chapter, you should be able to:

1. Define key terms introduced in this chapter.
2. Explain the importance of rapidly recognizing patients with external and internal bleeding.
3. Describe the four major causes of shock.
4. Explain the relationship between the body's attempts to compensate for shock and signs and symptoms that occur in early stages of shock.
5. Explain the transition between compensated and decompensated shock.
6. Explain the significance of a drop in blood pressure in the patient in shock.
7. Describe the progression of shock to irreversible shock.
8. Recognize signs and symptoms of shock in the primary assessment.
9. Describe the characteristics of arterial, venous, and capillary bleeding.
10. Given a description of a patient's presentation and history, identify signs and symptoms of internal bleeding.
11. Explain the importance of ensuring an open airway and adequate ventilation and providing a high concentration of oxygen to patients in shock.
12. Given a scenario in which a patient has external bleeding, including a nosebleed, demonstrate appropriate steps to control the hemorrhage.
13. Compare and contrast the characteristics of anaphylactic shock with those of hemorrhagic shock.
14. Given a variety of scenarios involving patients in shock, demonstrate appropriate assessment and patient care.

NAVIGATION GUIDE *(continued)*

Key Terms Page numbers indicate first major use in this chapter. The Margin Glossary in this chapter provides definitions as you read.

circulatory system, p. 432

perfusion, p. 434

shock, p. 434

compensated shock, p. 437

hypoxia, p. 437

decompensated shock, p. 437

decompensation, p. 437

hypotension, p. 438

internal bleeding, p. 440

exsanguinating hemorrhage, p. 443

direct pressure, p. 443

Media Resources Please go to **www.bradybooks.com** to access mykit for this text. You will find quizzes, critical thinking scenarios, weblinks, animations, and videos related to this chapter—and much more. Look for online information on bleeding and the stages of shock. You will also find animations and video clips on types of shock and ways to control bleeding.

ASK YOURSELF

- Can you define key terms introduced in this chapter?
- What is the importance of rapidly recognizing patients with external and internal bleeding?
- What is the relationship between the body's attempts to compensate for shock and signs and symptoms that occur in early stages of shock?

INTRODUCTION

Uncontrolled bleeding, both internal and external, rapidly leads to shock and patient death and continues to be a leading cause of death in trauma patients. External bleeding may be obvious, but often major bleeding occurs internally with little to no evidence visible on the outside of the body. A thorough patient assessment is the key to recognizing and stopping the progression of shock. Learn to identify this life-threatening condition and to act *quickly* to interrupt its downward spiral (See The Big Picture: Bleeding and Shock).

CASE STUDY

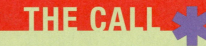

THE CALL

It is a very warm, humid evening in May. The temperature at 9:30 p.m. is 80 degrees. You receive a call to assist the police for a man bleeding. They report that the scene is safe. You arrive at a street corner to find a patient lying in a pool of blood, surrounded by police officers. He appears to be breathing. The police officers wave you in.

- Discussion: *How do you know the scene is safe? What is your general impression?*

The Downward Spiral of Shock

It is helpful to think of blood as the transportation system for the body. Just as trucks follow roads and deliver the necessary food and supplies we rely on, blood travels through vessels and carries oxygen and vital nutrients our cells require. The pumping of the heart powers the system and together with the blood and the blood vessels makes up the **circulatory system**. Also review Chapter 5, "Anatomy and Physiology."

When the system works correctly, the heart pumps bright red, oxygenated blood into arteries, which carry the blood to the small capillaries to supply oxygen and nutrients to the cells. From there, waste products are picked up and the veins transport the dark

circulatory system body system that delivers oxygen and nutrients to the cells, removes waste products, and consists of the heart, blood, and blood vessels.

The Big Picture
Bleeding and Shock

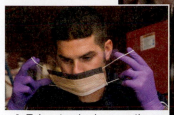

1 Take standard precautions for bleeding patient (gloves and face shield).

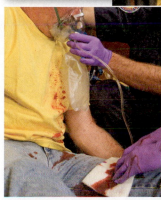

2 Initial assessment. Bleeding control—direct pressure, oxygen.

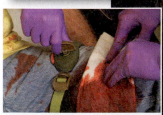

3 If bleeding continues use tourniquet or …

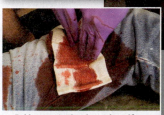

4 Hemostatic dressing if allowed by protocol.

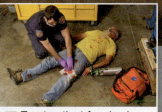

5 Treat patient for shock.

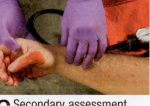

6 Secondary assessment and vital signs.

perfusion the consistent delivery of blood to adequately oxygenated cells.

shock inadequate oxygenation (perfusion) of the body at a cellular level.

ASK YOURSELF

■ What are the three major causes of shock?

colored, deoxygenated blood back to the heart to repeat the cycle. The consistent delivery of adequate oxygen to the cells is called **perfusion**. Adequate perfusion is essential for cells to survive and perform the functions that keep us alive.

When this system is interrupted, cells become *hypoperfused* due to the inadequate delivery of oxygenated blood and they begin to die. The progression of this condition is referred to as **shock**. If left uninterrupted, cellular hypoperfusion will progress to cell death, organ failure, and eventually patient death.

There are four major causes that lead to disruption of the circulatory system and shock:

1. Failure of the heart
2. Inability to control the size of blood vessels (abnormal dilation of the blood vessels)
3. Blood loss
4. Obstruction of the blood from reaching vital organs

As a result, shock is generally divided into four main types: hypovolemic, distributive, obstructive, and cardiac (cardiogenic).

Shock can occur in both trauma patients and medical patients (Figures 18-1a and 18-1b ■).

Consider the following patients and think about how each of their problems leads to cellular hypoperfusion and shock:

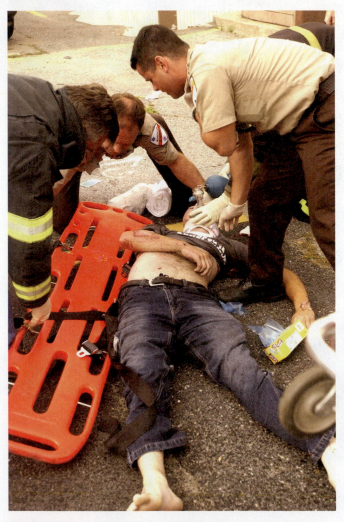

■ **Figure 18-1a** Trauma scene. (© *Mark C. Ide*)

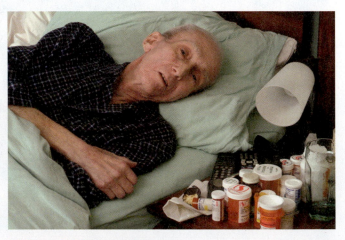

■ **Figure 18-1b** Medical scene.

1. A 52-year-old man has a massive heart attack. Because of muscle damage caused by the heart attack, his heart can no longer pump an adequate amount of blood to circulate and perfuse his cells (Figure 18-2a ■).

FOUR TYPES OF SHOCK

(a)

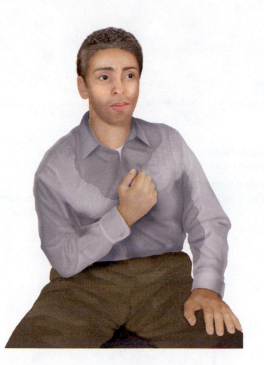

Cardiogenic shock is a pump problem. The heart isn't pumping the blood properly or efficiently.

■ **Figure 18-2a** Cardiogenic shock—a pump problem.

(b)

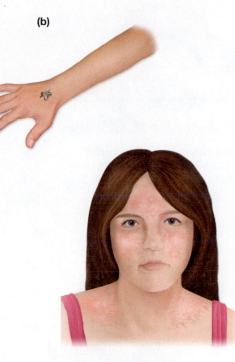

Distributive shock is a vascular tone problem. The blood isn't allocated properly.

■ **Figure 18-2b** Anaphylactic shock—a tone problem.

(c)

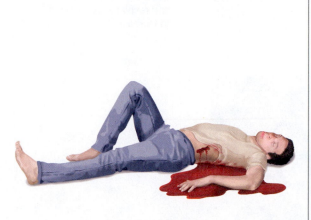

Hypovolemic shock is related to extreme blood loss or too little volume.

■ **Figure 18-2c** Hypovolemic shock—a volume problem.

(d)

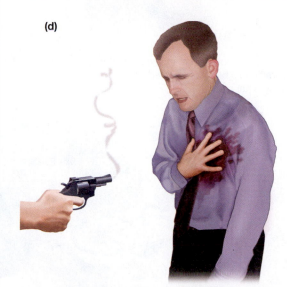

Pressure builds up causing an obstruction in his chest to the point his vena cava is partially collapsed, causing less blood to be pumped by his heart.

■ **Figure 18-2d** Obstructive shock—an obstructive problem.

(a)

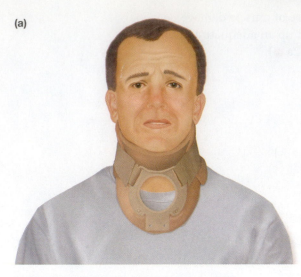

The patient will experience anxiety and mental status changes. The brain begins to feel the effect of decreased oxygen.

(b)

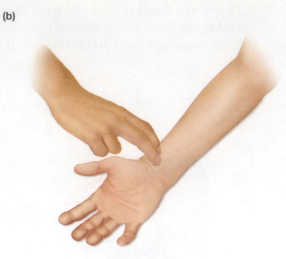

The patient will have cool, pale, sweaty skin and an increased pulse and respirations.

• Blood is shunted from the skin to the vital areas.
• Pulse and respirations increase to compensate for shock.

(c)

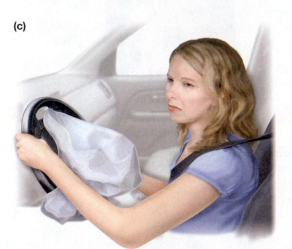

In addition to sweating, the patient may also experience nausea and vomiting as blood is shunted from the abdomen to more vital areas.

(d)

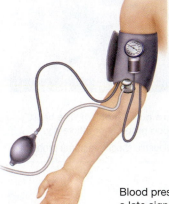

Blood pressure drops as a late sign of shock. Pulse and respirations continue to increase.

(e)

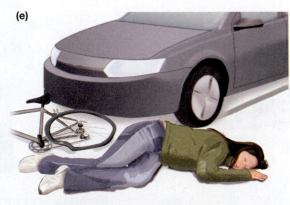

Uncorrected shock leads to death.

■ **Figure 18-3** Uncontrolled bleeding, both internal and external, can rapidly lead to shock and patient death.

2. An 8-year-old female is stung by a bee. As a result of the venom and her body's allergic response, she loses her ability to control the size of her blood vessels and they dilate (enlarge). Because of the change in size of the vessels, the pressure inside them drops and blood can no longer be efficiently transported to the cells (Figure 18-2b ■).
3. A 33-year-old male is stabbed in the abdomen. The knife cuts part of his liver. Blood rapidly leaves the circulatory system and accumulates in the abdominal cavity. Because there is now more blood outside the circulatory system than inside it, oxygen can no longer be delivered to the cells (Figure 18-2c ■).
4. A 50-year-old man is shot in the chest. Pressure builds up in his chest causing an obstruction to the point his vena cava is partially collapsed, causing less blood to be pumped by his heart (Figure 18-2d ■).

ASK YOURSELF
■ How would you describe the transition between compensated and decompensated shock?

Recognizing Shock

Shock is a series of events that occur over time. It is called progression of shock (Figures 18-3a and 18-3e ■). When the circulatory system fails, the body has predictable responses called compensation mechanisms. Compensation or **compensated shock** occurs as the body reacts to the hypoperfusion and takes steps to stay alive (Table 18-1).

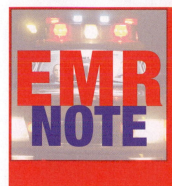

Despite compensation when in shock, the body is still underoxygenated at the level of the cell **(hypoxia)**. The brain is particularly sensitive to an inadequate supply of oxygen. As a result it is common to see evidence of this in a patient's mental status. As hypoxia increases, you can expect to see changes such as *restlessness and/or anxiety, combativeness, or even unconsciousness*. You should realize that these changes, even if they are subtle, are early signs of shock.

compensated shock the early stages of shock where minimum perfusion is maintained through compensatory actions of the body such as increased heart rate and constriction of blood vessels.

hypoxia inadequate oxygenation of the tissue.

decompensated shock the later stages of shock where compensation methods begin to fail due to the increasing lack of oxygen being delivered to vital organs.

decompensation the failure of the body's steps to compensate for insult or injury.

If left untreated, a shock patient's condition will become worse, and the patient will eventually **decompensate** (Table 18-2). In this stage, the body can no longer make up for the increasing lack of oxygen delivered to vital organs, and the methods of compensation

TABLE 18-1 Compensatory Shock	
THE BODY'S RESPONSE	**PHYSICAL SIGNS**
Increased Heart Rate With oxygen and valuable nutrients in short supply, the body takes steps to move what supply is left faster.	Rapid Pulse
Constriction (decreasing the diameter) of Blood Vessels The body attempts to make the container smaller to temporarily sustain a normal blood pressure. This process also takes blood away from the outer areas of the body (like the skin) and moves it toward the core, essential organs (like the heart and brain).	Pale, Sweaty Skin Delayed Capillary Refill

TABLE 18-2 Decompensated Shock

THE BODY'S RESPONSE	PHYSICAL SIGNS
Progressive Lack of Perfusion The problem continues to worsen and eventually overcomes the body's ability to compensate for the challenge.	Worsening Mental Status/Profound Changes (potentially a drop in AVPU from A to V, P, or U) Thirst
Failure of Blood Vessel Constriction Blood vessel constriction can only be sustained temporarily. As the deoxygenated smooth muscle that controls blood vessels tires, the constriction fails and blood pressure drops.	Gray, Blue, and/or Mottled Skin Decreased Blood Pressure

begin to fail. In addition to the signs of compensated shock, you may also expect to see the following issues:

hypotension low blood pressure.

■ *Drop in blood pressure.* A drop in blood pressure (**hypotension** or low blood pressure) is a sign of the late stages of shock; the body can no longer maintain compensation. Either the mechanisms of compensation have tired due to inadequate perfusion or the problem causing shock is progressing too rapidly for the body to keep up. When you find hypotension, your patient is in serious trouble.

ASK YOURSELF

■ What is the significance of a drop in blood pressure in the patient in shock?

■ How would you describe the progression of shock to irreversible shock?

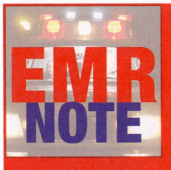

EMR NOTE

Blood pressure is not the best indicator of shock. Many people, especially children, can maintain a normal blood pressure despite massive blood loss and serious shock. Learn to identify shock through the larger patient presentation and never rely solely on blood pressure to indicate shock.

■ *Organ/system failure.* As shock progresses, the decreased perfusion causes cells, organs, and organ systems to begin to die. Decompensated shock will rapidly lead to death unless the patient receives definitive care at the hospital to treat the underlying cause of the shock.

Let's look at the following patients' signs and symptoms and consider what stage of shock each one is in:

PATIENT	SIGNS AND SYMPTOMS
A 10-year-old male who was just struck by a car. He complains of abdominal pain.	Pain, anxiety, pale skin, pulse 134, respirations 28, blood pressure 110/80
A 26-year-old male who was recently shot in the chest. He is unconscious.	Unconscious, pale skin, blue at lips, pulse 110, respirations 6, blood pressure 68/30. See Figure 18-4 ■ for an example of shock in a dark-skinned patient.

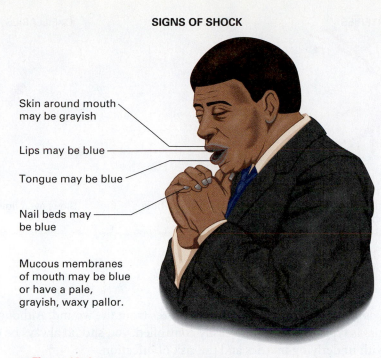

Skin around mouth
may be grayish

Lips may be blue

Tongue may be blue

Nail beds may
be blue

Mucous membranes
of mouth may be blue
or have a pale,
grayish, waxy pallor.

■ **Figure 18-4** Shock in a dark-skinned patient.

In the 10-year-old, the fast heart rate and relatively normal blood pressure indicate that his system is compensating for his injuries. How long this compensation will continue is difficult to predict, but he is compensating. Therefore, we would categorize him as in compensated shock.

The 26-year-old is clearly no longer compensating. He has a serious mental status change and a decreased blood pressure. His system is no longer meeting his needs. Therefore, we would categorize him as in decompensated shock.

EMR Patient Assessment: Bleeding

When assessing patients with life-threatening bleeding, it is easy to be distracted by the blood and inadvertently miss other potential emergencies such as airway compromise or inadequate breathing. Although it is important to control the bleeding, always be thorough in your primary assessment and remember to immediately treat any and all problems with airway, breathing, or circulation (see Chapter 10, "Patient Assessment: The Primary Assessment").

Primary Assessment

After you are sure the patient has an intact airway and adequate breathing, the next step in a primary assessment is to evaluate problems with circulation such as bleeding.

1. Look for obvious external bleeding.

    You can generally categorize external bleeding into one of three categories (Figure 18-5 ■):

    - *Arterial bleeding.* Bright red (oxygenated) blood spurts from the wound as the heart beats. Blood loss is rapid and often difficult to control. As bleeding continues and the patient's blood pressure drops, the pressure of the spurting may decrease.
    - *Venous bleeding.* Dark red (deoxygenated) blood flows steadily from the wound. Although venous bleeding is under less pressure than arterial bleeding, blood loss may be significant.

ASK YOURSELF

■ How can you recognize signs and symptoms of shock in the primary assessment?

■ What are the characteristics of arterial, venous, and capillary bleeding?

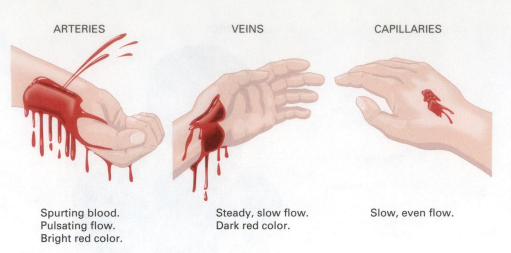

ARTERIES	VEINS	CAPILLARIES

Spurting blood. | Steady, slow flow. | Slow, even flow.
Pulsating flow. | Dark red color.
Bright red color.

■ **Figure 18-5** Types of external bleeding.

■ *Capillary bleeding.* Dark red blood oozes from the wound. Although blood loss is typically minor and easily controlled, you should always be concerned with underlying injuries and the risk of infection.

2. Recognize the potentially subtle signs of internal bleeding. Not all bleeding will be visible on the outside. **Internal bleeding** is caused when internal organs are injured and/or bones are fractured and bleed beneath the skin. Because there are natural spaces in the body, such as the abdominal cavity, large amounts of blood may accumulate without showing signs on the outside. This type of bleeding may be massive and often is life threatening. The assessment of internal bleeding requires careful consideration of mechanism of injury. What forces were exerted and what area of the body could we expect injury in? Consider anatomy as well. Knowing what lies beneath external injuries, such as bruising, often assists us in anticipating the potential internal injury. However, even without being able to find a specific injury, always consider the fact that the most significant, life-threatening bleeding may not be visible on the outside.

Other signs and symptoms of internal bleeding are:

- Penetrating injuries to the skull, chest, abdomen, or pelvis
- Puncture wounds
- Pain (especially abdominal and chest pain resulting from trauma)
- Tenderness (especially tenderness in the abdomen, chest, or pelvis resulting from trauma)
- Rigid or distended abdomen
- Fractures (especially pelvis, thigh, or other large, long bones)
- Nausea/vomiting bright red blood or blood that resembles dark coffee grounds
- Dark tarry stools or stools that contain blood
- Dizziness, fainting, or weakness
- Signs and symptoms of shock including:
  - Altered mental status (anxiety, restlessness, or combativeness)
  - Increased pulse and respirations
  - Pale, cool, moist skin
  - Delayed capillary refill

internal bleeding
bleeding that occurs under the skin and is not visible externally; often occurs into the cavities of the body such as the abdominal cavity.

ASK YOURSELF
■ Given a description of a patient's presentation and history, how would you identify signs and symptoms of internal bleeding?

Multiple Choice

Place a check next to the correct answer.

1. Venous bleeding is characterized by:

    _____ a. bright red spurting blood.

    _____ b. dark red oozing blood.

    _____ c. dark red steadily flowing blood.

    _____ d. bright red oozing blood.

2. Blood delivering an adequate oxygen supply to the cells is called:

    _____ a. perfusion.

    _____ b. hemorrhage.

    _____ c. shock.

    _____ d. hypoxia.

3. Which of the following is a major cause of disruption of the circulatory system and shock?

    _____ a. Abnormal dilation of blood vessels

    _____ b. High blood pressure

    _____ c. Abnormal constriction of blood vessels

    _____ d. Increased blood volume

4. Which of the following findings would specifically indicate decompensated shock?

    _____ a. A fast heart rate

    _____ b. Sweaty skin

    _____ c. Low blood pressure

    _____ d. Anxiety

5. A 55-year-old woman was involved in a serious motor vehicle crash. She complains of shoulder pain. She is anxious and her vital signs are pulse 116, respirations 20, and blood pressure 128/88. These findings indicate:

    _____ a. decompensated shock.

    _____ b. anaphylactic shock.

    _____ c. compensated shock.

    _____ d. neurogenic shock.

Emergency Medical Responder Practice

Identify the source of the following bleeding:

1. _____ Bleeding is dark red and flows steadily from the wound.

2. _____ Bleeding is bright red and spurts from the wound.

3. _____ Bleeding is dark red and oozes from the wound.

Short Answer

1. Explain the term *hypoperfusion*.

    _____

    _____

    _____

2. Explain why a person in compensatory shock might have pale skin.

    _____

    _____

    _____

    _____

3. Explain the difference between decompensated and irreversible shock.

_____

_____

_____

EMR Emergency Care: Bleeding

As an emergency responder you will take a series of steps to treat a patient with serious bleeding. As always, keep yourself safe, but act aggressively to control bleeding and prevent the onset of shock (Scan 18-1).

SCAN 18-1 | Controlling Bleeding

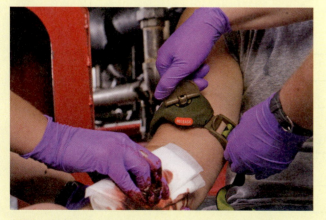

18-1a Use Standard Precautions.

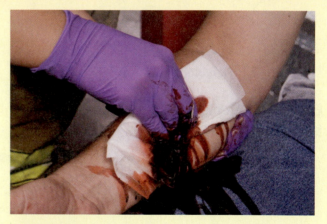

18-1b Apply direct pressure.

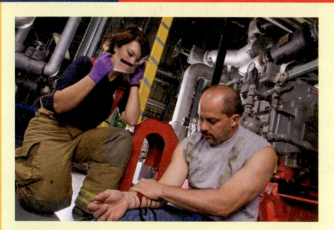

18-1c If bleeding does not stop, apply a tourniquet.

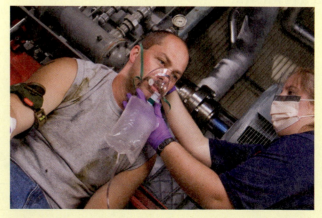

18-1d Administer oxygen and monitor patient. Assess for shock.

Standard Precautions and Personal Protective Equipment

Your first priority is to keep yourself safe. A patient's blood and other body fluids can transmit any number of dangerous diseases. It is important to take steps to protect yourself from harm, especially when treating a patient with severe external bleeding. Recall that in previous chapters we have discussed Standard Precautions. Standard Precautions place a barrier between you and your patient's blood and body fluids. The *minimum* protection is a pair of protective gloves. However, you may need a higher level of protection if the situation calls for it. Airway management requires eye/face protection, and severe bleeding (spurting blood) requires additional face protection and may require a gown and shoe protection. Use common sense, exercise good clinical judgment, and follow local protocol to determine the level of protection you need.

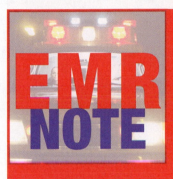

Because **exsanguinating hemorrhage** (uncontrolled severe bleeding in massive volume) kills rapidly, when you have additional resources it may be necessary for one rescuer to attempt to stop the bleeding while you are working through the first steps of airway and breathing. That said, such a circumstance is rare. You should always conduct your primary assessment in a systematic manner, treating any primary assessment problem immediately.

exsanguinating hemorrhage uncontrolled severe bleeding in massive volume that quickly leads to loss of total circulating blood volume.

Open the Airway and Ensure Adequate Breathing

Ensure your patient has an open airway and is breathing appropriately to help compensate for the circulatory challenge. If necessary, open the airway and manage breathing with a bag-valve mask.

Apply High-Concentration Oxygen

Any patient who shows signs and symptoms of a low perfusion state will benefit from high-concentration oxygen applied through a nonrebreather mask.

Control External Bleeding

Controlling external bleeding can be thought of as a series of steps. Although most external bleeding can be controlled with simple direct pressure, it is helpful to know there are additional, more aggressive steps if your plan does not work.

Direct pressure is application of pressure on a wound designed to stop bleeding or slow bleeding to aid clotting of blood. As soon as serious bleeding is discovered, apply direct pressure. Ideally use a sterile gauze pad or dressing, but when unavailable, a gloved hand placed directly over the wound might be enough until other more appropriate measures are available. Direct pressure should cover as much of the wound as possible. You may need to pack the area around a large wound with gauze. Make sure the pressure is steady, firm, and constant for a minimum of 5 minutes. Often it will take longer. A common mistake is removing the dressing to check if the bleeding has stopped.

If bleeding continues and soaks through a dressing, do not remove it. You may remove clots that have formed and restart bleeding. Simply add additional dressings on top of the original and continue direct pressure. If this problem persists, additional dressings may actually hurt your effort of applying pressure. It is important that your

ASK YOURSELF

- What is the importance of ensuring an open airway and adequate ventilation and providing a high concentration of oxygen to patients in shock?

- Given a scenario in which a patient has external bleeding, including a nosebleed, what are the appropriate steps to control the hemorrhage?

direct pressure pressure placed directly onto a wound to slow or stop bleeding.

fingertips actually press deeply into the wound to compress the vessel that is bleeding. If excess dressings prevent this, remove outer dressings but be sure to leave the dressing contacting the wound in place.

If you are treating bleeding from an extremity you may elevate the wound while you apply direct pressure. This elevation is not a step in bleeding control itself but may help when added to direct pressure. Do not delay methods listed below to elevate the wound in such cases as massive hemorrhage from an amputation at the mid-thigh. Do not elevate the wound or limb if extremity fracture is suspected.

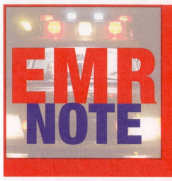

EMR NOTE

Do not be surprised if direct pressure does not completely stop bleeding. The important thing to learn is that it may slow otherwise uncontrolled bleeding.

Additional steps to control bleeding are the following:

- If local protocols allow, consider the use of a hemostatic agent. A hemostatic agent is a substance that contains drying properties that help slow bleeding and aid clotting. It may be applied directly to the wound to help control bleeding. Commercially available hemostatic agents are typically found either as a powder that is applied directly to a wound or a powder contained within a prepackaged dressing (also known as a contained hemostatic agent). A contained hemostatic agent is applied to a wound the way you would apply any other dressing. Use fingertip pressure to press the dressing into the wound to get the full effect for bleeding control.

- A tourniquet should be used (if local protocol allows) when direct pressure fails to control life-threatening bleeding in an extremity. You should use a tourniquet only when you cannot control bleeding any other way and only if you consider the bleeding life threatening.

  - To effectively control bleeding, a tourniquet should be placed between the wound and the heart. You should place it as close to the wound as possible while still keeping it off the wound itself.

  - If you are using a commercially available tourniquet, follow the manufacturer's instructions for application (Figure 18-6 ■).

  - If you do not have access to a commercially available tourniquet, you may be able to make one from materials available in the field. Ideal tourniquets are flat and wide (1 to 4 inches wide) and constructed of materials that will not cut into the patient.

  - A blood pressure cuff may be utilized as a tourniquet. However, if you choose this device, you should constantly monitor pressure in the cuff and take steps, like securing it with tape, to ensure it does not accidentally pop off.

  - To apply a tourniquet, wrap the material around the extremity. Use a stick or a rod (even a pencil or pen may work) to twist the tourniquet until the bleeding

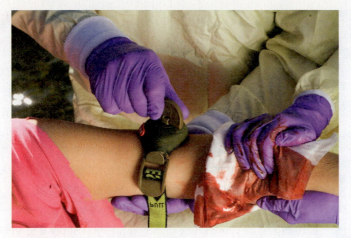

■ **Figure 18-6** Commercial tourniquet.

stops. (Note: Only tighten the tourniquet until the bleeding stops.) Once the bleeding has stopped, secure the stick in place and note the time.

- The tourniquet should be left in place to be removed at the hospital.
- When transferring care to other providers, be sure to advise them that you have applied a tourniquet.

■ Splint fractures. Cover external wounds and splint fractures. Keeping bone ends in place and restricting movement may help control bleeding.

The following steps in bleeding control were previously taught and may still be utilized in your system. Always follow local protocol.

■ Elevate the extremity. Elevating the extremity above the level of the heart while applying direct pressure may slow bleeding.

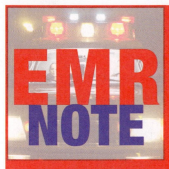

Elevating the extremity above the level of the heart while applying direct pressure may slow bleeding, but it should not be done routinely. Prior to splinting you should not elevate an extremity that you suspect has sustained a fracture or joint injury.

■ Apply pressure to pressure points. Slow bleeding by applying pressure to points where arteries lie close to the skin. You will be able to locate these points by feeling for a pulse.

- Slow bleeding in the arm by applying constant pressure to the area of the brachial artery (brachial pulse).
- Slow bleeding in the leg by applying constant pressure to the area of the femoral artery (femoral pulse).

THE RESPONSE ✳

The patient is lying on the ground supine in a large pool of blood. He is sweaty. When you call out to him, he barely picks his head up to respond. You assess that his airway is open and he is breathing rapidly. You cannot find a radial pulse. He does have a rapid carotid pulse around 120/minute. You immediately find a large laceration on the inner part of his upper thigh. The police tell you he was struck with a meat cleaver. When you examine the wound, you see that it is still slightly pumping blood.

You immediately apply direct pressure with your gloved hand. Your partner hands you a bulky dressing and you apply it to the wound. It soaks through rapidly so you decide to add a contained hemostatic agent and an additional dressing. The bleeding seems to be controlled.

You recognize that this person is in shock and alert the transporting ambulance of the priority patient. While you wait for their arrival, you place a blanket on your patient and deliver high-concentration oxygen through a nonrebreather mask.

■ Discussion: *What steps will you take in the secondary assessment before transporting the patient?*

✳ Stop, Review, Remember

Multiple Choice

Place a check next to the correct answer.

1. Personal protective equipment including face and eye protection would be most appropriate when providing care to which of the following patients?

    ____ a. A 6-year-old with a venous bleed from an ankle wound

    ____ b. A 26-year-old with abdominal pain and potential internal bleeding from a multiple-vehicle collision

    ____ c. An 18-year-old assault victim with severe bleeding in his airway

    ____ d. A 71-year-old with an amputated finger

2. A 13-year-old boy has been struck by a car. You find him unconscious/unresponsive with slow gurgling respirations and a serious arm wound that is steadily bleeding. After ensuring a safe scene, your first priority would be to:

    ____ a. suction the airway.

    ____ b. apply direct pressure to the wound.

    ____ c. elevate the patient's legs.

    ____ d. administer high-flow oxygen with a nonrebreather mask.

3. A 46-year-old male has accidentally cut his wrist. He tells you he is fine, but is having trouble controlling the bleeding. Your immediate treatment priority for this patient will be to:

    ____ a. administer high-flow oxygen with a nonrebreather mask.

    ____ b. keep the patient warm.

    ____ c. elevate his wrist above the heart.

    ____ d. apply direct pressure.

4. After applying a dressing to an arm wound, you notice that it has become soaked through and the bleeding continues. You should:

_____ a. remove the dressing and apply a fresh one.

_____ b. position the arm below the level of the heart.

_____ c. remove the original dressing and apply an occlusive dressing in its place.

_____ d. leave the dressing in place and add additional dressings on top.

5. Direct pressure to control bleeding on an isolated, lower leg wound has failed and the leg continues to bleed. The next most appropriate step would be to:

_____ a. elevate the extremity.

_____ b. apply pressure to pressure points.

_____ c. apply a tourniquet.

_____ d. continue direct pressure.

Emergency Medical Responder Practice

List in order the steps in controlling external bleeding:

1. _____

2. _____

3. _____

Critical Thinking

1. Explain why administering high-concentration oxygen to a person with a severe external bleed is important.

_____

_____

_____

_____

2. Explain why it would be important to splint the fractures of a person showing signs and symptoms of shock.

_____

_____

_____

_____

Special Situations

Nosebleeds

Nosebleeds are a common cause of bleeding. Although they are not usually life threatening, some situations can be serious.

- Extreme blood loss could theoretically lead to shock (although this is rare).
- Patients who take certain types of medications to "thin" the blood by reducing the blood's ability to clot may bleed seriously from relatively minor causes.

Nosebleeds in patients taking blood-thinning medications may be difficult to control and become more serious as the bleeding continues.

- Patients who have nosebleeds and have an altered mental status are at risk for airway compromise and aspiration of blood into the lungs. You should be prepared to aggressively suction to keep the airway open.
- Patients with nosebleeds often swallow blood, and vomiting of the blood is not uncommon due to irritation of the stomach.

Treating a Nosebleed

- Sit the patient in an upright and slightly forward position. This will decrease the likelihood of blood passing into the throat and threatening the airway. Continued ingestion of blood may also lead to nausea and vomiting.
- If there is no trauma to the nose, pinch the nostrils together to apply direct pressure. The same rules for direct pressure apply here as they do with any other wound. Maintain constant, steady, and firm pressure, and avoid "checks."
- Consider applying ice or a cold compress to the nose and face.
- When the bleeding stops, discourage the patient from blowing his nose and encourage only very gentle touching of the nose for the next few hours.
- If you are unable to stop the bleeding, prepare the patient for transport to the hospital as more aggressive measures may be necessary.

Internal Bleeding

As an EMR you will most commonly encounter patients with internal bleeding as a result of traumatic injuries. Occasionally you may also encounter internal bleeding from hemorrhage of the digestive tract. The patient may be vomiting blood or passing blood through the rectum.

A patient with serious internal bleeding must be transported as soon as possible. Often, trauma patients will require surgical intervention to stop internal bleeding, so the majority of your actions should be focused on facilitating transport of the patient to an appropriate facility.

Although arranging rapid transport is the most important treatment for a patient with internal bleeding, applying oxygen and taking steps to stop any additional external bleeding will help improve outcomes.

ASK YOURSELF

- Given a variety of scenarios involving patients in shock, what is the appropriate assessment and patient care?

EMR Emergency Care: Shock

In addition to maintaining airway and breathing and controlling external bleeding, you should consider the following interventions in patients with the signs and symptoms of shock:

- Lay the patient flat (supine).
- Administer high-concentration oxygen.
- Keep the patient warm. Remove wet clothing and use a blanket to prevent heat loss. Do not overheat.
- Administer supportive care. Reassure and comfort your patient while you wait for additional EMS personnel to arrive.

Anaphylactic Shock

Not all shock is caused by blood loss. As previously discussed, shock may be also caused by heart problems and by blood vessel problems. Anaphylactic shock is a blood vessel problem commonly encountered by EMRs. See also Chapter 16 for additional detail.

Obstructive Shock

In some cases shock can be caused by blood being blocked (obstructed) from reaching the lungs or the heart. For example, the pressure built up in the chest cavity as a result of a tension pneumothorax actually can squeeze the heart and the great vessels that fill the heart to the point where not enough blood is circulated. In the case of a pulmonary embolism, a clot blocks blood flow to a potentially large section of the lung and therefore stops the oxygen exchange in that area. In both these cases, shock is a result of the hypoperfusion caused by the obstructed blood flow. The treatment of obstructive shock is to remedy the specific condition causing the problem, and this may be above the scope of an EMR. Many of these specific conditions will be discussed in other chapters. However, it is critically important that you learn to recognize and treat the symptoms of the hypoperfusion (shock) and rapidly move these patients to a higher level of care.

ASK YOURSELF

■ How would you compare and contrast the characteristics of anaphylactic shock with those of hemorrhagic shock?

CASE STUDY

TRANSITION ✳

The patient is unconscious by the time the EMTs arrive. You decide to assist ventilations with a bag-valve mask. When the crew brings the stretcher, you assist in rapidly moving the patient to the ambulance. While loading the patient, you report your initial assessment findings, including the signs of shock, blood loss, and arterial bleeding. The patient is quickly loaded and transported to a local trauma center. You and your partner wash thoroughly and then complete your written documentation.

■ Discussion: *Do you think you have saved this patient? Why?*

THE LAST WORD

The key to treating serious bleeding and the progression of shock is recognition and action. Use your primary assessment to identify circulatory life threats and act to correct these problems. Although these findings will be in the context of a larger patient assessment, the time to act is when they are identified.

Multiple Choice

Place a check next to the correct answer.

1. Which of the following signs would specifically indicate *anaphylactic* shock?

    _____ a. Itchy skin

    _____ b. Hives

    _____ c. Anxiety

    _____ d. Stridor

2. Which of the following patients is potentially most serious?

    _____ a. A 5-year-old with an active nosebleed caused by bumping into a door

    _____ b. A 72-year-old patient who takes a blood thinner and has an active nosebleed

    _____ c. An intoxicated 21-year-old who had a nosebleed that is now controlled

    _____ d. A 50-year-old patient who has had a spontaneous onset of an active nosebleed

3. A 78-year-old man complains of severe nontraumatic chest pain and shortness of breath. He notes the pain began while sitting in his chair. He is anxious and pale. His vital signs are pulse 48, respirations 36, and blood pressure 66/40. This patient's condition could best be described as:

    _____ a. compensated shock.

    _____ b. anaphylactic shock.

    _____ c. decompensated shock.

    _____ d. respiratory shock.

4. A 62-year-old woman complains of severe chest pain and vomiting. She notes the pain began while walking to the bathroom. She is pale and sweaty. Her vital signs are pulse 100, respirations 36, and blood pressure 72/50. Her shock is most likely being caused by:

    _____ a. failure of the heart.

    _____ b. abnormal dilation of the blood vessels.

    _____ c. blood volume loss.

    _____ d. abnormal constriction of the blood vessels.

5. In treating a patient with suspected internal bleeding and shock, which of the following would be the most important priority?

    _____ a. Arrange rapid transport to an appropriate facility.

    _____ b. Administer high-concentration oxygen.

    _____ c. Keep the patient warm.

    _____ d. Elevate the patient's legs.

Short Answer

1. Describe the position in which you would place the patient with an active nosebleed, and explain why you would place him in that position.

    _____

    _____

    _____

    _____

2. Explain why it is important to control external bleeding in a patient with potential internal bleeding.

    _____

    _____

    _____

    _____

3. Explain why you are likely to find a rapid pulse in a patient in compensatory shock.

_____

_____

_____

_____

Critical Thinking

1. Recent battlefield information has led many to consider that treating severe external bleeding may be even more important than initially treating airway and breathing. Can you make an argument for this conclusion? If so, why?

_____

_____

_____

_____

2. You are first to respond to a patient who is bleeding severely. You have no equipment or even personal protective devices. What should you do for this patient?

_____

_____

_____

_____

3. A patient tells you that he accidentally ate peanuts and is very allergic to them. Although he is not having a serious reaction yet, what would you expect to see if and when the reaction progresses to anaphylaxis?

_____

_____

_____

_____

Case Study

You are the EMR called to assist a 36-year-old male who has cut his leg badly with a chain saw while cutting trees. You arrive to find him seated with his leg wrapped in a blood-soaked T-shirt. There is a great deal of blood on the ground. As you approach him, he calls out to you for help.

1. Describe the steps of your primary assessment.

_____

_____

_____

2. Are there immediate actions required in the primary assessment? If so, what are they?

_____

_____

_____

As you assess the T-shirt dressing, you note that spurting blood is clearly soaking through the shirt, and the bleeding is *not* controlled.

3. What does spurting blood indicate in this patient?

_____

_____

_____

4. Describe the steps you would take to control this bleeding.

_____

_____

_____

Once bleeding is controlled, you continue your assessment. You note that the patient is anxious and pale and has a heart rate of 128.

5. This patient is exhibiting signs and symptoms of what condition?

_____

_____

_____

6. Describe the ongoing steps to care for this patient.

_____

_____

_____

Chest and Abdominal Emergencies

NAVIGATION GUIDE

The following items provide an overview to the purpose and content of this chapter. The Education Standard and Competency are from the National EMS Education Standards.

Education Standard Trauma (Bleeding, Chest Trauma, Abdominal and Genitourinary Trauma)

Competency Uses simple knowledge to recognize and manage life threats based on assessment findings for an acutely injured patient while awaiting additional emergency medical response.

Knowledge Areas Bleeding, Chest Trauma
- Blunt vs. penetrating mechanisms
- Open chest wounds
- Open abdominal wounds
- Impaled object

Abdominal and Genitourinary Trauma

Anatomy, presentations, and management of shock associated with abdominal emergencies, including:
- Gastrointestinal bleeding
- Abdominal pain
- Evisceration

Objectives After reading this chapter, you should be able to:

1. Define key terms introduced in this chapter.
2. Discuss the relationship between chest and abdominal emergencies, and shock.
3. Explain the basic processes of inhaling and exhaling.
4. Explain how each of the following conditions interferes with breathing:
   a. Open chest injuries
   b. Pneumothorax
   c. Hemothorax
   d. Rib fractures
   e. Flail chest

5. Recognize signs and symptoms of each of the following during the primary and secondary assessments:
   a. Open chest injuries
   b. Pneumothorax
   c. Hemothorax
   d. Rib fractures
   e. Flail chest
   f. Traumatic asphyxia
   g. Open abdominal injuries, including evisceration
   h. Closed abdominal injuries
   i. Gastrointestinal bleeding

6. Demonstrate the management of patients with open and closed chest injuries.
7. Demonstrate the treatment of patients with open and closed abdominal injuries, including evisceration.
8. Demonstrate the management of patients with an impaled object in the chest or abdomen.

Key Terms Page numbers indicate first major use in this chapter. The Margin Glossary in this chapter provides definitions as you read.

diaphragm, p. 455

sucking chest wound, p. 455

pneumothorax, p. 456

occlusive dressing, p. 456

tension pneumothorax, p. 458

spontaneous pneumothorax, p. 458

hemothorax, p. 458

crepitus, p. 458

flail segment or flail chest, p. 459

paradoxical breathing, p. 459

traumatic asphyxia, p. 461

evisceration, p. 465

gastrointestinal (GI) bleeding, p. 467

abdominal distention, p. 467

Media Resources Please go to **www.bradybooks.com** to access mykit for this text. You will find quizzes, critical thinking scenarios, weblinks, animations, and videos related to this chapter—and much more. Look for online information on rib fractures and flail chest.

ASK YOURSELF

- What is the relationship between chest and abdominal emergencies, and shock?

INTRODUCTION

Many people lock away their valuables in a safe. Its sturdy construction provides protection and security to the items they are concerned the most about keeping safe. If something were to happen to the safe, such as a fire, that person would not worry so much about the safe itself, but rather the contents. You should think of the chest and abdominal cavity as the body's vault. The muscles and the bones protect and secure our most valuable organs, those that are vital in keeping us alive. Just as the owner of a safe is more concerned about the contents than the safe itself, in the event of an injury to the abdomen or chest, you should be more concerned about the contents than the container. Although soft tissue injuries of the chest and abdomen may be serious, the vital organs inside must be your first concern. Injuries to the heart, lungs, and great vessels housed within the chest can be immediately life threatening. Always assume an underlying injury to vital organs when assessing and treating abdominal and chest injuries (Figure 19-1 ■). You must understand the relationship between these emergencies and shock and include the possibility in your assessment.

CASE STUDY

THE CALL

It is a clear fall afternoon. The temperature is a comfortable 60 degrees and the weather is dry. Your team is called to respond to a telephone company line worker who has fallen off a pole. The dispatcher tells you that the patient is lying on the ground, not moving.

As you and your partner approach the scene, you notice a small crowd has gathered. One of the bystanders tells you that he witnessed him fall. The bystander says, "He hit the ground hard, bounced a bit, but did not get up."

■ Discussion: *After you determine the scene is safe, what is your initial reaction and impression?*

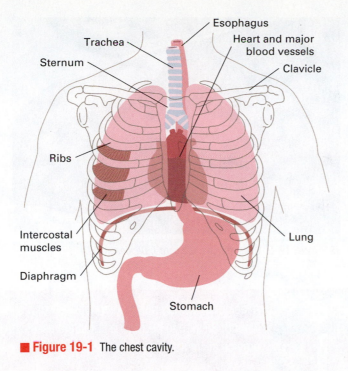

Figure 19-1 The chest cavity.

Labels: Trachea, Sternum, Esophagus, Heart and major blood vessels, Clavicle, Ribs, Intercostal muscles, Diaphragm, Lung, Stomach

The Chest

We use the chest to move air in and out of the lungs. An injury to the soft tissue and/or bone in this area can seriously threaten the ability to breathe. The lungs occupy much of the chest cavity. Under normal circumstances, the lungs elastically expand and contract with the movement of the chest wall. We use both the muscles of the chest wall and a large muscle called the **diaphragm** to draw air into and push air out of the lungs.

To inhale, we expand the chest and drop the diaphragm and air is pulled into the lungs. To exhale, we reverse the process. Think of the chest cavity as a syringe. In a syringe when the plunger is pulled back (dropped down) a negative pressure is created to draw fluid into the chamber through the needle. In the same way, the downward movement of the diaphragm creates a negative pressure in the chest that is used to pull air in through the airway. To push fluid out of the syringe, the plunger is pushed forward (moved upward) to create a positive pressure in the chamber and push the fluid out through the needle. To exhale we similarly move the diaphragm upward and contract the chest muscles to create a positive pressure and push air out through the airway. Under normal circumstances, this process works quite well at moving air. However, injuries can seriously impact this process.

Open Chest Injuries

In an open chest injury, the chest wall has been penetrated and at least theoretically has a hole in it (Figure 19-2 ■). Although the pain alone from such an injury may make breathing more difficult, the most serious concern may be the breakdown in the breathing process discussed earlier. If the hole is big enough, air may actually be pulled in through it when the diaphragm drops and negative pressure is created. This is called a **sucking chest wound** and you may actually hear a sucking noise or see bubbles as air is pulled in or pushed out.

ASK YOURSELF

- How would you explain the basic processes of inhaling and exhaling?
- How do the following conditions interfere with breathing?
  - Open chest injuries
- What are the signs and symptoms of each of the following during the primary and secondary assessments?
  - Open chest injuries
- Can you define key terms introduced in this chapter?

diaphragm   the large muscle that separates the chest from the abdomen and plays a major role in the mechanical function of breathing.

sucking chest wound   an open wound in the chest where air is pulled in and pushed out as the patient breathes.

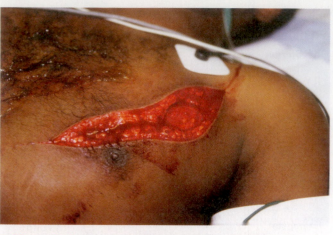

■ Figure 19-2 Chest trauma. *(Edward T. Dickinson, MD)*

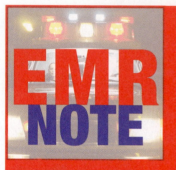

EMR NOTE

A lack of a sucking noise does not rule out a sucking chest wound. Be sure to perform a complete assessment and provide all information to the responding EMS.

pneumothorax air in the space between the lung and chest wall (the pleural space).

Not only does this problem make the breathing process far less efficient, it may also create a condition called a **pneumothorax** where air works its way in between the chest wall and the lung and causes the lung to collapse.

EMR Emergency Care: Open Chest Injury

occlusive dressing a dressing that is made of material that is airtight and is designed to create a seal over certain types of wounds.

An open chest injury must be stopped from allowing air into the chest cavity. The best way to do this is to apply an airtight seal over the wound. An **occlusive dressing** is made of plastic, Vaseline gauze, or a similar airtight material. You would apply this directly over a suspected open chest wound. By sealing the hole you stop air from entering the chest cavity and increase the diaphragm's ability to move air. Ready-made, commercial occlusive dressings are available; however, an occlusive dressing may be improvised by using any airtight material such as a plastic bag. The dressing should be at least 2 inches larger than the wound on all sides and should be made of material heavy enough to stay in place against the relatively high pressures of breathing.

ASK YOURSELF
■ How do the following conditions interfere with breathing?
 ■ Pneumothorax
■ What are the signs and symptoms of each of the following during the primary and secondary assessments?
 ■ Pneumothorax

You should apply an occlusive dressing over the wound and tape it on three sides. The fourth side is typically left untaped to allow air to escape if pressure builds in the chest cavity. Remember that air can build up in the chest between the chest wall and lung and collapse the lung. If you notice that your patient's condition has gotten significantly worse since the application of an occlusive dressing (increased shortness of breath, mental status changes), you should consider opening the dressing to release pressure (Scan 19-1).

Pneumothorax

As noted earlier, pneumothorax occurs when air gets into the space between the lung tissue and the chest wall. Under ordinary circumstances, the lung is essentially adhered to

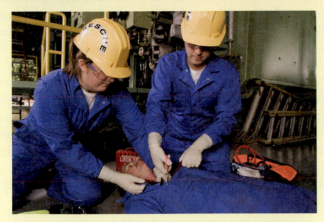

19-1a Use Standard Precautions. Cut away clothing.

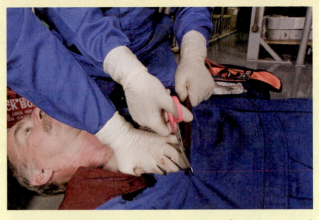

19-1b You may continue to cut clothing. Seal the wound immediately with a gloved hand.

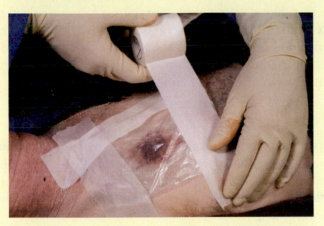

19-1c Place a three-sided occlusive dressing over the wound.

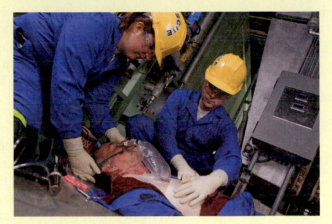

19-1d Administer oxygen.

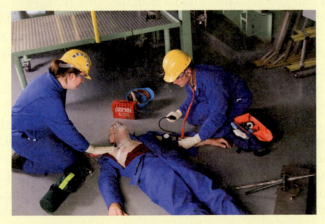

19-1e Continue assessing and monitoring the patient.

the chest wall and moves with the movement of the chest. If a hole is created in the chest wall or in the lung itself, air can leak and accumulate in that space forcing the lung away from the chest wall. As the lung collapses, air flow in and out is seriously decreased. Although the person may be breathing, little or no air may be passing into the affected lung. If the volume of the accumulated air becomes great enough, the collapsed lung can actually put pressure on the heart and great vessels of the chest and cause profound shock in a life-threatening condition known as **tension pneumothorax**.

A pneumothorax may be caused by chest trauma, such as someone being shot or stabbed through the chest wall, or it may be caused by a nontraumatic medical problem. Those with a tall, thin build, chronic obstructive pulmonary disease (COPD) patients, and longtime smokers may be prone to developing a small hole in their lung tissue that causes a **spontaneous pneumothorax**. Although the chest wall is intact, air leaks from the lung itself and can collapse the lung in the same manner as a traumatic wound. In the case of a spontaneous pneumothorax there is no open wound to seal, but you should recognize that this condition can be life threatening.

Hemothorax

Just as air can accumulate in the space between the chest wall and lung, so can blood. The chest contains a number of very large blood vessels, and chest trauma can cause them to rupture and leak. A **hemothorax** occurs when leaking blood builds up and collapses the lung in the same manner as a pneumothorax. In addition to air movement interruption and the potential to develop a tension hemothorax, remember that this patient also is experiencing internal bleeding that may rapidly progress to shock.

Closed Chest Injuries

In a closed chest injury the chest wall is intact. Although these injuries may seem less dramatic on your assessment, you must always be aware of the organs that lie beneath. The chest wall may be intact, but there may be serious injuries to vital organs that you cannot see. You should always assume that the vital organ is injured when the mechanism of injury and your knowledge of anatomy make you suspicious.

Rib Fractures

A person has twelve sets of ribs that give structure and form to the chest wall. The top ten sets are connected in the back to the spinal column and in the front to the sternum. The bottom two sets are connected in the back only and are commonly referred to as "floating ribs." As with any other bone, external trauma can fracture ribs. Your assessment may reveal deformity of the chest wall where ribs have been displaced and you may feel **crepitus**, the grating of bone ends rubbing together, when you palpate the chest. If the integrity of the lung is compromised by the trauma, air may leak into the soft tissues of the chest wall resulting in subcutaneous emphysema. On chest wall palpation, subcutaneous emphysema feels like crushing popcorn beneath the skin. Both of these findings should help you identify rib fractures. However, because the chest wall is extremely muscular, deformity associated with rib fractures is relatively rare and a lack of deformity or crepitus does not mean that there are definitely not rib fractures. Mechanism of injury will help you anticipate fractures even if they are not obvious on inspection.

Pain may be the most significant problem with rib fractures. When the chest wall is injured, it is extremely painful to breathe and as a result the amount of air your patient moves may be seriously decreased. Although this may be only a minor change for a healthy person, be especially concerned with those patients who have underlying breathing difficulties such as COPD as this minor change in the amount of air they breathe may have a serious effect on their already fragile system. Often rib fracture patients will favor an upright position of comfort and try to splint the chest by raising their arms up against their ribs. They may also breathe with very shallow breaths.

You should consider providing your patient with a pillow to hold close to his chest. This may actually improve breathing. You should not attempt to externally splint rib fractures as this may further restrict chest wall movement.

Flail Chest

When two or more adjacent ribs are broken in two or more places, a free-floating section called a **flail segment or flail chest** may be created (Figure 19-3 ■). This may also be caused by fracturing the sternum or by detaching the cartilage that connects the ribs to the sternum. Regardless of where it occurs, this free floating segment may disrupt the process of breathing. When the diaphragm drops and a negative pressure is created in the chest, the flail segment may be pulled in, decreasing the amount of air that can be moved. On exhalation the flail segment may be pushed out, causing the same decrease in air movement. This process is called **paradoxical breathing** and may significantly impact the body's ability to move air in and out of the chest.

A flail chest may seriously affect your patient's ability to move air. You should assess his breathing carefully and intervene with a bag-valve mask if you identify respiratory failure. In addition to managing ventilations, the positive pressure of mechanical breathing may benefit your patient.

Most current thinking recommends against splinting or restricting movement of the chest wall in a flail chest. As always, follow local protocol (Scan 19-2).

Rib Fractures Revisited

Although we have already discussed the pain and decreased air movement associated with fractured ribs, these issues may be the least serious of your patient's problem. Always use your assessment to think not just about the fracture of the rib itself, but also of the damage caused to the underlying structures by the fracturing force. When rib fractures are identified, you should always consider life-threatening injuries to the heart and lungs as well as the potential for severe internal bleeding from the liver or the spleen in the upper abdominal cavity that are also partially covered by the ribs. The movement of jagged bone ends associated with rib fractures (and flail chest in particular) can cause major internal damage. Bleeding, pneumo- and hemothorax, and a variety of other injuries may be caused by broken ribs and may or may not be apparent just by looking.

flail segment or flail chest two or more adjacent ribs that are broken in two or more places, creating a free-floating section.

paradoxical breathing one side or section of the chest rising while the other side falls (as in a flail chest).

FLAIL CHEST

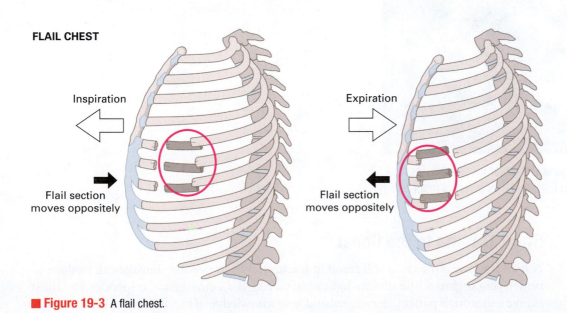

Inspiration

Flail section moves oppositely

Expiration

Flail section moves oppositely

■ **Figure 19-3** A flail chest.

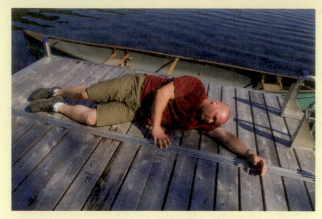

19-2a Consider mechanism of injury in the scene size-up.

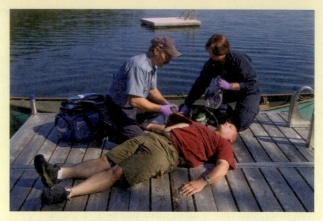

19-2b Perform a primary assessment. Expose the chest and administer oxygen.

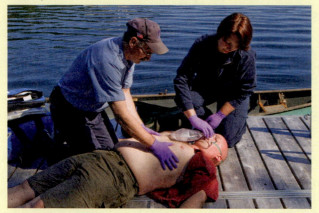

19-2c Assess the chest for injury.

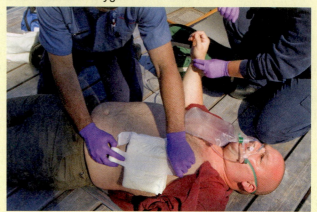

19-2d Apply a bulky dressing.

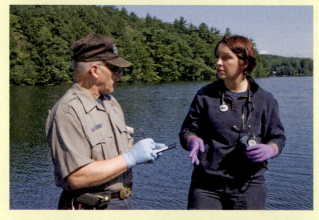

19-2e Continue to assess and monitor the patient. Prepare to hand off the patient to EMS and give a verbal report.

Blunt Trauma to the Chest

Not all trauma to the chest will result in fractures. Often massive damage can be done to underlying organs while ribs are left unfractured. As an emergency responder you must utilize a thorough patient assessment and your knowledge of mechanism of injury to predict underlying chest injuries.

Traumatic asphyxia occurs when massive blunt trauma is applied over a large portion of the chest. This massive compression forces blood out of the heart and other blood vessels in the chest and pushes it in an opposite direction. Signs of this include distended neck veins, blue skin (particularly in the head and neck), and bulging eyes. Traumatic asphyxia is also often associated with pneumothorax (often involving both lungs).

traumatic asphyxia
massive blunt trauma applied over a large portion of the chest forcing blood out of the heart and in an opposite direction.

EMR Emergency Assessment: Chest Injuries

In Chapter 10 we noted that the "breathing" portion of your primary assessment must ensure that all patients are breathing—and breathing adequately. In the assessment of a patient with a chest injury, this will be especially true. Examine both respiratory effort and rate. You should always think about how this injury is affecting your patient's ability to breathe. Concerning signs and symptoms may include (Figure 19-4 ■):

- Shortness of breath
- Painful breathing
- Cyanosis and other signs of hypoxia
- Coughing up blood
- Signs and symptoms of shock

Remember that a trauma patient has four sides. See Chapter 5, "Anatomy and Physiology." A thorough examination of the chest should include looking (observation) and touching (palpation) of all areas. Look at the bare chest for obvious injuries and deformities and feel to find crepitus and paradoxical movement. When palpating, place your hands on both sides of the chest at the same time to assess for equal rise. Concerning signs and symptoms upon examination of the chest wall may include:

- Pain and tenderness
- Poor chest expansion or decreased ability to move air

ASK YOURSELF

- What are the signs and symptoms of each of the following during the primary and secondary assessments?
  - Traumatic asphyxia

SIGNS AND SYMPTOMS OF CHEST INJURY

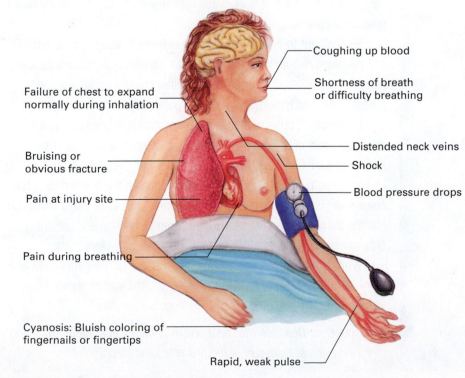

Coughing up blood

Shortness of breath or difficulty breathing

Failure of chest to expand normally during inhalation

Distended neck veins

Shock

Bruising or obvious fracture

Blood pressure drops

Pain at injury site

Pain during breathing

Cyanosis: Bluish coloring of fingernails or fingertips

Rapid, weak pulse

■ **Figure 19-4** Signs and symptoms of chest injury.

- Penetrating trauma (especially sucking chest wounds)
- Reduced or absent lung sounds
- Distended neck veins
- Chest wall deformity

Chest injuries may progress rapidly or slowly and may or may not have visible external injuries. Constant reassessment is critical. Be on the lookout for signs that your patient's injuries have led to deterioration in his condition (mental status changes, shock) and always assume chest injuries are life threatening.

ASK YOURSELF

- How would you demonstrate the management of patients with open and closed chest injuries?

EMR Emergency Care: Chest Emergencies

- Recognize the potential for underlying problems and arrange transport accordingly.
- Recognize airway and breathing failure and treat aggressively. If the patient cannot maintain his own airway or breathe adequately on his own, you must take steps to do it for him. Consider using a bag-valve mask.
- Place the patient in a position of comfort (if cervical spine stabilization is not a concern). Sitting upright may aid breathing.
- Provide high-concentration oxygen. Frequently, chest injuries affect the patient's ability to adequately oxygenate. Supplemental oxygen lends additional support.
- Apply occlusive dressings to penetrating wounds. If you are concerned that the chest wall may have been penetrated, you must seal the wound with an occlusive

CASE STUDY

THE RESPONSE

As you approach the patient, you take Standard Precautions and size up the scene. The patient is lying on his left side on the pavement and is not moving. You note that a 20-foot ladder lies on the ground next to him, and you see a tool bucket still hanging at the top of the telephone pole. There are no low hanging wires.

You call out to the patient, and he responds with a groan. You can see his chest rise as you get closer. After checking to make sure there are no downed wires, your partner applies manual cervical spine precautions, and together you roll the patient over.

His airway is open, and he is breathing rapidly. You count a quick respiratory rate of 38. When you look at his chest, you notice a small section of the left rib cage is moving paradoxically. You hear breath sounds on both sides but notice less air moving on the affected side. His chest is very tender, and you feel crepitus and the flail segment when you palpate the chest. Because of the mental status change and breathing difficulty, you elect to ventilate the patient with a bag-valve mask.

While bagging, you visually inspect the rest of the patient. He is awake, but responds only with groaning sounds and tolerates the bag-valve mask. There is no obvious bleeding.

- Discussion: *Describe the mechanism of injury. In addition to calling for immediate transport, what are your next steps?*

dressing. Be aware that potential lung injuries extend from the shoulders below the clavicles to the area around the belly button. You should always consider occlusive dressings for any penetrating trauma to the chest or abdomen.

- Reassess, reassess, reassess.

✳ Stop, Review, Remember

Multiple Choice

Place a check next to the correct answer.

1. The large muscle that helps move air in and out of the chest is called the:

    ____ a. quadriceps.

    ____ b. bicep.

    ____ c. hamstring.

    ____ d. diaphragm.

2. A chest injury in which the chest wall is intact would be considered a(n) _____ injury.

    ____ a. open

    ____ b. compound

    ____ c. closed

    ____ d. sealed

3. A chest wound that bubbles with the patient's breathing would best be described as a(n):

    ____ a. evisceration.

    ____ b. sucking chest wound.

    ____ c. closed chest wound.

    ____ d. hemothorax.

4. After applying an occlusive dressing to your patient's chest wound, his mental status significantly decreases and his shortness of breath becomes worse. You should next:

    ____ a. release the occlusive dressing.

    ____ b. apply pressure to the dressing.

    ____ c. apply additional dressings on top of the original.

    ____ d. place the patient in the shock position.

5. A 25-year-old man was involved in a serious motor vehicle crash. He is unconscious and blue from the neck up. You note distended neck veins. These findings would best indicate:

    ____ a. traumatic asphyxia.

    ____ b. spontaneous pneumothorax.

    ____ c. open chest injury.

    ____ d. flail chest.

Matching

Match the following descriptions with the correct term.

1. _____ Painful breathing, crepitus on palpation of the chest

2. _____ Bleeding in the chest that collapses the lung

3. _____ Air escaping from lung tissue without external injury

4. _____ Air in the chest cavity putting pressure on the heart and great vessels and causing shock

5. _____ Two or more ribs broken in two or more places

a. Hemothorax

b. Tension pneumothorax

c. Flail chest

d. Spontaneous pneumothorax

e. Rib fracture

1. Explain why an open chest injury impairs the diaphragmatic breathing process.

   _____

   _____

   _____

   _____

2. Explain why an occlusive dressing should only be sealed on three sides.

   _____

   _____

   _____

   _____

3. Explain the difference between a simple pneumothorax and a tension pneumothorax.

   _____

   _____

   _____

   _____

The Abdomen

The abdomen is the space that lies between the diaphragm and the pelvis. Housed within this cavity are many vital organs such as the liver and spleen, and large blood vessels such as the descending aorta. Unlike the chest, whose contents are protected by ribs and other bony structures, the abdomen is relatively unprotected, making its contents vulnerable to injury.

Your knowledge of abdominal anatomy will help identify potential underlying injuries. See Chapter 5, "Anatomy and Physiology." When you consider mechanism of injury, think about where the force impacted and what organs are positioned in the path of the force. When mechanism of injury threatens vital organs, always assume they have been injured. Consider the following situations:

- You assess an 8-year-old boy after a bicycle crash. He tells you his handlebars hit his belly in the crash. He complains of upper left quadrant abdominal pain and has tenderness in that area. By applying basic abdominal anatomy, you would know that the spleen lies generally in the upper left quadrant. You could predict that external trauma to that area could cause life-threatening internal bleeding.

- You assess a 16-year-old male who complains of lower right abdominal pain. He notes there was no trauma. The pain began earlier today and has gradually worsened. He also has a fever. By applying basic abdominal anatomy, you could conclude that the appendix lies in the lower right quadrant, and pain in that region could be originating in that organ.

Although it is helpful to have a working knowledge of abdominal anatomy, a specific diagnosis is not always possible, nor is it your role. Always err on the side of caution and

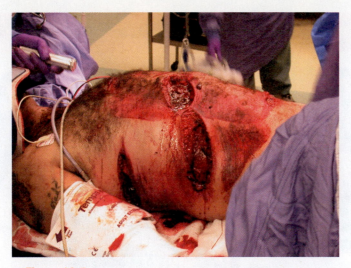

■ Figure 19-5 Open abdominal injury. *(Edward T. Dickinson, MD)*

assume the worst. Use mechanism of injury and anatomy to help you focus your assessment, but do not forget the global presentation and situation.

Abdominal Pain

Abdominal pain is a frequent complaint of people seeking emergency medical help. Whether the pain is caused from trauma or from a medical problem, abdominal pain can indicate a very serious problem. Finding the specific problem may not be possible, but given the many vital organs contained in the abdomen, you should treat all abdominal pain seriously and arrange transport for further evaluation.

Open Abdominal Injuries

In an open abdominal injury, the abdominal wall has been penetrated. Open abdominal injuries are very serious as they may spill abdominal contents, be a route for infection, and even disguise a chest injury (Figure 19-5 ■).

When treating penetrating abdominal trauma, seal wounds with an occlusive dressing in the same way you would seal an open chest wound. The occlusive dressing helps keep the abdominal vault protected from infection but also keeps out air in the event lung tissue is involved. Remember that the diaphragm can drop as low as the belly button on inhalation. Therefore, even midabdominal trauma poses a risk for lung injuries such as pneumothorax.

Evisceration

An **evisceration** occurs when abdominal organs, such as intestine, protrude from an open wound. If abdominal organs are exposed they need to be protected (Scan 19-3). Follow local protocol. General treatment guidelines are to:

- Clean away large debris.
- Cover the organs with a moist sterile dressing and then an occlusive dressing.
- Prevent heat loss.
- Never allow the exposed organs to dry out. It may be necessary to reapply sterile saline to keep the exposed abdominal contents moist.
- Never push organs back into the cavity.

ASK YOURSELF

- What are the signs and symptoms of each of the following during the primary and secondary assessments?
  - Open abdominal injuries, including evisceration

evisceration an open wound of the abdomen where abdominal organs, such as intestine, protrude.

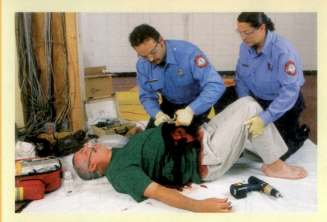

19-3a Cut away clothing.

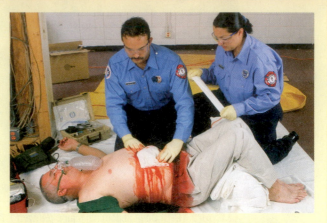

19-3b Cover the exposed organ with a moist bulky dressing.

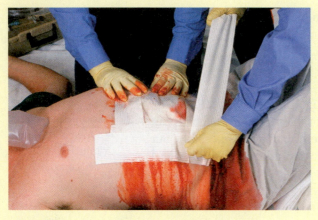

19-3c With your partner, close up the wound by securing an occlusive dressing over the bulky one.

ASK YOURSELF

- How would you demonstrate the management of patients with an impaled object in the chest or abdomen?

- What are the signs and symptoms of each of the following during the primary and secondary assessments?
  - Closed abdominal injuries

Impaled Objects to the Chest and Abdomen

In general, you should never remove an impaled object from the chest or abdomen. In many cases the object itself may be preventing bleeding and if removed may cause rapid deterioration and shock. Follow local protocol. In general, it is recommended you secure the impaled object by padding around the object with bulky dressings and tape. The goal of this padding is to keep the object from moving during transport. Never apply direct pressure on top of or to the object itself.

Closed Abdominal Injuries

Blunt trauma to the abdomen is a serious life threat. Often blunt trauma hides serious injury by damaging internal organs while showing very little evidence on the outside (Figure 19-6 ■). The abdominal cavity can hold an enormous amount of blood. If the injury is left untreated, your patient could bleed to death without losing a drop of blood externally. You must always consider the risk of internal bleeding and shock when treating an abdominal injury. Signs and symptoms that might indicate internal abdominal injury include:

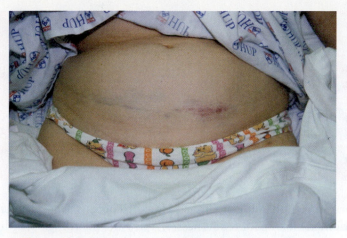

■ Figure 19-6 Contusions of the abdomen may indicate serious internal injuries. (*Copyright Edward T. Dickinson, MD*).

- Pain
- Tenderness (pain on palpation)
- Distended abdomen
- Rigid or guarded abdomen
- Bruising to the abdomen, back, or flanks
- Pain radiating to shoulders
- Nausea and vomiting
- Blood in vomit, urine, or stool
- Signs and symptoms of shock

Gastrointestinal Bleeding

For a variety of reasons, bleeding can occur within the esophagus, the stomach, and/or the intestines. This is called **gastrointestinal (GI) bleeding**. It can be minor or severe and can in some cases be a serious life threat to the patient. GI bleeding presents as bleeding from either end of the GI tract as bloody vomit or stool. Rectal bleeding or vomit from GI bleeding can be seen as typical (frank) blood. Blood in the vomit may also look like coffee grounds. GI bleeding may or may not be accompanied by abdominal pain. Be aware that the GI tract can hold large quantities of blood, and shock can progress rapidly as a result.

EMR Emergency Assessment: Abdominal Injuries

Your primary assessment will likely reveal clues to internal bleeding. Signs and symptoms of shock will quickly reveal a need to aggressively treat, transport, and further assess a patient with an abdominal injury. When assessing breathing, remember that abdominal injuries may involve lung tissue and therefore can lead to pneumothorax, hemothorax, and other related problems. Always look for signs of lung involvement such as difficulty breathing. When assessing circulation, look for signs of internal bleeding and shock such as rapid pulse, delayed capillary refill, and external bleeding.

Like the chest, assessment of the abdomen itself requires examination and palpation of four sides: front, back, and two sides. Look at the abdomen for external injuries, especially penetrating trauma and open wounds. Remember that even small punctures may have serious consequences internally. Look for a bulging belly, known as **abdominal distention**. This may be a sign of an abdominal cavity filling with blood.

ASK YOURSELF

- What are the signs and symptoms of each of the following during the primary and secondary assessments?
  - Gastrointestinal bleeding

gastrointestinal (GI) bleeding bleeding that occurs within the gastrointestinal tract (as in the stomach and/or intestines).

abdominal distention enlargement of the patient's abdomen due to pressure from within; typically a result of internal bleeding.

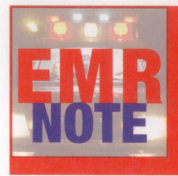

Look for bruising, protruding organs, and impaled objects. Gently touch all four quadrants of the abdomen looking for tenderness, rigidity, and guarding. Guarding is the involuntary spasm of abdominal muscles to protect injured internal organs (Figure 19-7 ■). It is important to understand the concepts of both voluntary and involuntary guarding. Areas that the patient notes are painful should be touched last and carefully.

ASK YOURSELF

- How would you demonstrate the treatment of patients with open and closed abdominal injuries, including evisceration?

EMR Emergency Care: Abdominal Injuries

- Recognize the potential for underlying problems and arrange transport accordingly.
- Recognize airway and breathing failure and treat aggressively. If the patient cannot maintain his own airway or breathe adequately on his own, you must take steps to do it for him. Consider using a bag-valve mask.
- Provide high-concentration oxygen.
- Recognize and treat shock.
- Control external bleeding. Although internal bleeding may be present, controlling external bleeding helps preserve necessary blood.
- Apply sterile dressings to open wounds. If abdominal contents are exposed (evisceration), moisten the dressings.
- Consider placing the patient in a position of comfort (if cervical spine stabilization is not a concern). Often a knee-flexed position (knees drawn up toward the chest) is helpful to alleviate abdominal pain.
- Reassess, reassess, reassess. Abdominal injuries may be severe despite minimal external signs. Recognize that changes may occur rapidly and anticipate the possibility of deterioration.

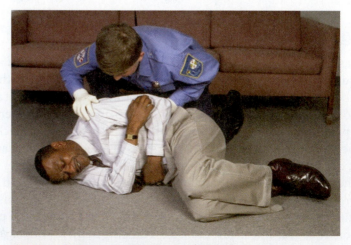

■ **Figure 19-7** A patient guarding a painful abdomen.

Multiple Choice

Place a check next to the correct answer.

1. The upper superior border of the abdomen is the:

____ a. pelvis.

____ b. belly button.

____ c. diaphragm.

____ d. rib cage.

2. A 55-year-old male involved in a snowmobile crash has an open abdominal evisceration. After ensuring a normal airway and breathing, you should next:

____ a. apply a moistened, sterile dressing.

____ b. apply direct pressure to the wound.

____ c. elevate the patient's legs.

____ d. flush the wound with sterile saline.

3. Abdominal organs protruding through an open wound is called a(n):

____ a. flail segment.

____ b. impalement.

____ c. distention.

____ d. evisceration.

4. A 25-year-old female has been involved in a motor vehicle crash. She complains of only shoulder pain but you cannot locate any tenderness in that area. You should be most concerned about:

____ a. abdominal injury.

____ b. anxiety.

____ c. chest injury.

____ d. arm injury.

5. The position of comfort most likely to help alleviate abdominal pain is the:

____ a. prone position.

____ b. knee-flexed position.

____ c. left lateral recumbent position.

____ d. standing position.

Emergency Medical Responder Practice

1. Describe the steps in treating an abdominal evisceration.

_____

_____

_____

_____

Critical Thinking

1. A 45-year-old woman complains of abdominal pain from her seat belt after a high-speed motor vehicle crash. She has no external injuries. She has pain and tenderness in her lower two abdominal quadrants. Her vitals are pulse 124, respirations 20, and blood pressure 122/80. Does this patient have the potential for life-threatening injuries and if so what type of injuries?

_____

_____

_____

_____

2. Explain why you should not remove an impaled object from someone's abdomen.

_____

_____

_____

_____

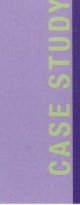

CASE STUDY

TRANSITION

The EMTs arrive and you transfer patient care to them. You report that you needed to assist ventilations, and they continue bagging. You also alert them to the mechanism of injury and the bystander report. You and your partner assist them as they place the patient onto a long board. You follow up your verbal report with written documentation of the event.

■ Discussion: *Would you have done anything differently than what was done in this case study?*

THE LAST WORD

Both the chest and abdomen contain many vital organs vulnerable to injury. Understand how to assess and recognize potential life-threatening injuries and treat aggressively. Beware that a lack of external findings may mask major internal injuries so a thorough patient assessment is essential to identify all life-threatening injuries.

✳ *Chapter Review*

Multiple Choice

Place a check next to the correct answer.

1. When the diaphragm contracts and a negative pressure is caused in the chest, _____ occurs.

   _____ a. inhalation

   _____ b. exhalation

   _____ c. hyperventilation

   _____ d. apnea

2. A gunshot wound to the chest would best be described as what type of injury?

   _____ a. Closed

   _____ b. Blunt force

   _____ c. Impaled object

   _____ d. Open

3. Which of the following would be the best choice for an improvised occlusive dressing to cover an abdominal evisceration?

_____ a. Sterile gauze

_____ b. Foil

_____ c. A plastic bag

_____ d. A roller bandage

4. On inhalation, lung tissue can be found as low as the:

_____ a. lowest rib.

_____ b. xiphoid process.

_____ c. pelvis.

_____ d. belly button.

5. The most appropriate treatment for an impaled object in the abdomen would be to:

_____ a. remove the object and apply direct pressure to the wound.

_____ b. remove the object and seal the wound with an occlusive dressing.

_____ c. leave the object in place and secure for transport.

_____ d. leave the object in place and apply direct pressure over it.

Short Answer

1. Your partner notes he has found crepitus on his exam of your patient's chest. What does that mean?

_____

_____

_____

_____

2. Explain why it is important to apply an occlusive dressing to penetrating abdominal trauma.

_____

_____

_____

_____

3. What does the term "closed" abdominal injury mean?

_____

_____

_____

_____

Critical Thinking

1. A hemothorax can cause shock two ways. Explain both of those mechanisms.

_____

_____

_____

_____

2. You are the first to respond to a patient who has been struck by a vehicle. He is unconscious and has a massive open abdominal wound with organs protruding from it. His vital signs are pulse 124, respirations 8 (snoring), and blood pressure 90/60. Describe the immediate steps you would take to treat this patient.

_____

_____

_____

_____

3. You find a patient in a motorcycle crash impaled through the abdomen by a branch from a tree. The branch is still attached to the tree and the patient is still impaled by the branch. Describe the steps you would take to appropriately treat this patient.

_____

_____

_____

_____

Case Study

You are the EMR called to assist a 36-year-old male who was punched in the abdomen during a fight. Before your arrival, the patient complained of pain in his abdomen and vomited blood. He is now unconscious with gurgling respirations.

1. Describe the steps of your primary assessment.

_____

_____

_____

_____

2. Are there immediate actions required in the primary assessment and, if so, what are they?

_____

_____

_____

_____

His vital signs are pulse 130, respirations 7, and blood pressure 88/58. Your assessment of his abdomen reveals distention.

3. What is the most likely cause of unconsciousness in this patient?

_____

_____

_____

_____

4. What is the most likely cause for the alteration of his vital signs?

_____

_____

_____

_____

5. Specifically, what does his blood pressure indicate?

_____

_____

_____

_____

EXPLORE PEARSON **mybradykit**™

Please go to **www.bradybooks.com** to access mykit for this text. You will find quizzes, critical thinking scenarios, weblinks, animations, and videos related to this chapter— and much more. Look for online information on rib fractures and flail chest.

Register your access code from the front of your book by going to **www.bradybooks.com** and selecting the mykit links.

CHAPTER 20

Soft Tissue Injuries

NAVIGATION GUIDE

The following items provide an overview to the purpose and content of this chapter. The Education Standard and Competency are from the National EMS Education Standards.

Education Standard Trauma (Orthopedic Trauma, Soft Tissue Trauma)

Competency Uses simple knowledge to recognize and manage life threats based on assessment findings for an acutely injured patient while awaiting additional emergency medical response.

Knowledge Areas

Orthopedic Trauma
- Open fractures
- Closed fractures
- Dislocations
- Amputations

Soft Tissue Trauma
- Wounds
- Thermal, electrical, and chemical burns
- Chemicals in the eye and on the skin

Objectives After reading this chapter, you should be able to:

1. Define key terms introduced in this chapter.
2. Explain the relationship between soft tissue injuries and more serious injuries the patient may have suffered.
3. Describe each of the various types of open and closed soft tissue injuries presented in the text.
4. Demonstrate the proper sequence of assessment and treatment of patients with soft tissue injuries.
5. Recognize situations in which a patient's injuries call for the EMR to use a higher level of Standard Precautions, such as face and eye protection, gowns, and shoe protection.
6. Given a scenario involving a patient with an open soft tissue injury or burn, apply an appropriate dressing and bandage for the situation.
7. Demonstrate special dressing, bandaging, and other care techniques required for patients with each of the following injuries:
   a. Impaled objects
   b. Neck wounds
   c. Amputations
8. Describe special considerations in the care of patients suffering from animal or human bite wounds.
9. Given a description of the characteristics of a burn injury, classify the injury according to depth and amount of body surface area affected.
10. Describe anatomical locations and other factors related to burns that are cause for increased concern.
11. Given a scenario in which a patient has received burns, demonstrate the proper sequence of patient assessment and treatment.

NAVIGATION GUIDE *(continued)*

12. Explain special considerations in the management of patients with the following burn injuries:

    a. Burns of the airway
    b. Chemical burns
    c. Electrical burns

Key Terms Page numbers indicate first major use in this chapter. The Margin Glossary in this chapter provides definitions as you read.

open wound, p. 475
closed wound, p. 475
blunt trauma, p. 476
contusion, p. 476
ecchymosis, p. 476
hematoma, p. 476
abrasion, p. 477

laceration, p. 478
avulsion, p. 478
puncture, p. 478
dressing, p. 482
trauma dressing, p. 483
bandage compress, p. 483

occlusive dressing, p. 483
hemostatic agent, p. 483
roller bandage, p. 484
triangle bandage, p. 484
air embolism, p. 487
amputation, p. 487

Media Resources Please go to **www.bradybooks.com** to access mykit for this text. You will find quizzes, critical thinking scenarios, weblinks, animations, and videos related to this chapter—and much more. Look for online information on tourniquets and bleeding.

INTRODUCTION

"Soft tissue" refers to the skin, muscle, nerves, blood vessels, and connective tissue—the body's external protective layer. Injuries, otherwise known as **wounds**, can be **open** or **closed**, and although they are not commonly life threatening, under the right circumstances they can be. Soft tissue injuries to the face, airway, and chest can interfere with breathing, and injuries to large blood vessels can lead to major bleeding. Your primary assessment and your knowledge of anatomy will help you identify these potential life threats.

Soft tissue injuries will often be terrible to look at and may initially attract your attention. They may also be the focus of the patient's cries for help. Although these injuries may be dramatic, they may be the least significant of the patient's problems. Regardless of the obvious injury, a thorough primary assessment is always the best starting point.

ASK YOURSELF

■ Can you define key terms introduced in this chapter?

open wound a wound in which the skin has been broken.

closed wound a wound in which the skin has not been broken.

CASE STUDY

THE CALL

It is late evening in May. It is warm, with low humidity. You respond to a house fire in a hilly, open area that has few trees. Soon after your arrival you are requested by the fire chief to evaluate a firefighter with burns. You respond to the front of the engine where you find a firefighter seated on the front bumper surrounded by the rest of his crew. The firefighter tells you he was working in the house when he lost his glove. He tells you his right hand has been burned.

■ Discussion: *What are your first steps in the assessment of this patient?*

ASK YOURSELF

■ What is the relationship between soft tissue injuries and more serious injuries the patient may have suffered?

Although you may find that a wound is not life threatening, a soft tissue injury may be a major concern to the patient. A good emergency medical provider always stays aware of the patient's emotional needs.

Closed Wounds

A closed wound means the skin has not been broken. Although there may be severe injury to soft tissue beneath the skin, the force of the injury has not actually penetrated it. *Never underestimate the seriousness of closed wounds.* Closed wounds are often difficult to assess as you cannot see the extent of the damage beneath the skin. Massive internal injuries can be hidden by intact skin. Consider the following example:

> An 8-year-old boy has crashed his bicycle and has been poked in the abdomen with one of the handlebars. Your patient assessment finds only a small bruise in the upper right quadrant of the abdomen. He complains of pain and will not let you touch that area. On the outside, his only injury appears to be a small bruise on his belly, but remember he may have more serious injuries beneath the skin. Consider the anatomy of the abdomen (see Chapter 5, "Anatomy and Physiology"). Basic anatomy reminds us that his liver lies underneath the area he injured. His skin may be intact, but he may be bleeding severely from his injured liver.

blunt trauma trauma (force) applied over a large area.

Typically closed wounds are caused by **blunt trauma**, that is, trauma or force applied over a large area. This force can be high energy such as a high-speed car/pedestrian crash or low energy such as a punch to the face. Either way intact skin often hides deeper injuries.

contusion a bruise often caused by blunt force trauma; typically seen as a discolored and swollen area of soft tissue.

Blunt trauma often results in a **contusion**. Common signs of a contusion include pain at the site of impact, tenderness (pain to the touch) at and around the site of impact, and swelling.

ecchymosis bleeding beneath the skin; typically seen as "black and blue" discoloration as in a bruise.

Ecchymosis occurs when the force breaks open small blood vessels beneath the skin and results in bluish discoloration (black and blue bruising).

A **hematoma** is seen when a large amount of bleeding occurs beneath the skin, enough to raise a bluish discolored lump.

hematoma a large amount of bleeding beneath the skin; typically enough to raise a bluish discolored lump.

EMR Patient Assessment: Closed Wounds

You will perform a thorough primary assessment to identify and treat immediate life threats. Due to the presence of many vital organs, be especially suspicious of airway and breathing problems when dealing with closed injuries to the neck and chest.

EMR Emergency Care: Closed Wounds

There is really little prehospital treatment for closed wounds. The most important aspect of your treatment will be to suspect problems that have occurred beneath the skin.

- Recognize the potential for internal bleeding. Use your knowledge of anatomy to think about what organs and bones lie beneath the area of impact and how they may have been injured. Be particularly suspicious of closed injuries to the abdomen and pelvis as both those areas contain many vital organs (see Chapter 19, "Chest and Abdominal Emergencies").

- Recognize and treat the onset of shock. Be watchful for signs and symptoms of shock, especially with a mechanism of injury and a closed wound in a life-threatening area (see Chapter 18).

- For a truly minor closed injury, apply ice or a cold pack to help reduce swelling and pain. Note: Ice or a cold pack should not be applied directly against the skin. Wrap the pack in a towel or similar material to prevent a cold-related injury to the skin.

OPEN WOUNDS

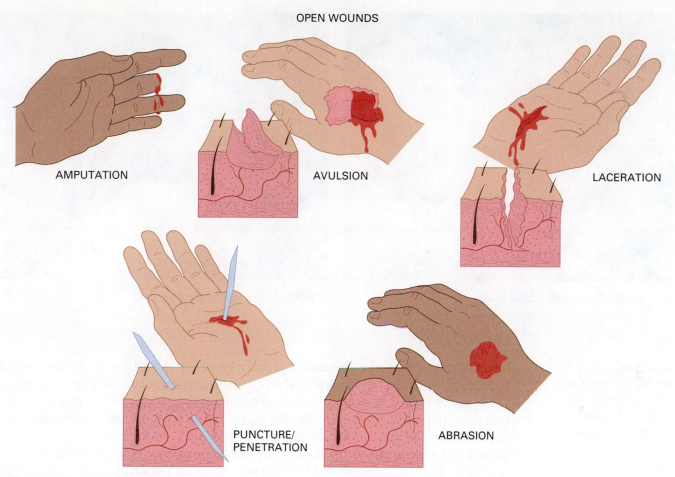

AMPUTATION

AVULSION

LACERATION

PUNCTURE/
PENETRATION

ABRASION

■ **Figure 20-1** Types of open wounds.

Open Wounds

An open wound means the injury has broken the skin. In this case the force involved has actually penetrated the skin. Open wounds are often more visible than closed wounds as you can actually see the trauma; but even open wounds can hide large, underlying injuries. Open wounds also defeat the skin's protective layer in the fight against infection and pose a significant risk of allowing in foreign objects (including bacteria) that can cause infection (Figure 20-1 ■).

Open wounds may be caused from the inside out. Fractures can cause bone ends to penetrate through the skin and even at times retract back beneath the skin, leaving an open wound. Consider any open wound on an extremity with a concerning mechanism of injury as a potential sign of fracture.

Abrasions

Abrasions are caused by a rubbing or scraping force that penetrates and destroys the outermost layers of skin. A "skinned knee" typically comes to mind when picturing an abrasion, but abrasions may be far more severe (Figure 20-2a ■). Think of a motorcycle rider thrown to the pavement. His abrasion might be full body. Although abrasions are rarely life threatening, they can pose a serious risk of infection and can be extremely painful to the patient. As always consider the underlying damage (Figure 20-2b ■).

ASK YOURSELF

■ How would you describe the various types of open and closed soft tissue injuries presented in the text?

abrasion a rubbing or scraping force that penetrates and destroys the outermost layers of skin.

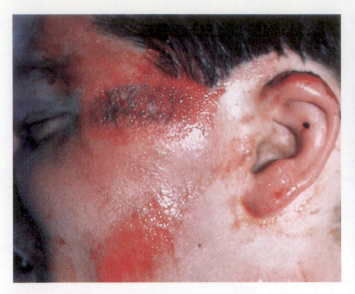

■ **Figure 20-2a** Example of facial abrasions.

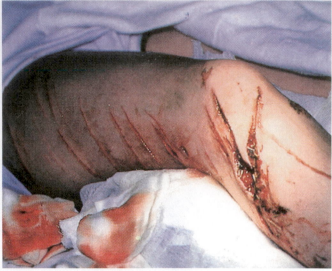

■ **Figure 20-2b** Lacerations of the leg.

Lacerations

laceration a cut to the skin and/or to the layers of soft tissue beneath the skin caused by a sharp object.

avulsion an injury in which the force completely tears away large pieces of soft tissue.

A **laceration** is a cut to the skin and/or to the layers of soft tissue beneath the skin caused by a sharp object. It may be smooth and precise such as an incision from a razor, or jagged and irregular such as from force from blunt trauma or from a blunt object that shears the skin open (Figure 20-2c ■). An **avulsion** occurs when the force completely tears away large pieces of soft tissue. An example is when a ring tears loose a large section of the finger in hand trauma. Beware of bleeding in lacerations as these cuts can involve veins or arteries (or both). Lacerations and bleeding are also visually dramatic (Figures 20-2d and 20-2e ■). Remember they *may not* be the most life-threatening problem. Do not let them distract you from airway or breathing priorities.

Punctures and Perforations

puncture a penetration of the skin that damages the soft tissue in the path of the penetrating object.

In a **puncture** wound, a sharp object has penetrated the skin and damaged the soft tissue (and anything else) in its path. Because often the path of a penetrating object damages vital organs, a puncture wound can be the most dangerous of open wounds. With a puncture wound, you will often see only a small entry wound with little or no external

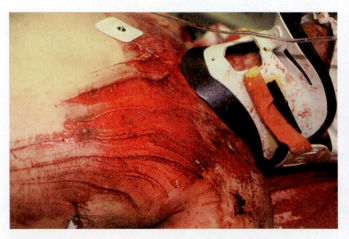

■ **Figure 20-2c** Deep abrasion and laceration. (© Edward T. Dickinson, MD)

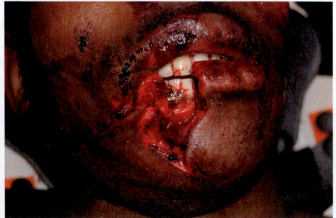

■ **Figure 20-2d** Trauma to the mouth. (© Edward T. Dickinson, MD)

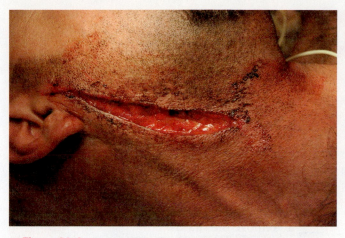

■ **Figure 20-2e** Laceration to the neck. *(© Edward T. Dickinson, MD)*

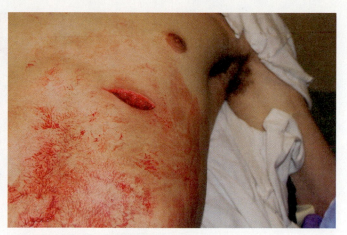

■ **Figure 20-2f** Gunshot wound. *(© Edward T. Dickinson, MD)*

bleeding. This can result from minor force (stepping on a nail) or major force (a stab wound). In some cases, it may even have an exit wound (a second wound where the puncturing object has left the body) (Figure 20-2e).

EMR Patient Assessment: Open Wounds

It is very difficult to know the extent of internal damage from just looking at a puncture wound. The outside of the body may have only a small wound, but remember the damage beneath that wound will include the entire path of the penetrating object. For example, a small bullet wound may only show you a small hole in the skin, but tissue, bone, and organs will be damaged as far throughout the body as that bullet traveled (Figure 20-2f ■). You would be making a serious mistake if you judged the seriousness of such a wound only by the size of the entrance wound.

As an emergency responder, you should consider all puncture and perforating wounds serious, especially if they occur in the head, neck, chest, or abdomen/pelvis. If safe to do so, consider gathering information about the penetrating object as well. For example, knowing the length and size of a knife often can help predict the amount of damage it caused along its pathway. Use your primary assessment to identify and treat immediate life threats. Be especially suspicious of airway and breathing problems when dealing with open injuries to the neck and chest.

EMR Emergency Care: Open Wounds

- Control bleeding (see Chapter 18, "Bleeding and Shock"). Open injuries can result in massive bleeding. You should immediately take the appropriate steps to control it. Remember that bleeding can occur internally in addition to externally. Use mechanism of injury, a thorough patient assessment, and your knowledge of anatomy to help identify potential internal injuries.
- Recognize and treat the onset of shock (see Chapter 18). Be watchful for signs and symptoms of shock, especially with a significant mechanism of injury or an open wound in a life-threatening area.
- Prevent infection. Remove or cut away clothing from the area of the wound. Clear loose debris. Note: Never remove embedded objects from a wound.
- Dress and bandage the wound. Apply a sterile (or as clean as possible) dressing over the wound and secure it using a bandage. Note: This topic will be discussed in greater detail later in this chapter.

ASK YOURSELF

- How would you demonstrate the proper sequence of assessment and treatment of patients with soft tissue injuries?

Stop, Review, Remember

Multiple Choice

Place a check next to the correct answer.

1. A 22-year-old man complains of a large cut on his forearm as a result of accidentally breaking a window. You could characterize this injury as:

    _____ a. an open wound.

    _____ b. a closed wound.

    _____ c. blunt trauma.

    _____ d. a hematoma.

2. Blunt trauma rupturing blood vessels beneath the skin and creating a bluish discoloration would best be described as a(n):

    _____ a. amputation.

    _____ b. laceration.

    _____ c. ecchymosis.

    _____ d. avulsion.

3. A 33-year-old man was cut by a razor blade during a fight. His wound is even and precise. This would best be described as a(n):

    _____ a. hematoma.

    _____ b. abrasion.

    _____ c. contusion.

    _____ d. laceration.

4. After assessing a large laceration, you note large shards of glass embedded in the wound. You should:

    _____ a. remove the shards.

    _____ b. leave the shards in place and apply a loose dressing.

    _____ c. use high-pressure water to flush the shards out.

    _____ d. leave the shards in place and apply direct pressure.

5. A 28-year-old woman involved in a motor vehicle crash has a wound on her leg in which a large flap of skin has been removed. This wound would best be described as a(n):

    _____ a. puncture.

    _____ b. avulsion.

    _____ c. incision.

    _____ d. abrasion.

Emergency Medical Responder Practice

Identify the patient's type of wound and whether it's open or closed.

1. A 13-year-old male fell off his skateboard and scraped and skidded his exposed leg across the pavement. He has "road rash" on his upper thigh.

    a. Type of wound _____

    b. Open or closed _____

2. An 18-year-old male was struck in the head with a baseball bat. He has pain, tenderness, and edema on the left side of his head.

    a. Type of wound _____

    b. Open or closed _____

3. A 9-year-old boy was struck by a baseball in his upper thigh. He has pain, and a raised, bluish lump in the area where he was struck.

    a. Type of wound _____

    b. Open or closed _____

4. A 31-year-old woman involved in a motor vehicle crash has a jagged cut on her face from hitting the rearview mirror.

    a. Type of wound _____

    b. Open or closed _____

5. A 43-year-old male was stabbed in the chest with an ice pick. He has a small entrance wound in his upper left chest.

    a. Type of wound _____

    b. Open or closed _____

Short Answer

1. A 55-year-old male was involved in a car crash. He has pain, bluish discoloration, and tenderness in his lower abdomen in the area where the seat belt was placed across him. What would your chief concerns be regarding the nature of this patient's injury?

    _____

    _____

    _____

    _____

2. A 24-year-old woman was slashed on the side of her neck in a domestic dispute. She tells you the wound is large, but she has it covered with a kitchen towel. What would your chief concerns be regarding the nature of this patient's injury?

    _____

    _____

    _____

    _____

3. A 20-year-old male was shot in the upper right chest. What would your chief concerns be regarding the nature of this patient's injury?

    _____

    _____

    _____

    _____

THE RESPONSE ✳

The burning process has been stopped. The hand was initially rinsed with water from the hose. Your assessment notes that the patient has a clear airway, he is talking, and he has normal breathing. He has moist, flushed skin. He is alert and oriented.

You assess the patient's hand and find red skin with blisters on the posterior wrist. He notes it is very painful. You do not find any further burn. He says he was wearing full protection, including self-contained breathing apparatus, at the time of the injury.

You bandage the burn with a dry sterile dressing, per your local burn protocols, and continue a full secondary assessment. Although the firefighter does not wish to be transported, you encourage him to go due to the location of the burn.

■ Discussion: *Should the depth of the burn be assessed? How would you handle the fact that the firefighter refuses transport?*

ASK YOURSELF

■ Can you recognize situations in which a patient's injuries call for the EMR to use a higher level of Standard Precautions, such as face and eye protection, gowns, and shoe protection?

■ Given a scenario involving a patient with an open soft tissue injury or burn, would you know how to apply an appropriate dressing and bandage for the situation?

dressing a covering for a wound designed to absorb blood and wound drainage, control bleeding, and protect and cover the wound to prevent infection.

EMR Emergency Care: Soft Tissue Injuries

The purpose of treatment in soft tissue injuries is to control bleeding, prevent infection, and promote healing. Immediate life threats must be treated first, but appropriate treatment of lower priority injuries may improve the overall outcome of the patient and certainly improves overall care.

Standard Precautions

Your first priority is always to keep yourself safe. A patient's blood and other body fluids can transmit any number of dangerous diseases. It is important to protect yourself from harm especially when treating a patient with severe external bleeding. Standard Precautions place a barrier between you and your patient's blood and body fluids. Standard Precautions include at a *minimum* a pair of protective gloves. However, you may need a higher level of protection if the situation calls for it. Airway management additionally requires eye/face protection, and severe bleeding (spurting blood) may require the addition of a gown and shoe protection. Use common sense, exercise good clinical judgment, and follow local protocol to determine the level of protection you need.

Dressings

A **dressing** is a covering for a wound. It is designed to absorb blood and wound drainage, control bleeding, and protect and cover the wound to prevent infection. A dressing should be sterile and opened in a manner that prevents touching it before application. However, in an unpredictable world of the emergency responder, this may not always be possible. If a sterile dressing is not readily available, think "as clean as possible." Attempt to choose a material that has the least amount of dirt and foreign bodies on it. Gauze pads are ideal as they are nonstick (that is, they are made to avoid sticking to the wound), "bulky" (providing many layers of material), absorbent, and frequently packaged in a

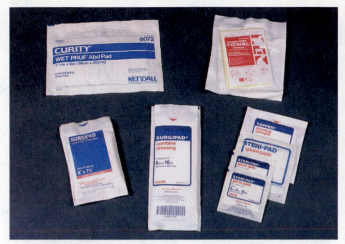

Figure 20-3a Sterile gauze pads.

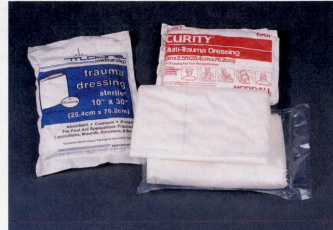

Figure 20-3b Multi-trauma dressing.

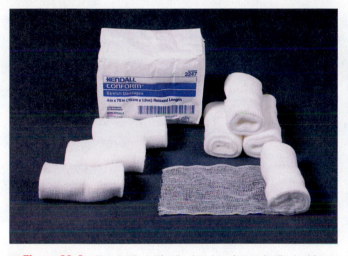

Figure 20-3c Nonelastic, self-adhering dressing and roller bandage.

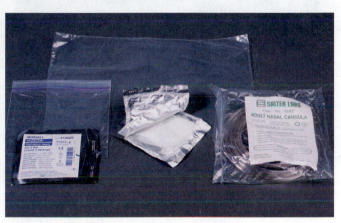

Figure 20-3d Occlusive dressings.

sterile container (Figure 20-3a ■). When gauze is not available, other household items such as feminine sanitary napkins, paper towels, or clean cloth will work. When choosing an alternative, keep in mind what makes gauze ideal and use the closest substitute.

Types of Dressings

Commercially available dressings come in many shapes and sizes. Choose the correct one considering size of the wound. The dressing must completely cover the wound.

- A **trauma dressing** is typically a large and absorbent dressing designed for major wounds (Figure 20-3b ■).
- A **bandage compress** is a dressing with a bandage attached (Figure 20-3c ■).
- An **occlusive dressing** is made of material that is airtight and is designed to create a seal over certain types of wounds (Figure 20-3d ■).
- There are also dressings that have **hemostatic agents** contained in them (sometimes referred to as contained hemostatic agents). In addition to the traditional role of a dressing, these types allow the addition of a drying agent to the wound to help control bleeding.

trauma dressing a large and absorbent dressing designed for major wounds.

bandage compress a dressing with a bandage attached.

occlusive dressing a dressing that is made of material that is airtight and is designed to create a seal over certain types of wounds.

hemostatic agent a drying agent applied to a wound to help control life-threatening bleeding.

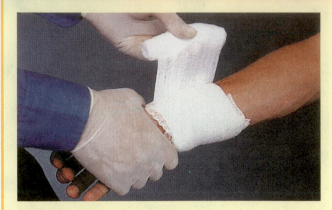

20-1a Applying a roller bandage.

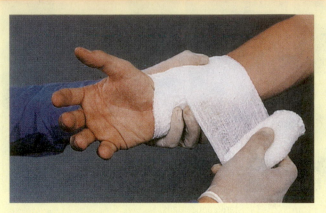

20-1b Roll bandage firmly.

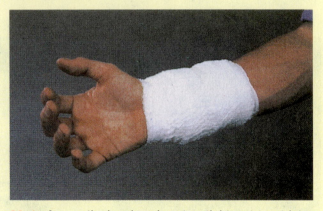

20-1c Assure the bandage is not so tight as to restrict blood flow.

Bandages

Material used to hold a dressing in place is known as a bandage. Theoretically, anything could be a bandage as long as it holds the dressing in place, but ideally the material used should be sterile or as clean as possible. Different types of bandage material include:

roller bandage a type of bandage commonly made from nonelastic material and packed in rolls; tends to cling together when rolled out onto itself.

triangle bandage a bandage made from a large piece of unbleached cotton cut to form a triangle.

- ■ **Roller bandage.** Roller bandage is commonly made from nonelastic material and comes packaged in rolls. It tends to cling together when rolled out onto itself (Scan 20-1).
- ■ **Triangle bandage.** A traditional triangle bandage is a large piece of unbleached cotton cut to form a triangle. It can be used for a variety of tasks, including fashioning a sling, forming a tourniquet, or bandaging. To use a triangle bandage to hold a dressing in place, you would fold it into a wide strip to form what is called a *cravat*.

Applying a Dressing and Bandage

- ■ Completely cover the wound with a dressing. No area of the wound should be left uncovered. Cover more area than necessary.
- ■ Apply the bandage over the dressing. Completely cover the dressing with the bandage (Figures 20-4a to 20-4f ■). Under ideal circumstances, the bleeding

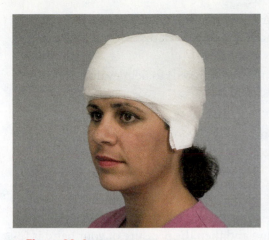

■ **Figure 20-4a** Head or ear bandage.

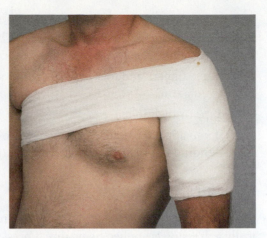

■ **Figure 20-4b** Shoulder bandage.

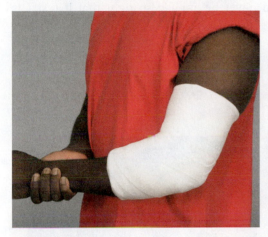

■ **Figure 20-4c** Elbow bandage.

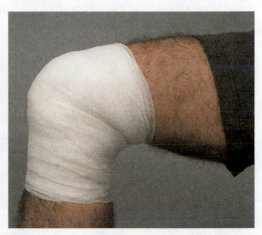

■ **Figure 20-4d** Knee bandage.

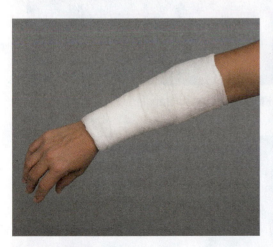

■ **Figure 20-4e** Lower arm bandage.

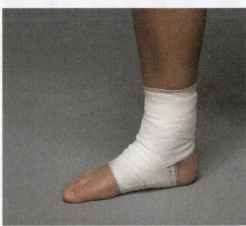

■ **Figure 20-4f** Foot or ankle bandage.

should be controlled prior to bandaging to allow for additional bulky dressings. (A pressure dressing used to control bleeding would be an exception to this rule.)

■ Apply the bandage over a wide area. Be careful not to create a tourniquet with your bandage. Even if the wound is small, apply bandages over an area wide enough to distribute pressure equally and allow good circulation.

- A bandage should be tight, but not restrict blood flow. It should be reasonably comfortable for the patient, and you should always check distal circulation after bandaging to ensure blood flow to the extremity.

- Leave fingers and toes exposed (unless they are injured) to help evaluate circulation.

- Tape or tuck in loose ends.

- If you apply a bandage over a joint, do not bend that joint after application. Bending the joint could tighten bandages enough to cut off blood flow.

Pressure Dressings

A pressure dressing is the application of a dressing and bandage to control bleeding. Typically a dressing is applied using direct pressure and then the pressure of your hand is replaced by the pressure of a bandage. Bandaging can be an effective means of continuing some direct pressure, but a bandage should never be applied so tight that it restricts blood flow.

SCAN 20-2　Care of an Impaled Object

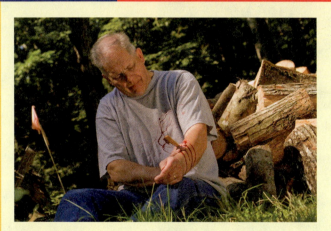

20-2a Treating an impaled object.

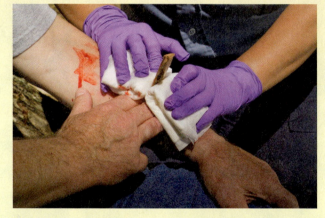

20-2b The EMR stabilizes an impaled object with a dressing.

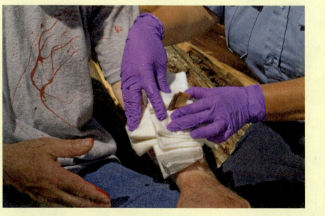

20-2c Add bulky dressings.

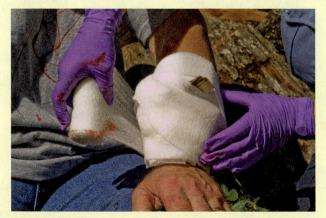

20-2d Bandage.

Special Circumstances

Some circumstances will require you to change what you would ordinarily do to control bleeding and dress and bandage a wound. As an EMR, you must be adaptable and use good clinical judgment to treat unusual situations.

Impaled Objects

As discussed in Chapter 19, you should not remove impaled objects but keep them secured in place (Scan 20-2). Use bulky dressings, roller bandage, and/or tape to secure and protect the object during transport.

The exception to this rule would be an impaled object through the soft tissue of the cheek. If bleeding from this type of wound interferes with breathing, you should remove the object if local protocol allows. Suction the airway when needed. You should remove the object in the direction it was inserted and then pack the area with sterile gauze. Use the space between the cheek and teeth to keep dressings in place. Be careful not to block the airway with the dressing. Consider positioning the patient on his side to promote drainage of the wound out of the mouth and continually reassess the airway.

Neck Wounds

Wounds to the neck potentially threaten the airway and large blood vessels. Closed injuries like this not only cause immediate damage to the airway and blood vessels, but also may cause swelling that can partially or completely obstruct the patient's airway. Constant reassessment is critical when managing neck wounds. Dangerous signs include difficulty speaking or hoarseness and shortness of breath.

Open wounds to the neck and chest should be covered with an occlusive dressing to prevent air from entering the great vessels and causing an **air embolism**, or air bubble in the bloodstream. Apply direct pressure but beware applying direct pressure to both sides of the neck at once or applying pressure or a bandage that occludes or obstructs the airway.

Amputations

Treatment of amputations varies from system to system, so please follow local protocol. An **amputation** occurs when a body part has been completely detached from the rest of the body (Figures 20-5a to 20-5c ■). Bleeding may be severe, but oftentimes (especially in complete amputations) bleeding is controlled by the spasm and constriction of the severed

ASK YOURSELF

■ How would you demonstrate special dressing, bandaging, and other care techniques required for patients with each of the following injuries?
   ■ Impaled objects
   ■ Neck wounds
   ■ Amputations

air embolism air bubble in the bloodstream.

amputation complete detachment of a body part from the rest of the body.

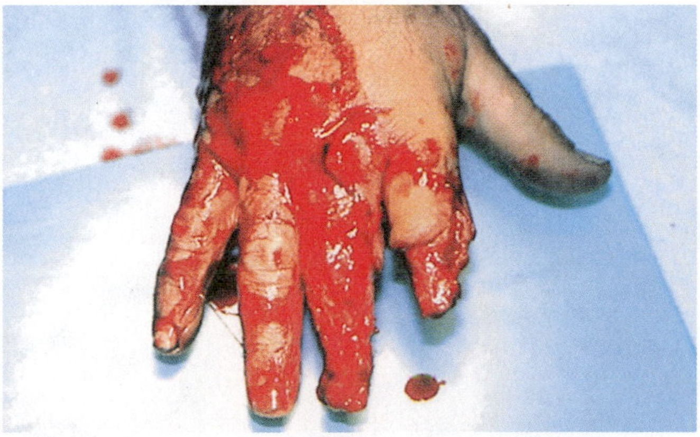

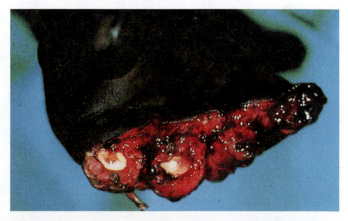

■ **Figure 20-5a** Finger amputation. (© Charles Stewart M.D. & Associates)

■ **Figure 20-5b** Fingers amputation. (© Charles Stewart M.D. & Associates)

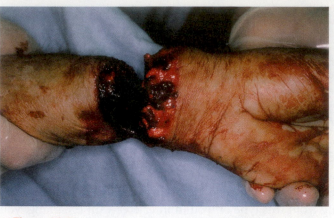

■ **Figure 20-5c** Amputation of hand at wrist. (© Charles Stewart M.D. & Associates)

SCAN 20-3 Emergency Care for an Amputated Part

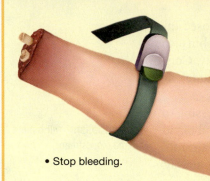

• Stop bleeding.

20-3a Locate the amputated part.

• Wrap amputated part in sterile dressing and place in plastic bag.

20-3b Keep the amputated part moist but do not submerge it.

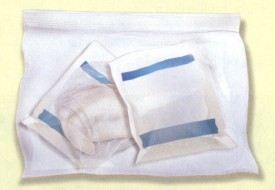

• Keep amputated part cool.
• Do not allow tissue to come directly in contact with ice or freeze.
• Do not submerge part in water.

20-3c Keep the amputated part cool. Do not allow it to freeze.

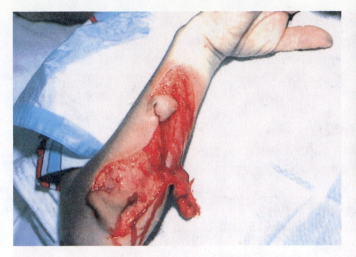

■ **Figure 20-6a** Avulsion to the forearm.

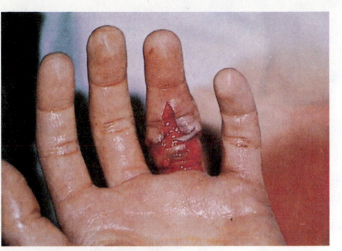

■ **Figure 20-6b** Ring avulsion.

blood vessels. You should control bleeding in the case of an amputation as you would any other open wound.

Medical technology has advanced to the point where many amputated parts can be reattached. Part of your responsibility as an emergency responder will be to arrange transport of the amputated part for potential reattachment (Scan 20-3). Always remember though that your first priority is the care of the patient.

Follow local guidelines to care for the amputated part. Typical care includes the following:

- Gently clean the amputated part by removing loose debris.
- Wrap the amputated part in gauze lightly moistened with sterile saline and place in a sealed plastic bag.
- Cool the amputated part by placing it in a container with ice (never use dry ice). Do not place the part directly on the ice and never immerse the amputated part in water.
- Label the part with the patient's name and arrange transport. Ideally the part will be transported with the patient. If it is found after the patient leaves the scene arrange for prompt transportation to the hospital (e.g., police cruiser).
- Never give false hope to a patient with an amputation that the amputated part will definitely be reattached at the hospital. Many amputated parts are not reattached after evaluation by a surgeon. It is better to inform the patient that you are carefully handling the amputated part for the *potential* that it *may* be reattached.

In many cases you will treat an avulsion in the same manner as an incomplete amputation (Figures 20-6a and 20-6b ■). Never complete an incomplete amputation. In the case of an avulsion, gently clean the avulsed part and (in the case of flaps of skin or tissue) replace the flap. Control bleeding and apply a dressing and bandage.

Animal and Human Bites

Although not typically life threatening, bite wounds pose a high risk for infection. In caring for a bite wound, scene safety is paramount. Do not attempt to capture or kill the offending animal, but rather record the description and location for later follow-up. It may be appropriate to help the patient clean with soap and water if the wound is small, such as to a finger or the hand. Manage larger bite wounds by appropriate control of bleeding, and applying a dressing and bandage.

ASK YOURSELF

- What are some special considerations in the care of patients suffering from animal or human bite wounds?

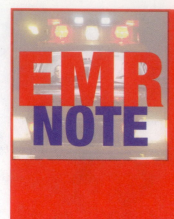

Although a non-life-threatening soft tissue injury may be low on your priority list, this injury may be a vastly different reality for the patient. The presence of blood and bleeding often has a dramatic effect on people. A patient's response may be more severe than the seriousness of the injury. This is especially true in children. Take time to consider the viewpoint of your patient and take steps to reassure and educate when reasonable to do so. Even though soft tissue injuries may not be a life threat, cosmetic injuries such as those to the face and neck may be life altering. Your concern and compassion may be the most important elements of care in these cases.

✳ Stop, Review, Remember

Multiple Choice

Place a check next to the correct answer.

1. Material you apply directly to the surface of a wound is called:

   _____ a. a dressing.

   _____ b. a bandage.

   _____ c. a cravat.

   _____ d. pressure points.

2. Which of the following impaled objects should you remove (if local protocol allows)?

   _____ a. a nail in a foot

   _____ b. a knife in the abdomen

   _____ c. a large shard of glass in the arm

   _____ d. a pencil through the cheek

3. A large and absorbent dressing designed for major wounds is called a(n):

   _____ a. occlusive dressing.

   _____ b. roller bandage.

   _____ c. trauma dressing.

   _____ d. cravat.

4. After bandaging an arm wound, your patient complains of numbness and tingling in her fingers. You should:

   _____ a. loosen the bandage.

   _____ b. have her breathe into a paper bag.

   _____ c. tighten the bandage.

   _____ d. treat her for shock.

5. The most appropriate treatment dressing for a laceration on the neck would be:

   _____ a. a Vaseline-impregnated gauze pad.

   _____ b. bulky sterile gauze.

   _____ c. a paper towel.

   _____ d. a contained hemostatic agent.

Emergency Medical Responder Practice

1. You find your patient with a pencil impaled in her leg. Describe the steps in treating this impaled object.

   _____

   _____

   _____

1. Discuss why a joint should not be bent after bandaging.

   _____

   _____

   _____

2. Explain why it is recommended to leave fingers and toes exposed when bandaging.

   _____

   _____

   _____

3. Identify at least two attributes of an effective dressing.

   _____

   _____

   _____

Burns

One of the most serious types of soft tissue injuries is the burn. A burn occurs when heat, electricity, or chemicals destroy the skin and soft tissue. A burn is always serious as the process not only damages tissue, but also destroys the protective ability of the skin and soft tissue. You should arrange transport for all burn patients for further evaluation by medical professionals. Burns may be minor or severe depending on the depth, area, and location of the burn. As always, you will use your primary assessment to identify and treat immediate life threats caused by burns.

EMR Patient Assessment: Burns

The severity of a burn is usually determined by looking at three factors: depth, surface area, and location.

Depth

The skin is divided into layers (Figure 20-7 ■). The epidermis is the outermost layer. The dermis contains blood vessels and nerves and is the middle layer. The deepest layer is the subcutaneous tissue, which is mostly fat. When assessing a burn you need to consider how deep (and to what layer) the burn has damaged the tissue. Typically, burns are categorized by depth into three classifications:

1. *Superficial.* In a superficial burn only the epidermis, or outermost layer of the skin, is involved. When assessing a superficial burn you will see redness and swelling. The burn may be very painful to the patient (Figure 20-8 ■). A severe sunburn is a good example of a superficial burn.
2. *Partial thickness.* In a partial-thickness burn, both the epidermis and dermis are involved. These burns are characterized by a moist appearance and blisters but may also be red and swollen (Figures 20-9a to 20-9e ■). Partial-thickness burns are also very painful to the patient.

■ Given a description of the characteristics of a burn injury, can you classify the injury according to depth and amount of body surface area affected?

■ Given a scenario in which a patient has received burns, can you demonstrate the proper sequence of patient assessment and treatment?

■ Can you describe anatomical locations and other factors related to burns that are cause for increased concern?

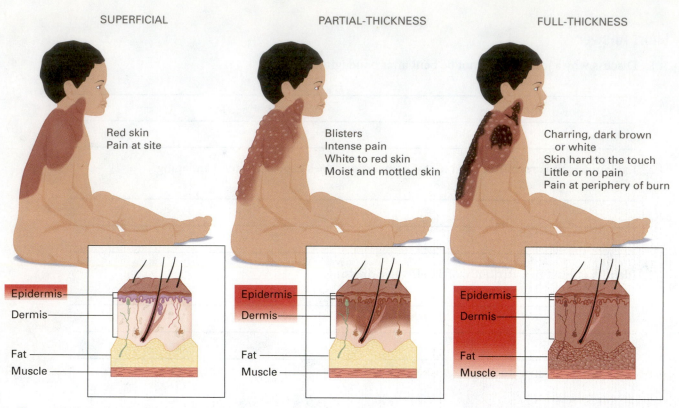

SUPERFICIAL	PARTIAL-THICKNESS	FULL-THICKNESS
Red skin Pain at site	Blisters Intense pain White to red skin Moist and mottled skin	Charring, dark brown or white Skin hard to the touch Little or no pain Pain at periphery of burn

Epidermis
Dermis
Fat
Muscle

Epidermis
Dermis
Fat
Muscle

Epidermis
Dermis
Fat
Muscle

■ **Figure 20-7** Classification of burns by depth.

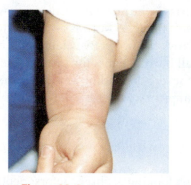

■ **Figure 20-8** Superficial burn.

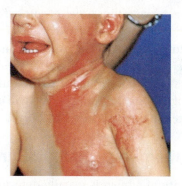

■ **Figure 20-9a** Partial-thickness burn.

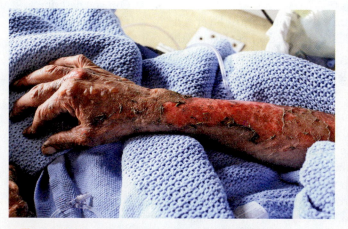

■ **Figure 20-9b** Partial-thickness burn. (© Daniel Limmer)

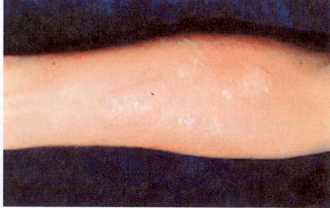

■ **Figure 20-9c** Partial-thickness burn.

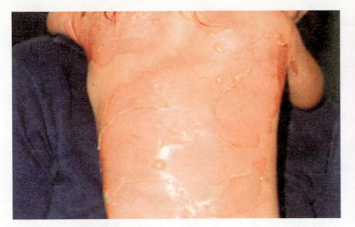

Figure 20-9d Partial-thickness burn.

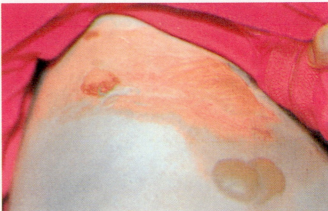

Figure 20-9e Partial-thickness burn.

3. *Full thickness.* A full-thickness burn involves all the layers of the skin and is the most serious of burns (Figures 20-10a to 20-10d ■). This type of burn often appears white and pale, and it has a leathery feel. Because they often destroy nerve pathways, your patient may note very little pain. But remember that partial-thickness burns often surround the areas of full-thickness burns, so pain is never a good indicator of the severity of a burn.

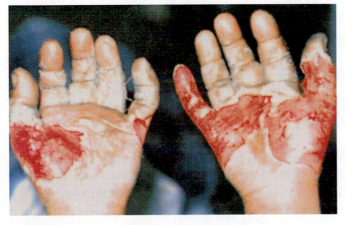

Figure 20-10a Full-thickness burn.

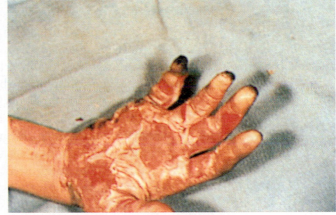

Figure 20-10b Full-thickness burn.

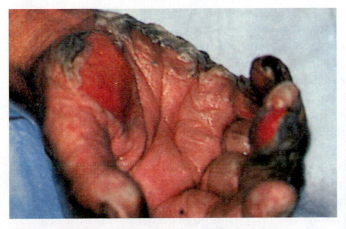

Figure 20-10c Full-thickness burn.

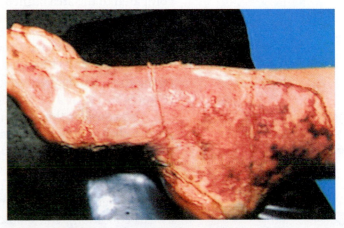

Figure 20-10d Full-thickness burn.

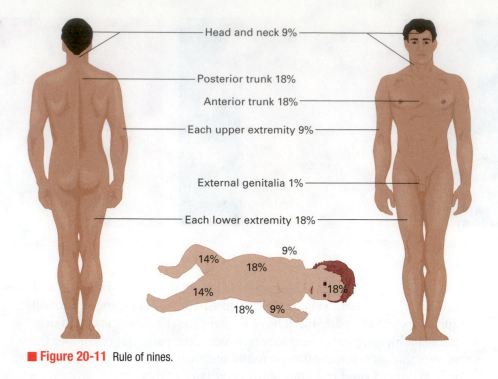

Head and neck 9%

Posterior trunk 18%

Anterior trunk 18%

Each upper extremity 9%

External genitalia 1%

Each lower extremity 18%

9%

14%

18%

14%

18%

18%

9%

■ **Figure 20-11** Rule of nines.

Surface Area

The severity of a burn is also judged by how much area of the body has been involved. The more area burned, the more severe the injury. Body surface area (BSA) burned is most commonly determined by using the "rule of nines" (Figure 20-11 ■). When using this formula on an adult, the body is divided into percentages and areas are assigned values. The rule of nines assigns 9 percent to the head and neck, 18 percent to the posterior trunk, 18 percent to the anterior trunk, 9 percent to each upper extremity, and 18 percent to each lower extremity. The groin area is 1 percent. These areas added together equal 100 percent of the body. Because an infant's body is anatomically different from an adult, the numbers need to be adjusted. In an infant the head and neck are 18 percent, the posterior trunk and anterior trunk are still 18 percent each, the upper extremities are still 9 percent each, and the lower extremities are 14 percent each.

An additional method used to estimate body surface area burned is to consider the area of the patient's palm to be 1 percent of his body surface area. The palm can then be compared to the area burned.

Location

The location of a burn is a major factor in considering how serious it may be. Burns of the face, neck, and chest all may potentially threaten breathing (Figure 20-12a ■). Burns of the eyes, hands, feet, or genitals may significantly impact the patient's way of life (Figures 20-12b and 20-12c ■). Burns in any of these areas need to be considered critical.

Also consider the age of the patient. The very young and the elderly tend to have a greater chance of death or disability as a result of the same BSA of burns as those not at the extremes of age (Figure 20-12d ■). Scene size-up will help you determine the method of burning (and potentially keep yourself safe). The mechanism of injury will help you consider other complicating injuries (such as fractures). A detailed patient history will help you identify underlying medical issues that may make a burn more serious (such as a heart condition). You should always complete a thorough patient assessment to see the "whole" patient.

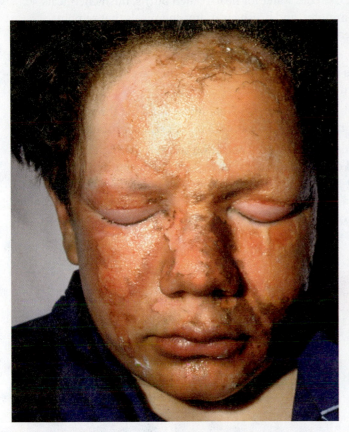

■ Figure 20-12a Burns to the face from an exploded gas cylinder. (© *Shout Picture Library*)

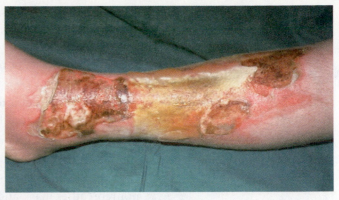

■ Figure 20-12b Petroleum burns to the foot and leg. (© *Shout Picture Library*)

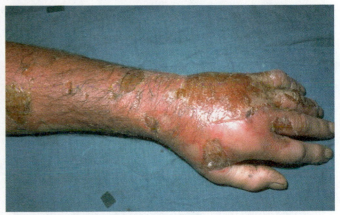

■ Figure 20-12c Cooking oil burns to the hand and arm. (© *Shout Picture Library*)

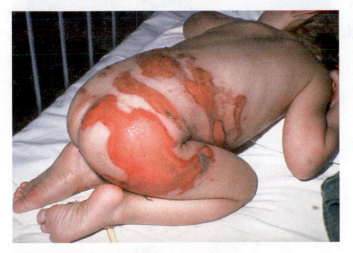

■ Figure 20-12d Scald burns encircling the torso of a child. (© *Shout Picture Library*)

EMR Emergency Care: Burns

■ Assess scene safety. What burned your patient could burn you! Always ensure that the scene is safe to proceed and request and await special resources (fire department, hazardous material teams, or others) if it is not. Be even more careful when the burning process is caused by electricity or chemicals.

ASK YOURSELF

■ What are the special considerations in the management of patients with the following burn injuries?
  ■ Burns of the airway
  ■ Chemical burns
  ■ Electrical burns

- Stop the burning process. If not done already, you should always take steps to stop the burning process. Use cold water for heat-related burns, flush chemicals with water for at least 20 minutes, and brush away any chemicals that remain (Scan 20-4a). Consider removing jewelry and any smoldering clothing (Scan 20-4b).

- Do not attempt to remove clothing and other items that may have melted to the wound. If it is difficult to remove items or if you find they are sticking to the wound, do not attempt further removal.

- Complete a thorough primary assessment. Treat immediate life threats and remember that the burn may not be the patient's most critical problem.

- Monitor breathing. Administer high-concentration oxygen through a nonrebreather mask and constantly reassess to make sure the patient is breathing adequately. If the patient inhaled superheated gases and potentially burned his airway, swelling may be a threat. Ominous signs include hoarseness, any difficulty speaking, and shortness of breath.

SCAN 20-4 BURN CARE

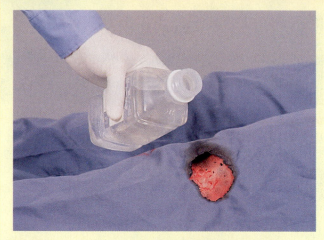

20-4a Stop the burning process with water . . .

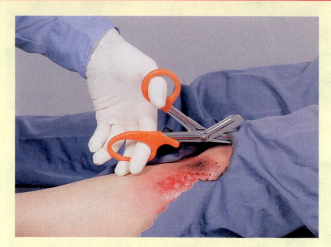

20-4b . . . and by removing all smoldering clothing.

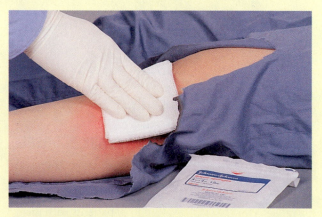

20-4c After you have treated life threats and completed a physical exam, cover the burn with dry sterile dressings.

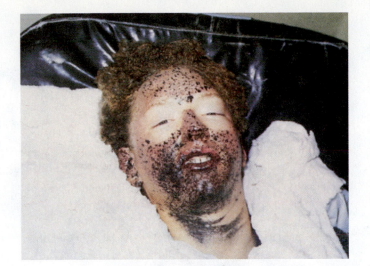

■ **Figure 20-13** Burns to the face.

- Cover the burns with a dry, sterile dressing (Scan 20-4c). This protects the burned tissue and helps prevent infection. Some EMS systems may allow the EMR to use moist sterile dressings for small body surface area burns. Follow your local protocol. You should never apply ointment or "burn cream." Do not pop blisters. If an eye is involved, you should cover both eyes to prevent movement.

- Keep the patient warm. Burn patients have difficulty regulating their temperature. Take steps to help them prevent heat loss.

Burns to the Airway

Burns to the airway or inhalation-related burns are particularly dangerous (Figures 20-13 ■ and 20-14 ■). These burns immediately damage tissue necessary to moving air. Later swelling can obstruct the airway, and even later the dangerous chemicals that were inhaled can threaten your patient's ability to oxygenate and ventilate (Table 20-1).

If any of these signs are present, consider your patient a true emergency and arrange transport to an appropriate facility as quickly as possible. Constantly reassess for airway and breathing difficulties and anticipate further problems to come. Consider humidified oxygen if local protocol allows.

Chemical Burns

Many chemical products can cause severe burns when they come in contact with skin and soft tissue. Your most important priority in the case of a chemical burn is to protect yourself. Handling a patient who has had a chemical exposure can put you at risk for the same exposure. Always wear gloves and appropriate eye protection. If you are not completely sure you can handle your patient safely, you should request expert rescue assistance such as a hazardous materials team and await their arrival.

TABLE 20-1 Signs of Inhalation/Airway Burns	
■ Burns to the face	■ Shortness of breath
■ Singed eyebrows and/or nose hairs	■ Noisy breathing or stridor
■ Soot in sputum	■ Restricted chest movement
■ Hoarseness or difficulty speaking	■ Cyanosis

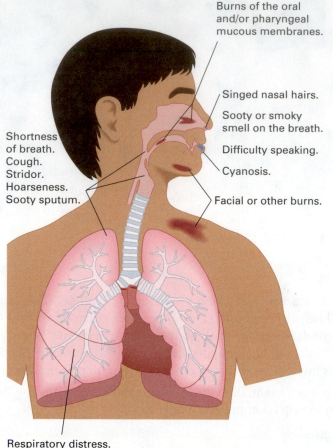

Burns of the oral and/or pharyngeal mucous membranes.

Singed nasal hairs.

Sooty or smoky smell on the breath.

Difficulty speaking.

Cyanosis.

Facial or other burns.

Shortness of breath. Cough. Stridor. Hoarseness. Sooty sputum.

Respiratory distress. Noisy breathing. Restricted chest movement.

■ **Figure 20-14** Signs and symptoms of inhalation burns.

At times you may be able to identify the specific chemical causing a burn, and this is always helpful. However, in a severe burn patient, identification may be secondary to the immediate treatment and transport you need to provide. You will have to use good clinical judgment to make the appropriate decision.

Stopping the burning process is particularly important with a chemical burn. Immediately brush away any remaining chemical and then flush the burn with copious amounts of water (Figure 20-15 ■). Any reasonably clean water would be appropriate (a garden hose, a sink, or a shower will do) and you should flush for at least 20 minutes if possible.

In the case of a chemical burn to the eye, flush with low-pressure water and be sure to flush away from an unaffected eye. Lay the patient on his side and flush the eye from the bridge of the nose outward to avoid the chemical running into the other eye (Figure 20-16 ■). It may be necessary to force open the patient's eye during the flushing process. Take care with burned tissue to avoid further damage.

Electrical Burns

When treating a patient with an electrical burn, you must ensure that the scene is safe before touching the patient. If the patient is still in contact with the electrical source, touching him could result in your own electrocution. If for any reason you are not sure that the source of electricity has been shut off, request expert rescue assistance and await their arrival.

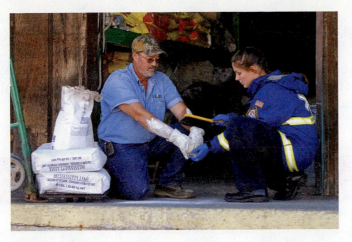

■ **Figure 20-15** Poison in powder form should be brushed off the skin before flushing.

Never approach a downed power line. Consider that no line is safe to touch. Also consider that the area around the downed power line may be energized. Always keep a safe distance. If a patient is in a vehicle in contact with a power line, advise that person to stay in the car until expert help arrives.

Electricity can cause severe burns in the same manner as heat. You may expect to see superficial, partial-thickness, and full-thickness burns. Often the patient will have two such wounds on his body, representing where the electrical current entered and exited the body. Treat these burns in the same manner you would other burns. Keep in mind, however, that an electrical burn is similar to a puncture wound in that the worst damage may not be visible from the outside. As electricity passes through your patient's body, severe damage can occur throughout its pathway. Small burns may be visible on the outside, but severe injury may have occurred internally. As an emergency responder, you should always consider a more severe internal injury in an electrical burn patient.

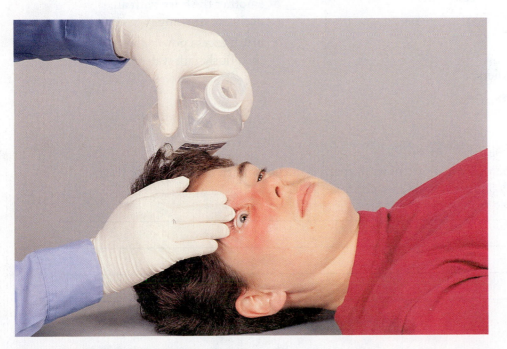

■ **Figure 20-16** Flush chemical burns to the eye.

Consider spinal precautions for patients with electrical burns because trauma can occur from the electricity itself or from the patient being thrown as a result of the electrical injury.

Electrical burns may also have a serious impact on the heart. Anticipate and be ready to address cardiac arrest and other heart-related complications in electrical burn patients. Request advanced life support.

Stop, Review, Remember

Multiple Choice

Place a check next to the correct answer.

1. The three most important factors in assessing the severity of a burn include area, depth, and:

    _____ a. time.

    _____ b. length.

    _____ c. type.

    _____ d. location.

2. The middle layer of skin that contains blood vessels and nerves is called the:

    _____ a. epidermis.

    _____ b. subcutaneous layer.

    _____ c. subdermis layer.

    _____ d. dermis.

3. A burn in which only the epidermis is damaged would be designated a _____ burn.

    _____ a. superficial

    _____ b. partial-thickness

    _____ c. full-thickness

    _____ d. secondary

4. In estimating the surface area of a burn, the patient's palm is considered to be _____ percent of his body surface area.

    _____ a. 4

    _____ b. 3

    _____ c. 2

    _____ d. 1

5. Your patient has been burned by a chemical powder. To stop the burning process you should:

    _____ a. flush immediately with copious amounts of water.

    _____ b. not flush with water.

    _____ c. smother the burn with an occlusive dressing.

    _____ d. brush excess powder away and then flush with water.

Emergency Medical Responder Practice

1. Describe the emergency care of a patient with a partial-thickness burn on his anterior thigh amounting to roughly 5 percent body surface area.

    _____

    _____

    _____

    _____

Short Answer

1. A 29-year-old patient has a superficial burn covering the anterior aspects of both legs (upper and lower). Using the rule of nines, what body surface area would be burned?

_____

_____

_____

_____

2. A 4-year-old patient has a partial-thickness burn covering his anterior chest and abdomen. Using the rule of nines, what body surface area would be burned?

_____

_____

_____

_____

3. Identify at least three signs of a potential inhalation injury/airway burn.

_____

_____

_____

_____

CASE STUDY

TRANSITION

When the EMTs arrive, you report your physical findings. You relate to them the body surface area of the burn and the fact that you believe it to be a partial-thickness burn. The patient is then transported as you complete your written documentation.

■ Discussion: *Why are you sure it is a partial-thickness burn? Using the rule of nines, what percentage of his body was burned?*

THE LAST WORD

Although many soft tissue injuries are not typically life threatening, you must never become complacent and let minor injuries distract you from underlying major issues. Be thorough with your patient assessment, treat major life threats first, and learn to recognize the signs and symptoms of critical burns or any underlying injuries. Remember that the treatment of minor issues helps increase the chances of a positive outcome. Finally, never forget to view the injury from the patient's perspective.

Multiple Choice

Place a check next to the correct answer.

1. A burn that affects only the outermost layer of the skin would be classified as:

    _____ a. superficial.

    _____ b. full thickness.

    _____ c. partial thickness.

    _____ d. critical.

2. A cut in the skin and underlying soft tissue is called a(n):

    _____ a. hematoma.

    _____ b. laceration.

    _____ c. abrasion.

    _____ d. contusion.

3. The most important priority in treating a chemical burn is to:

    _____ a. flush with water for at least 20 minutes.

    _____ b. constantly reassess the airway.

    _____ c. ensure scene safety.

    _____ d. brush away dry chemicals.

4. Closed wounds pose a lower risk of infection than open wounds because they:

    _____ a. tend to be caused by less force.

    _____ b. occur only in extremities.

    _____ c. are protected by intact skin.

    _____ d. swell and promote the immune response.

5. Which of the following would be the best choice to control bleeding?

    _____ a. Sterile gauze embedded with petroleum jelly

    _____ b. Sterile gauze lightly moistened with saline

    _____ c. Sterile gauze embedded with antibiotic cream

    _____ d. Sterile gauze embedded with hemostatic agent

Short Answer

1. Describe the steps in caring for an amputated body part.

    _____

    _____

    _____

2. Describe a full-thickness burn.

    _____

    _____

    _____

Critical Thinking

1. Why would it be important to recover the knife that inflicted a puncture wound?

    _____

    _____

    _____

2. A patient has been electrocuted while fixing a clothes dryer. You find him unconscious still lying on top of the dryer motor. Outline your treatment plan.

_____

_____

_____

3. A young woman has a large laceration on her face. The bleeding is controlled and you have effectively bandaged the wound. What additional issues regarding this type of wound should you consider?

_____

_____

_____

Case Study

You are the EMR called to assist a 39-year-old male who was stabbed in the back with an unknown object. He has a 1-inch puncture wound in the middle of his back just to the right of his spine and the bleeding is controlled on arrival.

1. Describe the steps of your primary assessment.

_____

_____

_____

2. Are there immediate actions required to treat this wound? If so, what are they?

_____

_____

_____

3. What concerns do you have with regard to the type and location of this wound?

_____

_____

_____

Injuries to the Head and Spine

NAVIGATION GUIDE

The following items provide an overview to the purpose and content of this chapter. The Education Standard and Competency are from the National EMS Education Standards.

Education Standard Trauma (Head, Facial, Neck, and Spine Trauma)

Competency Uses simple knowledge to recognize and manage life threats based on assessment findings for an acutely injured patient while awaiting additional emergency medical response.

Knowledge Area Head, Facial, Neck, and Spine Trauma
- Life threats
- Spine trauma

Objectives After reading this chapter, you should be able to:

1. Define key terms introduced in this chapter.
2. Describe the anatomy and physiology of the axial skeleton.
3. Describe the characteristics of each of the following types of conditions:
   a. Concussion
   b. Skull fracture
   c. Brain injury
   d. Increased pressure within the skull
4. Prioritize the steps of assessment and treatment in patients with suspected head injuries.
5. Explain special considerations in the assessment and management of each of the following:
   a. Penetrating wounds to the head
   b. Injuries to the face, ears, nose, and throat
   c. Injuries to the eyes
6. Recognize mechanisms of injury associated with risk of spinal cord injury.

7. Demonstrate the implementation of spinal precautions.
8. Recognize signs and symptoms of a spinal cord injury.
9. Prioritize the steps of assessment and management of patients with injuries to the spine.
10. Recognize indications that rapid extrication of a trauma patient is required.
11. If allowed in your scope of practice, demonstrate the following skills:
    a. Application of a rigid cervical immobilization device
    b. Spinal immobilization using a long backboard
    c. Spinal immobilization of a seated patient
    d. Rapid extrication of a trauma patient
    e. Removal of a helmet from a patient with a head or spinal injury

NAVIGATION GUIDE *(continued)*

Key Terms Page numbers indicate first major use in this chapter. The Margin Glossary in this chapter provides definitions as you read.

axial skeleton, p. 505

cerebrospinal fluid, p. 505

vertebrae, p. 506

articulation, p. 506

posturing, p. 508

foramen magnum, p. 508

herniation, p. 508

Cushing triad, p. 508

concussion, p. 508

battle sign, p. 510

raccoon eyes, p. 510

orbit, p. 514

rigid eye shield, p. 515

unstable fracture, p. 519

secondary injury, p. 519

neutral position, p. 521

Media Resources Please go to **www.bradybooks.com** to access mykit for this text. You will find quizzes, critical thinking scenarios, weblinks, animations, and videos related to this chapter—and much more. Look for online information on spinal cord injuries. You will also find animations and video clips on cervical injuries and application of a cervical collar.

INTRODUCTION

The **axial skeleton** consists of the skull, spinal column, and rib cage. These components protect and house the most important parts of the body, including the nervous system, the brain, and the heart and lungs. Injuries to the axial skeleton and especially to the underlying vital organs are often among the most life threatening. Aside from immediate life threats, however, injuries to the brain and spine can have serious long-term consequences that can be made worse by improper prehospital care. As an EMR you must recognize and treat immediate problems but at the same time consider the potential for long-term disability and treat in a manner that prevents you from making such an injury worse (Figures 21-1a and 21-1b ■).

> **axial skeleton** the skull, spinal column, and rib cage.

CASE STUDY

THE CALL

It is a sunny day in July. The temperature is 90 degrees with high humidity. You are called to a local public pool for a "diving-related injury." Dispatch tells you the patient has been removed from the water by bystanders.

■ Discussion: *If dispatch does not have more information at this time, what will you assume from this information?*

ASK YOURSELF

- Can you define key terms introduced in this chapter?
- How would you describe the anatomy and physiology of the axial skeleton?

Anatomy

The brain is responsible for control of all body functions, and the spinal cord is the message pathway. The brain is housed in a closed container called the skull and surrounded by liquid called **cerebrospinal fluid**. The skull provides rigid protection, and the cerebrospinal fluid acts as a shock absorber. Although the skull protects the brain well, it is a

> **cerebrospinal fluid** the protective liquid that surrounds the brain and spinal cord.

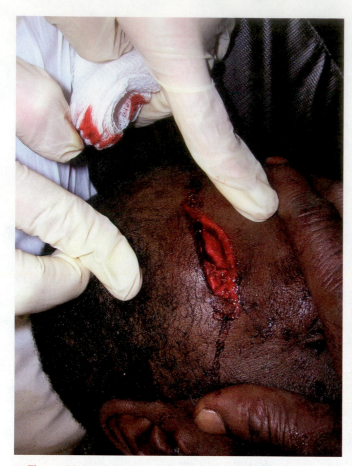

■ **Figure 21-1a** Serious head injury. (© Edward T. Dickinson, MD)

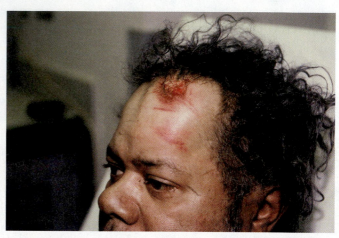

■ **Figure 21-1b** Minor head injury. (© Edward T. Dickinson, MD)

vertebrae the individual bones of the spinal column.

articulation two bones moving together (as in a joint).

closed container. Swelling or bleeding inside it can cause pressure to build and seriously injure the brain as a result.

The spinal cord extends from the base of the brain to the small of the back and is the primary route of travel for messages going to and from the brain. The cord itself is very fragile and would be easy to injure; however, it is extremely well protected by 33 stacked bones called **vertebrae**. These bones make up the spinal column. All 33 bones are connected by ligaments, padded in between by cartilage and protected by muscle. Although they are all connected, the individual bones are able to twist and bend together in a process called **articulation**. This allows for a person to twist, bend over, or lean back. Sometimes, however, excessive movement can cause injury. When major force (mechanism of injury) causes movement beyond the normal range or in an abnormal direction, the cord itself can be damaged by bones being shifted from their normal path of articulation. An example of this would be a hyperextension neck injury resulting from a rear-end motor vehicle crash. In this case the force of the crash throws the head backward as the body moves forward. If the force is great enough, the neck extends beyond the normal range it can articulate (hyperextend) and causes an injury.

The spinal column is commonly subdivided into five regions: the cervical, the thoracic, the lumbar, the sacral, and the coccygeal (Figure 21-2 ■).

The head is a large and heavy object, and the seven vertebrae of the cervical region bear its weight. Because of the relative weight of the head and the relatively small bones of this region, the cervical spine is especially vulnerable to outside force and is a common site of spinal injury. You should always consider forced movement of the head to be a potential mechanism of cervical spinal injury.

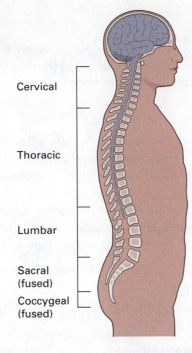

Cervical

Thoracic

Lumbar

Sacral
(fused)

Coccygeal
(fused)

■ **Figure 21-2** Regions of the spine.

There are 12 bones of the thoracic region, each connected to a right and left rib. These vertebrae are larger compared to the cervical bones and with the support of the rib cage provide excellent protection for the spinal cord. This area has the lowest frequency of blunt spinal injuries but can be threatened in penetrating trauma like gunshot wounds.

The lumbar region bears the weight of the body, and the five vertebrae that make up the region are the largest of the spinal column. This region is vulnerable to compression-related injuries such as when the bones of the spine are compressed together when a person lands after falling from a height. This area is also commonly responsible for long-term/chronic injuries (especially injuries related to the cartilage disks that pad the lumbar spine) that disable many EMS professionals each year as a result of poor lifting technique.

The sacral and coccygeal regions comprise the remaining nine vertebrae and form what we commonly refer to as the tailbone and posterior side of the pelvis. Under normal circumstances, these bones are fused together and move very little. However, they can be vulnerable to injuries from falls.

When you assess and treat major injuries to the head and neck, you should immediately think of the brain and spinal cord. However, you should also remember that this region contains other vital structures including the airway, major blood vessels, and the eyes.

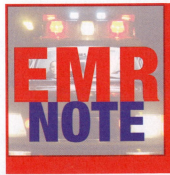

EMR NOTE

Although we do not typically consider an eye injury as life threatening, loss of vision is a major disabling injury and the possibility that an eye injury can lead to sight loss should be taken very seriously.

Head Injuries

Head injuries can be divided into two categories: open and closed. Unlike soft tissue injuries, however, closed or open does not refer just to the skin. Rather, closed or open head injuries refer to whether or not the skull has been fractured.

Closed Head Injuries

ASK YOURSELF

- How would you describe the characteristics of each of the following types of conditions?
  - Concussion
  - Skull fracture
  - Brain injury
  - Increased pressure within the skull

In a closed head injury the skull has not been fractured. Because the skull is a closed container, a closed injury is often the more serious and more life-threatening injury. Although the skull may still be intact, the force of injury may have damaged the brain tissue within the container. Injuries from the brain striking the inside of the skull include bruising, swelling, and even bleeding. The limited space available within the skull can be a serious threat to brain tissue if pressure builds. Even though the skull and even the scalp may look undamaged, injury to the brain itself may be severe. Signs of brain injury include:

- Altered mental status (Changes may include a range from confusion and anxiety to true unresponsiveness.)
- Weakness, numbness, or inability to move one side of the body
- Vision problems
- **Posturing**—involuntary movement (flexion or extension) of the patient's limbs that occurs either spontaneously or in response to pain
- Pupil changes—unequal, sluggish, or fixed in response to light
- Loss of balance or difficulty walking
- Nausea and vomiting after the injury

posturing involuntary movement (flexion or extension) of the patient's limbs that occurs either spontaneously or in response to pain.

foramen magnum the hole at the base of the skull where the spinal cord connects to the brainstem.

herniation pressure forcing the upper portions of the brain downward and through the foramen magnum.

Cushing triad the three trends in vital signs denoting increasing intracranial pressure: decreasing pulse rate, increasing blood pressure, and abnormal respiratory patterns.

concussion a blow to the head that temporarily interrupts the function of the brain.

If pressure inside the skull builds, the brain can be compressed. If unrelieved, this extreme pressure can force the upper portions of the brain downward and/or the brain to be forced through a hole in the base of the skull called the **foramen magnum** in a process called **herniation**. Because the area of the brain that sits atop the foramen magnum (the brainstem) is responsible for most of the involuntary and vital functions of the body including heart rate and breathing, damage to this area quickly causes death. Signs of herniation include:

- A profoundly altered and decreasing mental status
- A trend in vital signs known as the **Cushing triad**
  - Decreasing pulse rate
  - Increasing blood pressure
  - Abnormal respiratory patterns
- Posturing
- Changes to pupil response

When assessing a patient with a brain injury, you may not see all the signs immediately; however, multiple signs presenting together is truly an ominous finding. More often though a brain injury is progressive. That is, the signs develop and worsen over time. In fact, herniation is typically identified by assessing the patient over time and noticing changes or trends. You should constantly reassess a patient with a potential brain injury because the picture you see immediately may be very different from the one you see just a few minutes later.

EMR Patient Assessment: Concussion

ASK YOURSELF

- What are the steps of assessment and management of patients with injuries to the spine?

A blow to the head can temporarily interrupt the function of the brain. This condition is known as a **concussion**. Typical signs and symptoms include:

- Brief loss of consciousness
- Temporary confusion or altered mental status
- Amnesia (especially of the moments before or immediately after the event)
- Repetitive questioning
- Seizure
- Nausea and vomiting
- Incontinence

Signs of a concussion indicate brain injury and should therefore always be taken seriously.

Open Head Injuries

In an open head injury, skin has been broken and the skull has been fractured. In some cases it is actually better for a head injury patient to fracture his skull as this allows more room for the brain to swell or bleed. However, massive injuries can still occur.

EMR Patient Assessment: Open Head Injuries

Signs and symptoms of a fractured skull include (Figure 21-3 ■):

- Obvious deformity or visible fracture
- Pain or tenderness at the point of impact
- Cerebrospinal fluid (CSF) leaking from the ears, nose, mouth, or even the wound itself—presents as clear or blood-tinged (slightly pink) fluid
- Pupil changes

ASK YOURSELF

- What are the steps of assessment and treatment in patients with suspected head injuries?

SIGNS AND SYMPTOMS OF SKULL FRACTURE

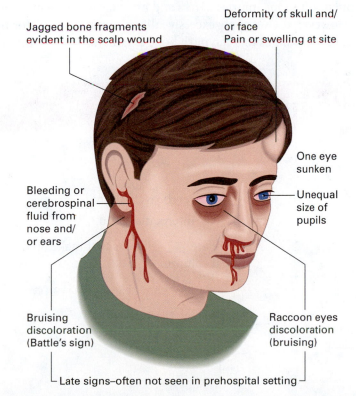

Jagged bone fragments evident in the scalp wound

Deformity of skull and/ or face
Pain or swelling at site

One eye sunken

Unequal size of pupils

Bleeding or cerebrospinal fluid from nose and/ or ears

Bruising discoloration (Battle's sign)

Raccoon eyes discoloration (bruising)

Late signs–often not seen in prehospital setting

■ **Figure 21-3** Signs and symptoms of a skull fracture.

- **Battle sign**—bruising behind the ears (a delayed sign)
- **Raccoon eyes**—bruising around the eyes (similar to black eyes, also a delayed sign)
- Signs and symptoms of a brain injury (Although the open head injury may be visually dramatic, the most significant injury may lie underneath. The brain is your ultimate concern when treating a head injury patient.)

EMR Emergency Care: Head Injuries

Your treatment priorities will focus on the vital organs and the functions that keep people alive. The most important aspect of head injury treatment is airway and breathing management.

- Beware of airway and breathing problems and treat accordingly. Secondary hypoxia (low oxygen related to airway and breathing problems) is a leading killer of head injury patients. Remember that injuries to the brain can affect the control centers for airway and respiration. Your first priority is to make sure your patient has an airway and is breathing adequately. If you find a problem with either of these areas, you might take action immediately.
- Suspect and stabilize potential spinal injuries. Injuries that apply force to the head often also apply force to the spine. We will discuss stabilization and treatment of spinal injuries later in this chapter.
- Reassess, reassess, reassess. Your patient can often deteriorate over time—sometimes rapidly, sometimes gradually. Your constant reassessment will help identify patterns and trends that will allow you to recognize ominous signs of pressure building in the skull (rising intracranial pressure, or ICP). Additionally, some signs of head injury occur later than the immediate event. Mental status changes, raccoon eyes, Battle sign, and even some pupil changes can occur long after the initial injury and will require your ongoing attention to find.
- Care for open soft tissue injuries. Dress and bandage wounds and control bleeding. However, do not apply excessive direct pressure to a deformity or depression of the skull as this can push bone fragments into the brain.

✳ Stop, Review, Remember

Multiple Choice

Place a check next to the correct answer.

1. Which of the following bones is a component of the axial skeleton?

    ____ a. Skull

    ____ b. Pelvis

    ____ c. Femur

    ____ d. Radius

2. The liquid that surrounds the brain and spinal cord and acts as a shock absorber is called:

    ____ a. amniotic fluid.

    ____ b. serous fluid.

    ____ c. cerebrospinal fluid.

    ____ d. interocular fluid.

3. There are ____ bones that make up the spinal column.

    ____ a. 22

    ____ b. 33

    ____ c. 37

    ____ d. 11

4. The _____ region of the spine bears the weight of the body and has the largest vertebrae.

_____ a. cervical

_____ b. thoracic

_____ c. lumbar

_____ d. sacral

5. A large laceration to the scalp that has an associated fractured skull would be considered a(n):

_____ a. open head injury.

_____ b. contusion.

_____ c. abrasion.

_____ d. closed head injury.

Emergency Medical Responder Practice

1. List three signs or symptoms of a brain injury:

   a. _____

   b. _____

   c. _____

2. List three signs or symptoms of a skull fracture:

   a. _____

   b. _____

   c. _____

Short Answer

1. Explain the term *herniation* and describe how you would identify the process in a head injury patient.

   _____

   _____

   _____

   _____

2. Explain specifically why airway and breathing are often threatened in a brain injury patient.

   _____

   _____

   _____

   _____

3. Explain why constant reassessment is particularly important when dealing with a brain injury patient.

   _____

   _____

   _____

   _____

Special Circumstances

Certain types of head injuries require special attention and treatment. In the following section we will review some specific situations that require special care.

ASK YOURSELF

- What are the special considerations in the assessment and management of each of the following?
  - Penetrating wounds to the head
  - Injuries to the face, ears, nose, and throat
  - Injuries to the eyes

EMR Patient Assessment and Care: Penetrating Wounds

Penetrating wounds to the head are always a serious emergency. Just as with penetrating trauma in other places in the body, it is not the wound itself that concerns us, but rather the damage done beneath the wound. In the case of penetrating trauma to the head, the damage is inflicted upon the brain and therefore can have both immediate and long-term life-threatening consequences. If the wound is bleeding, allow blood to drain. If there is an impaled object, do not remove it. Stabilize the object in place using bulky dressings and arrange for immediate transport.

EMR Patient Assessment and Care: Face, Ears, Nose, and Throat

Injuries to the face can be both life threatening and life altering. Immediate life threats include threats to the airway and large blood vessels of the neck. Although other injuries to the face may not be life threatening, you should consider the concerns of a patient who has injured a part of his body that defines who he is. These types of injuries are often more emotionally traumatic than physically traumatic. Your empathy and attention to the emotional side of the call may be the most important treatment.

EMR Patient Assessment and Care: Soft Tissue Injuries of the Face

Beware that soft tissue injuries of the face may be a sign of a brain injury. Although we generally think of the rest of the head when we assess for fractures and brain injuries, the face is the front part of the skull and injuries to it can pose a serious risk to the underlying brain tissue. Do not allow visually dramatic injuries to distract you from more life-threatening primary assessment problems or more potentially serious brain injuries (Figures 21-4a to 21-4c ■).

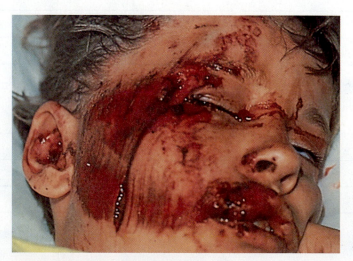

■ Figure 21-4a Injury to the face.

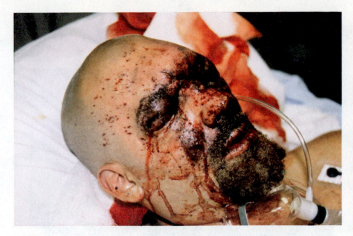

■ Figure 21-4b Blast injury to the face. *(© Edward T. Dickinson, MD)*

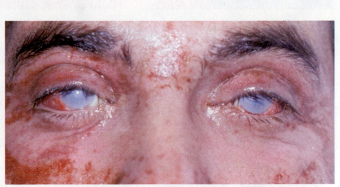

■ Figure 21-4c Injury to the face with damage to both eyes. *(© Chris Barry/PhototakeUSA)*

Soft tissue injuries to the mouth, tongue, and cheek can threaten the airway. Cheek injuries are rarely life threatening but bleeding can obstruct air movement. Suction appropriately and remove objects that have penetrated through the cheek.

Ear injuries often include major and even simple amputations. Treat such injuries as you would any other soft tissue injury (see Chapter 20).

The nose is a commonly broken bone in the face. Remember that the nose is part of the airway and bleeding can threaten air movement. When possible, position your patient sitting forward to promote drainage of blood. Do not attempt to remove foreign objects from the nose.

The jaw can be broken or dislocated, and injuries to this area are often an immediate threat to the airway. Suction appropriately. Signs of injury to the jaw include:

■ Difficulty opening or closing the mouth

■ Difficulty swallowing

■ Difficulty speaking

■ Difficulty closing the jaw properly (misaligned teeth on closing the mouth)

■ Pain, tenderness, or deformity in the area around the ears

■ Missing or dislodged teeth

If a tooth has been knocked out, transport it with the patient as often it can be replaced. Do not touch the roots. If necessary, rinse off debris with tap water and place the tooth in a glass of milk (if available). If milk is not available, wrap the tooth in gauze moistened with sterile saline.

Dentures should be left in place unless they are broken or their alignment causes a threat to the airway. If they are causing a problem, remove them and transport them with the patient.

EMR Patient Assessment and Care: Neck Injuries

Neck injuries pose the risk of severe bleeding. Major blood vessels are close to the surface and relatively exposed in the neck, and injury to them can be a major life threat. Large neck veins, when lacerated, can also pull air in and form a bubble in the bloodstream. This condition is called a pulmonary embolism. To avoid air entering a wound, you should apply an occlusive dressing followed by a protective bulky dressing. Apply direct pressure to one side at a time (to avoid cutting off blood flow to the brain) and never wrap a pressure dressing around the neck (Scan 21-1).

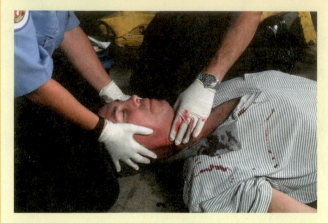

21-1a Apply pressure and seal wound with a gloved hand. Do not apply pressure on both sides of the neck at the same time.

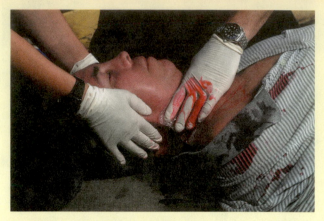

21-1b Place an occlusive dressing.

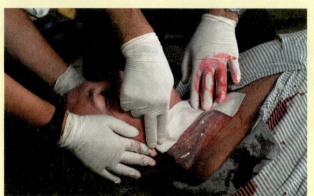

21-1c Seal the wound with tape on all four sides.

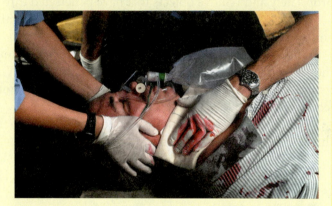

21-1d Cover the occlusive dressing. Continue to apply pressure.

Blunt trauma can also cause serious injuries to the neck. Swelling as a result of the injury can be a major threat to the airway immediately or even later on. Ominous signs include difficulty speaking or hoarseness, stridor, or any partial or complete airway obstruction. Transport should be an immediate concern.

EMR Patient Assessment: Eye Injuries

Although rarely life threatening, eye injuries pose a serious risk to vision and are potentially life altering. Therefore, you should consider them a true emergency. Injuries can occur to the soft tissue surrounding the eye (including the eyelid), to the bony structure that houses the eye (called the **orbit**), or to the eyeball itself. Your assessment should check for the following:

orbit the bony structure that houses the eye.

- Tenderness or deformity of the orbits
- Soft tissue injuries around the eye, including the eyelid (Note that soft tissue injuries to the eyelid may include injuries to the globe itself.)
- Foreign objects in the mucous membrane surrounding the eye or on the eye itself
- Injuries to the globe (the eyeball)

- Pupil reactivity
- Double vision
- Inability to move the eye normally

EMR Emergency Care: Eye Injuries

- If you need to dress or cover one eye, cover the other as well. Eyes move together, and covering the unaffected eye will help prevent unnecessary movement of the affected eye.
- Apply only enough gentle direct pressure to control bleeding of soft tissue injuries around the eye or injuries of the eyelid.
- Never apply direct pressure to the eyelid if the globe is affected or to the globe itself.
- Do not remove blood clots from the eye if they have formed.
- Do not force open an eye unless you need to flush out chemicals.
- Do not flush out an eye unless you are flushing out chemicals. Follow local protocol, but significant damage to the eye can be done by flushing if the eye has been perforated.

EMR Patient Assessment and Care: Foreign Objects in the Eye

Small particles and foreign objects in the eye can cause pain, tearing, and sensitivity to light as well as put the eye at risk for infection and even scarring of the cornea. Some EMS systems allow for removal of foreign objects. Always follow local protocol. The following steps may be helpful in removing foreign objects:

- Flush the eye with clean water (follow local protocol).
- Visualize the foreign object (either under the lower lid or under the upper lid) and remove the object with the corner of a piece of sterile gauze. Consider turning the upper lid over a cotton swab to provide better access.
- Use the lashes of the lower lid to clear a foreign object on the upper lid. Gently grasp the upper lid and draw it down over the lower lid.

If a foreign object cannot be removed, use a **rigid eye shield** (a special cup designed to protect the eye) to cover the eye and arrange transport. Also, consider covering the unaffected eye to minimize movement. *Never* allow a patient to rub the affected eye.

rigid eye shield
a special cup designed to protect the eye.

EMR Patient Assessment and Care: Impaled Objects in the Eye

An impaled object is a major threat to function of the eye including vision (Figure 21-5a ■). You should take extreme care to minimize further damage. Never remove an impaled object in the eye. Stabilize the object in place, but be very careful not to move the object. Use bulky dressings, a cone, a cup, or a rigid eye shield to protect the impaled object and bandage both eyes to prevent movement.

Always consider the emotional impact of an eye injury or even the impact of having to bandage both eyes. In this situation, your patient will be unable to see the procedures and will rely upon you to keep calm. Consider this emotional care as an essential component of your treatment.

EMR Patient Assessment and Care: Globe Injuries and Extruding Eyeballs

If the eyeball itself is injured, gently cover the eye with a sterile dressing and arrange transport. Do not apply direct pressure. Cover both eyes to limit movement.

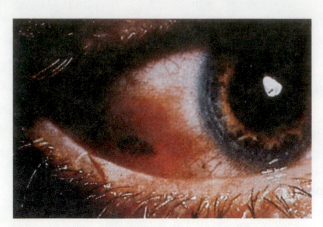

■ **Figure 21-5a** Foreign object lodged in the eye.

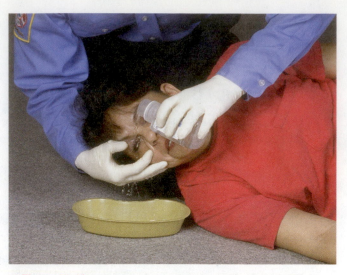

■ **Figure 21-5b** Flushing a foreign object from the eye.

In certain injuries, an eyeball can actually be extruded from the orbit (knocked out of the socket). Do not attempt to replace it. You should cover it with a dressing moistened with sterile saline and arrange for immediate transport.

EMR Patient Assessment and Care: Orbit Injuries

Injuries to the orbit may be recognized by obvious deformity of the bones surrounding the eye, or when a patient complains of difficulty moving his eye, double or impaired vision, or even numbness around the eye.

EMR Patient Assessment and Care: Chemical Burns to the Eye

A burning chemical in the eye is causing damage every minute it is in place. Your immediate action is essential in stopping this injury. When you treat a chemical burn to the eye, remember that timing is everything. Immediately flushing the affected eye removes or dilutes the offending chemical and stops or at least lessens the burning process (Figure 21-5b ■).

Use personal protective equipment to protect yourself from the burning chemicals. Remember that what is burning your patient probably could burn you. Flush the eye with sterile or clean water. If sterile water is not available, use ordinary tap water. Flush from the bridge of the nose outward and away from the unaffected eye. (Note that flushing in the opposite direction will carry the chemicals into the other eye.) Flush continuously for 30 to 60 minutes. If the patient cannot open his eye, you may have to assist (unless there is soft tissue damage to the eye itself). Opening the eye may be painful, but flushing the chemical away is very important (Figure 21-6 ■). You may also consider removing contact lenses if local protocol allows.

EMR Patient Assessment and Care: Removing a Contact Lens

In some cases of chemical burns, removing a contact lens is extremely important to avoid trapping the chemical between it and the eye. Follow local protocol as to when to remove lenses.

To remove a contact lens:

- Open the eyelid.
- Gently press down and forward on the edges of the lens to free it from the surface of the eye. Note: Applying drops of saline may help if you are not already flushing.
- Slide the lens out of the eye.
- Remove the lens and put it in a safe place.

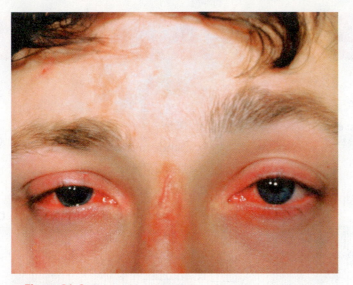

■ **Figure 21-6** Chemical burns to the eyes.

THE RESPONSE

You arrive to find a crowd gathered around an 18-year-old boy lying on the concrete deck of the pool. He does not appear to be moving. As you approach, bystanders tell you that he dove into a shallow part of the pool and had to be assisted out.

Your partner assumes manual spinal stabilization, and you begin your assessment.

You find the patient wet and shivering. He is responsive and answers your questions. He tells you his neck hurts. Your assessment finds a patent airway, normal breathing, and a rapid radial pulse. He is alert and oriented and did not lose consciousness.

His vital signs are pulse 116, respirations 24, and blood pressure 118/76.

Your secondary assessment finds tenderness in his posterior neck along the spinal column and good distal circulatory, sensory, and motor function in all four extremities.

Although he appears stable, the mechanism of injury concerns you. He tells you when he dove into the pool he struck his head and hurt his neck. He notes he had a difficult time swimming and needed help getting out. You decide to continue holding manual stabilization and await the responding EMT transport crew.

■ Discussion: *What should you say to this patient if he asks if he'll become paralyzed?*

Multiple Choice

Place a check next to the correct answer.

1. The bony structure that houses the eye is otherwise known as the:

   _____ a. mandible.

   _____ b. maxilla.

   _____ c. orbit.

   _____ d. hyoid.

2. When dealing with a head injury patient with dentures, you should:

   _____ a. remove the dentures only if they are broken or obstruct the airway.

   _____ b. never remove the dentures.

   _____ c. always remove the dentures.

   _____ d. leave the dentures in place as they provide splinting of the jaw.

3. Which of the following would be the most concerning sign following blunt trauma to the neck?

   _____ a. Pain

   _____ b. Tenderness

   _____ c. Difficulty speaking

   _____ d. Redness

4. The bony structure that forms the socket of the eye is called the:

   _____ a. globe.

   _____ b. maxilla.

   _____ c. orbit.

   _____ d. cornea.

5. When treating an extruded eyeball you should:

   _____ a. replace it in the socket.

   _____ b. apply direct pressure.

   _____ c. wrap the eyeball in a dry dressing.

   _____ d. never replace it in the socket.

Emergency Medical Responder Practice

1. List three signs or symptoms of jaw injury:

   a. _____

   b. _____

   c. _____

2. List three signs or symptoms of a fractured orbit:

   a. _____

   b. _____

   c. _____

Short Answer

1. Explain the steps in transporting a tooth that has been forcibly knocked out.

   _____

   _____

   _____

2. Explain the steps in dealing with a large neck laceration.

_____

_____

_____

_____

3. Describe a method of removing a foreign body from a patient's eye.

_____

_____

_____

Spinal Injuries

ASK YOURSELF

- How do you recognize mechanisms of injury associated with risk of spinal cord injury?

When dealing with spinal injuries, you must consider not only the immediate life threats the injury may pose but also the need to prevent further injuries, especially injuries that may be worsened by movement and handling of the patient. A severe spinal injury is a tragic event. Even if the patient survives, the injury may forever impact the patient's life. We must take every possible precaution to prevent further injury and ensure the best possible outcome.

The spinal cord is well protected but truly a fragile organ. When significant force is applied, major injury can occur. The spinal cord can be completely severed (transected), partially severed, or even damaged by swelling. In any of these cases, the injury may have a major impact on the body's ability to transmit and receive messages through the nervous system. Paralysis, disruption of the nervous system, and even death can occur.

On occasion, the force applied may break the bones of the spinal column (vertebrae) but not initially impact the spinal cord. If the broken bones are loose and uncontrolled, this injury would be referred to as an **unstable fracture**. The concern with an unstable fracture is that broken bone ends may be jagged, and movement of the spinal column may push those jagged bone ends into the soft and fragile spinal cord tissue, resulting in a **secondary injury** (an injury that occurs as a result of movement after the injury). With this in mind, you must handle potentially spinal injured patients very carefully and protect against secondary injury.

unstable fracture broken bones that are loose and uncontrolled.

secondary injury an injury that occurs as a result of movement after the original injury.

Assume Spinal Cord Injury

It is very difficult for an emergency responder to definitively rule out a spinal cord injury. As a result, you should always assume the presence of such an injury and err on the side of caution. Overtreating a patient rarely causes more harm than undertreating.

Mechanism of Injury

Not every injured patient has a spinal cord injury. Certain mechanisms of injury make spinal injuries more likely. Learn to assess the scene in addition to the patient to help predict the potential for spinal injury (Figure 21-7 ■).

ASK YOURSELF

- With another student, how would you demonstrate the implementation of spinal precautions?
- What are the signs and symptoms of a spinal cord injury?

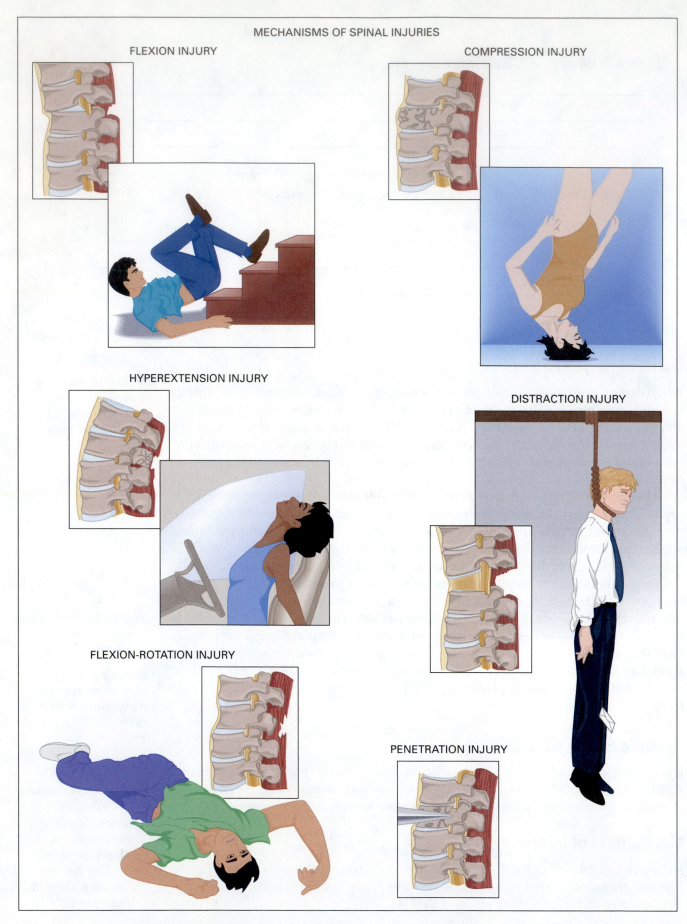

Figure 21-7 Common mechanisms of spine injury.

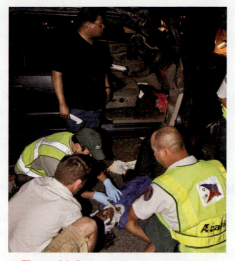

Figure 21-8 Maintain manual stabilization.

Spinal Precautions

The general principle of preventing a secondary spinal injury is the idea of in-line neutral position. That means we desire to keep the 33 bones of the spinal column aligned in an anatomical position so that jagged bone ends are not moving. Keep in mind, however, that while all 33 bones are considered connected, moving one may have the potential to move another bone even in another region of the spinal column.

The most immediate concern is to stabilize the head (recall that the head is a heavy object supported by the small bones of the cervical region). To stabilize a patient's head, first tell the patient to not move his head. Next, describe what you are about to do. Then you should place both your gloved hands on either side of the patient's head. This will immediately prevent movement. With spread fingers, hold the head in an in-line, neutral position (Figure 21-8 ■). **Neutral position** means that the head is neither flexed forward nor extended back, and *in line* means that the patient's nose is in line with the belly button. This position is natural and anatomical and keeps the bones aligned properly. Stabilization must be maintained until another trained provider takes over or until the patient is fully secured to a spinal immobilization device. If you find a patient's head in a position other than neutral and in line, you should gently return the head to the appropriate position. Stop movement if resistance is met or if a conscious patient complains of a severe increase in pain.

In addition to the head, always think of neutral, in-line position when moving or handling a spinal injury patient. All movements should be designed to minimize any alignment other than neutral, in-line position. That means the spine should always move as a single unit and the patient should avoid flexion/extension, lateral bending, and twisting.

neutral position the head is neither flexed forward nor extended back.

EMR Patient Assessment: Spinal Cord Injury

Besides mechanism of injury, your assessment may reveal signs of potential injury. These signs and symptoms may include:

- Pain or tenderness over the area of the spinal column
- Pain with movement (Do *not* ask the patient to move, however.)
- Numbness or tingling in the arms or legs
- Paralysis or difficulty moving any of the extremities
- Loss of sensation in the extremities
- Incontinence (loss of bowel or bladder control)

- Priapism (a constant erection of the penis)
- Deformity of the spine (Because of significant muscle support, this finding is very rare.)

Injuries to the head and neck can also indicate spinal injury. If the force was great enough to injure the head, it was probably great enough to injure the spine.

Keep in mind that other injuries may distract the patient from subtle signs of a spinal cord injury. Because of the potential consequences, in suspicious mechanisms of injury, even patients without assessment findings should be treated for a spinal injury.

ASK YOURSELF

- If allowed in your scope of practice, what are the steps of each of the following skills?
  - Application of a rigid cervical immobilization device
  - Spinal immobilization using a long backboard
  - Spinal immobilization of a seated patient
  - Rapid extrication of a trauma patient
  - Removal of a helmet from a patient with a head or spinal injury

EMR Emergency Care: The Spinal Cord Injury

- Treat the immediate life threats. Although spinal precautions are important, immediate life threats must be dealt with at the highest priority. Most of the time, however, multi-tasking is possible. For example, an airway can be opened using a jaw thrust as opposed to a head-tilt, chin-lift maneuver to account for spinal precautions. Unless you are alone, other providers can hold in-line stabilization while other procedures are performed.

- Take spinal precautions. In-line, neutral position should be the rule of thumb. Plan movements in advance to preserve this position.

- Utilize a thorough assessment to identify subtle signs of spinal injury.

- Immobilize if local protocol allows.

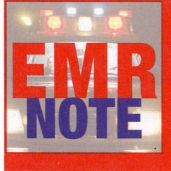

EMR NOTE

Not all systems allow emergency responders to immobilize a suspected spinal injury. In some situations, you can provide immobilization. In others, you may assist. Know your local protocol before you are on scene to make sure you are providing the correct care.

Spinal Immobilization

The principles of spinal immobilization follow the same ideas of stabilizing the head. Neutral, in-line position is desired and steps are taken to keep the patient in that position throughout transport. In this case, however, devices are used to assist in maintaining neutral, in-line position.

When assisting with immobilization, the key concept is keeping that in-line, neutral position. Always consider the entire spine. Spinal immobilization begins with neutral, in-line stabilization, and this manual immobilization needs to be continued until the patient is fully secured to a spinal immobilization device.

It is important to check circulatory, sensory, and motor function in four extremities before and after applying spinal immobilization to your patient (Scan 21-2). This check allows you to see initial problems (deficits) and can help identify problems caused by movement. To complete this exam, check pulses and/or capillary refill in the arms and feet. Check sensory function by touching the patient and asking him if he feels your touch. You might choose a lightly painful stimulus such as pinching for a patient with a decreased mental status. Finally ask the patient to wiggle his fingers and toes to assess motor function.

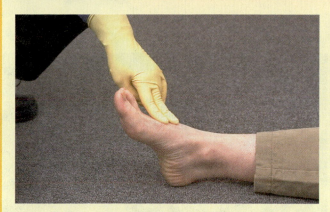

21-2a Feel for a pulse in all extremities.

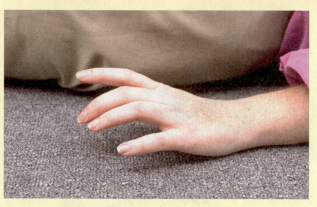

21-2b Ask the patient if she can move her hands.

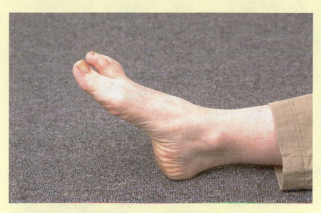

21-2c Ask the patient to move her foot.

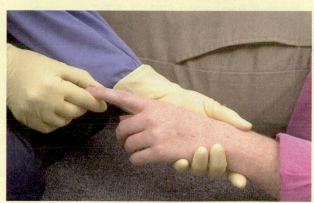

21-2d Touch a finger to assess sensation.

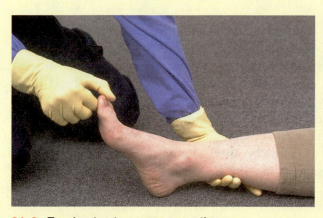

21-2e Touch a toe to assess sensation.

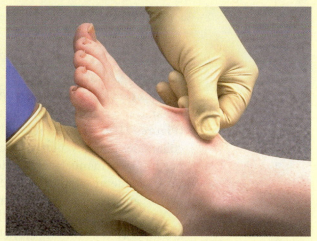

21-2f Pinch the top of a foot in an unresponsive patient to assess sensation through painful stimuli.

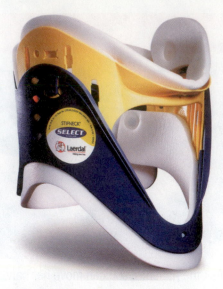

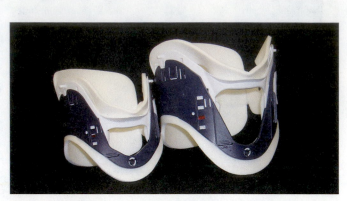

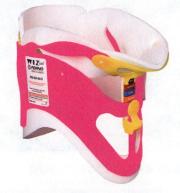

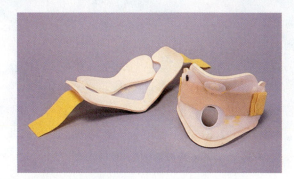

■ **Figure 21-9a** STIFNECK SELECT. *(Photography courtesy of Laerdal Medical Corporation)*

■ **Figure 21-9b** Philadelphia Cervical Collar.

■ **Figure 21-9c** WIZLOC Cervical Collar.

■ **Figure 21-9d** NEC-LOC rigid extrication collar.

Cervical Collars

A rigid cervical immobilization device also known as an extrication collar, a cervical collar (or c-collar) is applied to the neck to help splint the neck and head in place (Figures 21-9a to 21-9d ■). Only rigid cervical collars should be used in EMS. A cervical collar does not prevent movement but rather restricts movement, so even after it has been put in place, manual stabilization must be maintained. Be sure to follow the manufacturer's guidelines to properly fit all collars because an improper fit will render the collar useless and in some cases aggravate spinal injuries.

Application should also follow the manufacturer's guidelines, but in general, collars are supported by the jaw, clavicles, and shoulders. Placing a C-Collar on a supine patient generally requires you to pass the posterior portion of the collar through the natural gap behind the patient's neck. Once this is accomplished, the anterior portion can be positioned under the chin and the Velcro strap adjusted to secure the device. On a seated or standing patient, the collar is generally applied by seating the anterior portion first under the chin and then wrapping the posterior portion around the neck. Never tug or pull so forcefully as to threaten in-line, neutral position. Again, the manufacturer's recommendations should be followed (Scan 21-3).

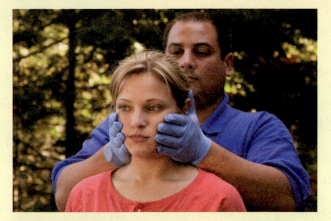

21-3a Stabilize the head.

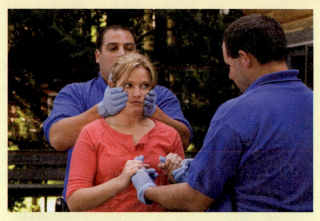

21-3b Check circulation, sensation, and movement.

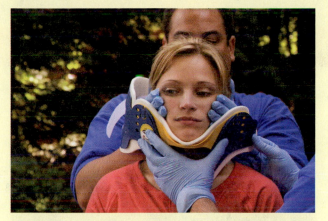

21-3c Apply collar—standing.

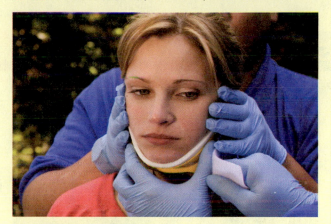

21-3d Fasten the collar.

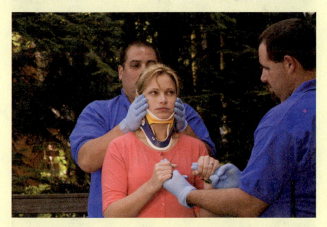

21-3e Check circulation, sensation, and movement.

Long Backboard Immobilization

A long backboard is a rigid, boardlike device designed for the transport of patients with suspected spinal injuries. The idea of the board is to provide a rigid splint to stabilize the entire length of the patient's body in order to keep all 33 bones of the spinal column from moving. The following are key concepts of successful long board immobilization:

- Maintain in-line position while moving the patient onto the device (see "Log Roll," which follows).

- Pad the void spaces. The spine is not naturally flat when a patient is lying down. Typically there are spaces created by the natural curvature of the spine. Apply simple padding (towels, blankets, and bulky dressings) to occupy these spaces and increase comfort for the patient.

- Secure the patient to eliminate flexion, extension, and lateral movement. Typically straps are used to secure the patient to the device. The order of strapping should be as follows: First secure the torso/pelvis. Next (and only after securing the torso) secure the head. Finally, secure the legs. Some systems recommend immobilization in the order: torso, legs then head. This is acceptable as long as the most important principle is followed: the head is always secured after the

SCAN 21-4 Application of Cervical Spine Collar on a Supine Patient

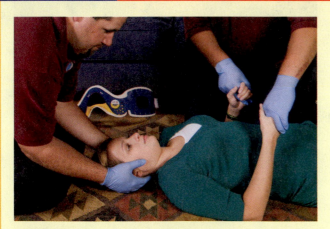

21-4a Stabilize the head and check circulation, sensation, and movement.

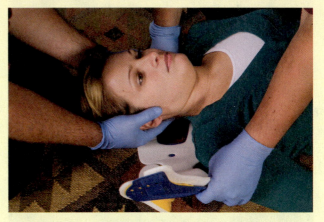

21-4b Begin by sliding the back of the collar under the patient's neck.

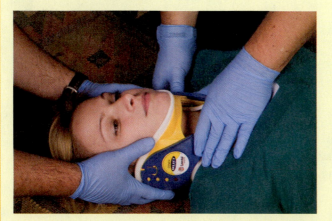

21-4c Move the front of the collar in place and fasten the Velcro strap(s).

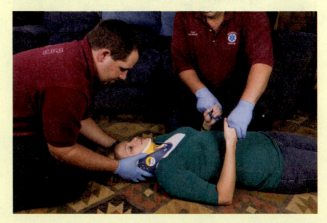

21-4d Check circulation, sensation, and movement with the collar on.

torso. Consider the idea that you are securing each of the centers of mass of the body (that is, the heaviest areas of the body). Proper immobilization needs to ensure that the chest, pelvis, and head are not capable of bending forward or back or shifting from side to side on the board. Often padding between the body and the connection points of the straps is required to eliminate the side-to-side movement. Chest straps should never be tight enough to impair breathing and the jaw should never be restricted in securing the head.

■ You should always check circulation, sensation, and movement in all four extremities prior to and after immobilization. This check allows you to see any initial deficits and to observe any changes that have resulted from immobilization (Scan 21-4).

Log Roll

The log roll is a technique used to move a patient onto a long board while maintaining in-line, neutral position. In this technique, the patient's body is moved as a single unit onto its side, the immobilization device is positioned, and then the patient's body is lowered back down onto the device, again as a unit (Scan 21-5).

Follow these steps to log roll a patient:

1. Manually stabilize the patient's head and apply a rigid cervical collar.
2. Assess circulation, sensation, and movement in all four extremities.
3. Position your team. One provider should continue to hold in-line stabilization of the head. This provider will direct the team's movements in order to keep the head in line with the rest of the body during movement. Two other providers should position themselves on the same side of the patient and reach across to grab the opposite side of the patient. One provider should grab the patient's shoulder and hip, and the other provider should grab the patient's upper thigh and lower leg. Coordinated movement is critical, so communication must be effective.
4. Upon the signal of the provider holding manual stabilization of the head, the team should roll the patient onto his side while keeping the body in line as a unit. The patient should be held in this position. This is an excellent time to assess the posterior surface of the patient if it has not been done already.
5. Position the device under the patient.
6. Upon the signal of the provider holding manual stabilization of the head, the team should roll the patient back down as a unit onto the immobilization device and onto his back.
7. Reassess circulation, sensation, and movement in all four extremities.

Never push a patient onto the backboard and never adjust your patient by pushing or pulling one section of the body. All movements must be done with the body in an in-line position and moving as a single unit.

EMR Emergency Care: The Seated Patient

A short backboard or short extrication device may be used to assist movement of a potentially spinal injured patient onto a long backboard. Follow the manufacturer's guidelines, but in general the following steps are utilized to apply a short backboard or extrication device:

1. Manually stabilize the patient's head and apply a rigid cervical collar.
2. Assess circulation, sensation, and movement in all four extremities.
3. Position the device behind the patient. Be careful not to jostle the patient while placing the device. Use the natural void spaces to gently shift the device into place. The bottom end of the device should be placed as far down into the seat as possible and the top should be level with the patient's head. If the device has body flaps, they should be positioned just below the armpits of the patient.

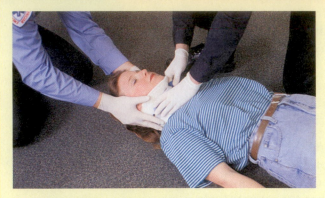

21-5a Stabilize the head and neck. Apply a cervical collar.

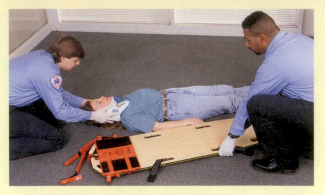

21-5b Place the board parallel to the patient.

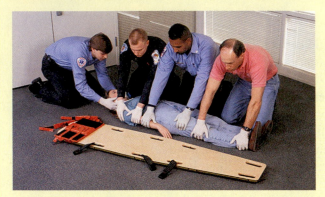

21-5c Place providers at the shoulder, waist, and knee. Continue to stabilize the head.

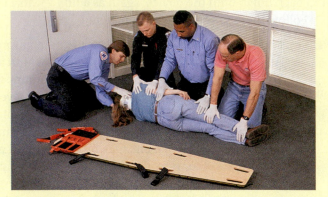

21-5d The person at the head and neck directs the others to roll the patient as a team.

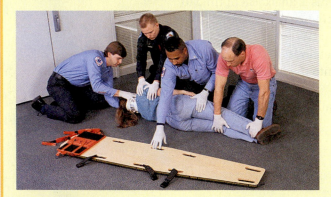

21-5e Position the board.

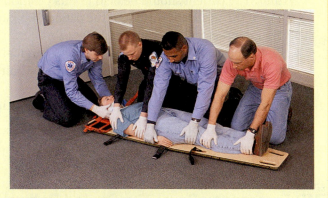

21-5f Roll the patient as a team onto the board.

4. Secure the device to the patient. Secure the torso first. If the device has leg straps, next secure the legs. Then, and only after the torso is secured, secure the head. Neutral alignment of the head may require you to place some padding between the device and the head.

Under normal circumstances the patient would next be moved to a long board. The long board is generally positioned next to the patient's buttocks and the patient is rotated and tilted back onto the board. If the extrication device has leg straps, they should be removed at this point. The patient should then be secured to the long board.

Rapid Extrication

Rapid extrication should only be performed when there is a critical need to remove the patient and using a short backboard or extrication device would take too much time. Examples of such situations would be an unsafe scene, a critical/unstable patient who needs immediate extrication, or a patient who is blocking access to other critical or unstable patients. Rapid extrication does not utilize a short board or extrication device, but rather uses only manual stabilization and teamwork to extricate the patient using short coordinated movements (Scan 21-6). This technique is generally performed with a minimum of three rescuers. To perform rapid extrication, follow these steps:

ASK YOURSELF

■ What are the indications that rapid extrication of a trauma patient is required?

1. Manually stabilize the patient's head and apply a rigid cervical collar.
2. The provider holding manual stabilization of the head will coordinate short, in-line movements to position the patient for extrication. The team will execute these short movements keeping the body as a whole in line and eventually rotate the patient so that his back faces the open door.
3. A long backboard is placed at the patient's buttocks so that the patient can be tilted back onto the board.
4. Using coordinated in-line movements, at the command of the provider holding manual stabilization of the head, the patient is lowered onto the backboard. (At this point it may be necessary to hand off in-line stabilization of the head to a provider outside of the vehicle.)
5. Secure the patient to the backboard.

Helmet Removal

Occasionally you will encounter a patient wearing a helmet. There is no absolute indication to remove a helmet unless it is interfering with assessment or treatment of the airway. In some cases, a sports helmet may have a face shield that can easily be unscrewed or snapped off to access the airway, so always check before you remove. At times a helmet may interfere with in-line spinal immobilization; however, often the combination of shoulder pads and a helmet provides very good in-line, neutral position. Always assess the need to remove a helmet carefully.

If a helmet must be removed from a suspected spinal injured patient, use the following steps (note this procedure requires at least two providers):

1. Stabilize the helmet. Place your gloved hands on either side. If possible, reach your fingers down to the lower areas of the head and jaw to ensure that the head is stabilized within the helmet.
2. Loosen and remove the chin strap.
3. Transfer manual stabilization to a second provider. The second provider should place his hands on the patient's jaw and on the back of the patient's head. It may be difficult, but the second provider should be able to maintain reasonable stabilization beneath the helmet.
4. Begin to remove the helmet. The provider removing the helmet should spread the sides of the helmet to clear the patient's ears and slide the helmet off until it is about halfway off.
5. Adjust in-line stabilization. At this point, the second provider should adjust his hand position to achieve better in-line stabilization. As the helmet is removed, the weight of the head will be increasingly transferred to the second rescuer. He must be prepared.
6. Remove the helmet completely.

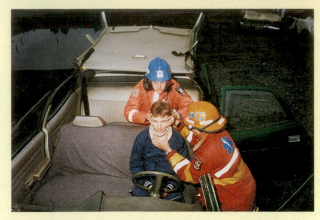

21-6a Stabilize the patient's head and neck. Apply a cervical collar.

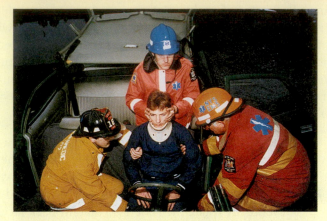

21-6b Carefully lift the patient enough to slide a long spine board between the patient and the seat.

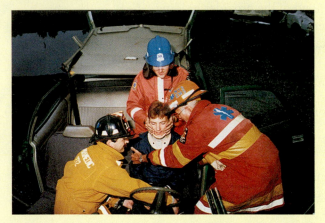

21-6c The rescuers reposition their hands so that one holds the patient's legs and pelvis while the other holds the upper chest and arms.

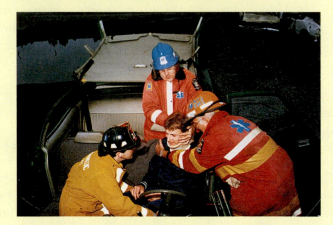

21-6d At the direction of the one stabilizing the head and neck, carefully turn the patient so his back is toward the door of the vehicle.

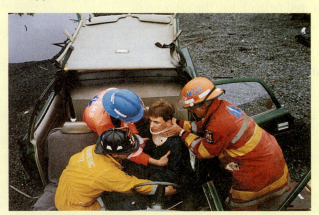

21-6e The team should reposition their hands but continue head and neck stabilization.

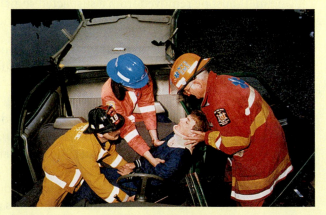

21-6f Gently lower the patient to the spine board.

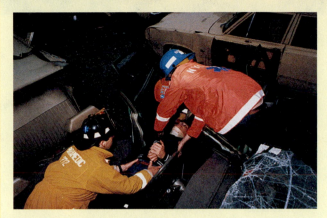

Scan 21-6g As an additional rescuer holds the end of the board, slide the patient on the board.

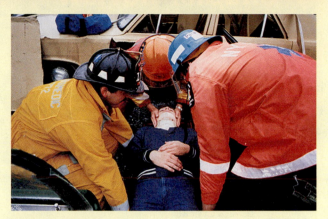

Scan 21-6h Apply straps and move the patient to a stretcher. Immobilize the head.

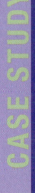

CASE STUDY

TRANSITION

When the EMTs arrive, you summarize the mechanism of injury and detail your physical findings. You alert them to the pain and tenderness in his neck. They decide to fully immobilize the patient prior to transport, and you assist moving the patient to a long board. You then detail the call in your written documentation.

■ Discussion: *After helping to calm the patient's fears, what is your role at this stage?*

THE LAST WORD

When dealing with injuries to the axial skeleton, take care to assess and treat not only the immediate life threats, but also the potential complications that can cause long-term damage. Assume brain injury. Also assume spinal injury and treat accordingly. Use mechanism of injury to predict injury patterns and always err on the side of caution to prevent secondary injuries.

Multiple Choice

Place a check next to the correct answer.

1. The _____ region of the spine has seven bones and supports the weight of the head.

    _____ a. lumbar

    _____ b. cervical

    _____ c. thoracic

    _____ d. coccygeal

2. Battle sign is best described as:

    _____ a. bruising around the eyes.

    _____ b. bruising on the neck.

    _____ c. bruising behind the ears.

    _____ d. bruising around the mouth.

3. "Posturing" would best be described as:

    _____ a. involuntary flexion or extension of the patient's limbs.

    _____ b. accessory muscle use to promote breathing.

    _____ c. the tripod position.

    _____ d. voluntary movement of the patient's limbs after a head injury.

4. A spinal injury caused by movement of the patient after the initial trauma would best be described as a:

    _____ a. primary injury.

    _____ b. tertiary injury.

    _____ c. secondary injury.

    _____ d. disqualifying injury.

5. Upon assuming manual stabilization of the head of a suspected spinal injury patient, you note that the head is not positioned in an in-line neutral position. You should:

    _____ a. stabilize the head in the position found.

    _____ b. move the head to a neutral position even if it causes an increase in pain.

    _____ c. move the head to a neutral position even if it is met with resistance.

    _____ d. move the head to a neutral position unless it causes an increase in pain.

Short Answer

1. Describe what is meant by in-line, neutral position.

    _____

    _____

    _____

    _____

2. Describe the signs and symptoms of a concussion.

    _____

    _____

    _____

    _____

3. List four of the signs or symptoms of a spinal injury.

   a. _____

   b. _____

   c. _____

   d. _____

4. List in order the three centers of mass that must be secured to the long board to achieve proper spinal immobilization.

   a. _____

   b. _____

   c. _____

5. Ideally, three team members would be used to complete a log roll. Describe the position and responsibility of each member as they conduct this skill.

   _____

   _____

   _____

   _____

Critical Thinking

1. Why would a closed head injury potentially be more dangerous than an open head injury?

   _____

   _____

   _____

   _____

2. Why might a patient who has sustained a soft tissue injury to the face consider this injury "life altering"?

   _____

   _____

   _____

   _____

3. Describe a specific scenario where rapid extrication would be the method of choice for removing a patient from a vehicle.

   _____

   _____

   _____

   _____

Case Study

You are the EMR called to assist a 22-year-old male who was shot in the neck. He is unresponsive on arrival and bleeding from a small neck wound.

1. Describe the steps of your primary assessment.

   _____

   _____

   _____

2. What immediate life threats should you suspect with penetrating trauma to the neck?

   _____

   _____

3. Describe the steps you would take to control the bleeding from this puncture wound in the neck.

   _____

   _____

   _____

Upon further assessment, you notice a larger exit wound in the middle of the patient's posterior neck.

4. What additional concerns does the location of this exit wound bring up?

   _____

   _____

5. Describe any additional treatment steps (beyond treating immediate life threats) you would consider in treating this patient.

   _____

   _____

Musculoskeletal Injuries

NAVIGATION GUIDE

The following items provide an overview to the purpose and content of this chapter. The Education Standard and Competency are from the National EMS Education Standards.

Education Standard Trauma (Orthopedic Trauma)

Competency Uses simple knowledge to recognize and manage life threats based on assessment findings for an acutely injured patient while awaiting additional emergency medical response.

Knowledge Area Orthopedic Trauma
- Open fractures
- Closed fractures
- Dislocations
- Amputations

Objectives After reading this chapter, you should be able to:

1. Define key terms introduced in this chapter.
2. Describe the common types of force that cause musculoskeletal injuries.
3. Differentiate between open and closed musculoskeletal injuries.
4. Differentiate between the terms *strain, sprain, dislocation*, and *fracture*.
5. Describe the typical findings associated with musculoskeletal injuries.
6. Explain the principles of caring for patients with musculoskeletal injuries.
7. Given a variety of scenarios involving patients with musculoskeletal injuries, apply the principles of splinting.
8. Demonstrate the application of a variety of splints, such as:
   a. Soft splints
   b. Rigid splints
   c. Traction splints
   d. Circumferential splints
   e. Improvised splints
9. Recognize potential complications of musculoskeletal injuries, including hemorrhage and damage to nerves and blood vessels.
10. Demonstrate the assessment and management of patients with amputations.

NAVIGATION GUIDE *(continued)*

Key Terms Page numbers indicate first major use in this chapter. The Margin Glossary in this chapter provides definitions as you read.

Media Resources Please go to www.bradybooks.com to access mykit for this text. You will find quizzes, critical thinking scenarios, weblinks, animations, and videos related to this chapter—and much more. Look for online information on fractures and sprains. You will also find video clips on applying splints.

INTRODUCTION

ASK YOURSELF

■ Can you define key terms introduced in this chapter?

orthopedic injury an injury to the skeletal system and/or associated muscles, joints, tendons, and ligaments.

An **orthopedic injury** is an injury to the skeletal system and/or associated muscles, joints, tendons, and ligaments. According to the American Academy of Orthopedic Surgeons, musculoskeletal injuries in the United States account for nearly 150 million lost days of work and over 20 million missed days of school, and cost the country nearly $250 billion annually. Although a broken bone is rarely life threatening, clearly this type of injury can have a serious impact. Think about the effect a broken leg would have on your own life: how many days of work you would miss, the simple tasks that would become much more difficult, and even the ability to get around. As an EMR, you will play a key role in helping your patient overcome an orthopedic injury. You will have immediate responsibilities in the case of life-threatening injuries; you will have secondary responsibilities to ensure no further harm. You also will have emotional responsibilities to help ease the impact of a potentially life-altering event. Careful and compassionate actions that occur in the prehospital stage will help maximize the potential for a positive outcome.

CASE STUDY

THE CALL

It is a cold January day. A recent snowstorm has clogged the sidewalks with snow. While walking down the street, you notice an elderly woman stumble and fall into the street. She attempts to get up, but promptly falls back to the ground. She yells for help as she struggles to sit up. You instruct another bystander to go into a nearby store and call 911. You then approach the patient to offer assistance.

■ Discussion: *How do you begin your assessment? How do you think this elderly woman is feeling?*

The Musculoskeletal System

There are 206 bones in the human body. These bones work together with muscles and with specialized tissue that connect bone to bone (ligaments) and muscle to bone to form the musculoskeletal system. This combination of bone and muscle allows us to walk and stand upright. It also provides protection for internal organs. The core of the body is protected by the **axial skeleton** (the skull, rib cage, and spinal column) while the arms and legs (upper and lower extremities) form the **appendicular skeleton**.

Musculoskeletal injuries can be life threatening. Large blood vessels often run alongside large bones, and breaking those bones frequently causes damage to the vessels. Significant bleeding can occur. In particular, injuries to the pelvis and femur are often associated with life-threatening bleeding.

Musculoskeletal injuries may be considered open or closed. An **open injury** means that the skin overlying the injured bone is broken, usually by a broken bone that has perforated the skin from the inside out (Figures 22-1a to 22-1c ■). A **closed injury** means that the skin is intact (Figure 22-2 ■).

Mechanism of Injury

A variety of different forces cause musculoskeletal injuries. By assessing the mechanism of injury, you can evaluate the way the force was applied and in some cases predict injury. Common forces that cause musculoskeletal injury include:

■ *Direct force.* Injury is caused by an impact with another object. The object might strike the body (for example, a bat striking a head) or the body might strike an object (for example, being thrown against a tree after being ejected from a vehicle).

axial skeleton the skull, rib cage, and spinal column.

appendicular skeleton the arms and legs (upper and lower extremities).

open injury (fracture) a broken bone that has perforated the skin overlying the injury.

closed injury (fracture) a broken bone that has intact skin overlying the injury.

ASK YOURSELF

■ How do you differentiate between open and closed musculoskeletal injuries?

■ What are the common types of force that cause musculoskeletal injuries?

OPEN INJURY

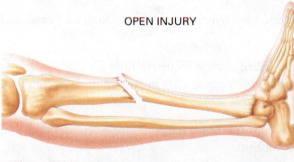

■ **Figure 22-1a** Open injury.

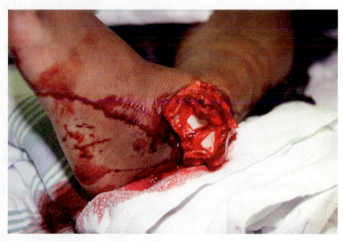

■ **Figure 22-1b** Open injury. (© Edward T. Dickinson, MD)

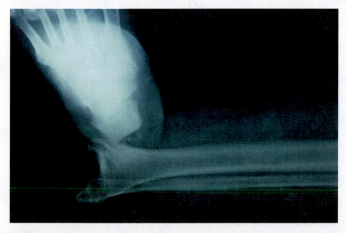

■ **Figure 22-1c** X-ray of the injury showing broken bones and joint dislocation both above and below the surface of the skin. (© Edward T. Dickinson, MD)

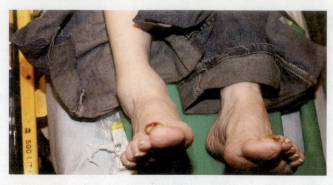

■ **Figure 22-2** Closed injury. (© Daniel Limmer)

■ *Indirect force.* Injury is caused away from the site of impact as the force is transferred to other parts of the body. For example, when a person falls from a height and lands on his feet he may have direct force injury to his feet, but also indirect force to his hips, pelvis, or spine as the force of impact is transferred up his legs.

■ *Twisting force.* This type of force occurs when one part stays stationary as the other part is twisted. An example is an ankle that breaks because a foot is caught as the body is thrown forward.

Specific Musculoskeletal Injuries

Not all musculoskeletal injuries involve broken bones. In fact, more often the soft tissue that connects structures is injured. It is always difficult to be sure if a bone is broken or not. For the most part, you will assume it is a fracture and treat accordingly.

Strain

A **strain** occurs when muscles and tendons are overworked or stretched and extended beyond their normal range of motion.

■ Example: A basketball player "pulls" a leg muscle while running for the ball. In this case, her burst of speed to the ball has caused a leg muscle to be overstretched.

Sprain

A **sprain** occurs when ligaments that connect bone to bone are overextended and stretched beyond their normal range of motion.

■ Example: A football player is hit in the leg and overextends his knee.

Dislocation

A **dislocation** occurs when a joint is disrupted—that is, when a bone (or bones) that makes up part of a joint is forced out of place (Figure 22-3 ■). This extremely painful injury can cause serious nerve damage and damage to the blood vessels that typically are seated close to bones. If not corrected, a dislocation can result in long-term loss of function or even loss of the limb itself. The force that causes the dislocation often causes fractures in nearby bones (indirect force).

■ Example: A volleyball player falls and lands hands first on the gym floor. The indirect force pushes her upper arm out of the shoulder joint.

Fracture

A **fracture** occurs when a bone is cracked or actually broken.

■ Example: A runner twists and breaks his ankle when he accidentally steps off the curb while running.

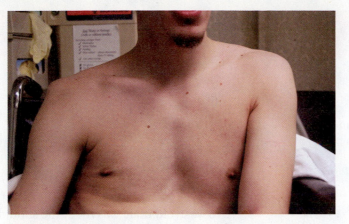

■ **Figure 22-3** An example of a right shoulder dislocation. (© Edward T. Dickinson, MD)

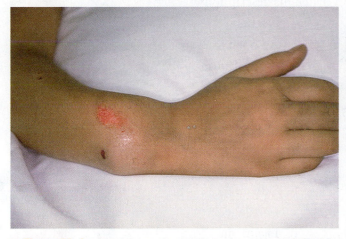

■ **Figure 22-4a** Exterior view of a closed angulated injury. (© Charles Stewart, M.D. & Associates)

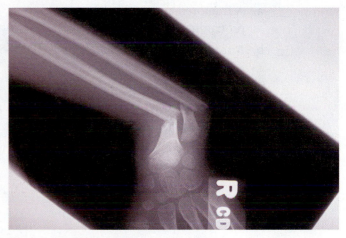

■ **Figure 22-4b** X-ray of a closed angulated injury. (© Charles Stewart, M.D. & Associates)

A fracture can be as simple as a crack or as severe as to actually move bones out of place. An example of a severe fracture would be an **angulated fracture**. In this case a normally straight bone is bent due to the fracture (Figures 22-4a and 22-4b ■). Angulated fractures can be serious threats to circulation and to nerves in the affected extremity. Recognize them as true emergencies.

angulated fracture a normally straight bone that is bent due to a fracture.

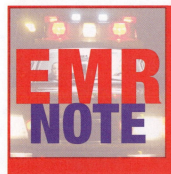

EMR NOTE

Although these are all different types of injuries, the signs and symptoms are often the same. It is almost impossible to distinguish a fracture from a less severe injury in the field. As an emergency responder you should always assume the worst and treat all musculoskeletal injuries as if they were a fracture.

Stop, Review, Remember

Multiple Choice

Place a check next to the correct answer.

1. Which of the following is a component of the appendicular skeleton?

    _____ a. Upper arm bone

    _____ b. Skull

    _____ c. Fourth rib

    _____ d. Pelvis

2. Which of the following would be considered a closed fracture?

    _____ a. A fractured arm with a bone protruding through the skin

    _____ b. A fractured leg beneath a large laceration

    _____ c. A fractured rib beneath a puncture wound

    _____ d. A fractured arm beneath bruised skin

3. Which of the following would best describe the injury that occurs when ligaments are overextended and stretched beyond their normal range of motion?

    _____ a. Strain

    _____ b. Sprain

    _____ c. Fracture

    _____ d. Contusion

4. A 16-year-old male was hit in the shoulder while playing football. He says that he feels like his arm "popped out of the socket." Which of the following injuries would best match his description?

    _____ a. A strain

    _____ b. An open fracture

    _____ c. A dislocation

    _____ d. A hematoma

5. Which of the following would be an example of specialized tissue that connects bone to bone?

    _____ a. Muscle

    _____ b. Skin

    _____ c. Cartilage

    _____ d. Ligaments

Emergency Medical Responder Practice

Indicate which type of force caused the injury that is described.

Direct force

Indirect force

Twisting force

1. A man catches his arm in a railing as he falls down the stairs. His body moves forward as his arm is held in place.

    _____

2. The bumper of a car strikes and breaks an upper leg bone of a person crossing the street.

    _____

3. A woman falls forward and lands on her hands. She complains of shoulder pain.

    _____

4. A man falls off a roof and lands feet first. You assess that he has fractured his pelvis even though he did not actually strike it. _____

5. A falling tree limb strikes and breaks a man's collar bone.

    _____

Short Answer

Discuss at least three reasons why an orthopedic injury that is not life threatening might be life altering.

1. _____

   _____

   _____

   _____

2. _____

   _____

   _____

   _____

3. _____

   _____

   _____

   _____

THE RESPONSE

You observe the patient seated on the road. Traffic has stopped in both directions. It is a bit icy but it is safe to walk to the patient. As you walk up, the patient calls to you and asks for your help. She says, "I think I broke my leg."

As she is talking, you assume her airway is patent. She has no obvious trouble breathing. Her skin is warm and dry, and she has a good radial pulse. She seems to be alert and oriented.

You notice her right lower leg is bent at an unusual angle. She complains that it hurts a great deal and notes that she heard a "snap" as she fell.

The other bystander returns and tells you that an ambulance is on the way.

In the meantime, you offer the patient your coat, and stabilize the leg by placing your hands above and below the fracture.

■ Discussion: *What do you think was forgotten as part of the assessment of this elderly person?*

EMR Patient Assessment: Musculoskeletal Injuries

Musculoskeletal injuries may easily distract you from more life-threatening problems. It is easy to pay a great deal of attention to an angulated fracture but not enough to the subtle signs of respiratory failure. It is critical to remember that the same force that broke a bone has acted on the organs beneath that bone. Although the broken bone may be the most dramatic sight, the more severe injuries may require careful assessment to find. Always complete a thorough primary assessment and aggressively treat primary assessment problems.

Consider mechanism of injury when assessing a patient for a musculoskeletal injury. Think of where the force impacted the patient and think of how much force was involved. Use a thorough patient assessment to prove your hunches and to find the injuries that are not readily apparent.

Typical findings will include:

■ Pain, particularly at the site of impact (but remember indirect force can injure areas away from the site of impact).

■ Tenderness, or pain on touching an area.

■ Deformity. Compare injured limbs with uninjured limbs and look for changes in shape, size, or even angulations.

■ Open wounds and exposed bone ends. Often you will be able to see a bone end protruding from the skin (Figures 22-5a and 22-5b ■).

crepitus the grating sound made when broken bone ends rub together.

■ Crepitus. **Crepitus** is the grating sound made when broken bone ends rub together. You should not purposefully move an extremity to look for this, but often it is found on simple palpation.

■ Loss of range of motion. A patient may complain of being unable to move a joint (a joint locked into position) or being unable to move an extremity.

■ Swelling.

■ Bruising or discoloration.

■ Loss of sensation. A patient may complain of numbness or tingling in the affected extremity.

■ Loss of circulation. An injury may cut off circulation to the affected extremity. Always assess pulses and capillary refill and compare them to the uninjured side.

■ "I heard it snap." The patient may tell you he heard the sound of bone breaking.

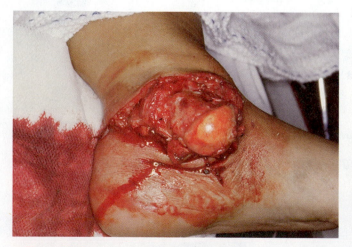

■ Figure 22-5a Open injury with bone exposed.

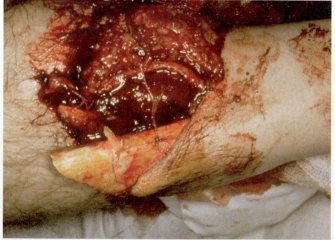

■ Figure 22-5b Open injury with bone exposed.

EMR Emergency Care: Musculoskeletal Injuries

Treatment of musculoskeletal injuries focuses on immobilizing the fracture—that is, to keep the broken bones from moving and causing more damage.

1. Treat life threats first. Always perform a thorough primary assessment before treating musculoskeletal injuries. Do not be distracted from more significant injuries that are not as visually dramatic. Be especially aware of underlying injuries in patients with musculoskeletal injuries to the head, chest, pelvis, and thighs. The bones of the thighs have very large arteries and veins running along the bones. Injuries to these bones can result in serious internal and external bleeding.
2. Consider manual stabilization of the spine. Use mechanism of injury to weigh the possibility of spinal injury. When appropriate, take spinal precautions.
3. Manually stabilize the injured extremity. The goal is to prevent movement and in particular prevent broken bone ends from moving and damaging surrounding tissue. When possible, you should place your hands above and below the site of the injury to stabilize both bone ends. Do not attempt to replace protruding bone ends.
4. Expose the wound. Cut away clothing to allow for assessment of the injured site. Consider removing jewelry if swelling may pose a risk to circulation.
5. Treat open wounds. Control external bleeding but be careful not to apply direct pressure to protruding bone ends. Cover open wounds with a sterile dressing and bandage appropriately.
6. Assess circulation, sensation, and motor function in the affected extremity. This will not only give you a picture of the extent of the injury, but also provide a baseline if things change later.
7. Apply ice or cold packs. Cold will help reduce swelling and decrease pain. (Note: Ice should never be applied directly to the skin.)
8. Place the patient in a position of comfort. When spinal precautions are not a concern, allow the patient to remain in whatever position makes him most comfortable.

Principles of Splinting

Splinting is the process of using an object or device to restrict movement of an injured area. Although there are many different types of commercially available splints, any object that effectively immobilizes a body part could be considered a splint. Reasons for splinting include the following:

- Stopping bone ends from damaging tissue. Jagged bone ends can do serious damage to blood vessels, muscle, and nerves that lie close to the injury site. Limiting motion prevents further damage.
- Managing pain. Limiting the movement of bone ends reduces pain, and the immobilization of the extremity helps limit muscle spasm (which can cause severe pain).
- Controlling bleeding. Often splinting is an effective way to control both external and internal bleeding related to a fracture.
- Preventing circulatory and nerve damage. Splinting often keeps an extremity in the position of function. Proper positioning helps limit restricted blood flow and nerve damage.

ASK YOURSELF

- What are the principles of caring for patients with musculoskeletal injuries?

ASK YOURSELF

- What are the general principles of splinting?

Rules of Splinting

- Communicate with the patient. Often the process of applying the splint will hurt. Good communication will make the process easier for everyone involved (Scan 22-1).
- Maintain manual immobilization until the splint is completely applied. Manual immobilization will help limit movement during application of the splint.
- Expose the injury prior to splinting. Remove restricting clothing and jewelry (be sure to account for all patient belongings).
- Dress open wounds before applying the splint.
- Straighten angulated injuries. If the injury is severely angulated or has evidence of decreased blood flow below the injury (absent pulse, delayed capillary refill, severe cyanosis), consider gently pulling on the extremity (applying traction) and moving it back to a normal position (anatomical position). Stop movement if pain significantly increases or if you meet resistance.

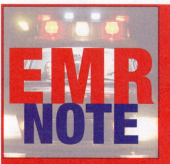

EMR NOTE

Not all EMS systems allow for straightening of a deformed injury. Regardless, it's important to learn the principles of care for these patients. In all cases, however, always follow local protocol.

- Assess circulation, sensation, and motor function.
- Consider padding a splint before applying it to increase patient comfort.
- Immobilize above and below the injury. In a long bone injury, the joint above and the joint below should be immobilized. In a joint injury, the bone above and the bone below should be immobilized.
- Reassess circulation, sensation, and motor function after the splint has been applied.

ASK YOURSELF

- How do you apply a variety of splints, such as:
  - Soft splints?
  - Rigid splints?
  - Traction splints?
  - Circumferential splints?
  - Improvised splints?

sling and swathe   an immobilization technique formed by the combination of a sling (triangle bandage) around the affected arm and triangle bandages securing the arm to the rest of the body.

Splinting Materials

Splints come in many shapes and sizes, and anything could be a splint as long as it does the desired job of immobilization. However, there are typical types of splints that are worthwhile to review (Figure 22-6a ■).

Soft Splints

A soft splint is made from soft materials. Examples would be a pillow or **sling and swathe** (triangle bandages). A sling and swathe is formed by the combination of a sling around the affected arm and triangle bandages securing the arm to the rest of the body (Figure 22-6b ■). To attach a sling and swathe you would first apply the sling to the affected arm. Gently pass the sling around the arm so that the point of the triangle points to the elbow. Note a small knot in the point of the triangle bandage will help hold the elbow. The other sides will be passed around the arm and tied. Attempt to keep the knot off the patient's

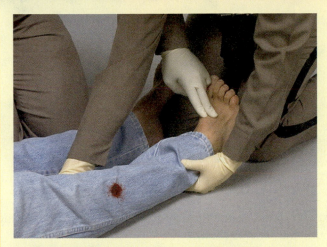

22-1a Assess pulse, movement, and sensation below the injury site.

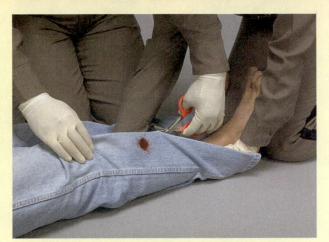

22-1b Cut away clothing to expose the injury.

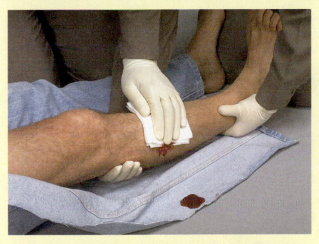

22-1c After controlling bleeding, place a dressing over open wounds, if any.

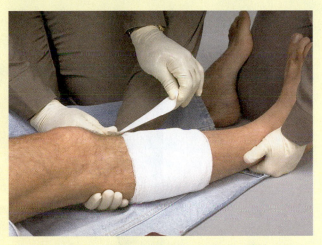

22-1d If there is severe deformity, align it with gentle traction.

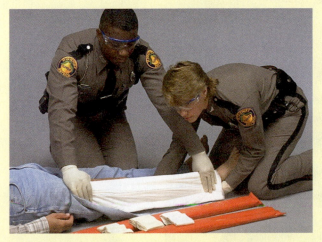

22-1e Pad the splint.

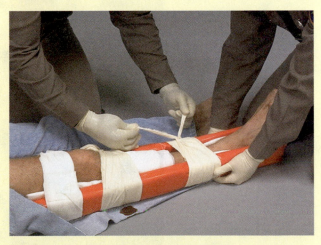

22-1f Secure the limb to the splint and reassess pulse, movement, and sensation.

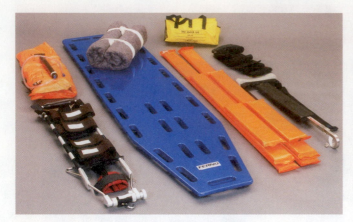

■ **Figure 22-6a** Splinting materials.

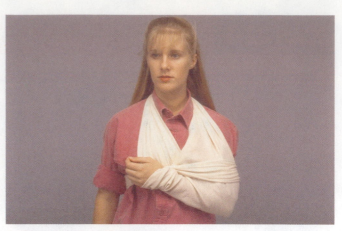

■ **Figure 22-6b** Sling and swathe.

neck or pad underneath it. Next you would secure the arm to the rest of the body using two to three cravats that wrap around the patient's chest.

Rigid Splints

A rigid splint is made from a solid object (wood, metal, plastic) and secured to an extremity to limit movement (Figure 22-6c ■).

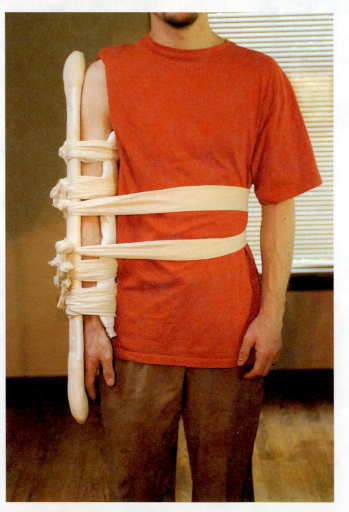

■ **Figure 22-6c** Rigid splint with swathe.

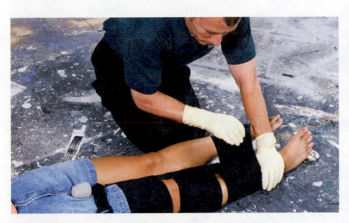

■ **Figure 22-6d** Traction splint.

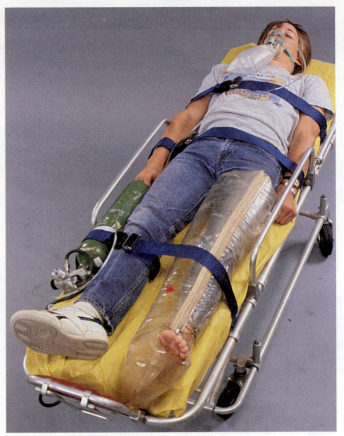

■ **Figure 22-6e** Air splint.

Traction Splints

A **traction splint** is a mechanical device that, when attached to an extremity, provides gentle pulling (traction) to help decrease pain and prevent muscle spasm (Figure 22-6d ■).

Circumferential Splints

Air splints are designed to be positioned around an extremity (like a sleeve) and then inflated to provide immobilization (Figure 22-6e ■). Vacuum splints are similar to air splints in that they surround an injured extremity. However, with a vacuum splint, air is evacuated to create a semirigid splint.

Improvised Splints

Depending on your situation and available equipment, it may be necessary to improvise a splint. Be creative. Many household and readily available items could be used as a splint. Wood, broom handles, sporting equipment such as shin guards, cardboard, rolled up magazines, and even pillows could all be used. Consider patient comfort and pad appropriately.

traction splint a mechanical device that, when attached to an extremity, provides gentle pulling (traction) to help decrease pain and prevent muscle spasm.

Multiple Choice

Place a check next to the correct answer.

1. The grating sound made when broken bone ends rub together is called:

   ____ a. crepitus.

   ____ b. subcutaneous emphysema.

   ____ c. crackles.

   ____ d. subdermal grinding.

2. When manually immobilizing a suspected musculoskeletal injury you should:

   ____ a. apply firm pressure below the injury site.

   ____ b. apply pressure above and below the injury site.

   ____ c. replace protruding bone ends.

   ____ d. apply firm pressure above the injury site.

3. You are treating a patient with an open fracture that has bone ends protruding through the skin. The wound is bleeding. To control the bleeding you should:

   ____ a. replace protruding bone ends.

   ____ b. apply direct pressure to protruding bone ends.

   ____ c. dress the wound and apply a splint.

   ____ d. apply a dressing only.

4. Which of the following is an indication to stop straightening a severely angulated fracture?

   ____ a. Pain increases slightly.

   ____ b. Bleeding is observed.

   ____ c. Bone ends disappear.

   ____ d. Resistance is met.

5. A mechanical device that, when attached to an extremity, provides gentle pulling to help decrease pain and prevent muscle spasm is otherwise known as a(n):

   ____ a. traction splint.

   ____ b. air splint.

   ____ c. vacuum splint.

   ____ d. sling and swathe.

Emergency Medical Responder Practice

1. List at least four signs or symptoms of a musculoskeletal injury.

   _____

   _____

   _____

   _____

2. List at least four rules of splinting.

   _____

   _____

   _____

   _____

EMR Patient Assessment and Emergency Care: Specific Circumstances

Upper Extremity Injuries

- *Shoulder injuries.* Shoulder dislocations are a common injury to the upper extremity. Mechanism of injury will often be indirect force (pushing or pulling). The most common dislocation occurs when the bone of the upper arm pops forward out of the joint. You may notice a bulge (deformity) in the front (anterior) portion of the joint. Other signs and symptoms include "dropped shoulder" (one shoulder that droops lower than the other), pain, and reduced range of motion in the affected arm. The patient often will be seen holding the arm close in to the chest. Joint injuries should always be splinted in the position found. Never attempt to straighten a joint injury. To splint this injury you would apply a sling and swathe if possible (Figure 22-7a ■). Be sure to assess circulation, sensation, and motor function before and after splinting as joint injuries frequently threaten those functions.

- *Elbow.* Apply the same rules as you used for the shoulder. Splint in the position found; never attempt to straighten. If the position found is straight, consider using a rigid splint. If it is bent or severely deformed, consider using a sling and swathe or a pillow to wrap around and immobilize (Figure 22-7b ■). Reassessment is important as with any joint injury.

- *Upper arm (humerus).* The bone in the upper arm is known as the humerus. Suspected fractures of this bone can be managed by applying a rigid splint to the

ASK YOURSELF

- What are the potential complications of musculoskeletal injuries, including hemorrhage and damage to nerves and blood vessels?

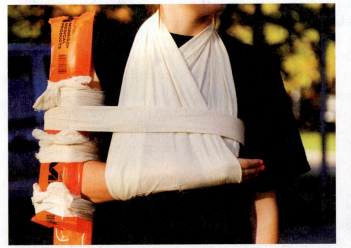

■ **Figure 22-7a** Fixation or rigid splint with a sling and swathe.

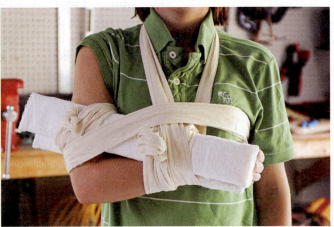

■ **Figure 22-7b** Injured elbow immobilized in a bent position.

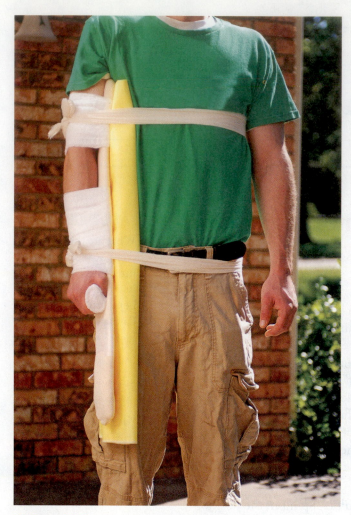

■ **Figure 22-7c** Injured elbow immobilized in a straight position.

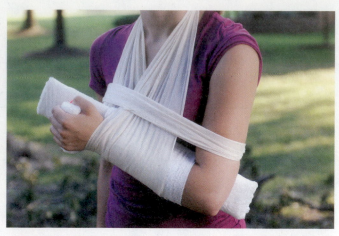

■ **Figure 22-7d** Immobilization of an injury to the forearm, wrist, or hand.

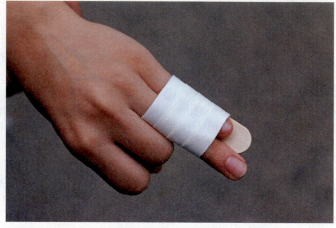

■ **Figure 22-7e** A tongue depressor used as a splint and then taped to an adjoining finger for stabilization.

upper arm and then securing the arm to the rest of the body using a sling and swathe (Figure 22-7c ■).

■ *Lower arm (radius and ulna).* Rigid splints or circumferential splints work well with lower arm injuries. Apply the splint but be sure to leave the fingers exposed to enable reassessment of circulation, sensation, and movement. Remember that with long bones you must immobilize the joint above and the joint below, so a sling and swathe should be used after application of the rigid splint to best immobilize the elbow (Figure 22-7d ■). Patient comfort will be improved by keeping the hand in an anatomical position. This can be accomplished by having the patient hold a small roll of gauze while you splint the arm.

■ *Fingers.* Fingers can be immobilized with a rigid splint such as a tongue depressor or by taping the injured finger to the next uninjured finger (Figure 22-7e ■). If multiple fingers or the entire hand is involved, consider using a soft splint such as having the patient hold a roll of gauze and wrapping the entire hand with roller bandage.

Lower Extremity Injuries

■ *Pelvis.* Pelvic injuries can cause life-threatening bleeding. Assess carefully for signs and symptoms of shock. Pelvic fractures can be managed by placing the patient on a long board and padding between the patient's legs and on either side of the pelvis.

You may also consider using a commercially available device called a pelvic binder. This device is specifically used to immobilize the pelvis. Some EMS systems also allow use of the pneumatic antishock garment (PASG) to treat unstable pelvic fractures when they are associated with shock. This device works in a similar manner to an air splint. Local protocols should be followed. It requires a great deal of force to fracture a pelvis. Be aware that serious underlying injuries may be present with any force great enough to break a large bone such as the pelvis.

■ *Upper leg (femur).* The bone in the upper leg is called the femur, and it is a large long bone that has large blood vessels running along its length. Because of those blood vessels and their potential for severe bleeding, any femur fracture should be considered a true emergency. Just as with the pelvis, consider that any force great enough to break the femur is great enough to cause more serious and potentially life-threatening injuries in other parts of the body. In an isolated femur injury (that is, the only injury is the femur), a traction splint is used to reduce pain and muscle spasm (if local protocol allows). You might also consider immobilizing the leg using one or two rigid splints applied to the affected leg. Remember that you must immobilize the joint above and below the injured bone, so rigid immobilization of a femur usually requires either a backboard (to immobilize the hip) or a long board to account for both the knee and the hip (Figure 22-7f ■).

■ *Hip.* A hip injury is usually an injury to the end of the femur closest to the joint of the pelvis. Fractures and dislocations are both relatively common. A sign of a hip fracture is often a rotated foot or a shortening of one leg compared to the other. If the leg is bent, consider padding beneath the knees with blankets or pillows and immobilize to a long board.

■ *Lower leg (tibia/fibula).* Like the lower arm, lower leg injuries are usually easy to splint using either a rigid splint (or splints) or a circumferential splint. Remember to immobilize the joint above and the joint below. Be sure to leave the toes exposed to reassess circulation, sensation, and motor function.

■ *Knee.* Splint the knee in the position found. A pillow can work or two rigid splints placed on the inside and outside of the leg can provide sturdy support (Figure 22-7g ■). Remember that joint injuries often have circulatory, sensory, or motor problems, so be watchful and constantly reassess.

■ *Foot.* The simplest splint to use for a foot is the pillow. Wrap the pillow around the foot and tie with cravats (Figure 22-7h ■). Similar soft padded items such as a blanket roll could also be substituted. Do not cover the toes if possible.

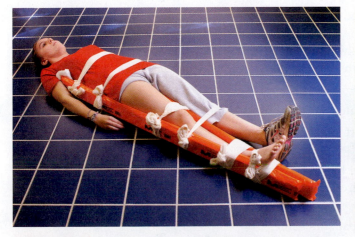

■ **Figure 22-7f** A high femur fracture immobilized in a fixation splint.

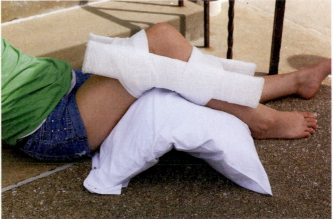

■ **Figure 22-7g** A splinted knee.

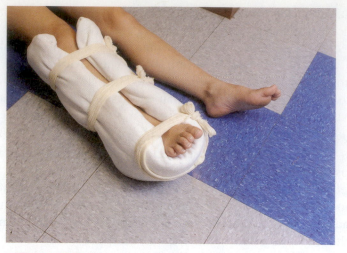

Figure 22-7h Blanket-roll splint of the ankle and foot.

ASK YOURSELF

■ What are the assessment and management steps for a patient with an amputation?

Amputations

See Chapter 20 where care for an amputation was first covered. An amputation means that a body part has been completely detached from the rest of the body. Bleeding may be severe, but oftentimes (especially in complete amputations) bleeding is controlled by the spasm and constriction of blood vessels. Control bleeding in the case of amputation as you would any other open wound.

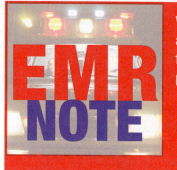

We have provided guidelines for typical care of amputations. Treatment of amputations, however, varies from system to system. Always check and follow your local protocol.

Medical technology has advanced to the point where many amputated parts can be reattached. When possible the amputated part should be transported with the patient Note: Your first priority will always be the patient.

Follow local guidelines to care for the amputated part. Typical care includes the following:

■ Gently clean the amputated part by removing loose debris.

■ Wrap the amputated part in gauze lightly moistened with sterile saline and place in a plastic bag.

■ Cool the amputated part by placing it in a container with ice (never use dry ice). Do not place the part directly on the ice and never immerse the amputated part in water.

■ Label the part with the patient's name.

TRANSITION

When the EMTs arrive, you caution them about the slippery sidewalk and describe the fall you witnessed. You summarize your initial assessment and turn over stabilization of the leg to the crew. As they have decided to straighten the angulated leg, you stay with the patient and assist her through this painful process. The EMTs then apply a splint and prepare the patient for transport.

■ Discussion: *Has the treatment been handled properly?*

THE LAST WORD

Musculoskeletal injuries often distract us from the more serious, underlying injuries. Always remember that the same force that broke the bone was also applied to the vital organs under and around the bone. Use a thorough primary assessment to identify and treat life threats, and deal with musculoskeletal concerns only after the life threats have been managed.

Even if the musculoskeletal injury is not life threatening, emergency responders should always be aware of the life-altering consequences of an orthopedic injury and provide appropriate emotional support.

✳ *Chapter Review*

Multiple Choice

Place a check next to the correct answer.

1. A 35-year-old male has fallen off a ladder. You find him holding his left arm against his body and notice one shoulder is drooping lower than the other. Which of the following injuries would these signs specifically indicate?

_____ a. Broken rib

_____ b. Broken radius

_____ c. Dislocated elbow

_____ d. Dislocated shoulder

2. A sling and swathe would be an appropriate splint for which of the following injuries?

_____ a. Dislocated shoulder

_____ b. Dislocated femur

_____ c. Fractured tibia

_____ d. Fractured ulna

3. In which of the following injury sites would you be most concerned about circulatory or sensory damage?

_____ a. Humerus

_____ b. Tibia

_____ c. Ulna

_____ d. Elbow

4. A 17-year-old has injured his knee playing football. You find the knee in a bent position. You should:

_____ a. apply a circumferential splint.

_____ b. straighten the knee prior to splinting.

_____ c. splint in the bent position.

_____ d. apply a sling and swathe.

5. Patient comfort can be improved by splinting a patient's hand in the _____ position.

_____ a. rotated

_____ b. flexed

_____ c. anatomical

_____ d. straight

Short Answer

1. Describe the signs and symptoms of a hip fracture.

_____

_____

_____

2. Describe a method of splinting an unstable pelvic fracture.

_____

_____

_____

3. List the steps you would take in applying a sling and swathe.

_____

_____

_____

Critical Thinking

1. Why is it important to check circulation, sensation, and motor function in the affected extremity both before and after splinting?

_____

_____

_____

2. In a patient with suspected internal bleeding in the abdomen, why is it important to splint an angulated femur fracture?

_____

_____

_____

3. What is the purpose of keeping an amputated part cool and transporting it in moistened dressings?

_____

_____

_____

Case Study

You are the EMR called to assist a 25-year-old female who has been involved in a motor vehicle crash. As you assist in her extrication, you notice she has an angulated, closed fracture of the right femur and complains of severe pain in her pelvic area.

1. Does your general impression indicate any potential life threats? If so, what are they?

_____

_____

_____

_____

2. Are there immediate actions required? If so, what are they?

_____

_____

_____

_____

Her vital signs are pulse 124, respirations 24, and blood pressure 90/60. She is anxious.

3. Given her vital signs, would you consider this patient stable or unstable? Why?

_____

_____

_____

_____

4. What is the most likely cause for the alterations of her vital signs?

_____

_____

_____

_____

 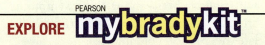

✳ NAVIGATION GUIDE

The following items provide an overview to the purpose and content of this chapter. The Education Standard and Competency are from the National EMS Education Standards.

Education Standard Trauma (Environmental Emergencies)

Competency Uses simple knowledge to recognize and manage life threats based on assessment findings for an acutely injured patient while awaiting additional emergency medical response.

Knowledge Area Environmental Emergencies
- Submersion incidents
- Temperature-related illness

Objectives After reading this chapter, you should be able to:

1. Define key terms introduced in the chapter.
2. Discuss how environmental temperatures can impact health.
3. Explain how the body produces and loses heat.
4. Give examples of each of the following means of heat loss from the body:
   a. Convection
   b. Conduction
   c. Radiation
   d. Evaporation
   e. Respiration
5. List factors that may interfere with the body's ability to compensate for changes in environmental temperature.
6. Given a variety of scenarios, recognize the signs and symptoms of:
   a. Generalized cold emergencies (hypothermia)
   b. Local cold emergencies (frostbite)
   c. Heat-related emergencies (heat cramps, heat exhaustion, heatstroke)
7. Given a variety of scenarios, demonstrate the management of patients with:
   a. Cold-related emergencies
   b. Heat-related emergencies
8. Differentiate between the signs, symptoms, and management of mild and severe hypothermia.
9. Differentiate between the signs, symptoms, and management of early (superficial) and late (deep) local cold injuries.
10. Describe several ways of preventing drowning.
11. Discuss guidelines for determining how to respond in a water rescue situation.
12. Given a scenario, demonstrate the assessment and management of patients with a submersion emergency.

NAVIGATION GUIDE (continued)

Key Terms Page numbers indicate first major use in this chapter. The Margin Glossary in this chapter provides definitions as you read.

metabolism, p. 558

convection, p. 558

conduction, p. 558

radiation, p. 558

evaporation, p. 558

respirations, p. 558

hypothermia, p. 559

frostbite, p. 559

gangrene, p. 564

hyperthermia, p. 568

drowning, p. 574

suffocation, p. 574

boil line, p. 575

Media Resources Please go to **www.bradybooks.com** to access mykit for this text. You will find quizzes, critical thinking scenarios, weblinks, animations, and videos related to this chapter—and much more. Look for online information on hypothermia and hyperthermia.

INTRODUCTION

ASK YOURSELF

■ Can you define key terms introduced in the chapter?

■ How do environmental temperatures impact health?

When we think of the environment, we think of the world around us. Whether we live and work in a rural, suburban, or urban setting, we are constantly interacting with our environment. While most of these interactions are pleasant, some may create an emergency situation. As an Emergency Medical Responder (EMR) you may be called upon to respond to emergencies resulting from the heat or cold. As you render assistance, keep in mind that the same situation creating the emergency situation might also affect you or your crew.

Remember that your responsibility as an EMR will be to ensure safety, perform a patient assessment, and provide appropriate emergency medical care based on that assessment until EMS personnel arrive to continue care and transport.

CASE STUDY

THE CALL

You are dispatched to a local park to assist with a female patient who appears to have "overexerted herself." While en route, you and your partner discuss some possibilities and assign duties.

It is a hot, sunny day with temperatures in the mid-90s. Temperatures are expected to reach near 100 degrees. The humidity is approximately 83 percent and the barometric pressure is on the rise.

As you approach the scene, you perform a scene size-up and determine it is safe to proceed. You and your partner have donned the appropriate Standard Precautions. You grab your gear and proceed toward the patient. You find your patient sitting under a shade tree with several bystanders fanning her.

■ Discussion: *What's your first impression of the patient's situation? Why is it still important to perform a primary assessment, even if the patient's condition seems obvious to you?*

metabolism all the physical and chemical changes that occur in the body, including digestion.

ASK YOURSELF

■ What are some examples of each of the following means of heat loss from the body?
■ Convection
■ Conduction
■ Radiation
■ Evaporation
■ Respiration

convection heat loss through moving air or water passing over the body.

conduction heat loss through direct contact with an object.

radiation heat loss involving the transfer of heat to an object without physical contact.

evaporation the process by which sweat changes to vapor and has a cooling effect on the body.

respirations heat loss through breathing.

Temperature Regulation

To better understand how the body responds to cold or heat emergencies, let us start by looking at the normal process of temperature regulation. The body produces heat mainly through the process of **metabolism** (all the physical and chemical changes that occur in the body, including digestion). This process is regulated in the brain by the hypothalamus, which acts like the body's thermostat to maintain a normal body temperature of 98.6°F (37°C).

In cold, the body retains heat by constricting blood vessels near the surface of the skin. Hair also erects, thickening the layer of warm air trapped near the skin. The body can produce more heat, if needed, by shivering and by producing certain hormones such as epinephrine that at least temporarily increase metabolism.

The body eliminates heat by dilating blood vessels near the surface of the skin and increasing heat elimination. There are generally five ways the body gives off heat (Figure 23-1 ■):

■ **Convection** occurs when moving air passes over the body and carries heat away from the body (Figure 23-2 ■). An example of convection is sitting in front of a fan on a warm afternoon or the effects of the wind on the temperature.

■ **Conduction** occurs when direct contact with an object carries heat away. For example, a swimmer is in direct contact with the water. If the water is cooler than the body, the water will take away the swimmer's body heat. The heat loss in water can be 25 times faster than heat loss in air.

■ **Radiation** involves the transfer of heat to an object without physical contact. For example, look down a stretch of roadway during a hot day. The visual distortion you see is a result of heat radiating off the pavement. Most body heat loss is from the head and neck, which are areas rich in blood and blood vessels.

■ **Evaporation** is the process by which sweat changes to vapor. It has a cooling effect on the body. For example, think about the difference you feel while working outside on a hot dry day versus a hot, humid day. Note that evaporation stops when the relative humidity of the air reaches 75 percent.

■ **Respirations** occur when a person breathes in cold air and breathes out air that was warmed inside the body. An example is when you walk outside on a cool morning and you "see your breath."

Through these normal processes of heat retention and heat loss, our bodies maintain a normal temperature. When we are sick, injured, under the influence of a variety of substances, or otherwise unable to compensate for the environment, we may not compensate appropriately and we fall victim to that environment.

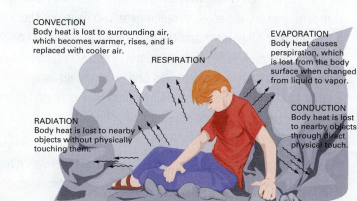

CONVECTION
Body heat is lost to surrounding air, which becomes warmer, rises, and is replaced with cooler air.

RESPIRATION

EVAPORATION
Body heat causes perspiration, which is lost from the body surface when changed from liquid to vapor.

RADIATION
Body heat is lost to nearby objects without physically touching them.

CONDUCTION
Body heat is lost to nearby objects through direct physical touch.

■ **Figure 23-1** Mechanisms of heat loss.

WIND SPEED (MPH)	WHAT THE THERMOMETER READS (degrees °F.)											
	50	40	30	20	10	0	−10	−20	−30	−40	−50	−60
	WHAT IT EQUALS IN ITS EFFECT ON EXPOSED FLESH											
CALM	50	40	30	20	10	0	−10	−20	−30	−40	−50	−60
5	48	37	27	16	6	−5	−15	−26	−36	−47	−57	−68
10	40	28	16	4	−9	−21	−33	−46	−58	−70	−83	−95
15	36	22	9	−5	−18	−36	−45	−58	−72	−85	−99	−112
20	32	18	4	−10	−25	−39	−53	−67	−82	−96	−110	−121
25	30	16	0	−15	−29	−44	−59	−74	−88	−104	−118	−133
30	28	13	−2	−18	−33	−48	−63	−79	−94	−109	−125	−140
35	27	11	−4	−20	−35	−49	−67	−82	−98	−113	−129	−145
40	26	10	−6	−21	−37	−53	−69	−85	−100	−116	−132	−148

Source: U.S. Army

Little danger if properly clothed | Danger of freezing exposed flesh | Great danger of freezing exposed flesh

■ **Figure 23-2** Wind-chill index.

Cold Emergencies

Cold emergencies can be divided into two major groups. The first group is those cold emergencies that affect the entire body. This group is called a generalized cold injury, or **hypothermia**. The second group is those cold emergencies that affect only a portion of the body. This group is called a localized cold injury, or **frostbite**.

Generalized Cold Emergencies

Exposure to extreme cold for a short period of time or moderate cold for a long period of time can cause hypothermia. Several risk factors impact how your patient responds to the cold. The first is the general condition of the patient. Any underlying medical condition (such as infection, diabetes, hypoglycemia, or circulatory problems) or traumatic condition (such as shock, head or spine injury, or burns) can weaken the body's responses to heat and cold.

The second risk factor is the use of drugs and alcohol or exposure to poisons. Any one of these can impede the body's ability to maintain body temperature. The momentary flush of warmth felt after an alcoholic drink actually increases the heat loss. That, along with impaired judgment, can quickly turn a canoe trip into a deadly excursion.

Finally, the third risk factor is the age of the patient. Very young or very old patients are especially at risk. Infants are at risk because of their anatomy. The infant's head is larger in proportion to the body than the adult's. The body surface is large compared to the mass. As a result, infants lose heat more rapidly than do adults. Infants also have an immature nervous system, which means they cannot shiver well enough to warm themselves when needed. Elderly people are also at risk. Sudden illness or injury can limit their ability to escape the cold. Impaired judgment due to medication or limited mobility due

hypothermia condition of lower than normal body temperature.

frostbite localized cold injury.

ASK YOURSELF

■ What are the factors that may interfere with the body's ability to compensate for changes in environmental temperature?

■ Given a variety of scenarios, how do you recognize the signs and symptoms of:
  ■ Generalized cold emergencies (hypothermia)?

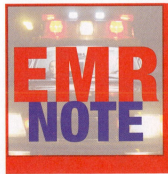

EMR NOTE

The body loses heat anytime the ambient temperature is less than body temperature. The patient does not have to be walking in a raging blizzard or falling into a near-frozen pond to be hypothermic. Your patient who wrecked his motorcycle at 3:00 a.m. on a cool spring morning may also be suffering from hypothermia, especially if alcohol or other substances are involved.

to a medical condition can also contribute to their risk for hypothermia. If they are on a fixed income, for example, they may not be able to heat their homes properly.

EMR Patient Assessment: Generalized Cold Emergencies

During scene size-up, notice the location of the patient. Does the environment suggest the possibility of generalized hypothermia? How long has the patient been exposed to those conditions? If scene size-up suggests the possibility of a cold emergency, put your hand on the patient's abdomen during the physical exam. If the skin is cool or cold, treat for hypothermia.

Hypothermia is a progressive condition. Without intervention, a patient may rapidly deteriorate. At first the patient will shiver. When shivering stops, he may appear clumsy, confused, and forgetful. He may even appear intoxicated. Often witnesses will say that the patient had mood swings, one moment calm and the next agitated or even combative (Figure 23-3 ■).

Finally, the patient's level of responsiveness decreases. He becomes less communicative and is difficult to rouse. He may display poor judgment and do things like remove his clothes while still in the cold. There may be muscle stiffness, a rigid posture, and loss of sensation. The most ominous sign of a life-threatening condition is unresponsiveness. As the patient becomes unresponsive, blood is shunted away from the skin and vital signs slow. The patient may have the appearance of death. These patients are unstable and need immediate transport to survive.

Signs and symptoms of a generalized cold emergency are listed in Table 23-1 and shown in Figures 23-4 ■, 23-5a, and 23-5b ■.

STAGES OF HYPOTHERMIA

Stage 1: Shivering is a response by the body to generate heat. It does not occur below a body temperature of 90°F.

Stage 2: Apathy and decreased muscle function. First, fine motor function is affected, then gross motor functions.

Stage 3: Decreased level of responsiveness is accompanied by a glassy stare and possible freezing of the extremities.

Stage 4: Decreased vital signs, including slow pulse and slow respiration rate.

Stage 5: Death.

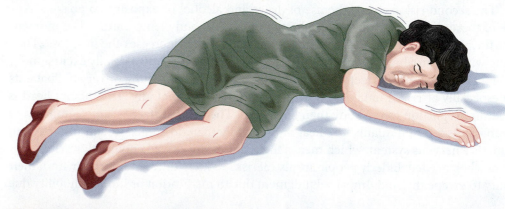

■ **Figure 23-3** Stages of hypothermia.

TABLE 23-1	Signs and Symptoms: Generalized Cold Emergency	
■ Cool or cold skin temperature	■ Initially rapid, then slow pulse	
■ Shivering	■ Lack of coordination	
■ Impaired judgment	■ Complaints of joint/muscle stiffness	
■ Decreased mental status	■ Stiff or rigid posture	

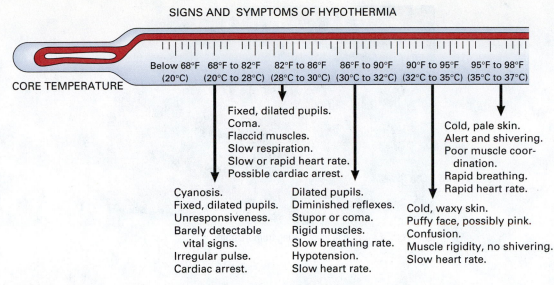

SIGNS AND SYMPTOMS OF HYPOTHERMIA

CORE TEMPERATURE

| Below 68°F (20°C) | 68°F to 82°F (20°C to 28°C) | 82°F to 86°F (28°C to 30°C) | 86°F to 90°F (30°C to 32°C) | 90°F to 95°F (32°C to 35°C) | 95°F to 98°F (35°C to 37°C) |

Fixed, dilated pupils.
Coma.
Flaccid muscles.
Slow respiration.
Slow or rapid heart rate.
Possible cardiac arrest.

Cold, pale skin.
Alert and shivering.
Poor muscle coor-
dination.
Rapid breathing.
Rapid heart rate.

Cyanosis.
Fixed, dilated pupils.
Unresponsiveness.
Barely detectable
vital signs.
Irregular pulse.
Cardiac arrest.

Dilated pupils.
Diminished reflexes.
Stupor or coma.
Rigid muscles.
Slow breathing rate.
Hypotension.
Slow heart rate.

Cold, waxy skin.
Puffy face, possibly pink.
Confusion.
Muscle rigidity, no shivering.
Slow heart rate.

■ **Figure 23-4** Signs and symptoms of hypothermia vary according to body temperature.

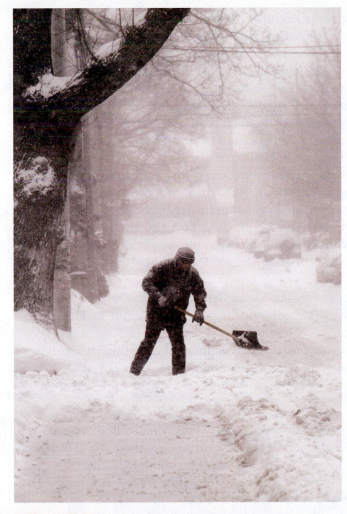

■ **Figure 23-5a** A patient at risk for developing generalized hypothermia. (© Scott Tysick/Masterfile)

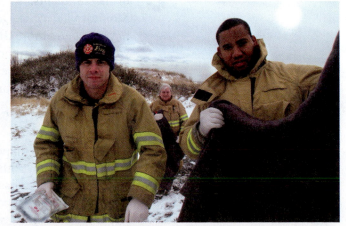

■ **Figure 23-5b** It is essential that you initiate care for generalized hypothermia as soon as possible.

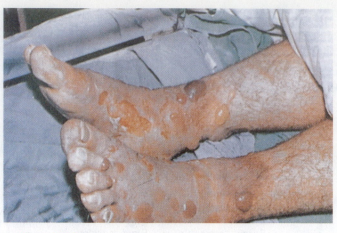

Figure 23-6a Patient suffering from frostbite.

ASK YOURSELF

- Given a variety of scenarios, how would you demonstrate the management of patients with:
  - Cold-related emergencies?

EMR Emergency Care: Generalized Cold Emergencies

If you suspect a patient has a generalized cold emergency, you should immediately notify the responding EMS personnel and take appropriate Standard Precautions. Steps to providing care for this patient include (Figure 23-6a ■):

1. Perform an appropriate scene size-up, including Standard Precautions. This may include donning specialized apparel for the environment.
2. Make sure the EMS system is activated, as appropriate.
3. Remove the patient from the cold environment. Move him to a shelter, away from the cold wind or water. If the patient is on the ground, get him off the ground or put a blanket or backboard between him and the ground.
4. Administer oxygen, if you are allowed to do so. If possible, it should be warm and humidified. You can warm the oxygen by wrapping the tubing around a hot pack or wrapping it in a warm blanket or towel.
5. Remove all wet clothing, and cover the patient with a blanket. A thin layer of dry clothing or even just a blanket is better than a thick layer of wet clothing. You can warm a blanket by using a vehicle defroster, if available.
6. Handle the patient very gently. Rough handling can make the patient's condition worse and even cause injuries. Do not massage the extremities. Do not allow the patient to walk or exert himself. Do not allow the patient to eat or drink stimulants.
7. Monitor vital signs. Depending upon the extent of the hypothermia, you may have to spend more time while assessing the vital signs. Be sure to document your findings for trends.
8. Comfort, calm, and reassure the patient. Tell him that everything that can be done will be done. Communicate with empathy.

ASK YOURSELF

- How would you describe the difference between the signs, symptoms, and management of mild and severe hypothermia?

Mild Hypothermia

As previously mentioned, hypothermia is a progressive condition without intervention. Patients suffering from hypothermia may be classified as suffering from mild hypothermia or severe hypothermia based upon the presenting signs and symptoms.

The patient with mild hypothermia will present with cold skin and shivering. He will still be alert and oriented. Signs and symptoms are listed in Table 23-2.

If the patient is alert and able, allow him to drink warm fluids. A good test of the patient's ability to protect his own airway is to have him hold the cup. If he drops the cup or

TABLE 23-2 Signs and Symptoms: Hypothermia

MILD HYPOTHERMIA	SEVERE HYPOTHERMIA
■ Increased breathing rate	■ Extremely slow breathing
■ Increased pulse rate	■ Extremely slow pulse rate
■ Increased blood pressure	■ Unresponsiveness
■ Slow, thick speech	■ Fixed and dilated pupils
■ Staggering or unsteady walk	■ Rigid extremities
■ Apathy, drowsiness, incoherence	■ Absence of shivering
■ Sluggish pupils	
■ Uncontrollable shivering	

is unable to get it to his mouth, for example, do not allow him to drink. Never give a confused or lethargic patient anything to drink as the danger of aspiration is too great. Never give coffee, tea, cola, or other caffeinated drinks. Do not allow the patient to smoke. Stimulants promote heat loss.

Remember that heat loss is greatest from the head and neck. An old sailor's saying is, "When your feet are cold, put on a hat." Cover the patient's head, and wrap a warm blanket around him.

If heat packs are available, consider using them (follow your local protocols). Apply the packs to the patient's neck, armpits, and groin. Remember that the patient may have a decreased sense of touch. Check the skin beneath the heat packs periodically to be sure they are not burning the patient. Placing gauze pads or a thin towel between the heat pack and the skin will help reduce possible burning.

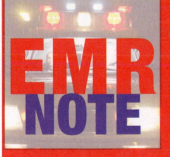

EMR NOTE

Some sources categorize hypothermia in three categories:

■ Mild hypothermia—90°F to 95°F (32°C to 35°C)
■ Moderate hypothermia—82°F to 90°F (28°C to 32°C)
■ Severe hypothermia—Less than 82°F (28°C)

Source: Zimmerman, J. Hypothermia, Hyperthermia, and Rhabdomyolysis. ACCP Critical Care Board Review 2003.

Severe Hypothermia

Patients with severe hypothermia may become unresponsive. This is a true medical emergency that can lead to death. Signs and symptoms are listed in Table 23-2.

Consider using an oropharyngeal airway to secure the airway of an unresponsive patient (follow your local protocols). Administer high-concentration oxygen. If breathing is adequate, administer oxygen with a nonrebreather mask. If breathing is not adequate, assist ventilations with a bag-valve mask and supplemental oxygen.

When assessing circulation, you might find no pulses in the patient's limbs. Remember that the body is a "metabolic icebox" at this stage. It does not need normal circulation to sustain life, because everything is slowed down. A slow pulse is not deadly and may actually be protective in nature.

Assess the carotid pulse for about one minute before starting cardiopulmonary resuscitation (CPR). If it is cold outside, remember that your sense of touch may be less than it should be. Consider putting your fingers in your armpits before taking a pulse. Handle the patient gently. Any rough handling can induce ventricular fibrillation or sudden cardiac death.

If the patient is breathless and pulseless, begin CPR. Even if he has all the signs of death—including fixed pupils and stiff extremities—begin CPR. The rule of thumb for EMS is: "You're not dead until you're warm and dead." This means you cannot consider resuscitation a failure until the heart has been given a chance to restart at a near normal temperature. There are many reports of patients with severe hypothermia who were thought to be dead who survived after receiving appropriate care.

Rewarming in the field is not recommended for patients with severe hypothermia. These patients need special attention in a hospital. Arrange for transport to the nearest medical facility as soon as possible (follow your local protocols).

Local Cold Emergencies

Cold emergencies can also result from the cooling of parts of the body, most commonly the face, nose, ears, hands, fingers, and toes. This type of cold emergency is called a local cold injury or frostbite. When a body part is exposed to intense cold, blood vessels constrict and circulation is limited. When this happens, tissues freeze. The body is made up of about 60 percent water. As the temperature in the affected part drops, this water can freeze forming ice crystals in the skin. In the most severe cases, **gangrene** (localized tissue death) can eventually set in and ultimately lead to the loss of a body part (Figure 23-6b ■).

Like general cold emergencies, local cold emergencies can be divided into two groups: early or superficial local cold injury and later or deep local cold injury.

EMR Patient Assessment: Local Cold Emergencies

Signs and symptoms you might see in a patient with an early or superficial local cold injury are listed in Table 23-3.

Signs and symptoms you might see in a patient with a late or deep local cold injury are listed in Table 23-3.

When the injured parts begin to thaw, skin color changes. It may appear flushed with areas of purple and blanching, or it may be mottled and cyanotic. The patient often will experience severe pain as the frozen part begins to thaw.

EMR Emergency Care: Local Cold Emergencies

The goal of patient care for the patient with a localized cold injury is to prevent further heat loss and improve circulation to the body part. Appropriate patient care includes the following:

1. Perform an appropriate scene size-up, including Standard Precautions. This may include donning specialized apparel for the environment.
2. Make sure the EMS system is activated, as appropriate.
3. Remove the patient from the cold environment. Move him to a shelter, away from the cold wind or water. If the patient is on the ground, get him off the ground or put a blanket or backboard between him and the ground.
4. Do not allow him to walk on a frostbitten limb.
5. Administer oxygen, if you are allowed to do so.
6. Remove all wet clothing.
7. Protect the frostbitten area from further injury.

gangrene localized tissue death.

■ Given a variety of scenarios, how do you recognize the signs and symptoms of:
  ■ Local cold emergencies (frostbite)?
■ How would you describe the difference between the signs, symptoms, and management of early (superficial) and late (deep) local cold injuries?

TABLE 23-3 Signs and Symptoms: Local Cold Injury

EARLY OR SUPERFICIAL	LATE OR DEEP
■ Light skin that reddens ■ Dark skin that turns pale ■ Skin that, when depressed gently, blanches and then returns to its normal color ■ Loss of normal feeling and sensation	■ Waxy skin ■ Skin that is firm to the touch ■ Mottled or blotchy skin ■ Swollen, blistered, and white skin

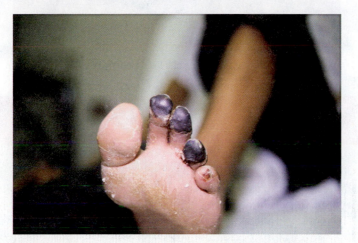

■ **Figure 23-6b** Patient suffering from a deep local cold injury, or frostbite, that has progressed to gangrene. (© Edward T. Dickinson)

8. If the injury is to an extremity, manually stabilize it.
9. If the injury is superficial, cover it with a blanket.
10. If it is late and deep, cover it with a dry cloth or dressings.
11. Do not rub or massage the area. Ice crystals under the skin could damage the fragile capillaries and tissues, making the injury worse.
12. Comfort, calm, and reassure the patient. Tell him everything that can be done will be done.
13. Monitor the patient for signs of hypothermia.

Rewarming

If transport will be delayed, consider rewarming the affected area. Never rewarm an area with late or deep frostbite. Never rewarm an area if there is a chance that it may refreeze. The injury from the second freezing would be much worse than the original one.

Warm the entire frostbitten area in tepid water (about 100°F–105°F). The water should feel comfortable to the normal hand. Be sure to pick a container that permits the entire area to be immersed (Figure 23-7 ■). Continue to support the injured area during rewarming. Do not allow the injured area to touch the bottom or side of the container. If the water starts to cool, remove the patient, then add more warm water. As the area rewarms, the patient may complain of tingling and shooting pains. In this case, some EMS systems allow EMRs to help an alert patient self-administer an analgesic such as Tylenol (follow your local protocol).

When the injured area is rewarmed, the tissues will be fragile. To protect them, cover the injury with dry, sterile gauze. If the injury is to the fingers or toes, place gauze between them to keep separated. Consider padding the entire area with a large bulky dressing.

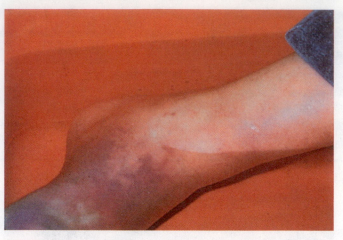

■ **Figure 23-7** Active rewarming of a local cold injury.

✴ Stop, Review, Remember

Multiple Choice

Place a check next to the correct answer.

1. The term used to describe all the physical and chemical changes that occur in the body is:

____ a. homeostasis.

____ b. metabolism.

____ c. digestion.

____ d. ingestion.

2. The term used to describe a generalized cooling of the body is:

____ a. hyperthermia.

____ b. hypovolemia.

____ c. hypervolemia.

____ d. hypothermia.

3. In a late or deep localized cold injury:

____ a. light skin will redden.

____ b. the skin will blanch, then return to normal color.

____ c. the skin will be waxy, mottled, or blotchy.

____ d. dark skin will turn pale.

Emergency Medical Responder Practice

You respond to a ski slope to find a 26-year-old patient injured his ankle. He had been out skiing for several hours before tripping and injuring his ankle.

1. List four signs and symptoms you might expect to see in this patient.

_____

_____

_____

2. What is your emergency care for this patient?

_____

_____

_____

3. When should you consider rewarming a local cold injury? At what water temperature?

_____

_____

_____

4. You are treating a patient who has been out shoveling snow for several hours without gloves. Your assessment shows his hands are waxy in appearance and you notice blistering. How would you treat this patient?

_____

_____

_____

Matching

Match the following descriptions with the appropriate term.

1. _____ Direct contact with an object

2. _____ Sweat changing to vapor

3. _____ Breathing out warm air

4. _____ Moving air passing over the body

5. _____ Heat transfer without contact

a. Convection
b. Conduction
c. Radiation
d. Evaporation
e. Respiration

Indicate whether each of the following signs or symptoms is seen in mild hypothermia (M) or severe hypothermia (S).

6. _____ Increased breathing rate

7. _____ Extremely slow pulse rate

8. _____ Increased blood pressure

9. _____ Drowsiness

10. _____ Fixed and dilated pupils

11. _____ Rigid extremities

12. _____ Shivering

13. _____ No shivering

Indicate whether each of the following is a type of generalized cold emergency (G) or localized cold emergency (L).

14. _____ Early or superficial frostbite

15. _____ Mild hypothermia

16. _____ Severe hypothermia

17. _____ Late or deep frostbite

1. What risk factors may contribute to a generalized cold emergency?

_____

_____

_____

_____

2. What is the EMS "rule of thumb" for a hypothermic patient?

_____

_____

_____

_____

Heat Emergencies

When a person cannot lose excessive heat, heat-related emergencies often develop. In severe cases left untreated, the body can lose its ability to control body temperature and the patient may develop an uncontrolled rise in body temperature (**hyperthermia**). Hyperthermia can lead to organ damage and death. There are three major heat-related medical conditions. These are commonly called heat exhaustion, heat cramps, and heatstroke. Heatstroke, the most serious, is life threatening.

hyperthermia condition of higher than normal body temperature.

Heat Cramps

Heat cramps involve acute spasms of the muscles of the legs, arms, or abdomen. This may be the result of losing too much electrolytes, including salt, during profuse sweating. Heat cramps usually follow hard work in a hot environment.

ASK YOURSELF

■ Given a variety of scenarios, how would you recognize the signs and symptoms of:
■ heat-related emergencies?

Heat Exhaustion

Heat exhaustion results from excessive sweat loss, resulting in a mild state of shock (hypoperfusion). Hard work in a hot, humid environment can lead to a decrease in blood flow. The resulting decrease in perfusion causes a state of shock.

Heatstroke

Heatstroke is a very serious condition and should be considered life threatening. The body becomes overheated and, in many patients, sweating stops. If left untreated, brain cells will die, causing permanent disability or even death. Think of your vehicle engine running without engine coolant to take away the excess heat. Eventually, the engine overheats and breaks down.

Contributing Factors

Several factors contribute to the risk of heat-related emergencies. One involves heat and humidity. High air temperature can reduce the body's ability to lose heat by radiation.

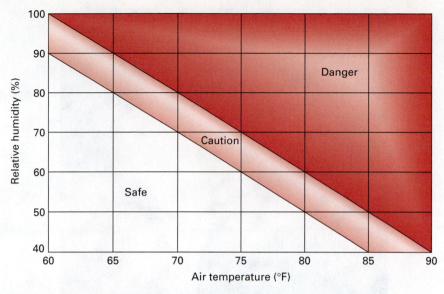

Figure 23-8 Heat and humidity risk scale.

High humidity can reduce its ability to lose heat by evaporation (Figure 23-8 ■). Exercise and strenuous activity also play a part. Each can cause a person to lose more than one liter of sweat (water and electrolytes) per hour.

Other risk factors for a heat emergency include age, medical condition, and certain drugs and medications. Very young and very old patients may be unable to respond to overheating effectively. Any number of medical conditions, such as heart or lung disease, diabetes, dehydration (fluid loss), obesity, fever, and fatigue, can inhibit heat loss. Alcohol, cocaine, barbiturates, psychiatric prescription medications, hallucinogens, and other drugs can affect heat loss in many ways, including through side effects such as dehydration.

EMR Patient Assessment: Heat Emergencies

When you suspect a heat emergency, feel the patient's abdomen to check the body temperature. The chief characteristics of heatstroke are hot skin and a change in mental status. General signs and symptoms of a heat emergency are listed in Table 23-4 and Figures 23-9 ■ and 23-10 ■.

TABLE 23-4 Signs and Symptoms: Heat Emergencies

- High body temperature
- Weakness, exhaustion
- Muscle cramps
- Dizziness, faintness
- Rapid pulse rate that is strong at first, but becomes weak as damage progresses
- Headache
- Seizures
- Loss of appetite, nausea, vomiting
- Altered mental status, possibly unresponsiveness
- Skin that may be moist, pale, and normal to cool in temperature (heat exhaustion or heat cramps) or hot and moist or hot and dry (heatstroke) (Figure 23-10)

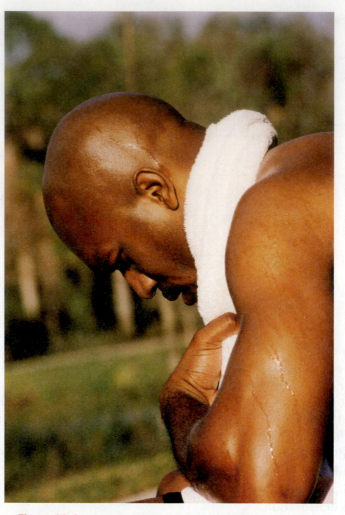

■ **Figure 23-9** Physical activity in extreme temperatures may cause heat-related emergencies. (© *Kevin Dodge/Masterfile*)

EMR Emergency Care: Heat Emergencies

If you suspect a patient has a heat emergency you should immediately notify the responding EMS personnel and take appropriate Standard Precautions (Scan 23-1). Steps to providing care for this patient include:

1. Remove the patient from the hot environment. Place him in a cool place, if possible. If the source of heat is the sun, place the patient in the shade.
2. Administer oxygen, if you are allowed to do so. If breathing is adequate, administer oxygen with a nonrebreather mask. If breathing is not adequate, assist ventilations with a bag-valve mask and supplemental oxygen.
3. Cool the patient. First, loosen or remove his clothing. Then:
   a. If the patient has moist, pale, and normal to cool skin, fan the surface of his body while applying a light mist of water.
   b. If the patient has an altered mental status and either hot and dry or hot and moist skin, apply cold packs to his neck, armpits, and groin. Keep the skin wet by applying water with wet towels or a sponge. Fan the patient aggressively or direct an electric fan toward him.
   c. Be careful not to cool the patient so fast that he becomes chilled and starts shivering. This will generate more internal heat. Do not let the patient fan himself, as this too will generate more internal heat.

NORMAL SKIN TEMPERATURE

HEAT STROKE

- High body temperature
- Heat stroke
- Rapid pulse and breathing (pulse may be bounding)
- Skin dry or only slightly moist
- Dilated pupils
- Altered mental status
- Seizures possible

HEAT EXHAUSTION

- Rapid pulse and breathing (pulse may be weak)
- Moist skin
- Weakness, exhaustion, muscle cramps

■ **Figure 23-10** Comparison of heat emergencies.

4. Position the patient. Place him in a supine position with legs elevated 8 to 12 inches, if there is no indication of spine or lower-extremity trauma.
5. Monitor the patient. Take vital signs frequently. Advise the incoming units if the patient develops signs of shock.

SCAN 23-1 | Caring for a Heat Emergency Patient

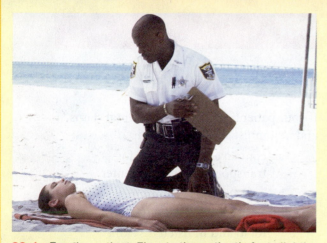

23-1a Fan the patient. Elevate the patient's feet slightly with a blanket.

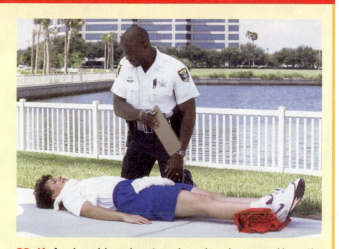

23-1b Apply cold packs at neck and groin areas. Keep the patient's feet slightly elevated with a blanket.

If the patient is alert and not nauseated, encourage him to drink about one-half glass of cool water or sport drink every 15 minutes or so (follow local protocol or consult with medical direction).

THE RESPONSE ✳

As you begin your assessment, you notice the patient is responding to verbal stimuli but is not very alert. Her airway appears clear, and she is breathing rapidly. Her pulse is rapid and weak. Her skin is hot to the touch and reddish in color. You notice that even though you and most people around you are sweating, your patient is not. The patient's initial vital signs are pulse of 136 and weak, respirations of 32, and blood pressure of 102/48.

The patient says she is extremely weak and feels like she might faint. Your partner brings your attention to a medical identification bracelet that states she has an allergy to penicillin. She states this has never happened to her before. When you ask what she was doing when the symptoms started, she states she was finishing her daily run when she suddenly became very exhausted and started having a headache. She sat down under the tree and doesn't remember much else.

You allow the patient to sit in a position of comfort while continuing to monitor her airway and breathing. You place the patient on oxygen at 15 lpm by nonrebreather mask. Following local protocol, you place cold packs to her neck, armpits, and groin. You request the bystanders to keep fanning her.

Reassessment shows a slightly improved mental status. Repeated vital signs are pulse of 112, respirations of 26, and blood pressure of 108/56.

■ Discussion: *Regarding medications and her allergy to penicillin, what else must you ask the patient?*

✳ Stop, Review, Remember

Multiple Choice

Place a check next to the correct answer.

1. A severe heat emergency that develops into an uncontrolled rise in body temperature is called:

   ____ a. hypothermia.

   ____ b. hyperthermia.

   ____ c. hypoventilation.

   ____ d. hyperventilation.

2. If your patient has an altered mental status and hot, moist skin you should:

   ____ a. contact air evacuation for transport to a trauma center.

   ____ b. cool the patient until they shiver.

   ____ c. apply cold packs to the patient's torso and moisten his skin.

   ____ d. Fan the body only. Do not apply cold or moisten the skin.

3. Which of the following statements in regard to heat emergencies is true?

_____ a. Do not apply oxygen in heat emergencies to prevent cellular damage.

_____ b. Care for heat emergencies is the same no matter the amount of heat or patient presentation.

_____ c. Nauseated patients should be encouraged to drink to eliminate the nausea.

_____ d. Patients should be moved immediately from areas where they are exposed to heat.

4. Which of the following is NOT a predisposing factor to heat emergency?

_____ a. Age

_____ b. Humidity

_____ c. Alcohol use

_____ d. Mental state

5. Heat cramps involve muscles in all of the following areas except the

_____ a. abdomen.

_____ b. head.

_____ c. arms.

_____ d. legs.

Matching

Match the heat emergency with the appropriate presentation.

1. _____ Spasms in legs, arms, or abdomen

2. _____ Mild state of shock

3. _____ Life-threatening overheating

a. Heat exhaustion
b. Heat cramps
c. Heatstroke

Emergency Medical Responder Practice

You respond to a construction site for a patient who has collapsed after working in the heat.

1. List four signs or symptoms you would expect to see.

_____

_____

_____

_____

2. What emergency care would you provide for this patient?

_____

_____

_____

_____

3. What risk factors may contribute to a heat emergency?

_____

_____

_____

_____

Submersion Emergencies

Water is a valuable compound that affects many aspects of our daily lives. It fills the oceans, lakes, ponds, rivers, creeks, swimming pools, drainage ditches, and the list goes on. In fact, 70 percent of the world we live on is covered with water. Water even makes up 60 percent of the human body. We use water to quench our thirst, prepare our food, wash our clothes, and provide us a source for recreation. Like so many aspects of life, water can enhance our daily lives or it can be a source of dangerous consequences, including death.

Drowning is defined as death from suffocation due to submersion. In 2005, the Centers for Disease Control and Prevention (CDC) reported over 3,500 fatal unintentional drownings in the United States and an additional 710 deaths from drowning and other causes in boating-related incidents. You may still hear responders using the term "near-drowning." However, its use is being phased out. A near-drowning is simply a patient who survived a drowning incident.

Keep in mind that a drowning patient dies from **suffocation**, the deprivation of air exchange, and not because his lungs filled with water. Autopsies have revealed that only a small percentage of patients who died from drowning had aspirated a significant amount of water.

There are many contributing factors involved in drownings and water-related incidents. Most of these are preventable:

- *Lack of barriers and supervision.* Children under 1 year of age most often drown in bathtubs, buckets, or toilets. Children 1 to 4 years of age most often drown in residential swimming pools. In most cases, children were left unsupervised for less than 5 minutes. Fencing and other access control measures can help prevent unsupervised pool access.

- *Age and recreation in natural water settings.* The percent of drownings in natural water settings (such as lakes, rivers, or the ocean) increases with age. Most drownings in those over 15 years of age occur in natural water settings.

- *Lack of appropriate choices in recreational boating.* In 2006, the U.S. Coast Guard reported 90 percent of those boaters who drowned were not wearing personal flotation devices (life jackets).

- *Alcohol use.* Alcohol use is involved in up to half of adolescent and adult deaths associated with water recreation and about one in five reported boating fatalities. Also, intoxicated adults may fail to properly supervise children who suffer drowning or submersion emergencies.

- *Seizure disorders.* For persons with seizure disorders, drowning is the most common cause of death from an unintentional injury, with the bathtub as the site of highest drowning risk.

General Guidelines for Water Rescue

When determining how to appropriately respond to a water emergency, you need to take several considerations into mind:

- Patient condition
  - *Mental status.* Is the patient responsive and able to assist in the rescue? If so, reaching out with a pole or throwing a rope may be the safest method of rescue.
  - *Position.* Is the patient on the surface or is he submerged? If submerged, he may need basic life support immediately. He may also be difficult to locate.
  - *Injuries.* Does the patient have any obvious injuries? Did the patient dive into the water and possibly suffer a neck injury? If so, you may have to properly extricate him from the water before beginning care.

---

drowning death from suffocation due to submersion.

suffocation the deprivation of air exchange.

ASK YOURSELF

- What are several ways to prevent drowning?

ASK YOURSELF

- What are the guidelines for determining how to respond in a water rescue situation?

■ Water conditions

■ *Visibility.* How deep can you see? Is the water clear, cloudy, or muddy? Can you see any potential hazards in or under the water? Can you see the patient and his injuries?

■ *Temperature.* For a cold water drowning, you must continue resuscitation until the patient is rewarmed at the hospital. Remember, "You're not dead until you're warm and dead." Also remember that a patient loses body heat 25 times faster in water than air.

■ *Moving water.* Will the location of the patient change? Is it safe for you to enter the water? Fast moving water can sweep you away or hold you under. Look for hazards specific to moving water:

■ Strainers are obstructions that allow water to pass through but catch people and larger objects.

■ Fixed obstructions such as bridge abutments may pin the patient or rescuer.

■ Holes created from the moving current where water recirculates may trap the patient or rescuer.

■ Low-head dams can be either man-made or a result of a horizontal obstruction (Figure 23-11 ■). Water flows over the dam and recirculates at the bottom. You may notice a **boil line** where the water below the dam divides, part continuing downstream and part recirculating in the boil.

boil line point where the water below a low-head dam divides; part of the water continues downstream and part recirculates back into the boil.

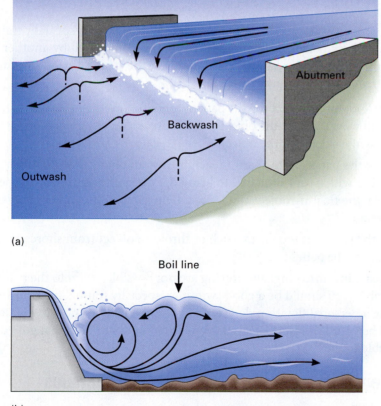

(a)

(b)

■ **Figure 23-11** A low-head dam (a) can form a large and uniform hole creating a boil line (b). If too close to the boil line, a boater can capsize and get pushed to the bottom.

- *Water depth.* Can your feet touch the bottom so you can stand? Will additional equipment be needed to reach the patient?
- *Other hazards.* Are there any hazardous materials present? Submerged vehicles may be leaking fluids. Are there any obstructions such as fallen trees, branches, or debris? Is there any chance of electrocution?
- Resources on hand
- *Number of personnel and abilities.* How many rescuers are on scene? Can they all swim? Are they trained in water rescue?
- *Equipment.* Do they have the appropriate equipment, including personal flotation devices (PFDs) for each rescuer?
- *Specialized teams.* Do you need assistance from specialized teams, such as a dive rescue team?

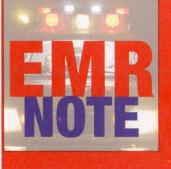

EMR NOTE

Everyone in or near the water during a rescue situation must wear a personal flotation device. Many well-intended rescuers have been injured or even lost their lives by not wearing this indispensable safety device.

Never attempt a water rescue unless you are a good swimmer, specially trained in water rescue, wearing a personal flotation device, and accompanied by another rescuer. If you can answer "yes" to these criteria, you should use the "reach, throw, row, and then go" strategy to attempt rescue (Figure 23-12 ■):

- *Reach.* Hold out an object for the patient to grab. Anything that will extend your reach will work. Be sure the object will not break. Make sure you maintain a solid footing while extending the object.
- *Throw.* If the patient is too far to reach, throw an object that floats (preferably something with a rope attached to bring the patient to shore). If a rope is not available, the floating object can at least help support the patient above water until rescue.
- *Row.* If the patient is too far to reach or throw an object from shore, use a boat to get closer to the patient.
- *Go.* If reaching, throwing, and rowing are not possible, swim to the patient. Remember, you should be a good swimmer, specially trained in water rescue, wearing a personal flotation device, and accompanied by another rescuer. This should be your last resort as it puts you in the same situation that got your patient in trouble in the first place.

EMR Patient Assessment: Submersion Emergencies

Any type of medical or traumatic emergency that occurs on land may occur in the water. If the mechanism of injury leads you to suspect a spine injury, you should use appropriate manual stabilization techniques throughout your assessment and care. General signs and symptoms of a submersion emergency are listed in Table 23-5.

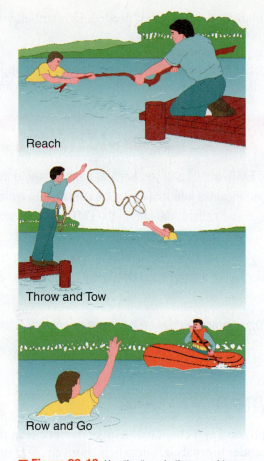

Reach

Throw and Tow

Row and Go

■ **Figure 23-12** Use the "reach, throw and tow, row and go" strategy when attempting a water rescue.

TABLE 23-5 Signs and Symptoms: Submersion Emergency

- Coughing
- Vomiting
- Difficulty breathing
- Respiratory arrest
- Cardiac arrest

EMR Emergency Care: Submersion Emergencies

The goal of patient care for the patient suffering from a submersion emergency is to safely rescue the patient from the water and provide appropriate care as follows:

1. Perform an appropriate scene size-up, including Standard Precautions. This may include donning specialized apparel for the environment.
2. Make sure the EMS system is activated, as appropriate.
3. Establish and maintain airway and breathing. This can be done in the water, if needed. Drowning patients frequently vomit, so be prepared to suction or turn the patient on his side. If there is a suspected neck injury, use the jaw-thrust maneuver to open the airway.
4. Remove the patient from the water. Use the "reach, throw, row, and then go" strategy.
5. Position the patient. If you suspect a spine injury, use manual stabilization and the jaw-thrust maneuver. If you do not suspect a spine injury and the patient is breathing, place him in the recovery position.

ASK YOURSELF

■ Given a scenario, how would you demonstrate the assessment and management of patients with a submersion emergency?

6. Maintain circulation. Begin CPR, if needed. Remember, your patient is not dead until he is warm and dead.
7. Administer oxygen, if you are allowed to do so.
8. Monitor the patient for signs of hypothermia and treat appropriately.
9. Notify responding EMS personnel of the patient's condition and any changes.

CASE STUDY

TRANSITION

The EMTs arrive, and you transfer patient care to them. Your verbal report includes information on the condition in which you found the scene and patient. You inform the EMTs that her skin was hot and nearly dry so you placed the ice packs to cool her.

After providing the EMTs with your verbal report, you proceed to restock your supplies and document the response in your written report.

■ Discussion: *What have you learned from this case? Would you recommend doing anything differently?*

THE LAST WORD

Metabolism is all the physical and chemical changes that occur in the body. This process generates heat which, under normal circumstances, is given off from the body by convection, conduction, radiation, evaporation, or respirations.

There are several risk factors that might not allow the body processes to function normally. These include the environment, medical conditions, medications or substances, and age.

Many contributing factors are involved in drownings and water-related incidents. Most of these are preventable by using safety devices around pools, using personal flotation devices in and around water, and avoiding substances that might impair judgment or abilities.

Keep in mind that the same situation creating the emergency might also affect you or your crew. Your care must be focused on scene safety, appropriate patient assessment, and providing support to the airway, breathing, and circulation. If your patient is experiencing a cold emergency, your goal is to stop further heat loss and possibly warm the patient. If your patient is experiencing a heat emergency, your goal is to cool the patient. If your patient is experiencing a submersion emergency, your goal is to safely remove the patient from the water and provide appropriate care.

As you render assistance, remember that the same situation that caused your patient's cold, heat, or submersion emergency may also affect you and your crew. You cannot help others if you, too, succumb to an environmental emergency.

Multiple Choice

Place a check next to the correct answer.

1. In which of the following situations is the patient losing body heat primarily by convection?

   _____ a. A 55-year-old male is found lying on the frozen ground without a coat.

   _____ b. A 24-year-old male is wearing wet clothing after falling out of his boat while fishing.

   _____ c. A 32-year-old female is outside in cool, windy weather.

   _____ d. A vapor cloud is created every time your 80-year-old female patient breathes into the cool night air.

2. Which of the following is *not* a significant risk factor for heat- and cold-related emergencies?

   _____ a. Old age

   _____ b. Gender

   _____ c. Circulatory problems

   _____ d. Very young age

3. If your patient is found in the cold, not shivering, with a diminished level of responsiveness, you should suspect:

   _____ a. mild hypothermia.

   _____ b. severe hypothermia.

   _____ c. mild hyperthermia.

   _____ d. severe hyperthermia.

4. Which of the following signs is *not* seen in severe hypothermia?

   _____ a. Rigidity or freezing of the extremities

   _____ b. Slow or irregular pulse rate

   _____ c. Increased respiratory rate

   _____ d. Dilated pupils

5. Your severely hypothermic patient is showing signs of death. What rule of thumb can guide you in your decision to continue, or stop, performing CPR on this patient?

   _____ a. You're not dead until you're warm and dead.

   _____ b. Rely on the chain of survival.

   _____ c. Airway! Airway! Airway!

   _____ d. OPQRST-ASPN.

6. All of the following are appropriate steps in the management of a patient with a generalized cold emergency except:

   _____ a. remove the patient from the cold environment.

   _____ b. protect the patient from further heat loss.

   _____ c. provide warm liquids to drink.

   _____ d. monitor his vital signs.

7. Emergency Medical Responder care for a late or deep local cold injury to an extremity includes:

   _____ a. rubbing and massaging the affected area.

   _____ b. covering the affected area with a dry dressing.

   _____ c. actively rewarming the part to prevent tissue damage.

   _____ d. allowing the patient to walk to maintain circulation.

8. A responsive patient who is suffering from a heat emergency has cool, moist skin. She is most likely suffering from:

   _____ a. mild hypothermia.

   _____ b. severe hypothermia.

   _____ c. heat exhaustion.

   _____ d. heatstroke.

9. Which of the following factors does *not* directly contribute to the risk of a heat-related emergency?

   _____ a. Patient's age

   _____ b. Strenuous activity

   _____ c. Patient's mental status

   _____ d. Patient's medication and drug use

10. In order, what are the steps in water rescue?

    _____ a. Throw, reach, row, go

    _____ b. Row, reach, throw, go

    _____ c. Row, go, throw, reach

    _____ d. Reach, throw, row, go

Emergency Medical Responder Practice

It's your summer vacation and you and your friend Pat are hiking through the state park. You are both in good physical condition. After a while, you notice that she is trailing behind. You backtrack and find her stopped and standing just to the side of the path.

1. As you approach her, what should you do first?

   _____

   _____

   _____

2. When you are at Pat's side, you ask her, "Are you okay? Why did you stop?" She looks you straight in the eye, smiles, and says, "I'm fine. I just want to rest for a second. I'm not used to trekking uphill with a full backpack." You notice that she is sweating a little harder than you'd like, but her breathing and color seem to be fine. As you observe your friend, you bring to mind the signs and symptoms of a heat emergency. What are they?

   _____

   _____

   _____

   _____

3. When Pat feels she has rested enough, you both continue on with your hike without any further incident. However, if Pat had been experiencing a heat emergency, what could you have done for her?

   _____

   _____

   _____

   _____

Matching

Match the following descriptions with the appropriate term.

1. _____ Point where the water below a low-head dam divides; part of the water continues downstream and part recirculates back into the boil
2. _____ Heat loss through breathing
3. _____ All the physical and chemical changes that occur in the body, including digestion
4. _____ Localized tissue death
5. _____ The process by which sweat changes to vapor and has a cooling effect on the body
6. _____ Death from suffocation due to submersion
7. _____ Heat loss involving the transfer of heat to an object without physical contact
8. _____ Heat loss through direct contact with an object
9. _____ Heat loss through moving air or water passing over the body
10. _____ Condition of lower than normal body temperature
11. _____ Localized cold injury
12. _____ Condition of higher than normal body temperature
13. _____ The deprivation of air exchange

a. Metabolism
b. Convection
c. Conduction
d. Radiation
e. Evaporation
f. Respirations
g. Hypothermia
h. Frostbite
i. Gangrene
j. Hyperthermia
k. Drowning
l. Suffocation
m. Boil line

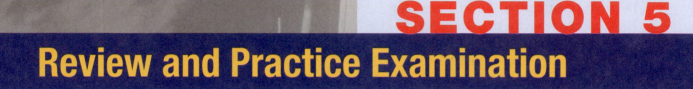

Review and Practice Examination

Assess what you have learned in this section by checking the best answer for each multiple-choice question. When you are done, check your answers against the key provided in Appendix B.

1. EMS systems initially developed from the desire to provide better care to victims of:
   _____ a. trauma.
   _____ b. heart attack.
   _____ c. choking.
   _____ d. environmental emergencies.

2. Hospitals that meet strict criteria set by the American College of Surgeons to properly care for trauma patients are known as:
   _____ a. EMS systems.
   _____ b. emergency departments.
   _____ c. accident and emergency rooms.
   _____ d. trauma centers.

3. The first step in the scene size-up on trauma calls is:
   _____ a. determining the mechanism of injury.
   _____ b. developing an index of suspicion for specific injuries.
   _____ c. determining scene safety.
   _____ d. determining the number of patients.

4. Your patient is a 40-year-old male who cut his hand while he was sharpening a lawn mower blade. He is alert and oriented, but has a 3-inch cut across the palm of his right hand. Which of the following best describes the appropriate EMR assessment for this patient?

   _____ a. Perform a primary assessment, examine the injured area, and take vital signs.
   _____ b. No assessment of this patient is required before the transporting EMS unit arrives.
   _____ c. Perform a primary assessment, take vital signs, and perform a head-to-toe exam.
   _____ d. Examine the injured area.

5. Strong consideration for transporting to a trauma center or using helicopter transportation should be given to patients who have a Glasgow Coma Scale score of less than:
   _____ a. 15.
   _____ b. 12.
   _____ c. 8.
   _____ d. 3.

6. While you are assessing a patient, he does not open his eyes to a verbal request or to a pinch of his trapezius muscle. His eye-opening score for the Glasgow Coma Scale is:
   _____ a. 0.
   _____ b. 1.
   _____ c. 2.
   _____ d. 3.

7. While you are assessing a patient, he complies with your request to roll up his pants leg so you can inspect his injured ankle. You would assign a Glasgow Coma Scale motor response score of:
_____ a. 6.
_____ b. 5.
_____ c. 4.
_____ d. 3.

8. A 25-year-old male was beaten with a metal pipe during a fight. Law enforcement is on the scene, and the patient is awake, sitting up against a wall when you arrive. He is angry and resisting the help of his friend, who is trying to hold an ice pack on his forehead. The patient is not wearing a shirt. You see no bleeding, but the patient has several bruises on his back, sides, and chest. The patient is sweating and cursing, and trying to get up from the floor. Which of the following is the highest priority in caring for this patient?
_____ a. Getting him to calm down so his friend can hold the ice pack on his forehead
_____ b. Giving the patient oxygen
_____ c. Inserting a nasal airway
_____ d. Checking the blood pressure

9. Which of the following is an early sign of shock?
_____ a. Unresponsiveness
_____ b. Low blood pressure
_____ c. Increased heart rate
_____ d. Blue or mottled skin

10. A 21-year-old female complains of severe lower abdominal pain. She is pale with cool, sweaty skin. Her radial pulse is very weak and rapid, her respirations are shallow and rapid, and her blood pressure is 100/78. Which of the following can you say for certain about this patient?
_____ a. She is in early shock.
_____ b. She is starting to decompensate.
_____ c. She is in irreversible shock.
_____ d. Her signs and symptoms are most likely due to her pain.

11. True or False: When blood loss occurs, a patient's tissue oxygenation remains normal until his blood pressure drops.
_____ a. True
_____ b. False

12. In which of the following patients should you be most concerned about shock?
_____ a. A 12-year-old male who has numerous scrapes on his hands, elbows, knees, and chin after falling off his skateboard
_____ b. A 25-year-old female who says she vomited once and that the vomit looked like what she ate for lunch
_____ c. A 75-year-old female who fainted in church and who still says she feels weak, dizzy, and nauseated
_____ d. A 35-year-old male who stepped on a nail, which remains stuck in his foot

13. A 19-year-old male has been stabbed in the neck, and has what appears to be significant blood loss. He does not respond to your voice and you can hear gurgling with each shallow breath that he takes. Bleeding from the wound continues. Which of the following should you do?
_____ a. Apply direct pressure to the wound while simultaneously opening the airway, and then apply oxygen with a nonrebreather mask.
_____ b. Open the airway with a jaw thrust, begin ventilations with a bag-valve mask, and then apply direct pressure to the wound.
_____ c. Apply direct pressure to the wound, turn the patient on his side, suction the airway, and communicate the situation to the responding ambulance crew.
_____ d. Apply direct pressure to the wound while simultaneously opening the airway, suction blood from the airway, and begin ventilations with a bag-valve mask.

14. Your patient is a 16-year-old male who was accidentally struck in the back of the head with a machete while cutting weeds. His mother is holding a cloth over the wound. The cloth is saturated with blood, but there does not seem to be a great deal of additional bleeding. The patient is awake and his skin is warm and dry. Which of the following should you do?
_____ a. Have the mother continue direct pressure while you assess the patient and get a history.
_____ b. Take over direct pressure and wait for the responding ambulance crew.
_____ c. Remove the cloth and place a sterile dressing over the wound.
_____ d. Lift the cloth to see how much bleeding is continuing, then continue direct pressure.

15. A 45-year-old male has a large laceration on the inside of his thigh from a mishap with a chain saw. He is sitting on a log and his neighbor is applying direct pressure to the wound. Direct pressure has failed to control the bleeding and the patient is pale, sweaty, and anxious. Which of the following should you immediately do?

_____ a. Inspect the wound, apply a pressure dressing, apply oxygen by nonrebreather mask, then have the patient lie down.

_____ b. Have the patient lie down, apply oxygen by nonrebreather mask, and then secure a tourniquet between his knee and the wound.

_____ c. Apply oxygen by nonrebreather mask, apply a pressure dressing, and then splint the extremity. Add more dressings as needed.

_____ d. Have the patient lie down, secure a tourniquet between the wound and the patient's groin, and then apply oxygen by nonrebreather mask.

16. Your patient is an 82-year-old female with a nosebleed. She states the nosebleed started about an hour ago and hasn't stopped. She is pale with moist skin. Her radial pulse is about 100 per minute and slightly weak. Her respiratory rate is 22. She says she feels a bit woozy and sick to her stomach. Which of the following should you do?

_____ a. Pinch the patient's nostrils together firmly, position her on her side, and be prepared to suction the airway.

_____ b. Pinch the nostrils together firmly, have the patient sit up, leaning slightly forward, and offer her a basin in case she needs to vomit.

_____ c. Place the patient supine and pinch the nostrils together firmly.

_____ d. Obtain a blood pressure before deciding what additional action should be taken.

17. Your patient is a 5-year-old boy who experienced dizziness, wheezing, and difficulty breathing after eating some of a friend's cookies at school. He seems very drowsy and has hives on his arms and body. His respirations are 40 per minute and shallow, and his radial pulse is weak, at about 130 per minute. Which of the following is the highest priority in the care of this patient?

_____ a. Immediately obtain the blood pressure to determine if the patient is in anaphylactic shock.

_____ b. Contact the parents for consent to treat the patient.

_____ c. Find out if the boy has any allergies and exactly what was in the cookies he ate.

_____ d. Start ventilations with a bag-valve mask and supplemental oxygen.

18. Which of the following would you do when caring for a patient who has a 1-inch diameter open wound just below the right shoulder blade?

_____ a. Cover the wound with airtight material and tape on three sides.

_____ b. Apply a cold pack to the wound.

_____ c. Use a thick, absorbent dressing to control bleeding.

_____ d. Pack the wound with petroleum gauze.

19. You have applied an occlusive dressing to a sucking chest wound. Your patient begins to deteriorate. His breathing is more labored and shallow, he is more anxious, and his heart rate is increasing. He is becoming mottled and sweaty. You should:

_____ a. replace the occlusive dressing with a thick, absorbent dressing to control bleeding.

_____ b. lift the occlusive dressing to release pressure building up in the chest.

_____ c. insert a needle into the chest to relieve pressure building up in the chest.

_____ d. apply firm direct pressure over the top of the occlusive dressing.

20. A hemothorax involves:

_____ a. air trapped in the chest cavity under pressure.

_____ b. an accumulation of air between the lung and chest wall.

_____ c. blood in the alveoli of the lungs.

_____ d. an accumulation of blood between the lung and chest wall.

21. A 21-year-old male patient was struck in the right side of his chest with a baseball bat. As you palpate the area, you feel a crackling, popping sound in the soft tissues around the area. This finding is known as:

_____ a. subcutaneous emphysema.

_____ b. pneumothorax.

_____ c. traumatic asphyxia.

_____ d. tension pneumothorax.

22. An 82-year-old female fell out of bed, striking the left side of her chest against a nightstand in the process. She is awake and has had no change in mental status. Her airway is open, she is breathing 20 times per minute, and she has a radial pulse of 88 per minute. Her skin is warm and dry. She complains of pain in the left side of her chest, difficulty breathing, and pain with breathing. Her breath sounds are present and equal bilaterally. After applying oxygen, which of the following is appropriate in the care of this patient?

_____ a. Wrapping the chest with an elastic bandage to splint the ribs

_____ b. Having the patient lie on her left side

_____ c. Having the patient hold a pillow against the painful area of her chest

_____ d. Performing positive pressure ventilation

23. A 50-year-old male was working in an industrial setting when a sealed 55-gallon drum of fluid fell onto him, striking him in the chest. He is lying supine on a concrete floor, and the barrel has rolled off to the side. It is not leaking, and there are no other hazards. The patient responds to your voice, but is anxious and confused. His skin is mottled, especially above the shoulders, and cool. He is sweating profusely. His airway is open, he is breathing 30 times per minute with shallow breaths, and he has a weak radial pulse of 124. An examination of the chest reveals bruising, but no deformity, crepitus, or abnormal motion. Which of the following is the best way of managing this patient until EMS arrives?

_____ a. Assist the patient into a semisitting position and have him hold a pillow against the injured area; apply oxygen by nonrebreather mask.

_____ b. Apply oxygen by nonrebreather mask, manually stabilize the spine, and secure a firm object such as a clipboard or book over the injured area to limit movement of the flail segment.

_____ c. Manually stabilize the spine, apply oxygen by nonrebreather mask, and elevate the legs 24 to 36 inches at the feet.

_____ d. Manually stabilize the spine, assist breathing with a bag-valve mask and supplemental oxygen, and perform continual reassessment.

24. An evisceration of the abdominal organs is best treated by:

_____ a. direct pressure over the affected organs.

_____ b. bulky, dry, sterile dressings.

_____ c. moist, sterile dressings covered by an occlusive dressing.

_____ d. repositioning the organs within the abdominal cavity.

25. A 35-year-old man who fell from a second-story roof landed on a garden stake, which is impaled in his abdomen, just below the right costal margin (lower border of the rib cage). The other end of the stake is protruding 3 to 4 inches from the body, just below the right scapula. There is surprisingly little bleeding around the entrance and exit wounds. Which of the following should be done in the care of this patient?

_____ a. Lay him supine and manually stabilize his head and neck.

_____ b. First use a hand saw to cut the protruding portions of the stake flush with the body, then lay the patient supine.

_____ c. Stabilize the patient's head and neck with the patient on his left side; use bulky dressings to stabilize both ends of the stake.

_____ d. Withdraw the stake by pushing it through the body in the same direction it entered.

26. Which of the following statements concerning soft tissue injuries is true?

_____ a. Soft tissue injuries are never life threatening.

_____ b. Soft tissues include skin, fatty tissue, muscle, and bone.

_____ c. Blunt mechanisms of soft tissue injury are not as concerning as penetrating mechanism.

_____ d. Soft tissue injuries may distract the patient and the EMR from other, more serious injuries.

27. An 11-year-old boy has a hematoma to the back of his head after falling out of the hayloft of a barn and striking his head on the concrete barn floor. Of the following, the most serious immediate concern for this patient is:

_____ a. potential injury to the brain.

_____ b. bleeding from the hematoma.

_____ c. the possibility of swelling around the wound.

_____ d. infection of the wound.

28. A 31-year-old female caught the back of her arm on a piece of metal while working around the barnyard. She describes the injury as a "three-corner tear." In your documentation, you could accurately refer to this injury as a(n):

_____ a. incision.

_____ b. laceration.

_____ c. avulsion.

_____ d. abrasion.

29. The first consideration in caring for a patient with an open soft tissue wound is:

_____ a. controlling bleeding.

_____ b. ensuring an open airway.

_____ c. preventing further contamination of the wound.

_____ d. performing a head-to-toe assessment.

30. Which of the following statements regarding wound dressings is true?

_____ a. The ideal dressing for most wounds is sterile, absorbent, and nonstick.

_____ b. A dressing is used to secure bandages in place.

_____ c. A dressing should be exactly the same size as the wound.

_____ d. Most dressings are made to stick to the wound to aid in bleeding control.

31. Which of the following is true concerning soft tissue injuries to the neck?

_____ a. Open wounds are more serious than closed wounds.

_____ b. Closed, but not open, wounds may compromise the airway.

_____ c. Open wounds should be covered with an occlusive dressing.

_____ d. A circumferential dressing is used for both open and closed wounds.

32. A 30-year-old factory worker's hand has been amputated after being caught in machinery. The first priority in this situation is:

_____ a. making sure the machinery has been shut down and no other uncontrolled hazards are present.

_____ b. retrieving the amputated hand for possible reimplantation.

_____ c. controlling bleeding from the wound.

_____ d. applying oxygen.

33. Upon arriving at the scene of an injured woman as a result of a dog attack, a large dog approaches your vehicle. He does not seem aggressive and it is not known if this is the dog that caused the injuries. You should:

_____ a. open your door slowly and see if the dog shows signs of aggression.

_____ b. check with dispatch to see if animal control is en route.

_____ c. park as close to the house as possible in order to make entrance with the least chance of contact with the animal.

_____ d. attempt to capture the animal so it can be checked for rabies.

34. A 14-year-old girl accidentally made contact with a hot iron on her forearm. She has two blisters surrounded by an area of reddened skin and complains that the burn is very painful. This injury is most likely a _____ burn.

_____ a. full-thickness

_____ b. partial-thickness

_____ c. serious superficial

_____ d. superficial

35. In addition to the depth of a burn injury, which of the following would make the burn be considered more severe?

_____ a. Burns of the lower leg

_____ b. Burns of 2 percent body surface area or more

_____ c. Burns of the face

_____ d. Burns caused by heat, rather than chemicals

36. A 28-year-old male received an electrical shock when he cut through an electrical line beneath a trailer with a power saw. The most critical concern for this patient should be:

_____ a. potential heart complications.

_____ b. extensive external burn injuries.

_____ c. finding an exit wound.

_____ d. long bone fractures.

37. Which of the following is a sign of increased pressure within the skull?

_____ a. Low blood pressure

_____ b. Abnormal respiratory patterns

_____ c. Increased heart rate

_____ d. Temporary memory loss for events occurring after the injury

38. A 55-year-old male who was not wearing a helmet was thrown from his motorcycle after colliding with a car. He is having seizure activity when you arrive. Your highest priority in caring for this patient is:

_____ a. examining the head for signs of injury.

_____ b. checking the pupils for signs of brain injury.

_____ c. doing your best to prevent movement of the neck and maintain an open airway.

_____ d. checking for an increase in blood pressure and decrease in heart rate.

39. A 51-year-old female fell off a ladder and struck her head on the sidewalk. You notice blood-tinged fluid in the right ear. This is an indication of:

_____ a. a skull fracture.

_____ b. concussion.

_____ c. increased intracranial pressure.

_____ d. herniation.

40. Which of the following principles should be followed when caring for an eye injury?

_____ a. Apply direct pressure to the eye.

_____ b. Irrigate the eye with water to remove blood in order to better examine the eye.

_____ c. Remove impaled objects from the eye.

_____ d. Bandage both eyes, even if only one is injured.

41. Which of the following statements is true concerning cervical collars?

_____ a. It is better to use a poorly fitting collar than not to use a collar if you do not have the right-sized collar for a patient.

_____ b. A cervical collar prevents movement of the neck.

_____ c. A properly fitting cervical collar allows neutral, in-line immobilization of the neck.

_____ d. A soft cervical collar can be used if the mechanism of injury is questionable.

42. In which of the following cases should a helmet be removed from a patient?

_____ a. The helmet interferes with airway management.

_____ b. The patient complains of head pain.

_____ c. Cervical spine injury is suspected.

_____ d. The patient is also wearing shoulder pads.

43. A strain is an injury of a:

_____ a. joint.

_____ b. muscle.

_____ c. bone.

_____ d. ligament.

44. The best way to immobilize a shoulder injury is a:

_____ a. traction splint.

_____ b. rigid splint.

_____ c. sling and swathe.

_____ d. pillow splint.

45. A traction splint is appropriate only for fractures of the:

_____ a. pelvis.

_____ b. femur.

_____ c. humerus.

_____ d. knee.

46. An amputated part is best managed by:

_____ a. placing it directly on ice.

_____ b. wrapping it in a dry, bulky dressing.

_____ c. soaking it in water.

_____ d. wrapping in sterile, saline-moistened gauze.

47. True or False: Shivering stops when patients become progressively more hypothermic.

_____ a. True

_____ b. False

48. Which of the following is appropriate in the treatment of a patient who is severely hypothermic?

_____ a. Warm fluids by mouth

_____ b. Vigorous massage of the extremities

_____ c. Having the patient move about

_____ d. Removing wet clothing

49. The most serious type of heat-related emergency is:

_____ a. heatstroke.

_____ b. heat exhaustion.

_____ c. heat cramps.

_____ d. hypothermia.

50. A 17-year-old high school athlete collapsed during practice in 90°F temperatures and 80 percent humidity. She responds only to painful stimuli, and has hot, flushed skin. Which of the following is most critical in the treatment of this patient?

_____ a. Administer sips of cool water or sports drink.

_____ b. Have the coaching staff bring as many bags of ice as possible and cover the patient with ice.

_____ c. Wet the skin and fan the patient aggressively.

_____ d. Begin CPR if a radial pulse cannot be felt.

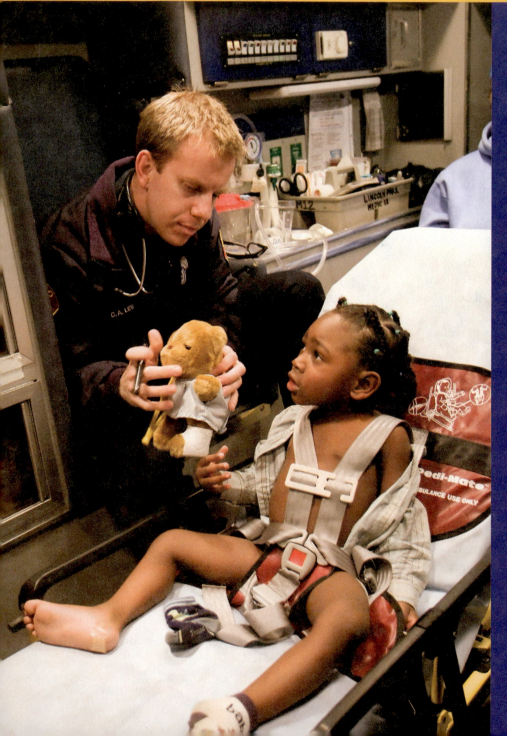

SECTION 6
Special Patient Populations

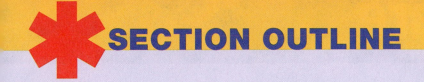

SECTION OUTLINE

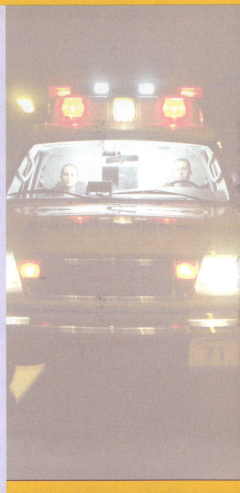

In this section you will cover the following EMS Education Standards:

■ Special Patient Populations

■ Trauma

Obstetrics and Neonatal Care

NAVIGATION GUIDE

The following items provide an overview to the purpose and content of this chapter. The Education Standards and Competency are from the National EMS Education Standards.

Education Standards Special Patient Populations (Obstetrics, Neonatal Care); Trauma

Competency Recognizes and manages life threats based on simple assessment findings for a patient with special needs while awaiting additional emergency response.

Knowledge Areas Obstetrics, Neonatal Care
- Normal delivery
- Vaginal bleeding in the pregnant patient
- Newborn care
- Neonatal resuscitation

Objectives After reading this chapter, you should be able to:

1. Define key terms introduced in this chapter.
2. Describe the functions of the uterus, cervix, placenta, umbilical cord, amniotic sac, and birth canal in pregnancy and childbirth.
3. Describe the events of each of the three stages of labor.
4. Discuss the indications that you should expect to assist with delivery on an emergency call.
5. Demonstrate patient positioning to manage or prevent supine hypotension syndrome.
6. Given a scenario, demonstrate preparation for and assistance in newborn delivery.
7. Select correct Standard Precautions for assisting with childbirth.
8. Given a scenario, demonstrate clearing the newborn's mouth and nose of meconium.
9. Given a scenario, demonstrate assessment and care of the newborn.

10. Given a scenario, demonstrate management of complications of delivery, including:
    a. Umbilical cord around the neck
    b. Prolapsed umbilical cord
    c. Abnormal presentations, multiple births
    d. Infant with inadequate breathing, heart rate below 100 per minute, or persistent central cyanosis
    e. Excessive maternal bleeding
11. Recognize the signs and symptoms of pregnancy complications, including preeclampsia, eclampsia, vaginal bleeding, and ectopic pregnancy.
12. Describe the pregnant patient's altered physiological response to trauma.
13. Discuss special considerations in the management of premature infants.

NAVIGATION GUIDE (continued)

Key Terms Page numbers indicate first major use in this chapter. The Margin Glossary in this chapter provides definitions as you read.

Media Resources Please go to **www.bradybooks.com** to access mykit for this text. You will find quizzes, critical thinking scenarios, weblinks, animations, and videos related to this chapter—and much more. Look for online information on pregnancy, labor, and delivery. You will also find video clips on the first stages of labor and newborn resuscitation.

INTRODUCTION

From time to time, an Emergency Medical Responder (EMR) will respond to a call where childbirth has just occurred, or where childbirth is about to occur and there is not enough time to transport the mother before the baby delivers. Most childbirth is uneventful, yet childbirth is painful for the mother and stressful for the family. It can also lead to anxious moments for the EMR. Each of these is an anticipated and appropriate response.

This chapter will provide guidance on making transport decisions, handling a normal delivery and postdelivery care, managing complications associated with pregnancy and childbirth, assessing and caring for the newborn, and providing newborn resuscitative techniques for the rare instances when they are needed. Almost all deliveries will go smoothly and you will have a second patient to care for. Regardless, providing support to the expectant mother is a key component of the obstetrical call. You can help by showing calm and taking control.

ASK YOURSELF

- Can you define key terms introduced in this chapter?

- What are the functions of the uterus, cervix, placenta, umbilical cord, amniotic sac, and birth canal in pregnancy and childbirth?

Anatomy of Pregnancy

The **uterus** is the organ that contains the developing fetus (unborn infant). A special arrangement of smooth muscles and blood vessels in the uterus allows for its expansion to accommodate a pregnancy and the forcible contractions necessary for labor and delivery. After delivery, it also allows for rapid contractions that help to constrict blood vessels and prevent excessive bleeding (Figure 24-1 ■).

During the course of the pregnancy, the wall of the uterus becomes thin. The **cervix**, which is the neck of the uterus that connects with the vagina, contains a mucous plug that is discharged during labor. The expulsion of this plug is known as the **bloody show** and appears as vaginal discharge that is pink-tinged mucus.

The **placenta** is a disk-shaped organ that develops during pregnancy on the inner lining of the uterus. Rich in blood vessels, it provides nourishment and oxygen to the fetus from the mother's blood. It also absorbs waste from the fetus into the mother's bloodstream. The mother's blood and the baby's blood do not

uterus the organ that contains the developing fetus.

cervix the neck of the uterus that connects to the uterus.

bloody show the plug of mucus that is discharged during labor.

placenta a disk-shaped organ on the inner lining of the uterus that provides nourishment and oxygen to a developing fetus.

THE CALL ✳

As your evening shift is about to start, the dispatcher sets off radio tones to tell you to stand by for a call. Shortly you are told to respond to the farmhouse on the corner of County Route 55 and Greenbush Road for a 33-year-old in labor and reporting her contractions to be 4 to 5 minutes apart. The time out is 1605 hours.

Your time to the scene is 12 minutes. When you arrive, you hear a dog barking. A woman's voice tells you she is home alone, the door is open, and the dog won't hurt you. As you enter the residence you see your patient sitting in a chair, and she announces her "water has broken." The dog is jumping up and while not a danger certainly is a significant distraction. Luckily the husband shows up, takes the dog into a room, and closes the door.

You turn all your attention to the patient because you need to find out if she is having contractions, ask numerous other pregnancy-related questions, do an assessment, and get a full set of vital signs. As you start asking the expectant mother questions, the dispatcher radios that the ambulance is still 10 minutes from the scene.

■ Discussion: *What questions should you ask the expectant mother at this point?*

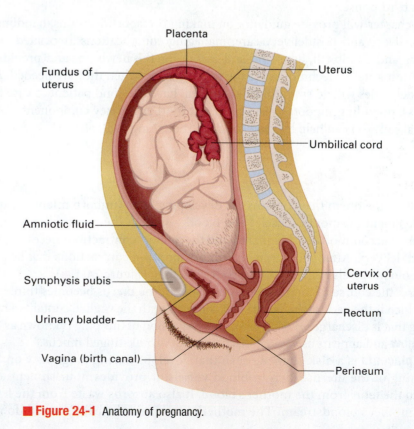

Figure 24-1 Anatomy of pregnancy.

mix. The placenta also produces hormones such as estrogen and progesterone that sustain the pregnancy.

After the baby is delivered, the placenta separates from the uterine wall and delivers as the **afterbirth**. It usually weighs about a pound or about one-sixth to one-seventh of the infant's weight.

The **umbilical cord** is the unborn infant's lifeline. It is an extension of the placenta through which the fetus receives nourishment. The umbilical cord contains one vein and two arteries. The vein carries oxygenated blood to the fetus. The arteries carry deoxygenated blood back to the placenta. When the baby is born, the cord resembles a sturdy rope about 22 inches long and 1 inch in diameter.

The **amniotic sac** is filled with a fluid in which the fetus floats. The amount of fluid varies. It usually ranges from 500 to 1,000 milliliters (from one pint to one quart). The sac of fluid insulates and protects the fetus during pregnancy. During labor, part of the sac usually is forced ahead of the baby, serving as a wedge to help dilate (expand) the cervix. The sac usually bursts during labor, resulting in a gush of fluid from the vagina. The patient will often say, "My water broke."

The **birth canal** is made up of the cervix and the vagina. The vagina is about 8 to 12 centimeters in length, which is approximately 3 to 5 inches. It originates at the cervix and extends to the outside vaginal opening. Its smooth muscle layer stretches gently during childbirth to allow the passage of the infant.

A full-term pregnancy lasts approximately 280 days (40 weeks). Toward the end, the baby usually is in a head-down position, which brings the uterus down and forward. Mothers often can feel the difference and may say that the baby has "dropped." This position is most favorable for the baby's passage through the birth canal.

afterbirth the placenta, after it separates from the uterine wall and delivers.

umbilical cord an extension of the placenta through which the developing fetus receives nourishment while in the uterus.

amniotic sac the sac of fluid in which the developing fetus floats; also called *bag of waters*.

birth canal an anatomical passage made up of the cervix and the vagina.

Stages of Labor

Labor is the term used to describe the process of childbirth. It consists of contractions of the uterine wall, which force the baby into the outside world and later aid the delivery of the placenta. Normal labor is divided into three stages: dilation of the cervix, expulsion, and delivery of the placenta. The length of each stage varies greatly in different women and under different circumstances (Figure 24-2 ■).

labor the term used to describe the process of childbirth

Stage One: Dilation of the Cervix

During this first and longest stage, the cervix becomes fully dilated (expanded). This allows the baby's head to progress from the uterus into the birth canal. Through uterine contractions, the cervix gradually stretches and thins until the opening is large enough for the baby to pass through.

The contractions may begin as an aching sensation in the small of the back. Within a short time, the contractions become cramplike pains in the lower abdomen. These reoccur at regular intervals, each one lasting about 30 to 60 seconds. At first, the contractions are usually 10 to 20 minutes apart and may not feel very painful. They may even stop completely for a while and then start again. Appearance of the mucous plug (bloody show) may occur before or during this stage of labor. Also before or during this stage, the amniotic sac may rupture, resulting in a gush of fluid from the vagina.

Stage one may continue for 18 hours or longer for a woman having her first baby. Women who have had a child before may have labor as short as 2 or 3 hours. By the end of the first stage of labor, contractions are at regular 3- to 4-minute intervals, last at least 60 seconds each, and feel very painful or intense. The patient may indicate that she is having a considerable amount of discomfort or even pain.

ASK YOURSELF

■ What are the events of each of the three stages of labor?

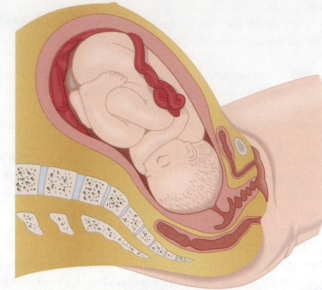

FIRST STAGE:
First uterine contraction to dilation of cervix

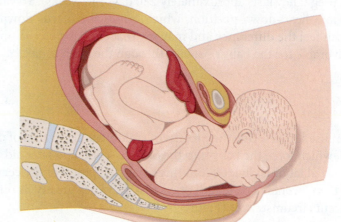

SECOND STAGE:
Birth of baby or expulsion

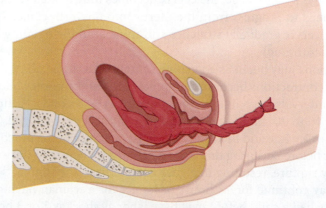

THIRD STAGE:
Delivery of placenta

■ **Figure 24-2** First stage: Uterine contraction to dilation of cervix.
Second stage: Birth of baby (expulsion). Third stage: Delivery of placenta.

Stage Two: Expulsion

During this stage, the baby moves through the birth canal and is born. Contractions are closer together and last longer, approximately 45 to 90 seconds each. As the baby moves downward, the mother experiences considerable pressure in her rectum, much like the feeling of a bowel movement, combined with the feeling that she wants to push, as with a bowel movement.

When the mother has this sensation, she should lie down and get ready for the birth of her child. The tightening and bearing-down sensations will become stronger and more frequent. The mother will have an uncontrollable urge to push down, which she may do. There probably will be more bloody discharge from the vagina at this point.

Soon after, the baby's head will appear at the opening of the birth canal. This is called **crowning**. The shoulders and the rest of the body follow. Helping the freshly delivered newborn will be discussed later in the chapter.

Stage Three: Delivery of the Placenta

During this stage, the placenta separates from the uterine wall. Usually, it is spontaneously expelled from the uterus, although it may not be immediately after the baby is born.

Assisting in Childbirth

Ideally, childbirth should take place in a hospital, so calls for emergency childbirth are rare. Unlike other emergencies, childbirth is not an illness or injury. When you are called to a scene where the delivery of a baby is imminent, remain calm. Make sure you have an obstetrics kit and keep in mind that you are assisting a natural, normal process. Remember that you have two patients: the baby and the mother.

EMR Patient Assessment: Labor

When you are called to the scene of childbirth, perform a scene size-up and initial assessment and treatment as you would for any patient. Give the mother calming reassurance. Then, assess her condition to see if there will be time for transport to the nearest medical facility or if she will have the baby in her present location. Update the responding transporting EMS unit. If you decide to deliver the baby on the scene, the assistance of other EMS personnel will be extremely helpful. This is a situation where teamwork will make a big difference. Generally, you should expect to assist in the delivery of the baby on scene if the event is going to happen immediately and there is no time to package the patient and transport, or if the patient cannot reach the hospital or physician due to a natural disaster, bad weather, or some kind of catastrophe. Follow local protocols, which may specify that if delivery of the baby can be expected within a certain time frame (such as 5 or 10 minutes) then prepare for an on-scene delivery.

To determine if delivery of the baby can be expected within a few minutes, time the contractions by following these steps:

1. Place your gloved hand on the mother's abdomen, just above her navel. Feel the involuntary tightening and relaxing of the uterine muscle.
2. Time these involuntary movements in seconds. Start from the moment the uterus first tightens until it is completely relaxed.
3. Time the intervals in minutes from the start of one contraction to the start of the next.

If the contractions are more than 5 minutes apart, the mother usually has time to be transported to a hospital safely, as long as traffic, weather conditions, or prolonged

crowning the appearance of the baby's head or other body part at the opening of the birth canal.

ASK YOURSELF

■ What are all the indications that you should expect to assist with delivery on an emergency call?

transport times are not a problem. If the contractions are 2 minutes apart, she probably does not have time. Prepare to help deliver the baby where you are.

If the contractions are between 2 and 5 minutes apart, you must make a decision based on the factors in the following list. The mother is usually nervous and apprehensive, so be gentle and kind, show confidence and support, and ask these questions:

- Have you had a baby before? (It is not uncommon for the mother to be in labor longer for the first pregnancy.)
- What is your due date? Have you seen a doctor during your pregnancy and received prenatal care? Did your doctor tell you that you are having more than one baby or that there may problems or complications?
- Are you having contractions? How far apart are they?
- Has the amniotic sac ruptured (or did your water break)? If so, when? What color was the fluid?
- Do you feel the sensation of a bowel movement? (If yes, the baby's head is pressing against the rectum and will soon be born. Do not let the mother sit on the toilet.)
- Do you feel like the baby is ready to be born?

Take Standard Precautions and examine the mother if you think there is a possibility based on the responses to these questions that delivery might be happening soon and you may need to deliver on the scene. In order to examine the mother to determine if there is crowning, she should be on her back with knees bent and legs spread. Inspect the vaginal area, but do not touch it except during delivery and, if possible, when another EMS person is present. If you can see bulging in the vaginal area, and either the head or other part of the baby is visible, prepare for delivery on the scene. It is possible, although a rare event, that you will see one of the baby's limbs or the umbilical cord when inspecting the vaginal area. Handling this type of special circumstance will be discussed later in the "Complications of Delivery" section. If the transporting ambulance has not yet arrived, provide an update to let them know you are preparing for an immediate delivery before transport or that there is a presentation of a limb or the umbilical cord.

EMR Patient Assessment: Supine Hypotension Syndrome

ASK YOURSELF
- How would you describe the patient positioning to manage or prevent supine hypotension syndrome?

Be alert to the possibility of a condition known as supine hypotension syndrome. This condition may occur in the last few months of pregnancy when the mother lies on her back. The combined weight of the uterus and the fetus presses on the great vein called the inferior vena cava. The inferior vena cava, which lies in the right side of the abdomen, collects blood from the lower body and delivers it back to the heart. Pressure on this thin-walled vein can limit (decrease) the blood returning to the heart and circulating through the body. You may observe signs of shock in your patient, including reduced blood pressure, increased pulse, and pale skin color. Also be alert for fainting, and ask if the patient thinks she is going to faint or has fainted recently.

To avoid supine hypotension syndrome, the patient should be in a sitting position, if appropriate, or lying on her left side. If you suspect the condition, position the patient on her left side and treat for shock. If the pregnant patient has experienced trauma, position her on the backboard, which can be tipped leftward as a unit to relieve the pressure of the baby on the inferior vena cava.

EMR Emergency Care: Preparation for Delivery

ASK YOURSELF
- Given a scenario, what are the steps of preparation for and assistance in newborn delivery?

Always act in a calm, professional manner. Reassure the mother; tell her that you are there to help with the delivery. Provide as much quiet and privacy for her as you can. If you have other EMS personnel present, decide who will be responsible for what tasks. Remember that you will have at least two patients to tend to and possibly more if there are multiple births. Also, dealing with family and friends may be a concern. Do your best to minimize any possible distractions. Consider holding the mother's hand and always speak encouragingly to her. Help the mother concentrate on breathing regularly with the contractions. The father, family member, friend, or another rescuer can help. Do your best to keep the scene calm and controlled. Teamwork among the EMS personnel on the scene of this potentially chaotic event is essential to get all the tasks accomplished during a delivery.

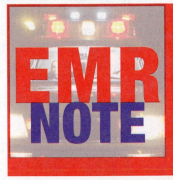

When childbirth occurs in the field, the scene can easily become chaotic. An important responsibility of the EMR is to keep the scene as calm and controlled as possible. Stay calm and be reassuring. When other EMS personnel are on the scene, help coordinate each team member's responsibilities. Teamwork is crucial!

At a minimum, the following materials and equipment should be included in your obstetrical (OB) kit (Figure 24-3 ■):

- Sheets and towels, sterile if possible
- One dozen 4-inch square gauze pads
- Two or three sanitary napkins
- Rubber suction syringe
- Baby receiving blanket
- Surgical scissors for cutting the umbilical cord
- Cord clamps or ties

ASK YOURSELF
■ What are the correct Standard Precautions for assisting with childbirth?

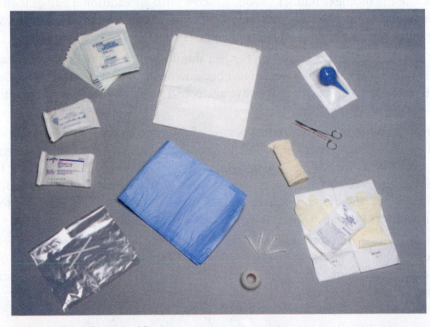

■ **Figure 24-3** Obstetrics kit.

- Foil-wrapped germicidal wipes
- Large plastic bags (one for the placenta and additional ones for waste)
- Sterile gloves and gown

All materials used during delivery should be sterile, or at least as clean as possible. This is to protect both the baby and the mother from contamination and infection.

In addition, because delivery results in exposure to a great deal of blood and other body fluids, you must take Standard Precautions. Put on a face shield (or eyewear and face mask), protective gloves, a disposable gown, and shoe coverings if possible. Handle soaked dressings, pads, and linens carefully. Place them in separate bags that will not leak. Then seal and label the bags. Try to scrub your arms, hands, and nails thoroughly before a delivery as time and resources permit. And, as with any EMS call, a careful and complete hand washing should be done after the delivery has been completed and contaminated material has been properly discarded.

Other guidelines include:

- Help the mother relax with each contraction. Inhaling causes muscles to tighten, so have her exhale with each contraction. Encourage her to keep her breathing slow but comfortable. Tell her not to strain or push during the first stage of labor.

- The amniotic sac may rupture, if it has not already done so. There also may be some blood-tinged mucus. These fluids increase as labor progresses. If you have a clean towel, place it under the mother's buttocks to absorb the fluids. Always wipe in a down-and-away direction to minimize contamination. Properly discard soiled towels or sheets used for this purpose. Replace them frequently with clean ones.

- If the patient feels more comfortable sitting, reclining, or in some other position during the first stages of labor, let her do so.

- As contractions become longer and closer together, the patient should lie down or get into a semisitting position on a flat, firm surface that she can push against. It is easiest for you if the mother is on an elevated surface. However, if the floor is the only firm surface available, use it. Pad it with folded sheets, towels, or blankets. Elevate the mother's buttocks about 2 inches with an additional pad of folded sheets or towels. The pad, which should extend about 2 feet in front of her, will help to support the slippery baby when he is born.

- When the mother is in position, her feet should be flat on the surface beneath her. Her knees will naturally spread apart because of the size of her abdomen. Do not pull them apart any further. Remove any constricting clothing, or push clothing above the mother's waist.

- Create a sterile field around the opening of the vagina. Place a sterile or clean sheet under the mother's hips. Touching only the corners of the sheet, have the mother lift her hips while you place one fold well under her hips. Unfold it toward her feet. If you have time, place another sheet or towel over the mother's abdomen and legs, leaving the vaginal area uncovered. Direct the best possible light toward the mother's genitals. Do not touch the vagina.

- During the second stage of labor, when the mother bears down, remind her not to arch her back. She should curve it and bring her chin to her chest to avoid excessive straining. Have her hold her breath for 7 to 10 seconds as she bears down. Holding the breath any longer will cause too much straining, broken blood vessels, and tearing of the vaginal area.

- ***Be prepared to provide basic life support to both the mother and the infant, including treatment for shock.***

EMR Emergency Care: Assisting in Childbirth

1. Place the palm of your hand gently on top of the baby's head, avoiding the **fontanels** (the soft spots at the top of the head). When the head crowns, apply *very gentle* pressure to prevent an explosive delivery (Scan 24-1).

2. Break open the amniotic sac if it has not already broken. Tear it or pinch it open with your fingers and push it away from the infant's head and mouth.

fontanel the soft spot between the cranial bones of the skull of an infant.

SCAN 24-1 | **Assisting in Childbirth**

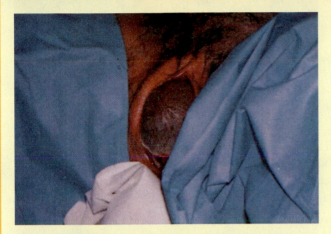

24-1a Crowning.

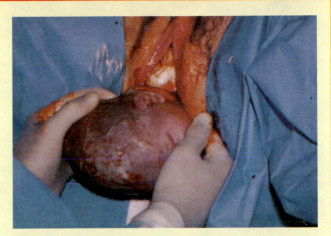

24-1b Head delivers and turns.

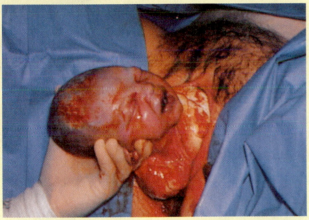

24-1c Shoulders deliver.

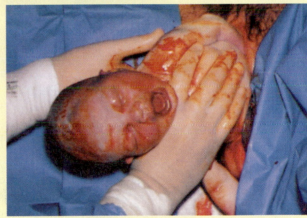

24-1d Chest delivers.

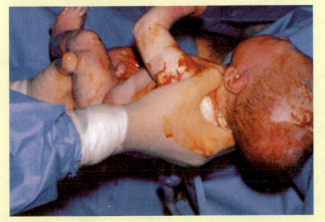

24-1e Legs and feet deliver.

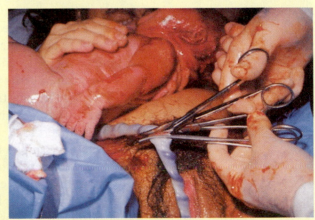

24-1f Clamp and then cut the cord.

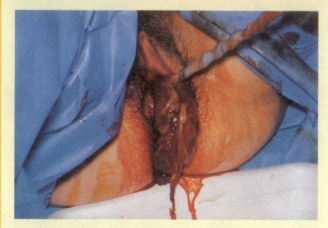

24-1g Placenta begins delivery.

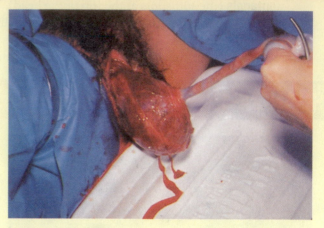

24-1h Placenta delivers.

meconium staining
greenish or brownish color to the amniotic fluid, which means the unborn infant had a bowel movement.

ASK YOURSELF

■ Given a scenario, how would you demonstrate clearing the newborn's mouth and nose of meconium?

Note that the baby can safely inhale clear amniotic fluid. However, if there is **meconium staining** (greenish or brownish fluid), the baby has had a bowel movement, which is a sign of fetal distress. If the baby inhales it, it could cause pneumonia.

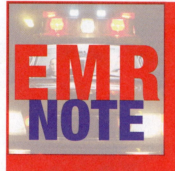

EMR NOTE

The presence of meconium is a serious condition indicating that the baby has had a bowel movement and may be in fetal distress. If you deliver the baby's head and see this greenish or brownish fluid, be sure to report its presence to the EMTs or Paramedics upon transition.

In the case of meconium staining, clean the area around the baby's mouth and nose once the head is delivered. Suction the mouth first, and then the nose, with a rubber suction syringe. Expel all air from the suction bulb prior to placing it in the baby's mouth or nose. Insert the syringe into the newborn's mouth and then release the bulb to create suction. Suctioning may need to be repeated to clear the airway. Note that meconium staining can be a life-threatening event. Consider requesting an advanced life support (ALS) unit to assist. If the responding ambulance is ALS and they haven't yet arrived on the scene, alert them if possible so they can be better prepared when they get to the patient.

3. Determine the position of the umbilical cord. When the baby's head delivers, check to see if the umbilical cord is around the baby's neck. If it is, use two gloved fingers to slip the cord over the shoulders. If you cannot dislodge it, attach two clamps a few inches apart. Then, cut between the clamps. Be extremely careful when cutting because of how close you are to the baby's skin.

4. Support the baby's head as soon as it appears. Place one hand below it. Spread the fingers of your other hand gently around it. Avoid touching the fontanels. In most normal presentations, the baby's head faces down. It then turns so that the nose is toward the mother's thigh. This position allows for the shoulders to deliver.

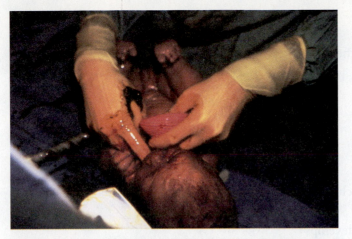

■ **Figure 24-4** Suctioning of the newborn's mouth, which is done before the nose is suctioned.

5. Remove fluids from the infant's airway with a rubber bulb syringe, mouth first and then the nose (Figure 24-4 ■). Remember to fully compress the syringe before you bring it to the baby's face. Insert the tip no more than an inch into the mouth, avoiding contact with the back of the mouth. Slowly release the bulb to allow fluid to be drawn into the syringe. If a syringe is not available, wipe the baby's mouth and then the nose with gauze.

6. Support the baby with both hands as the rest of the body is born. Once the shoulders are delivered, the rest of the body will appear rapidly. Note that you should never pull the baby from the vagina. Do not touch the mother's vagina or anus. Handle the baby's slippery body carefully. Do not put your fingers in the baby's armpits, because pressure on the nerve centers there can cause paralysis.

7. Grasp the feet as they are delivered. Be sure you don't pull on the umbilical cord.

8. Position the baby level with the mother's vagina until the umbilical cord is cut. The neck should be in a neutral position. Then note the time of birth. One way to do this is to radio dispatch and have them record the time of delivery.

9. Recognize that maternal bleeding is very common after childbirth.

10. Be prepared for the placenta to deliver.

✳ Stop, Review, Remember

Multiple Choice

Place a check next to the correct answer.

1. The "bag of waters" refers to the:
   ____ a. embryonic sac.
   ____ b. amniotic sac.
   ____ c. umbilical sac.
   ____ d. placental sac.

2. A full-term pregnancy lasts how many weeks?
   ____ a. 28
   ____ b. 32
   ____ c. 40
   ____ d. 48

3. To treat supine hypotension syndrome, how should you position the pregnant patient?
   ____ a. Prone
   ____ b. On her right side
   ____ c. Supine
   ____ d. On her left side

Matching

Match the following descriptions with the correct term.

1. _____ Extension of the placenta through which the fetus receives nourishment

2. _____ Neck of uterus

3. _____ Organ that contains the developing fetus

4. _____ Filled with a fluid in which the fetus floats

5. _____ Disk-shaped organ that develops during pregnancy

6. _____ Made up of the cervix and vagina

7. _____ The process of birth

a. Placenta

b. Umbilical cord

c. Amniotic sac

d. Birth canal

e. Labor

f. Uterus

g. Cervix

List

1. List the three stages of labor:

   1. _____

   2. _____

   3. _____

2. List seven of the items found in an OB kit:

   1. _____

   2. _____

   3. _____

   4. _____

   5. _____

   6. _____

   7. _____

Emergency Medical Responder Practice

1. You arrive on the scene of a 25-year-old pregnant patient with contractions 3 minutes apart. List five specific questions that you would ask her to help determine if delivery should be done on the scene.

   1. _____

   2. _____

   3. _____

   4. _____

   5. _____

2. What finding during the physical exam of a pregnant patient is used to determine if a delivery should be done on the scene?

_____

_____

_____

_____

Caring for the Newborn

Gently dry the infant with towels. Wrap him in a clean, warm blanket (Figure 24-5 ■). Place the baby on his side, head slightly lower than the trunk. Turn the baby's head slightly to one side to allow mucus and fluid to drain from the nose and mouth.

MAINTAINING WARMTH OF A NEWBORN

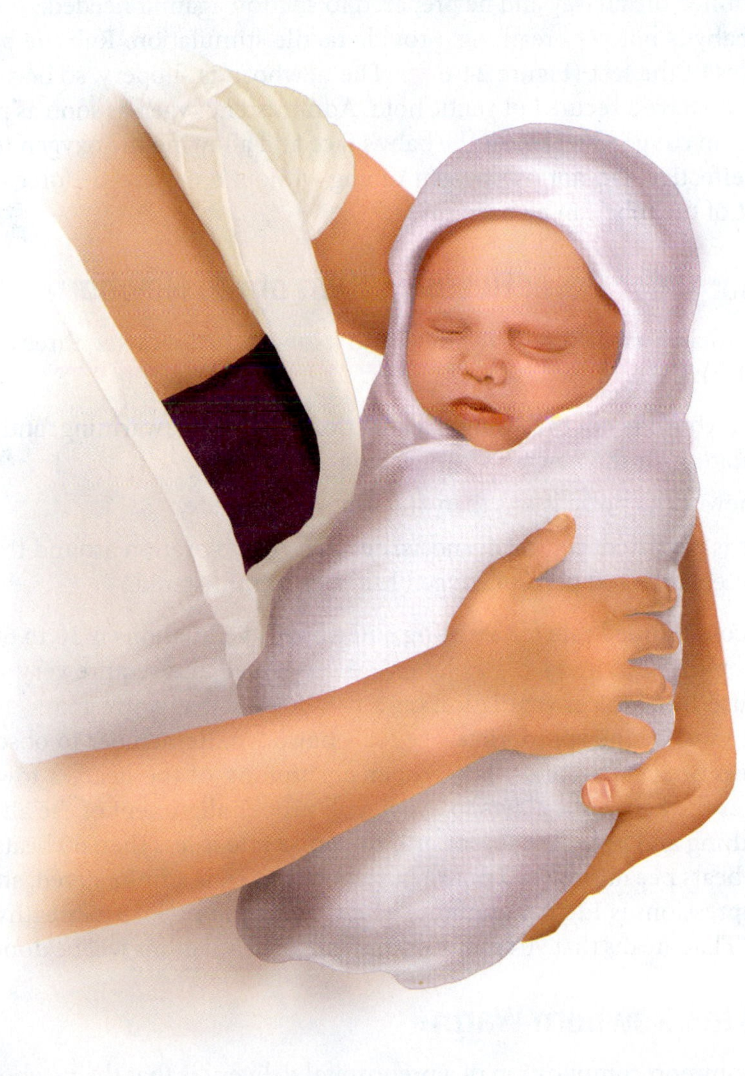

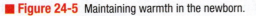

■ **Figure 24-5** Maintaining warmth in the newborn.

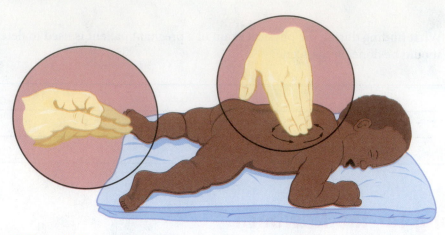

Then clean the newborn's mouth and nose. Wipe blood and mucus from the baby's mouth and nose with sterile gauze. Again, suction the mouth first and then the nose. The infant should cry almost immediately. The importance of suctioning the airway as soon as possible after the head is delivered can't be stressed enough. It is also essential to continually monitor the airway and be prepared to suction again if needed.

If the baby is not yet breathing, provide tactile stimulation. Rub the back gently or slap the soles of the feet (Figure 24-6 ■). The newborn is slippery, so be very careful to make sure you have a secure but gentle hold. Administer oxygen as soon as possible. Usually, placing an oxygen mask near the baby's face and allowing the oxygen to blow by the neonate is effective. Do not use oxygen tubing without a mask. The force of the oxygen coming out of the tube can be harmful.

EMR Emergency Care: Resuscitation of the Newborn

Perform artificial ventilation on the newborn if any of the following three conditions exist (Scan 24-2):

- The newborn is not breathing after suctioning, drying, warming, and tactile stimulating, or the newborn has gasping respirations.
- The newborn's pulse is less than 100 beats per minute.
- There is persistent central cyanosis, or bluish discoloration around the chest and abdomen after 100 percent oxygen has been administered.

The recommended rate for assisting a newborn's ventilations is 30 to 60 breaths per minute. Keep in mind that a baby's lungs are very small and require very small puffs of air. Never use mechanical ventilation on a newborn. A bag-valve-mask device may be used, but it must be the appropriate size for a newborn. Remember to observe for chest rise. Reassess after 30 seconds. For proper positioning of the head, a towel should be placed under the baby's shoulders to assist with proper alignment of the airway.

If breathing and pulse are absent or if the pulse rate is less than 60 beats per minute, or 60 to 80 beats per minute and not rising when oxygen is administered, start CPR. The rate of compressions is 120 per minute. The ratio of compressions to breaths for the newborn is 3:1. That means that 90 compressions and 30 ventilations will be done per minute.

Keeping the Newborn Warm

The most common complication of a prehospital delivery is that the newborn is allowed to become too cold. Prevention of newborn hypothermia is the next most critical part of

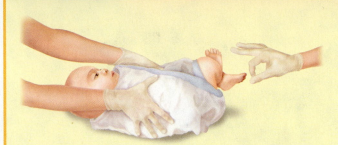

24-2a Stimulate, warm, and dry the baby.

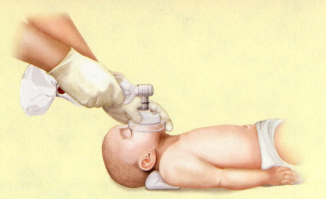

24-2b Ventilate if not breathing, pulse is less than 100/minute, or persistent cyanosis.

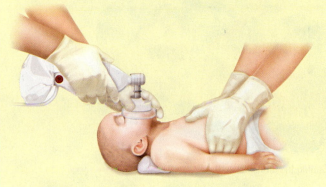

24-2c Perform CPR if the pulse rate is less than 60/minute.

the care of the newborn after you have ensured adequate breathing and heart rate. Follow these steps to prevent newborn hypothermia:

- Replace any wet blankets or towels from the delivery with ones that are clean and dry.
- Keep the newborn's head covered. Only the face should be exposed.
- Keep the newborn in a warm environment while awaiting the arrival of the transporting EMS crew.

Cutting the Umbilical Cord

Clamp, tie, and cut the umbilical cord when it stops pulsating (Figure 24-7 ■), if your EMS system allows you to do so. Place two clamps or ties on it about 3 inches apart. Position the first clamp about 6 inches from the infant. Use sterile surgical scissors to cut the cord between the two clamps or ties. Periodically check the end of the cord for bleeding, and control any that occurs.

Caring for the Mother

Further EMR care for the mother includes providing emotional support, assisting in the delivery of the placenta, and controlling vaginal bleeding.

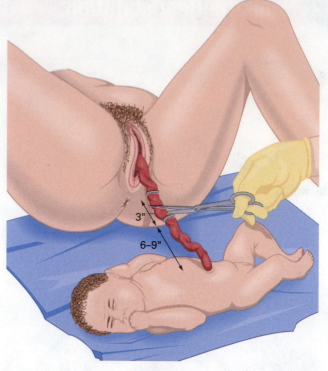

■ **Figure 24-7** Cutting the umbilical cord.

Delivering the Placenta

Observe for the delivery of the placenta. When it starts to separate from the uterus, the cord will appear to be longer. The uterus will also contract and feel like a hard, grapefruit-size ball. Encourage the mother to bear down as the uterus contracts. The placenta usually delivers within 10 minutes of the infant, and almost always within 30 minutes.

Normally, there will be some bleeding as the placenta separates. When the placenta appears, slowly and gently guide it from the vagina. Never pull on the umbilical cord to hasten the delivery of the placenta. Place the placenta in a plastic bag to be taken to the hospital where a physician can confirm the delivery is complete.

If the placenta does not deliver in 10 to 15 minutes after the baby is born, then package both patients and transport to the hospital. The placenta can be delivered there.

Controlling Bleeding After Birth

After the placenta delivers, check the mother's vaginal bleeding. Up to 500 mL (usually, less than a quart) of blood loss is normal and usually well tolerated by the mother. Place two sanitary napkins over the opening of the vagina. Touch only the outer surfaces of the pads. Do not touch the mother's vagina. At this time, ask the mother if she plans to breastfeed the infant. If so, now is a good time to encourage the mother to start. Breastfeeding helps the uterus to contract, which decreases the size of the uterus and helps to stop bleeding.

Make sure that the mother and the baby are covered and warm. The mother as well as the infant can chill easily following birth. Activate the EMS system if you have not already done so. The mother and the baby should be taken together to the hospital for evaluation by a physician.

If, after delivery of the placenta, bleeding appears to be excessive, assess and treat the mother for shock and arrange for immediate transport. Then massage the uterus by cupping a hand around the uterus and making a circular motion (Figure 24-8 ■). As mentioned

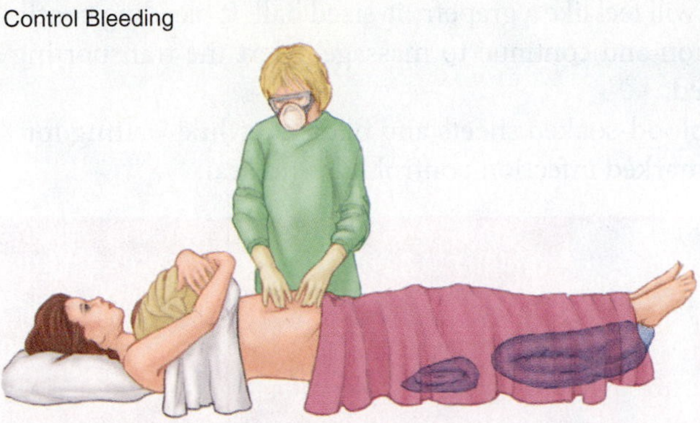

Control Bleeding

■ **Figure 24-8** Uterine massage—treating bleeding after delivery of the placenta.

THE RESPONSE

The patient tells you her "water broke" about 30 minutes ago and she immediately called 911. She experienced only one contraction before EMS arrived. This is her first pregnancy and she has received regular prenatal care. The due date is in 2 weeks. The patient reports that she has preeclampsia and that her blood pressure is being regularly monitored and is reported to be under control.

You take a set of vital signs and find that the pulse is 90, strong, and regular; respirations are 22 and regular; and blood pressure is 170/100. The blood pressure seems high and you notify the responding transporting ambulance, which is still 5 minutes from the scene, of the patient information including the vital signs. You place the mother on oxygen and make sure she is comfortable. She asks for a blanket.

You return to your patient to get a SAMPLE history and determine she has no past medical history to report and no known allergies. She ate her last meal of a turkey sandwich and a glass of milk about 3 hours ago.

The patient experiences another contraction that lasts 15 seconds. You ask if she feels like she needs to move her bowels and she says she doesn't. Based on the information you now have, you don't believe that delivery is imminent and you do not need to check for crowning.

You take another set of vital signs, which are just about the same as the initial set, and provide support for the expectant mother. The husband is busy preparing a bag for his wife to take to the hospital. You also ask him how he is doing and let him know the plan to transport his wife.

■ Discussion: *What is your priority for the patient at this time?*

earlier, the uterus will feel like a grapefruit-sized ball. If bleeding continues to be excessive, check hand position and continue to massage. Alert the transporting ambulance if they have not yet arrived.

Replace any blood-soaked sheets and blankets while waiting for transport. Place all soiled items in a marked infection control bag and seal.

ASK YOURSELF

■ What is the pregnant patient's altered physiological response to trauma?

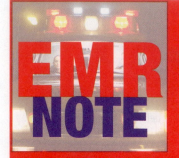

Trauma to a pregnant woman raises a number of important issues for the EMR to consider. For example, it may be difficult to determine shock because during pregnancy a number of changes occur, such as the following:

■ Blood volume increases by 30 to 45 percent.

■ Heart rate increases by 15 beats per minute.

■ Blood pressure falls by 10 to 15 mmHg.

All these factors can mask what are usually signs used to identify shock. In fact, a pregnant woman can lose 40 percent of her blood volume before the typical signs of shock are obvious. Basically, this means that shock can be missed when evaluating a pregnant patient. Continually assessing a pregnant patient, including taking frequent vital signs, is extremely important. If the mother goes into shock, it affects the fetus. Be suspicious that an expectant mother is in shock even when signs and symptoms are not clearly apparent. Any subtle indications need to be monitored closely and care started immediately.

ASK YOURSELF

■ Given a scenario, what are the management steps of the possible complications of delivery, including:
  ■ Umbilical cord around the neck?
  ■ Prolapsed umbilical cord?
  ■ Abnormal presentations and multiple births?
  ■ Infant with inadequate breathing, heart rate below 100 per minute, or persistent central cyanosis?
  ■ Excessive maternal bleeding?

Complications of Delivery

Although most births follow a similar pattern, you need to be prepared and knowledgeable about possible complications and the care you may provide.

Prolapsed Umbilical Cord

In some situations, the umbilical cord comes out of the birth canal before the infant. When this happens, the baby is in great danger of suffocating. The cord is compressed against the birth canal by the baby's head, which cuts off the baby's supply of oxygenated blood from the placenta. Emergency care is extremely urgent. Arrange for immediate transport.

While you wait for additional medical help to arrive to transport, position the patient. Have her lie down on her left side, if possible. Knees should be drawn to her chest, or her hips and legs should be elevated on a pillow. Administer high-flow oxygen. Next, free the umbilical cord. That is, with your gloved hand, gently push the baby up the vagina far enough so that the baby's head is off the cord. Place pressure around the outside of the head to avoid putting pressure on the anterior fontanel. (Another option recommended in some systems is to use two fingers between the baby's face and the cord to gently lift the baby from the cord. Follow your local protocols.) Finally, cover the cord with a sterile towel moistened with clean water, preferably sterile. Do not try to push it back into the vagina.

Breech Birth

In a breech birth, the baby's feet or buttocks are delivered first (Figure 24-9 ■). Whenever possible, the mother should be taken to the hospital for the birth. If that is not possible,

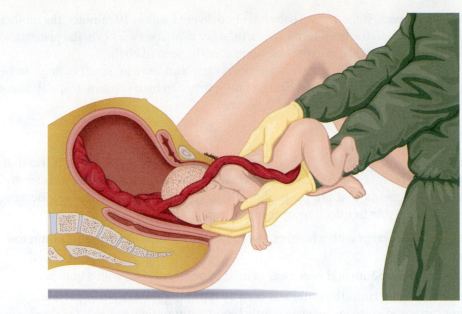

Figure 24-9 In a breech birth, the baby's feet or buttocks are delivered first.

prepare the mother for a normal delivery, letting the baby's buttocks and trunk deliver on their own. (Never try to pull the baby from the vagina by the legs or trunk.) Then place your arm between the baby's legs, letting the legs dangle astride your arm. Support the baby's back with the palm of your other hand. Let the head follow on its own, which usually occurs within 3 minutes.

If the head does not deliver within 3 minutes, the baby is in danger of suffocating when the head compresses the umbilical cord and prevents the flow of oxygenated blood from the placenta. To prevent that, clear the baby's face. That is, place the middle and index fingers of your gloved hand alongside the infant's face. Your palm should be turned toward the face. Form an airway by pushing the vagina away from the baby's face until the head is delivered. Hold the baby's mouth open a little with your finger so that the baby can breathe.

Limb Presentation

If the baby's arm or leg comes out of the birth canal first, it means that the baby has shifted so much in the uterus that a normal delivery may not be possible. Delay can be fatal. Never pull on the baby by the arm or leg. The mother must be taken immediately to a hospital. Transport without delay.

Multiple Births

Twins are delivered the same way as single babies, one after the other. In fact, since twins are smaller, delivery is often easier. Identical twins have two umbilical cords coming out of a single placenta. If the twins are fraternal (not identical) there will be two placentas.

The mother may not be aware that she is carrying twins. You should suspect them if one or more of the following conditions exists:

- The abdomen is still very large after one baby is delivered.
- The baby's size is out of proportion with the size of the mother's abdomen.
- Strong contractions begin again about 10 minutes after one baby is born. The second baby is usually born within minutes and almost always within 45 minutes.

To manage a multiple birth, follow these guidelines: After the first baby is born, clamp and cut the cord to prevent bleeding, which will affect the second baby. About one-third of second twins are breech. If the second baby has not delivered within 10 minutes, the mother should be transported to the hospital for the birth. After the babies are born, the placenta(s) should deliver normally. You can expect bleeding after the second birth.

Keep the babies warm. Twins are often born early and may be small enough to be considered premature. Guard against heat loss until they can be taken to a hospital. Make sure they are wrapped well and the head is covered.

Premature Birth

If a woman gives birth before the 36th week of pregnancy, or if the baby weighs less than 5 1/2 pounds, the baby is considered to be premature. Premature babies are smaller and redder. They have heads that are proportionally larger than full-term babies. Because they are very vulnerable to infection, special care must be taken:

- Keep the baby warm with a blanket. If you lack other supplies, use aluminum foil as an outer wrap.
- Keep the baby's mouth and nose clear of fluid by gentle suction with a bulb syringe.
- Prevent bleeding from the umbilical cord by clamping it securely. A premature infant cannot tolerate losing even a little blood without being at risk for shock.
- Administer oxygen, if you are permitted, by blowing it gently across the baby's face. Never blast oxygen directly into the face.
- Since premature babies are so vulnerable to infection, do not let anyone breathe into the baby's face. Do everything you can to prevent contamination.

ASK YOURSELF

- What are some special considerations in the management of premature infants?

Complications of Pregnancy

Some of the changes that occur during pregnancy are not always favorable for the mother. One of these conditions is called **preeclampsia** and affects between 5 and 8 percent of pregnancies. An affected expectant mother may also refer to her condition as *pregnancy-induced hypertension* or *toxemia*.

EMR Patient Assessment: Preeclampsia

Preeclampsia presents with the following signs and symptoms:

- High blood pressure
- Swelling on the face and extremities
- Headache
- Nausea or vomiting
- Abnormal weight gain

Some expectant mothers affected by preeclampsia will go on to develop **eclampsia** as a more serious problem. Eclampsia has the same signs as preeclampsia, but in addition seizures develop. It is possible that the patient could go into a coma. Eclampsia is an emergency situation that can threaten the life of both the mother and fetus.

EMR Emergency Care: Seizure and Preeclampsia

Treatment is the same as for any patient for a seizure in that you need to protect the patient from harm. Once the seizure has ended, provide applied high-flow oxygen, if you are allowed, and position the patient on her left side. Constantly monitor the airway and take vital signs frequently. Take extra care to be quiet around these patients, dim lighting, and avoid any rough motions. Also avoid the use of emergency lights and sirens as these disturbances can potentially trigger seizures. If the patient is in a coma, place her on her left side and treat as any other unconscious patient. Make sure you monitor closely.

ASK YOURSELF

- What are the signs and symptoms of pregnancy complications, including preeclampsia, eclampsia, vaginal bleeding, and ectopic pregnancy?

preeclampsia a complication of pregnancy where the woman retains large amounts of fluid and has high blood pressure.

eclampsia a severe complication of pregnancy that produces seizure and possibly coma.

EMR Emergency Care: Vaginal Bleeding

There are many reasons for vaginal bleeding. Common reasons for vaginal bleeding include local trauma and abnormal menstrual bleeding. Vaginal bleeding that occurs in a pregnant woman is of particular concern. The following are a few of the more common pregnancy-related conditions where there may be vaginal bleeding.

Spontaneous Abortion

Sometimes called a **miscarriage**, a spontaneous abortion is the loss of pregnancy before the 20th week. It occurs naturally, unlike abortions deliberately performed in either legal or criminal settings. Signs and symptoms include vaginal bleeding that often is heavy, pain in the lower abdomen similar to menstrual cramps or labor contractions, and passage of tissue from the vagina.

    To provide EMR care, arrange for immediate transport. Treat the patient for shock. Save any passed tissue by packaging it in a sealed bag. The bag should then be transported with the patient for evaluation by a physician.

> **miscarriage**   the natural loss of pregnancy before the 20th week; also called *spontaneous abortion.*

Ectopic Pregnancy

A woman has two **fallopian tubes**. Each one extends up from the uterus to a position near the **ovary**. Each month an egg is released from an ovary into a fallopian tube. The fallopian tube then conveys the egg to the uterus, and sperm from the uterus toward the ovary.

    In a normal pregnancy, a fertilized **ovum** (egg) is implanted in the uterus. In an ectopic pregnancy, a fertilized ovum is implanted outside the uterus. It could be in the abdominal cavity, on the outside wall of the uterus, on the ovary, or on the outside of the cervix. In 95 percent of ectopic cases, the ovum is implanted in a fallopian tube.

    An ectopic pregnancy is a severe medical emergency. The expanding fertilized ovum eventually causes rupture of the fallopian tube and severe internal bleeding. It is the leading cause of death in pregnant women in their first trimester (first 3 months).

    Signs and symptoms include:

> **fallopian tube**   one of the two tubes or ducts that extend up from the uterus to a position near an ovary.
>
> **ovary**   one of two almond-shaped glands in the female that produce the reproductive cell (the ovum).
>
> **ovum**   the reproductive cell, or "egg."

- Sudden, sharp abdominal pain in one side (If internal bleeding is extensive, pain will become more diffuse.)
- Pain under the diaphragm, or pain radiating to one or both shoulders
- Tender bloated abdomen
- Vaginal spotting or bleeding
- Missed menstrual periods
- Signs of shock

    Suspect ectopic pregnancy in any woman of childbearing age when these signs and symptoms are present, even if the patient is unaware that she is pregnant. To provide EMR care, arrange for immediate transport. Place the patient on her back with knees elevated. Keep the patient warm. Administer oxygen, if you are allowed.

Placenta Previa

Placenta previa occurs later in pregnancy when the placenta is positioned in the uterus in an abnormally low position. When the cervix dilates (expands), the fetus moves, or labor begins, the placenta begins to bleed as it is pushed into the birth canal. This puts both the mother and the baby in danger.

    Signs and symptoms include severe usually painless bleeding from the vagina and signs of shock.

    To provide EMR care, arrange for immediate transport. Elevate the patient's legs. Maintain body temperature. If possible, administer 100 percent oxygen by mask.

Abruptio Placentae

Another major cause of bleeding during pregnancy is *abruptio placentae*. It is the leading cause of fetal death after blunt trauma. Life threatening for both the mother and the baby, it needs to be recognized and treated rapidly.

There are several causes, including toxemia and trauma. Whatever the cause, the normally implanted placenta begins separating from the uterus sometime during the last 3 months of pregnancy. Bleeding begins, but it is often behind the placenta and the mother is unaware of it. Shock then develops in the mother, and the baby does not get enough oxygen.

Signs and symptoms include bleeding from the vagina but not usually in great quantities, severe abdominal pain, rigid abdomen, and signs of shock.

To provide EMR care, arrange for immediate transport. Monitor vital signs carefully and treat for shock. Administer 100 percent oxygen by mask, if you are allowed.

✳ Stop, Review, Remember

Multiple Choice

Place a check next to the correct answer.

1. Artificial ventilation on a newborn should be performed:

    ____ a. when the pulse is less than 100 beats per minute.

    ____ b. before suctioning, drying, warming, and tactile stimulation.

    ____ c. when there is mild cyanosis of extremities.

    ____ d. when the newborn does not immediately breathe after nasal suctioning.

2. When the umbilical cord comes out of the birth canal before the infant, it is called:

    ____ a. reversal delivery.

    ____ b. breech birth.

    ____ c. prolapsed umbilical cord.

    ____ d. abruptio placentae.

3. Ectopic pregnancy should be suspected in which of the following patients?

    ____ a. A woman of childbearing years with abdominal pain

    ____ b. A woman with a confirmed pregnancy with severe bleeding and no pain

    ____ c. A woman with swelling and hypertension during pregnancy

    ____ d. A woman in her third trimester with abdominal pain

Emergency Medical Responder Practice

1. You arrive on the scene where another EMR has already assisted with a baby that was just delivered before you arrived. The other EMR informs you that she suctioned the mouth and nose when the head came out. You are asked to assist with care of the infant. What steps should you take? (Assume the newborn does not need to be resuscitated.)

    1. _____

    2. _____

    3. _____

    4. _____

    5. _____

    6. _____

2. The baby starts to show signs of stress after all the initial care is provided. The pulse rate falls below 100 beats per minute to about 70 beats per minute. What care should be provided?

_____

_____

_____

3. The heart rate does not improve with artificial ventilation. What should be done next?

_____

_____

_____

Matching

Match the following definitions with the appropriate term.

1. _____ Loss of pregnancy before the 20th week

2. _____ Separation of the placenta from the uterus during the last 3 months of pregnancy

3. _____ A complication of pregnancy with fluid retention and high blood pressure

4. _____ Placenta positioned in the uterus in an abnormally low position

5. _____ Severe complication of pregnancy that produces seizures

6. _____ Implantation of a fertilized egg outside the uterus

a. Preeclampsia

b. Eclampsia

c. Ectopic pregnancy

d. Spontaneous abortion

e. Placenta previa

f. Abruptio placentae

Place in Order

Arrange in order how the EMR should provide care to a patient who is giving birth.

_____ Support the baby with both hands as the rest of the body is born.

_____ Break open the amniotic sac if it has not already broken.

_____ Be prepared for the placenta to deliver.

_____ Support the baby's head as soon as it appears.

_____ Grasp the feet as they are delivered; be sure you don't pull on the umbilical cord.

_____ Remove fluids from the infant's airway with a rubber bulb syringe, mouth first and then the nose.

_____ Place the palm of your hand gently on top of the baby's head to prevent an explosive delivery.

_____ Position the baby level with the mother's vagina until the umbilical cord is cut.

_____ Determine the position of the umbilical cord. When the baby's head delivers, check to see if the cord is around the baby's neck.

TRANSITION ✳

The ALS transporting ambulance arrives on the scene. You provide an updated report. You give them the time sequences for the breaking of the amniotic sac and the contractions. As part of the SAMPLE history report, you inform the ambulance crew about the preeclampsia and provide the vital signs you obtained. You assist with packaging the patient and ask if they want any assistance during transport. The ambulance crew declines as they feel, as you did, that the patient will not deliver en route.

You return to service and make sure that all your equipment is ready for the next call. You are just about to call back in service when the dispatcher radios and asks if you are available for another call. You tell the dispatcher you are ready for another call and realize that cup of coffee will have to wait.

■ Discussion: *Should you have accompanied the patient to the hospital with transport?*

THE LAST WORD

Most deliveries are normal events that occur uneventfully without difficulties, but occasionally problems may present and the EMR needs to provide specific care. The following are important points for dealing with calls for pregnant patients:

■ The three stages of labor are dilation of the cervix, expulsion, and delivery of the placenta. Assessment of a patient in labor begins with a scene size-up and initial assessment and treatment, as you would for any patient.

■ Prepare the mother for delivery. Do not touch the vagina.

■ Care for the mother includes assisting in delivery of the placenta, which usually occurs within 10 to 30 minutes of the infant. Address all complications of pregnancy and delivery.

✳ *Chapter Review*

Multiple Choice

Place a check next to the correct answer.

1. During pregnancy, the developing fetus is in the:

_____ a. cervix.

_____ b. uterus.

_____ c. vagina.

_____ d. symphysis pubis.

2. During which of the following does the infant's head progress from the uterus into the birth canal?

_____ a. Dilation stage of labor

_____ b. Passage of the placenta

_____ c. Expulsion stage of labor

_____ d. Passage of the bloody show

3. Contractions are 2 minutes apart. Which other indicators would signal an imminent delivery?

_____ a. Meconium staining

_____ b. A first pregnancy

_____ a. Placental dilation

_____ d. Urge to move bowels

4. Meconium is:

_____ a. a normal pregnancy.

_____ b. the covering of the placenta.

_____ c. a fetal bowel movement.

_____ d. the "bloody show."

5. When is the baby's actual time of birth?

_____ a. When the baby's head crowns

_____ b. After the umbilical cord is cut

_____ c. When the baby takes his first breath

_____ d. After the whole body delivers, including the feet

6. The compression rate for doing CPR on a newborn is:

_____ a. 100 per minute.

_____ b. 120 per minute.

_____ c. 140 per minute.

_____ d. 80 per minute.

7. Approximately how long should you wait for the placenta to deliver before transporting to the hospital, even if the placenta has not delivered?

_____ a. 10–15 minutes

_____ b. 20–30 minutes

_____ c. 30–45 minutes

_____ d. 45–60 minutes

8. How far away from the infant should the first clamp be placed on the umbilical cord before it is cut?

_____ a. 3 inches

_____ b. 9 inches

_____ c. 6 inches

_____ d. 12 inches

9. When timing a contraction, the starting and stopping of each contraction is determined how?

_____ a. When the patient indicates she is no longer feeling pain

_____ b. From when the uterus first tightens until it is completely relaxed

_____ c. Based on the expectant mother's pulse rate

_____ d. From the start of one contraction until the start of the next contraction

10. A pregnant patient who presents with vaginal bleeding, severe abdominal pain, a rigid abdomen, and signs of shock is most likely having what complication of pregnancy?

_____ a. Placenta previa

_____ b. Abruptio placentae

_____ c. Preeclampsia

_____ d. Uterine inversion

Matching

Match the following descriptions with the appropriate term.

1. _____ Appearance of the baby's head at the opening of the birth canal
2. _____ The plug of mucus that is discharged during labor
3. _____ An indication that an unborn infant had a bowel movement
4. _____ One of two almond-shaped glands in the female that produce the reproductive cell
5. _____ The result of the combined weight of the uterus and the fetus pressing on the inferior vena cava
6. _____ The natural loss of pregnancy before the 20th week
7. _____ The soft spot between the cranial bones of the skull of an infant
8. _____ The reproductive cell
9. _____ The placenta, after it separates from the uterine wall and delivers
10. _____ Ducts that extend up from the uterus to a position near an ovary

a. Supine hypotension syndrome
b. Bloody show
c. Fallopian tube
d. Crowning
e. Afterbirth
f. Fontanel
g. Ovary
h. Ovum
i. Miscarriage
j. Meconium staining

Emergency Medical Responder Practice

You arrive at a private residence where you ring the bell and a woman's voice tells you to come in. You do a quick check and determine the scene is safe. As you walk into the living room, you see the patient who appears to be in her late 20s sitting on the couch. She tells you that her "water broke" about 30 minutes ago.

1. Based on the presentation of the mother, what should you do next?

_____

_____

_____

_____

In response to questions concerning her pregnancy, the mother tells you this is her first delivery and that she has only had two contractions since her "water broke" about half an hour ago. The husband appears as you are talking with the mother-to-be and tells you that the baby isn't due for another 2 weeks and asks if anything is wrong. You ask the patient if she feels like she needs to push down or feels like she wants to move her bowels. The patient responds no to both questions.

2. Based on the information, do you think you should transport or set up to deliver the baby on the scene? Explain.

_____

_____

_____

_____

3. You take a set of vital signs and obtain a SAMPLE history. The pulse is 90 and regular and respirations are 22, but you are concerned that the blood pressure is 190/110. During the history the mother tells you the doctor said she had pregnancy-induced hypertension. What condition can this lead to and what care should you provide for this patient?

_____

_____

_____

_____

4. The ALS ambulance is 5 minutes from the scene. What information should you communicate to the crew? (Write it as you would give the information in a radio report.)

_____

_____

_____

_____

5. Once you have assisted with packaging the patient for transport, including transitioning care to the transporting unit, you give a full patient update. As an EMR, what do you have left to do before you have completed this call?

_____

_____

_____

_____

Pediatric Emergencies

NAVIGATION GUIDE

The following items provide an overview to the purpose and content of this chapter. The Education Standard and Competency are from the National EMS Education Standards.

Education Standard Special Patient Populations (Pediatrics)

Competency Recognizes and manages life threats based on simple assessment findings for a patient with special needs while awaiting additional emergency response.

Knowledge Area Pediatrics
- Upper airway obstruction
- Lower airway reactive disease
- Respiratory distress/failure/arrest
- Shock
- Seizures
- Sudden infant death syndrome

Objectives After reading this chapter, you should be able to:

1. Define key terms introduced in this chapter.
2. Describe the key differences in the anatomy and physiology of pediatric patients.
3. Relate the anatomical and physiological differences of pediatric patients to modifications in patient assessment and management.
4. Use milestones in physical and developmental maturity to estimate the age of pediatric patients.
5. Demonstrate effective techniques of approaching and communicating with pediatric patients.
6. Respond appropriately to the needs of the pediatric patient's caregivers.
7. Given a scenario, select the properly sized equipment for pediatric patients.
8. Involve caregivers in the care of pediatric patients as appropriate to the situation.
9. Adapt your scene size-up to pediatric calls.
10. Use the pediatric assessment triangle to determine the severity of a pediatric patient's condition.
11. Discuss the role of respiratory compromise and upper airway obstruction in pediatric cardiac arrest.
12. Recognize indications of airway compromise and inadequate breathing in the pediatric patient.
13. Recognize the indications for CPR in infants and children.
14. Describe the ability of pediatric patients to compensate for hemorrhagic shock, relative to that of adults.

NAVIGATION GUIDE (continued)

15. Given a scenario, compare a pediatric patient's vital signs to the expected vital signs for a patient of that age.
16. Given a scenario, recognize and manage pediatric patients with the following conditions:
    a. Croup
    b. Epiglottitis
    c. Asthma
    d. Cardiac arrest
    e. Seizures
    f. Shock
    g. Trauma
    h. Special health care needs
    i. Sudden infant death syndrome
    j. Abuse or neglect

Key Terms   Page numbers indicate first major use in this chapter. The Margin Glossary in this chapter provides definitions as you read.

pediatric patients, p. 619

pediatric assessment triangle (PAT), p. 625

retractions, p. 629

croup, p. 638

epiglottitis, p. 639

febrile seizures, p. 640

sudden infant death syndrome (SIDS), p. 646

child abuse, p. 647

child neglect, p. 647

nonaccidental trauma, p. 647

shaken baby syndrome, p. 647

Media Resources   Please go to **www.bradybooks.com** to access mykit for this text. You will find quizzes, critical thinking scenarios, weblinks, animations, and videos related to this chapter—and much more. Look for online information on infant dehydration, child maltreatment, and child behavior disorders. You will also find animations and video clips on communicating with toddlers, SIDS, and respiratory distress in children.

INTRODUCTION

Pediatric patients can be among the most challenging patients for many reasons. You will need to communicate differently with them than with adults and you need to be aware of the anatomy and physiology differences from adults. On the positive side, pediatric patients many times present with signs that make identifying acute problems relatively easy. They are resilient and can be fun and engaging.

pediatric patients
patients who are infants or children.

ASK YOURSELF

- Can you define the key terms introduced in this chapter?

CASE STUDY

THE CALL

As you sit down for a well-deserved coffee break, the dispatcher sends a call to 90 Autumn Place for a sick and vomiting 2-year-old. The caller reports the child is not "acting right." The closest intersection is Pine Tree Road, and the time out is 1022 hours.

When you arrive on the scene, you find a frantic mother holding her child. The scene is safe to enter, but you observe the living room is a mess with garbage and dirty dishes scattered about. You also observe full ashtrays. You ask the mother if you can move to an area where you can examine the child.

- Discussion: *Without rushing to judgment, what is your first impression of this child's living conditions? How will it affect your assessment?*

- Based on the anatomical and physiological differences of pediatric patients, what modifications would you make in patient assessment and management?

- What are the key differences in the anatomy and physiology of pediatric patients?

Pediatric Anatomical Differences

Pediatric patients (infants and children) are very similar to adult patients, but there are differences that the Emergency Medical Responder (EMR) must know when assessing and providing care to pediatric patients.

Infants and small children have proportionally larger tongues than adults do. When comparing the size of the mouth and tongue in an adult to the mouth and tongue of an infant or small child, you will find that the tongue takes up more space in the infant's or child's mouth. Therefore, when the pediatric patient's tongue relaxes, it can quite easily block the airway. The EMR must be diligent in monitoring the infant's or small child's airway and breathing at all times (Figure 25-1 ■). The following are some important considerations when providing treatment:

- Always support the head when you lift an infant. Before the age of 9 months, an infant usually cannot fully support his own head. Sudden movement can possibly cause injury.

- An infant has soft spots, called fontanels, between the cranial bones of the skull. The posterior fontanel turns into bone by the end of the first year, and the anterior fontanel does the same thing by the end of the second year. When examining or caring for the pediatric patient's head, do so very gently.

- Compared to an adult's head, the head of an infant or small child is larger in proportion to the rest of the body. It is also heavier, with less-developed neck structures and muscles. When you suspect an injury, provide in-line stabilization and, if possible, apply a cervical immobilization device.

The child's head is larger in proportion to the body than an adult's head.

The temperature control mechanism is immature and unstable in babies.

Children have smaller airways with more soft tissue and a narrowing at the cricoid cartilage. The openings of the trachea and esophagus are closer together.

Children have faster respiratory rates.

Children dehydrate easily.

Children have less blood and are therefore in greater danger of bleeding to death from a relatively minor wound or developing severe shock.

Children have faster heart rates.

Young children's extremities are likely to appear mottled. This may be a response to cold because of an immature temperature control mechanism — or may be the result of poor perfusion or shock.

■ **Figure 25-1** Age-specific differences in anatomy and physiology in the infant and child.

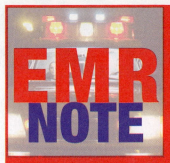

- Stop bleeding in a pediatric patient as quickly as possible. Blood loss that would be comparatively small in an adult would be significant in a child. Be alert to open fractures, which tend to bleed profusely.
- Injuries to the extremities can damage the growth plates, with long-term effects. When you assess extremities, be very gentle and careful not to cause any additional pain. Follow local protocols for splinting.
- A child's skin surface is large compared to body mass. This makes children more susceptible to dehydration and hypothermia. Response to burns also can be more severe. Watch closely for signs of shock as children tend to compensate for shock longer than adults. Children then show signs of shock rapidly.

Determining the Age of a Pediatric Patient

Sometimes knowing the age of a pediatric patient is important when giving care. For many years the age-related definition of infants was from birth to 1 year of age, and the definition of a child was 1 to 8 years of age. In recent years, the revised cardiopulmonary resuscitation (CPR) standards changed the definition of a child to 1 year of age to puberty. The age for infants remains the same.

Usually, a parent or caregiver on scene can tell you the age of a young patient. However, there are times when determining age can be difficult. Even though age is a common benchmark for certain types of treatments, not all young patients physically mature at the same pace (Table 25-1). The sign that a male child has reached puberty is facial, chest, or underarm hair. In females, breast development is the sign of puberty.

When the exact age of a patient is unknown, use your best judgment. Under normal circumstances, most children will act as one might expect for their age. Yet, when children are in a stressful situation, they may act younger or differently than they normally do. This can make it difficult for you to assess and provide care without knowing their normal behavior.

When possible, ask the parent or caregiver if the child is reacting to the pain or stress of the emergency as one may expect or in what way he is reacting differently.

Developmental Characteristics

Knowing the characteristics of children at each age can help when you are providing care. Strive to understand what to expect from them and how to best communicate. Review Chapter 6, "Life Span Development," to again familiarize yourself with the developmental characteristics of the pediatric patient.

ASK YOURSELF

- How do you estimate the age of a pediatric patient by using milestones in physical and developmental maturity?

TABLE 25-1 Childhood Development by Age

DEVELOPMENTAL STAGE	AGE	CHARACTERISTICS AND BEHAVIORS
Infant	Birth to 1 year	Knows the voice and face of parents. Crying may indicate hunger, discomfort, or pain. Will want to be held by a parent or caregiver. It will be difficult for you to identify the precise location of an injury or source of pain.
Toddler	1–3 years	Very curious at this age, so be alert to the possibility of poison ingestion. May be distrustful and uncooperative. Usually does not understand what is happening, which raises level of fear. May be very concerned about being separated from parents or caregivers. A stuffed toy may be helpful in gaining trust.
Preschooler	3–5 years	Is able to talk, but still may not understand what is being said. Uses simple words. May be scared or believe what is happening is his own fault. Sight of blood may intensify response. Sometimes a Band-Aid helps.
School-age child	6–12 years	Should cooperate and be willing to follow the lead of parents and EMS provider. Has active imagination and thoughts about death. Continual reassurance is important.
Adolescent	13–18 years	Is able to provide accurate information. Modesty is important. Fears permanent scarring or deformity. May become involved in "mass hysteria." Be tolerant and do not get caught up in it.

ASK YOURSELF

■ What are some effective techniques of approaching and communicating with pediatric patients?

Communication with the Pediatric Patient

As an EMR encountering children, you will be with them when they are ill or injured. They are apt to be upset before you arrive. When you arrive on scene, the presence of an unfamiliar person will add to what the patient already perceives as a frightening situation. This is a common and appropriate reaction to a stranger.

In addition, children pick up anxiety easily. It is very important for you to stay calm. Children, at any age, often take the lead from what they observe. If you stay calm, a pediatric patient is likely to stay calm, too.

When dealing with children younger than 10, the following tips will help you:

■ Get down to the child's eye level.

■ Do not stare. Include the child in your conversation.

■ Do not make sudden movements when performing an assessment or providing emergency care.

■ If a child is old enough to understand, ask permission to remove a piece of clothing or to touch his body.

■ If a child holds out a hand or allows you to examine some part, seize the moment. The rule in pediatric care is to examine what you can, when the opportunity presents itself.

With adolescents, it is important to be sensitive to their feelings of modesty. In many ways they are young adults.

■ Depending on the injury, the adolescent may have the concern of permanent disfigurement.

■ Also, adolescents are very sensitive to peer pressure and may need to be reassured that what they tell you will be held in confidence. In fact, it may not be possible to get answers to sensitive questions when parents or friends are close by. This is okay.

Most of the time, the patient's answers will not alter your care at the scene and can wait until the patient is in the hospital. Of course, you would still be required to include relevant information in your prehospital care report or in any report to emergency medical providers who have a need to know.

Dealing with Caregivers

With pediatric patients it is important to understand that caregivers, especially parents, may be very upset and understandably quite concerned. In fact, when a child is ill or injured, the EMR should view the situation as one that involves a family, not just the child. Anticipate a variety of responses from caregivers. A few of the more common ones are crying, emotional outbursts, anger, guilt, and confusion. Some of the emotion may be directed at you and other emergency responders. Do not take it personally. Caregivers need support and understanding.

As the assessment of the patient progresses, explain to the caregivers along with the child what is being done, and if time permits, tell them why. If appropriate, ask them to assist with the emergency care. For example, a parent can hold an oxygen mask near the infant's face. Unless it interferes with providing care, let the child stay with the parent (caregiver) whenever possible. Most children will be most comfortable being held or sitting on the parent's lap.

You may encounter a parent who will not let you help an ill or injured child. That parent may insist on remaining in control. Avoid becoming defensive. The parent's behavior has nothing to do with you. Remember, even though the parents may be coping in the only way they know how, ultimately the child is the patient and you must ensure that any needed emergency medical care is not delayed.

The following techniques may help in situations where parents are especially anxious:

- The first priority is to protect the health and safety of the patient. If parents are making unsafe demands, try an approach of reserved confrontation. Explain that the assessment and care being provided is based on sound medical knowledge and that their demands are obstructing what is considered appropriate and in the child's best interest.

- Realize that the parents may be offering sound advice. They usually know their child extremely well. A parent of a chronically ill child probably has a good grasp of what is happening.

- Regardless of how parents behave, treat them with courtesy, respect, and understanding. Avoid raising your voice. Tell them you know they want to help. Be as positive as you can, whenever it is appropriate to do so.

- Let parents stay as close to the patient as possible, as long as they are not interfering with care. If medically appropriate, a child can be held by a parent. Also, consider letting the parents do something for the child in order to help focus their attention away from you.

- Whatever you do, do not react with anger.

Using the Proper Equipment

Having the right equipment in the correct sizes for the pediatric patient is extremely important to make sure that quality care is delivered. With children, one size does *not* fit all. Having a wide variety of sizes is essential to fit the needs of each patient and ensure optimal care (Figure 25-2 ■).

The list of equipment in Table 25-2 can be used as a reference for needed pediatric supplies. This list is meant to complement the resources that are carried to provide emergency

ASK YOURSELF

- What are some examples of appropriate responses to the needs of the pediatric patient's caregivers?

ASK YOURSELF

- Given a scenario, how do you select the properly sized equipment for pediatric patients?

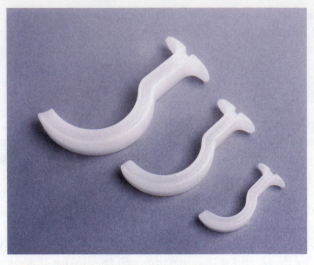

■ **Figure 25-2** Airways come in a variety of sizes.

TABLE 25-2 Essential Pediatric Equipment and Supplies
■ Airway adjuncts in pediatric sizes
■ Bag-valve masks with oxygen reservoirs in appropriate sizes for pediatric patients
■ Pediatric pocket mask with a one-way valve
■ Oxygen masks in pediatric sizes
■ Bulb syringes
■ Portable suction unit with regulator
■ Suction catheters, tonsil tips and 6 French and 14 French
■ Defibrillator (capable of pediatric settings) with pediatric size pads
■ Cervical immobilization devices in pediatric sizes
■ Backboards in pediatric sizes
■ Extremity splints in pediatric sizes
■ Pediatric stethoscope
■ Blood pressure cuffs in pediatric sizes
■ Obstetric (OB) pack
■ Thermal blanket
■ New, clean stuffed animals (optional)
■ Pediatric Glasgow Coma Scale and trauma references

care and is illustrative. Be sure to follow local or state requirements and standards regarding supplies and equipment for pediatric patients.

Pediatric Process

Assessment is the cornerstone of providing emergency medical care. Correctly identifying the patient's presenting problem is an obvious important step that leads to correctly treating the patient.

With children much of the assessment can be done "from the doorway," meaning the information you can gain even from a distance as you approach: general appearance, status of breathing, and skin color give the EMR a great deal of information about the patient's status and the need for urgent care.

When treating a child, usually a parent or other caregiver is present. Most of the time the parent can be beneficial and helpful to the EMR by providing information about the events that led up to EMS being called and the medical history. If the child has a recurring medical problem such as an asthma attack or a special need, the parent or caregiver should be very helpful in giving support to the EMR. Look to parents to help provide emotional support and, when needed, calm the child.

Children are different from adults in that they can become unstable very quickly rather than it being a slow process. Without keeping a very close eye on your young patient, you might miss a critical change. The need to continually provide ongoing assessment can't be emphasized enough. You must pay close attention to the airway and breathing, level of consciousness, and circulatory status of a sick or injured child.

EMR Patient Assessment: Pediatrics

There are some differences with the scene size-up between the pediatric patient and the adult. In addition to the general patient assessment, it is necessary to multitask and get a look at the big picture, which should only take a few seconds. As always, determine if the scene is safe. On pediatric calls that means making a mental note on how the child is interacting with parents or caregivers. Pay close attention to the environment in regard to health and safety. Be alert for such things as medicine bottles, chemicals, alcohol, or drug paraphernalia. Another issue of concern may be the possibility of child abuse (nonaccidental trauma).

Use the **pediatric assessment triangle (PAT)** when assessing your first impression. (Figure 25-3a ■). The PAT is a tool that allows for a rapid way to determine the severity of an injury or illness of a pediatric patient by reviewing the appearance, work of

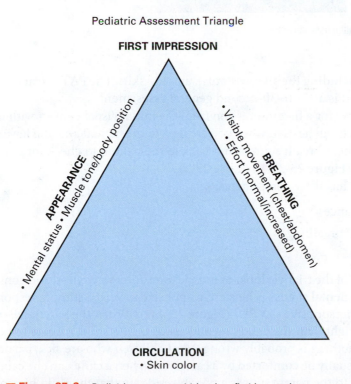

Pediatric Assessment Triangle

FIRST IMPRESSION

APPEARANCE • Mental status • Muscle tone/body position

BREATHING • Visible movement (chest/abdomen) • Effort (normal/increased)

CIRCULATION
• Skin color

■ **Figure 25-3a** Pediatric assessment triangle—first impression.
Used with permission of the American Academy of Pediatrics.

INITIAL ASSESSMENT

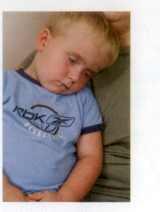

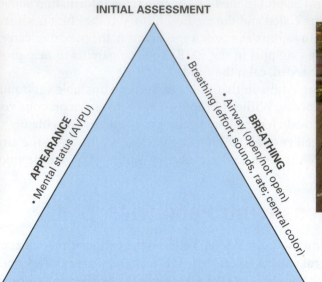

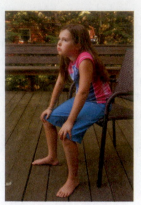

APPEARANCE
• Mental status (AVPU)

BREATHING
• Airway (open/not open)
• Breathing (effort, sounds, rate; central color)

CIRCULATION
• Pulse (rate/strength) • Skin color (extremities)/temperature
• Capillary refill time • Blood pressure

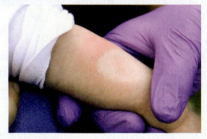

■ **Figure 25-3b** Pediatric assessment triangle—initial assessment.
(Used with permission of the American Academy of Pediatrics.)

breathing (including the airway status), and the skin. The PAT is usually used "from the doorway" and is a 15- to 30-second general assessment.

This allows for a first impression from the initial visual contact with the patient. The same approach can be used when you are next to the patient and you have a chance to not only see but hear breath sounds and palpate the patient to check for chest rise and skin temperature (Figure 25-3b ■) (Table 25-3).

The PAT has three components:

- ■ Appearance
- ■ Work of breathing
- ■ Skin

The first side of the triangle looks at muscle tone, interactiveness, and consolability. What is the child's mental status? Is he alert, responsive to verbal stimuli, responsive to painful stimuli, or unresponsive (AVPU) (Figure 25-4 ■)? When the parent tells you that something is not right with the child's mental status or the child appears to be drowsy, it is a clue that something is probably wrong. Most children who are sick, particularly the very young, can usually be comforted by a caregiver. When a child can't be calmed or does not respond well to the parent, this is a possible red flag that the child has considerable discomfort or acute pain (Figure 25-5 ■).

TABLE 25-3 First Impression of Pediatric Respiratory Emergencies

ASSESSMENT	RESPIRATORY DISTRESS	RESPIRATORY FAILURE	RESPIRATORY ARREST
Mental status	Alert or agitated	Very agitated or sleepy	Unresponsive
Muscle tone/ body position	Normal, able to sit	Somewhat limp	Completely limp
Breathing/visible movement	Present	Present	Slight or none
Breathing effort	Increased	Greatly increased with periods of weakness	Absent
Skin color	Pink or pale	Pale, mottled, or bluish	Blue
Actions	Work at moderate pace; help child into position of comfort; administer high-concentration oxygen without agitating patient.	Move quickly; open airway; suction; administer high-concentration oxygen; assist ventilations if needed.	Immediately open airway; suction; administer high-concentration oxygen; provide ventilations.

When assessing the mental status, take note of the child's posturing. If the child is "floppy," meaning he has no muscle tone, this is serious. If the patient is sitting forward to assist breathing, this is a sign of difficulty breathing. Basically, appearance is an important clue of a significant illness or injury.

Looking at each side of the PAT separately, remember that they are connected. As previously mentioned, position (the appearance side of the triangle) can be a sign of difficulty breathing (Figure 25-6 ■). The patient in a tripod is positioning himself to make breathing easier. Indications of breathing difficulty include:

- Wheezing, a sign of lower airway disease such as asthma
- Stridor, upper airway constriction or blockage
- Grunting, seen with infants in respiratory distress
- Use of accessory muscles to breathe (The muscles between the ribs are used to help the patient breathe. This effort is very visible, so it is important to be observant and look at the entire patient.)
- Nasal flaring

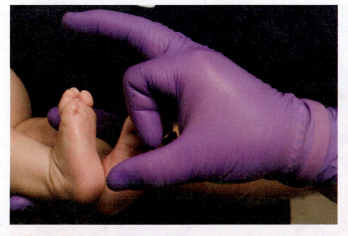

■ **Figure 25-4** Flick the infant's heels to stimulate for a response.

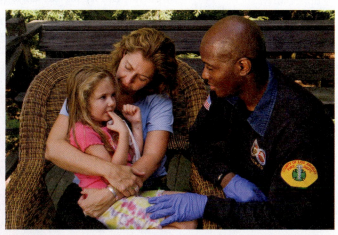

■ **Figure 25-5** Having the parent sit with the child can have a calming influence.

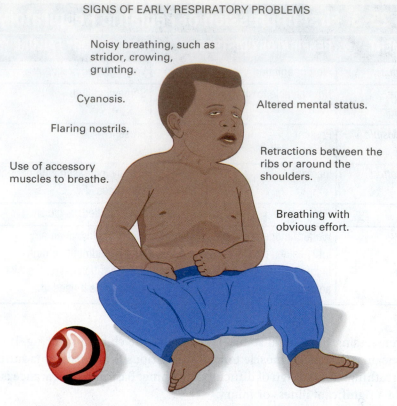

Noisy breathing, such as stridor, crowing, grunting.

Cyanosis.

Flaring nostrils.

Use of accessory muscles to breathe.

Altered mental status.

Retractions between the ribs or around the shoulders.

Breathing with obvious effort.

■ **Figure 25-6** Signs of early respiratory problems.

The bottom portion of the PAT is an evaluation of circulation by evaluating the skin. The following is a list of abnormal skin colors and what they indicate:

- Pale—poor perfusion (impaired blood flow)
- Cyanotic—inadequate oxygenation or poor perfusion
- Flushed—exposure to heat or fever

ASK YOURSELF

- What is the role of respiratory compromise and upper airway obstruction in pediatric cardiac arrest?

Airway and Breathing

Most life-threatening problems in the pediatric patient have to do with the airway and breathing issues. Making sure that the airway is open and the patient is breathing well is the highest priority for the emergency responder. Remember that maintaining the child's airway is different from the adult. The head is larger in proportion to the body. When the child is on his back, the head can flex forward resulting in airway compromise (Figure 25-7a ■). One way of keeping this from occurring is to place a folded towel under the shoulders (Figure 25-7b ■). Take note of this step with an infant.

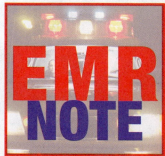

Making sure that the airway is open and your pediatric patient is breathing well is the EMR's highest priority. One study identified that 43 to 80 percent of cardiac arrests in children are the result of respiratory compromise, with upper airway obstructions and asthma being the leading causes.

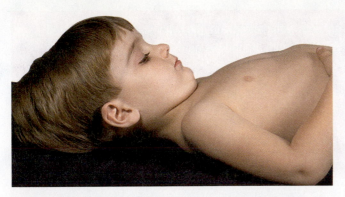

■ **Figure 25-7a** When a child is supine, the head tips forward, obstructing the airway.

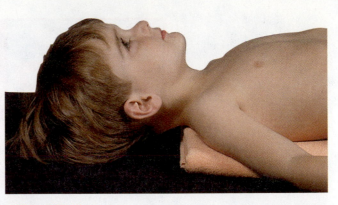

■ **Figure 25-7b** To keep the airway open, place a folded towel under the shoulders.

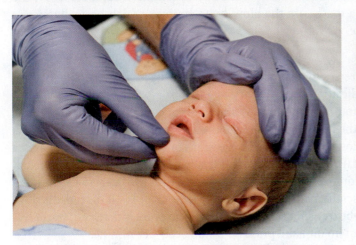

■ **Figure 25-7c** Use the head-tilt, chin-lift method to open the airway.

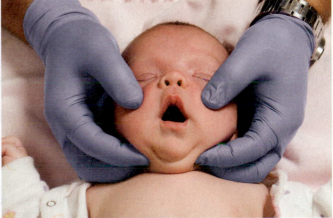

■ **Figure 25-7d** Jaw thrust in an infant.

As with the adult, a head-tilt, chin-lift method would be used to open the airway unless trauma is suspected and then a jaw-thrust maneuver should be used (Figures 25-7c and 25-7d ■). Be prepared, which means have a suction device close, as children can have abundant secretions. Besides secretions, be alert for a foreign body and vomiting. Consider performing an abdominal thrust.

Once the airway is open and maintainable it is essential to ensure the patient is breathing adequately. As the respiratory effort increases, the signs and symptoms change. There will be more use of accessory muscles, and initially the respiratory rate will increase. As breathing gets worse, the muscle tone will worsen and the skin color may become blue.

Common signs of respiratory distress are as follows:

- Noisy breathing (wheezing, stridor, crowing, grunting)
- Cyanosis (In the early stages, the lips and fingernails will appear blue. As it progresses, the central part of the body will appear cyanotic.)
- Flaring nostrils
- **Retractions** (drawing back) between the ribs or around the shoulders
- Using accessory muscles to breathe
- Breathing with obvious effort
- Extreme respiratory rate that is either too slow or too fast
- Altered mental status (This is a serious finding that should alert the EMR to be ready to support respiration with a bag-valve mask.)

ASK YOURSELF

■ What are the indications of airway compromise and inadequate breathing in the pediatric patient?

retractions   sucking in the skin between the ribs, above the sternum, and above the clavicles.

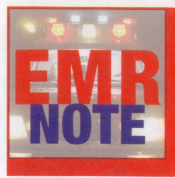

Any child showing signs of respiratory distress, no matter how minor, should receive oxygen. If the patient is moving air adequately, then an oxygen mask can be used. If the young child will not tolerate a mask, use the blow-by technique, which basically means to hold the mask near the face.

CPR Indication

If the respiratory distress progresses to respiratory failure or cardiac arrest, then ventilatory assistance is needed. A key indicator is a respiratory rate that is less than 20 per minute for infants and less than 10 per minute for children. With infants and children, hypoxia (an insufficiency of oxygen) causes the heart rate to slow and then cardiac arrest. Therefore, it is critical to evaluate the circulation whenever a child has signs of respiratory distress. Palpate the brachial artery of the infant. For the responsive child, palpate either the radial or brachial pulse. In infants and small children a stethoscope may be used over the heart to listen to the heart rate. If the child is unconscious, palpate the carotid or femoral pulse. If the pulse is slow, it is imperative that the patient be oxygenated immediately. If no pulse is detected, start CPR immediately. Perform CPR if an infant has a pulse below 60 beats per minute.

When assessing circulation, bleeding must also be checked. Any external bleeding must be stopped immediately. Children have the ability to compensate for blood loss longer than adults, but they decompensate quicker. This means that the heart will rapidly lose its ability to maintain sufficient circulation of blood. This is another reason that pediatric patients must be monitored closely. Their status can change quickly.

Patient History and Physical Examination

The patient history needs to ask about symptoms and durations. You must ask questions about the presence of a fever, how long it has lasted, whether the child's activity level has changed, and whether his eating habits have changed. Determine the frequency of urination, vomiting, diarrhea, and any indication of abdominal pain. Use the SAMPLE assessment:

S = signs and symptoms

A = allergies

M = medications

P = past medical history

L = last meal

E = events that led to the illness

To make the history taking more complete for a medical patient, consider expanding the questions to ask:

- When did signs and symptoms develop?
- How have they progressed?

- Is the problem a reoccurring one?
- Has the child been seen by a physician for the problem?
- Do you know the diagnosis?
- What treatment was received?

For trauma, patient history includes details of the incident such as the time it occurred, mechanism of injury, and emergency care given before EMS arrived.

Obtaining the patient history may be unnerving with the parent being anxious or upset, and the child possibly crying or screaming. When doing the interview, try to talk with the child and involve the caregiver. The exception to this may be when the patient is an adolescent. This interview should be done, if possible, out of range of parents and friends, particularly when asking sensitive questions about "risk behavior."

Avoid asking questions that only require a "yes" or "no" answer. If answers to your questions seem inconsistent or do not correspond to assessment findings, consider rephrasing questions and asking again.

As part of the assessment, there may be a need to expose the child to identify any additional injuries. Remember that children are prone to hypothermia. It is important to keep your patient covered or in a warm environment such as the back of the ambulance whenever possible. A child loses a significant amount of heat through the head, so keep the head covered too.

The physical examination should be organized, starting at the head and going to the toes (Table 25-4).

The following are tips for conducting a physical exam:

- If possible and appropriate, assess the child while he is on the parent's lap.
- It is not uncommon that young children don't like strangers. Being calm, reassuring, friendly, and confident can help.
- Try to get at the child's eye level, but do not stare.
- Describe what you are doing and why.
- Remember that younger children take statements literally.
- Talk to the child directly.
- Be gentle. Do whatever you can to reduce or minimize pain. Tell a child if you are going to do something that might hurt before you do it. Keep painful procedures to the end of the assessment or treatment.
- Do not lie to the patient.
- If the child isn't cooperating, ask his permission before you examine or treat.
- Do not separate the child from the parent unless it is required for emergency care.
- Only restrain a child when there is no other alternative and it is imperative for essential treatment.
- A stuffed animal may help win the confidence of a young child. It may also help to distract the child during assessment and treatment. The child may communicate through the stuffed animal, telling you where the animal hurts as a proxy for where he hurts.

The following is a list of things that should be looked at and palpated, when appropriate, during this part of the examination:

- Head—look for any bruising.
- Ears—observe for drainage (suggestive of trauma or infection).
- Pupils—determine if they are equal size and react to light.

TABLE 25-4 Impact of Anatomical Differences on Assessment and Treatment

ANATOMICAL DIFFERENCES	IMPACT ON ASSESSMENT AND TREATMENT
Larger tongue	Can block airway.
Reduced size of airway	Can become easily blocked.
Abundant secretions	Can block airway.
"Baby" teeth	Can easily dislodge and block airway.
Flat nose and face	Difficult to obtain good airway seal with face mask.
Proportionally large head	Must maintain neutral position to keep airway open and in-line stabilization of head and neck. Higher potential for head injuries in cases of trauma.
"Soft spots" on head	Bulging "soft spots" may indicate intracranial pressure; sunken ones may indicate dehydration.
Thinner and softer brain tissue	Consider head injury more serious than in adults.
Short neck	Difficult to stabilize and immobilize.
Shorter and narrower trachea, with more flexible cartilage	Can close off trachea with overextension of the neck.
Faster respiratory rate	Muscles fatigue easily, which can lead to respiratory distress.
Primarily nose breathers (newborns)	Airway more easily blocked.
Abdominal muscles used to breathe	Difficult to evaluate breathing.
More flexible ribs	Lungs are more easily damaged. May be significant injuries without external signs.
Faster heart rate sustained for longer period of time	Can compensate longer before showing signs of shock and usually decompensates more quickly than an adult.
More exposed spleen and liver	Significant abdominal injury more likely. Abdomen more often a source of hidden injury.
Larger body surface	Prone to hypothermia.
Softer bones	Can easily bend and fracture.
Thinner skin	Consider burns to be more serious than in an adult.

- Mouth—check for loose teeth, odors, and bleeding.
- Neck and spine—look for signs of injury such as bruising.
- Chest and back—check for bruises, injuries, and rashes.
- Extremities—observe for deformities, swelling, or pain on movement.

ASK YOURSELF

- Given a scenario, how do you compare a pediatric patient's vital signs to the expected vital signs for a patient of that age?

Vital Signs

The body of an infant or child can hide injury for some time. Only after compensatory abilities fail will you see changes in vital signs. The changes may occur very quickly, resulting in the patient deteriorating fast. That is why it is so important to continually monitor pediatric patients, and this includes frequent vital signs. Remember, vital signs are only one piece of the assessment information and should be combined with appearance, how the patient acts, the physical exam, and the patient history to get the complete picture (Table 25-5).

TABLE 25-5 Normal Vital Sign Ranges for Infants and Children

DEVELOPMENTAL STAGE	NORMAL PULSE RATES (BEATS PER MINUTE, AT REST)	
Newborn	120–160	
Infant 0–5 months	90–140	
Infant 6–12 months	80–140	
Toddler 1–3 years	80–130	
Preschooler 3–5 years	80–120	
School-age child 6–10 years	70–110	
Adolescent 11–14 years	60–105	
NORMAL RESPIRATION RATES (BREATHS PER MINUTE, AT REST)		
Newborn	30–50	
Infant 0–5 months	25–40	
Infant 6–12 months	20–30	
Toddler 1–3 years	20–30	
Preschooler 3–5 years	20–30	
School-age child 6–10 years	15–30	
Adolescent 11–14 years	12–20	
NORMAL BLOOD PRESSURE RANGES		
	Systolic	**Diastolic**
	Approximately 80 plus 2 x age	Approximately 2/3 systolic
Preschooler 3–5 years	Average 99 (78–166)	Average 65
School-age child 6–10 years	Average 105 (80–122)	Average 69
Adolescent 11–14 years	Average 114 (88–140)	Average 76

Note: Blood pressure is usually not taken in pediatric patients younger than 3 years of age. In cases of blood loss or shock, a child's blood pressure will remain within normal ranges until near the end and then fall rapidly.

When taking pediatric vital signs, keep the following in mind:

- *Pulse.* Use the brachial artery when checking the pulse in an infant. Use a radial or brachial pulse if the child is conscious. If the pulse is too rapid or too slow, immediately examine the patient for problems such as respiratory distress, shock, or head injury. A rapid pulse may indicate oxygen deficiency, shock, or fever, but it can be normal when a child is scared. A slow pulse must be assumed to be a sign of hypoxia. Other causes of slow pulse may include pressure in the skull or depressant drugs. A pulse below 60 beats per minute in an infant requires CPR.

- *Respiration.* Children sometimes breathe irregularly. Monitor respirations for a full minute to determine the rate and take it frequently. Young children are "belly breathers," so when counting the rate consider putting your hand over the abdomen. Pay close attention to rate changes.

  The rate and the quality of breathing are both important. To determine if breathing is adequate, observe to see if the child is working to breathe and using

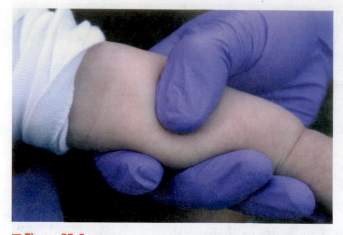

■ **Figure 25-8a** Assess the capillary refill by pressing the infant's arm.

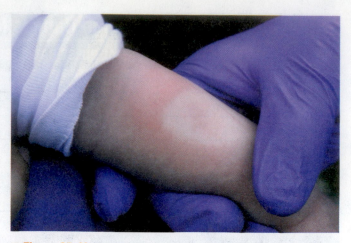

■ **Figure 25-8b** Release the arm to show the results.

accessory muscles. Look for retractions. Notice if breathing is noisy. Shortness of breath may indicate the need to assist ventilations.

■ *Blood pressure.* A falling pulse rate and low blood pressure on a pediatric patient can be a late indicator of shock. Be sure to use a blood pressure cuff that is the correct size for the patient and a pediatric stethoscope if available. Do not take a blood pressure in children under 3 years of age. Without the proper cuff size, an accurate reading is unlikely. Other signs of perfusion in infants and young children (capillary refill, pulse rate, respiratory rate mental status) provide more accurate information very easily.

■ *Temperature.* Feel the arms and legs of infants and children to see if they are cold. The torso may be warm in comparison. Cold hands and feet may indicate shock if a young patient is not in a cold environment.

■ *Skin condition.* Always look to see if the skin is pale or bluish, indicating cyanosis. Also check the skin for signs of injury.

■ *Capillary refill.* If the capillary refill time is more than 2 seconds, this may be a sign of shock, but capillary refill is not a stand-alone sign. In other words, if a pediatric patient has a delayed capillary refill, it is usually significant if there are other signs of shock present. Obtain capillary refill by pressing on the hand, foot or forearm. Infants and young children's fingers will be too small. It is also difficult to obtain a reliable capillary refill when the child's extremities are cold (Figures 25-8a and 25-8b ■).

EMR Emergency Care:
Pediatric Respiratory Emergencies

Once you have identified the respiratory emergency, it is extremely important that you take immediate action. If the child is choking, appropriate action must be taken quickly to free the foreign object. If the patient needs to be ventilated because he is not receiving enough oxygen, use the following technique for pediatric bag-valve-mask ventilation (Scan 25-1):

1. *Select the proper size mask.* It is critical to ensure the good seal of the mask on the face. Pick the smallest one that will cover the patient's mouth and nose without pressing down on the eyes. The top of the mask should rest on the bridge of the nose, and the bottom should rest on the crease of the chin.

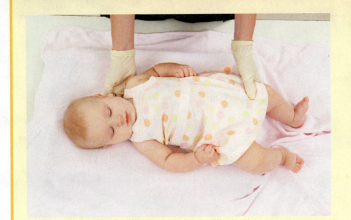

25-1a Infant in a supine position.

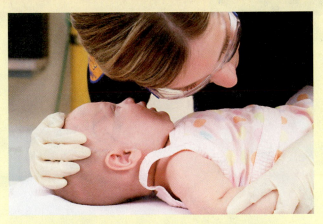

25-1b Assess the breathing by leaning close to the infant.

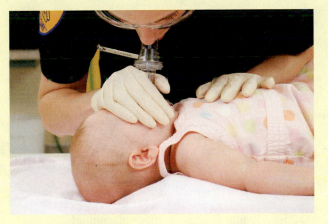

25-1c Ventilate the infant.

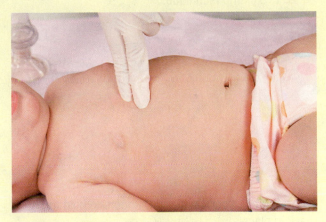

25-1d Begin CPR on the infant with chest compressions.

2. *Select the proper bag, attach the mask and tubing, and set the oxygen flow rate.* The oxygen flow rate for the supplemental oxygen should be 10–15 lpm. Be sure to maintain an open airway by checking that the patient's head and neck are in the proper position. Insert an airway adjunct if needed. *Only insert an oropharyngeal airway for a patient with no gag reflex.*

3. *Apply the mask to the patient using one of the following techniques:*

   a. *One-handed mask placement.* If you are alone and you do not suspect trauma in your patient, use this one-handed or "E-C clamp" mask placement technique (Scan 25-2).

      ■ Using your nondominant hand, apply the tips of your long, ring, and small fingers to the bony ridge between the chin and angle of the jaw. Your three fingers should form the "E."

      ■ Keeping your fingertips in place along the jaw, gently rest the palm of your hand against the patient's temple.

      ■ Place the clear plastic face mask with an inflatable rim over the patient's mouth and nose. Hold it in place by resting the tips of your thumb and index finger over the front of the chin and the bridge of the nose. This will

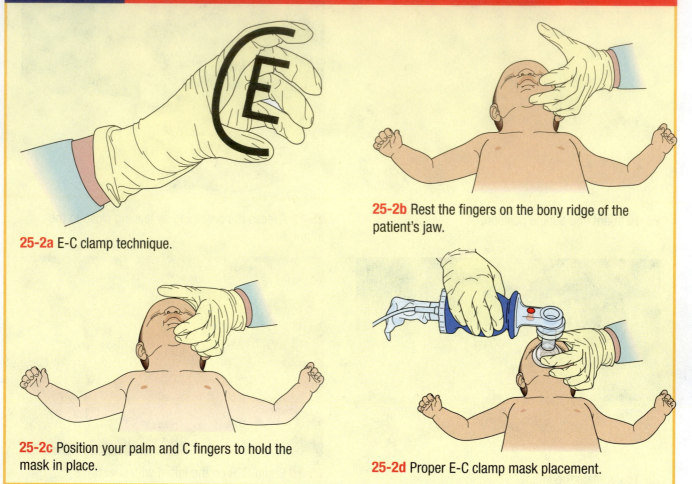

25-2a E-C clamp technique.

25-2b Rest the fingers on the bony ridge of the patient's jaw.

25-2c Position your palm and C fingers to hold the mask in place.

25-2d Proper E-C clamp mask placement.

form the "C" part of the technique. To avoid damaging or obstructing the patient's airway, avoid pressing on the soft tissue under the chin.

b. *Two-handed mask placement.* This technique requires two EMRs. It is the preferred technique if there is trauma (jaw-thrust technique is used) or if the one-handed technique does not create an effective seal.

■ If trauma is *not* suspected, the EMR at the patient's head holds the mask on the patient's face with the thumb and index finger of both hands, using the other fingers to lift the chin. The EMR at the patient's side squeezes the bag and watches for chest rise.

■ If trauma *is* suspected, the EMR at the patient's head performs a jaw-thrust maneuver, lifting the jaw into the mask while maintaining manual in-line stabilization. The rescuer at the patient's side holds the mask in place, using the one-handed technique previously described to squeeze the bag.

4. *Squeeze the bag.* Do so gently and only until chest rise is visible. Do not overinflate the lungs. Then release it, allowing time for the patient to breathe out. The chest will fall back into resting position.

Continue ventilating at a rate of 20 breaths per minute for infants and children (one breath every 3 seconds), or 12 breaths per minute for adolescents (one breath every 5 sec-

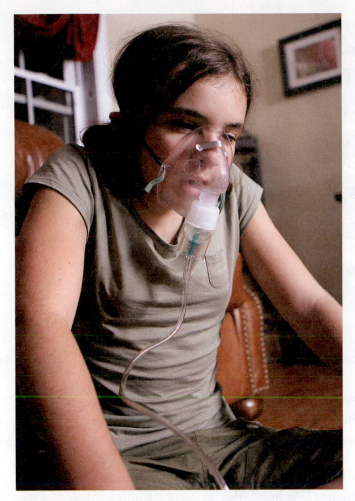

■ Figure 25-9 Child in respiratory distress.

onds). Be prepared to suction, if necessary. Watch the abdomen for signs of enlargement during ventilation. If this occurs, reposition the airway and decrease the force of ventilations. Gently squeeze the bag while watching for chest rise.

According to the National Pediatric Trauma Registry, 30 percent of all pediatric trauma deaths are related to inappropriate management of the airway. The American Heart Association reports that more than 90 percent of pediatric deaths from foreign body airway obstructions occur in children younger than 5 years of age and of these, 65 percent are infants. It has been speculated that most could have been saved with early intervention. Aggressive airway assessment and treatment are keys to the survival of infants and young children (Figure 25-9 ■).

Anatomical Care Considerations

There are differences in the anatomy of the child's airway that have an impact on treatment (Figure 25-10a ■):

■ *Children are more susceptible than adults to respiratory problems.* They have smaller airway passages and less reserve air capacity. Pay careful attention to ensure an open and clear airway.

■ *A child's airway structures are not as long or as large as an adult's.* A child's airway can close off if the neck is flexed or extended too far. The best position is neutral

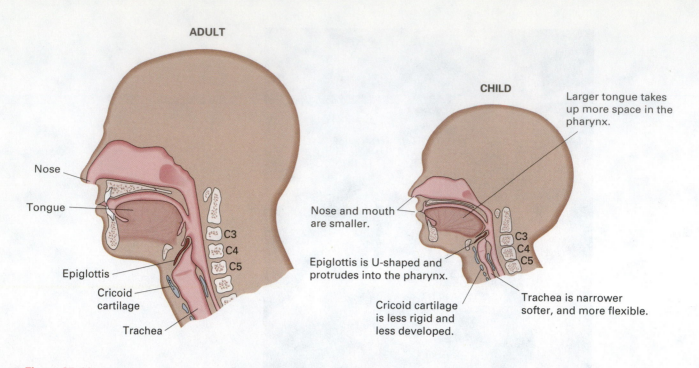

ADULT

Nose

Tongue

Epiglottis

Cricoid
cartilage

Trachea

CHILD

Larger tongue takes
up more space in the
pharynx.

Nose and mouth
are smaller.

Epiglottis is U-shaped and
protrudes into the pharynx.

Cricoid cartilage
is less rigid and
less developed.

Trachea is narrower
softer, and more flexible.

■ **Figure 25-10a** Comparison of the airways of an adult and an infant or child.

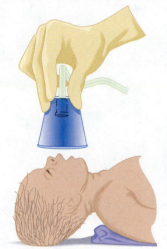

■ **Figure 25-10b** The use of
blow-by oxygen.

or slightly extended. If a child is flat on his back, place a thin pad or towel under
the shoulders to keep the head and neck properly aligned.

■ *Because of immature accessory muscles, children use the diaphragm to breathe.* If
there are no reasons to prevent you from doing so, place a child in a position of
comfort. That is usually the sitting position.

■ *Children have a large tongue that can block the airway.* Make sure the tongue is
forward. If you use a jaw-thrust maneuver, make sure your hand stays on the bony
part of the chin. If it falls below, the tongue could be pushed back to block the airway.

■ *Infants and children tend to breathe through the nose.* They also have abundant
secretions. Be prepared to suction to keep the nose clear. Only suction for short
periods of time (10 seconds for a child and 5 seconds for an infant). Provide oxygen
before and immediately after each suctioning whenever possible.

Apply oxygen by way of a mask. Humidified oxygen is preferred, but never withhold or
delay oxygen to have it humidified. If a child will not tolerate the mask, try the blow-by technique (Figure 25-10b ■). Hold the mask or oxygen tubing 2 inches away from the patient's
face. Some children respond well when the tubing is pushed through the bottom of a cup
(paper, not Styrofoam), especially if the cup is colorful or has a picture drawn inside of it.

If an infant or child is having a respiratory emergency, notify the incoming EMS unit
and be sure advanced life support (ALS) is en route, if available. Even if the signs and
symptoms of a respiratory emergency subside, it is still important for the child to be
transported to a hospital.

Croup

croup a common viral
infection of the upper airway,
most common in children
between the ages of 1 and 5
years.

Croup is a common viral infection of the upper airway. It is most common in children between the ages of 1 and 5. With croup, swelling progressively narrows the airway. As the
child breathes, he may produce strange whooping sounds or high-pitched squeaking.
There may be hoarseness, with the child's sound typically described as a "seal bark."
Episodes of croup generally develop slowly and occur more commonly at night.

As the child gets worse, he may experience the following signs of respiratory distress: breathing with effort, nasal flaring and retractions (pulling in of the sternum and ribs with each inhalation), rapid breathing, rising pulse, paleness or cyanosis, and restlessness or altered mental status.

Severe attacks of croup can be dangerous. About 10 percent of all children with croup need to be hospitalized. Treat a child with croup the same way you would treat any respiratory emergency. Arrange for transport to the nearest hospital as quickly as possible.

Epiglottitis

Epiglottitis is caused by a bacterial infection that inflames the epiglottis. It often resembles croup but is more serious. Thanks to vaccinations it does not occur often but, if left untreated, epiglottitis can be life threatening. Signs and symptoms include occasional noise while inhaling, anxious concentration on breathing (the child may need to stay very still), sitting up and leaning forward with the chin thrust forward (tripod position), pain on swallowing and speaking, drooling, changes in voice quality, and high fever (usually above 102°F).

If you suspect epiglottitis, keep the child calm. *Do not* ask the child to open his mouth. Do not try to examine the child's throat or place anything in the mouth. Touching the larynx can cause the airway to close completely. Treat the child as you would for any respiratory emergency. If you must move the patient, be very gentle. Arrange for transport to the nearest hospital as quickly as possible.

Asthma

Asthma is common among children, especially those with allergies. However, it should always be considered a serious medical condition. Most parents know their child's history and recognize an asthma attack. Determine if the child is taking medication such as using an inhaler with a spacer (Figure 25-11 ■).

An acute asthma attack occurs when the bronchioles spasm and contract. This causes the bronchial membranes to swell and congest with mucus, which interferes with the child's ability to exhale. As a result, air is trapped in the lungs, the chest gets inflated, breathing becomes impaired, and oxygen deficiency occurs.

Especially critical signs and symptoms include rapid irregular breathing (most common in younger children), exhaustion, changes in level of responsiveness or sleepiness, cyanosis, rapid pulse and dropping blood pressure, signs of dehydration, wheezing (high-pitched breathing sounds usually heard when the child exhales), and quiet or silent chest.

epiglottitis a bacterial infection that inflames the epiglottis; often resembles croup but is more serious.

ASK YOURSELF

- Given a scenario, how do you recognize and manage pediatric patients with the following conditions?
  - Croup
  - Epiglottitis
  - Asthma
  - Cardiac arrest
  - Seizures
  - Shock
  - Trauma
  - Special health care needs
  - Sudden infant death syndrome
  - Abuse or neglect

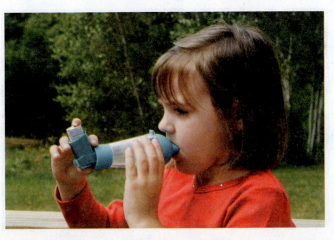

■ **Figure 25-11** Child with an inhaler and spacer.

In the late stages of respiratory distress, respirations may become so shallow that they no longer cause noise. Do not be fooled into believing that the child has gotten better. The condition has actually worsened.

EMR care is the same as for any respiratory emergency. Be sure to monitor the airway and breathing constantly. Arrange for transport to the nearest hospital as quickly as possible.

Cardiac Arrest

Most cardiac arrests in infants and children result from airway obstruction and respiratory arrest from an underlying medical problem or trauma. It is extremely important to ensure an open airway and adequate breathing in your patients.

Signs and symptoms of circulatory failure in the pediatric patient are increased or decreased heart rate, unequal central (femoral) and distal pulse rates, poor skin color, delayed capillary refill, and altered mental status.

In cases of cardiac arrest in infants and children, provide CPR for two minutes and then call for help if you are alone. Your goal is to keep your patient's brain alive. Remember that children have remarkable recuperative abilities. Cases of drowning, particularly cold-water drowning, and hypothermia may need an extensive resuscitation effort. Do not stop or interrupt CPR. Arrange for transport to the nearest hospital as quickly as possible.

For use of an automatic external defibrillator (AED) on pediatric patients, the American Heart Association recommends using pediatric-specific defibrillators and pads when available. These devices use energy levels corresponding to the size and weight of the child. If these items are not available, an adult defibrillator and pads may be used on patients of any age.

Seizures

febrile seizures seizures caused by a rapid rise in body temperature usually resulting in a high fever.

Febrile seizures are caused by a rapid rise in body temperature usually resulting in a high fever. They are the most common type of seizure in children. Some other causes include infection, poisoning, trauma, decreased level of oxygen, epilepsy, hypoglycemia, inflammation of the brain, and meningitis. However, all seizures, including febrile seizures, should be considered potentially life threatening.

During most seizures, a child's arms and legs become rigid, the back arches, muscles may twitch or jerk in spasm, the eyes roll up and become fixed with dilated pupils, breathing is often irregular or ineffective, and the child may lose bladder and bowel control. The child may become completely unresponsive (Figure 25-12 ■).

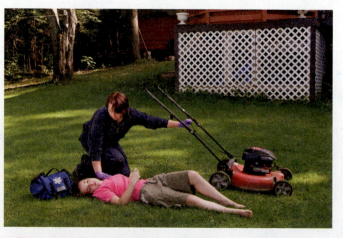

■ **Figure 25-12** Care for a child with a seizure.

If the seizure lasts long enough, the child will show signs of cyanosis. The spasms will prevent swallowing. Saliva will be pushed out of the mouth, which will appear to be frothing. If saliva is trapped in the throat, the child will make bubbling or gurgling sounds. This may mean the airway needs suctioning when the seizure has ended. After the seizure, the child often appears to be extremely sleepy.

To obtain a patient history, ask the parents the following questions:

- Has the child had a seizure before? How often? Is this the child's normal seizure pattern? Have the seizures always been associated with fever or do they occur when the child is well? Did others in the family have seizures when they were children?

- How many seizures has the child had in the past 24 hours? What was done for them?

- Has the child had a head injury, a stiff neck, or a recent headache? Does he have diabetes?

- Is the child taking a seizure medication? What has the doctor told you about the seizure disorder?

- Could the child have ingested any other medications?

- What did the seizure look like? Did it start in one part of the body and progress? Did the eyes go in different directions?

During the seizure, the tongue may relax and shift backward, decreasing the size of the airway passage. To prevent this, as well as to encourage draining of mucus and frothing, place the patient in the recovery position. But do so only if there is no possibility of spine injury. Do not put anything in the patient's mouth.

Do not restrain the child during a seizure. Place him where he cannot fall or strike something. An open space on the floor with furniture and other objects moved away is fine. If the child is on a bed that does not have sides, move him to prevent a fall, if necessary. Loosen any tight and restricting clothing, especially around the neck or face.

After the seizure, make sure the airway is open. The jaw may be relaxed, so consider gently pushing the mandible (the lower jawbone) forward. This should help keep the airway open. Be prepared to suction.

Administer high-concentration oxygen if local protocol allows. Hold the mask slightly away from the patient's face until the seizure is completely over. If breathing is diminished or absent and the airway is clear, assist ventilations with a bag-valve mask (BVM) or pocket face mask with oxygen enrichment attached. Follow local protocol in regard to cooling in the field if the child has a high fever. Only tepid water should be used. Never use rubbing alcohol. Be sensitive to cooling the child to the point where he becomes chilled. After cooling, dry if tepid water was used, and cover the child (Figures 25-13a and 25-13b ■).

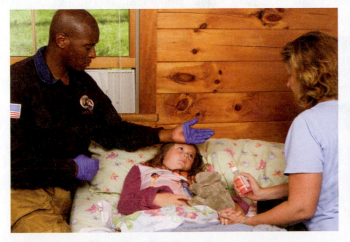

■ **Figure 25-13a** Care for a child with a fever by assessing the skin temperature.

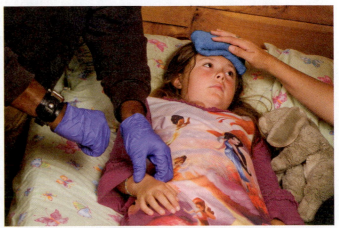

■ **Figure 25-13b** Cool the forehead with tepid water.

Be sure to assess for injuries that may have occurred during the seizure.

If the seizure lasts longer than a few minutes and reoccurs without a recovery period, the seizure may be status epilepticus. This condition is a true emergency. Notify the incoming EMS unit immediately.

CASE STUDY

THE RESPONSE

You observe the airway is open and breathing is rapid and shallow. Your young patient is lethargic and doesn't react to your presence or mind being touched. When you check capillary refill, it is delayed at 4 to 5 seconds.

The child has a blanket covering him but you also cover the head to ensure less body heat is lost. You set up oxygen to be given by blow-by. The mother has calmed down and she is willing to hold the oxygen mask near her son's face.

The next part of the assessment is to obtain a SAMPLE history. You find out that this is her first child. Along with her husband, they just moved into the area about a month ago and do not have a pediatrician. The patient has been vomiting since early morning and the diarrhea started last night. The child's diaper is dry and has not been changed for 3 hours. The mother informs you that her son is not taking any medications and has no allergies. She reports that she has been trying to get her son to drink fruit juice all morning with little success.

You continue to ask about previous illnesses and about the possibility that the child has ingested something he shouldn't have. The mother claims that she keeps a very close eye on her son. You then take a full set of vital signs.

The patient seems stable, but you want to make sure the responding ambulance is updated. You give a brief radio report of the history and the current status of a child who responds to verbal stimuli with delayed capillary refill. You conclude with information on the treatment you are providing.

You continue to monitor the patient, obtain another set of vital signs, and provide comfort and support to both the patient and his mother.

■ Discussion: *How would you ask the same question in different ways in situations such as these?*

Multiple Choice

Place a check next to the correct answer.

1. The three sides of the pediatric assessment triangle (PAT) are:

   _____ a. airway, breathing, and circulation.

   _____ b. assessment, breathing, and circulation.

   _____ c. airway, bleeding, and consciousness.

   _____ d. appearance, breathing, and circulation.

2. Which of the following is a true statement about a child's response to shock?

   _____ a. A child compensates only with severe bleeding.

   _____ b. A child decompensates rapidly.

   _____ c. A child decompensates slowly.

   _____ d. A child compensates for a shorter time than an adult.

3. Which of the following is an early sign of respiratory distress?

   _____ a. Cyanosis of the central part of the body

   _____ b. Severe altered mental status

   _____ c. Use of accessory muscles to breathe

   _____ d. Somewhat limp

4. Lungs of children are more easily damaged by trauma because:

   _____ a. ribs are more flexible.

   _____ b. ribs are less flexible.

   _____ c. ribs are smaller, giving less protection.

   _____ d. lungs are less dense.

Emergency Medical Responder Practice

You are called to a residence where a 1-year-old boy has been sick for 2 days. The mother tells you her son has been vomiting and has diarrhea, and the diaper was dry during the last changing.

1. What are five signs you expect to see with this patient?

   _____

   _____

   _____

2. What is the emergency care for this patient?

   _____

   _____

   _____

   _____

You are called to a school for a child having trouble breathing. Upon arrival, you find a 10-year-old having an asthma attack. He was given one puff of his inhaler and then ran out of his medication.

3. List five signs and symptoms you would expect this patient to have.

_____

_____

_____

_____

Matching

Match the characteristic and behavior to the age for the following pediatric patients.

1. _____ The child is very curious at this age (be alert to poison ingestion).

2. _____ Modesty is important at this age.

3. _____ The child has an active imagination.

4. _____ The child is likely to be scared and may believe what happened is his own fault.

5. _____ The child will want to be held by his parents.

a. Birth to 1 year (infant)
b. 1–3 years old (toddler)
c. 3–5 years old (preschooler)
d. 6–12 years old (school-age child)
e. 13–18 years old (adolescent)

Short Answer

1. Fill in the blanks in the following chart.

ANATOMICAL DIFFERENCE	IMPACT ON ASSESSMENT AND TREATMENT
Larger tongue	
	Difficult to obtain good airway seal with face mask
Shorter neck	
Larger body surface	
	Muscles fatigue easily, can lead to respiratory distress
	Can compensate longer before showing signs of shock

2. List five questions you would ask a parent of a seizure patient when taking a patient history.

_____

_____

_____

_____

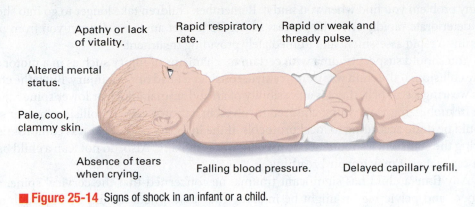

SIGNS OF SHOCK

Apathy or lack of vitality.

Rapid respiratory rate.

Rapid or weak and thready pulse.

Altered mental status.

Pale, cool, clammy skin.

Absence of tears when crying.

Falling blood pressure.

Delayed capillary refill.

■ **Figure 25-14** Signs of shock in an infant or a child.

Shock

Shock can be caused by blood loss as the result of trauma, but with children there is another common cause: dehydration. When children get sick, vomiting, diarrhea, and lack of oral intake lead to dehydration. When dehydration becomes severe enough, it can result in shock. As stated before, children compensate longer but decompensate very rapidly. You might think the patient is stable when, in fact, he is just about to decompensate. Therefore, diligence is crucial. You must continually monitor the patient as he can change so quickly. Part of the monitoring includes frequent vital signs and checking capillary refill.

EMR Patient Assessment and Emergency Care: Pediatric Shock

Signs and symptoms of shock (Figure 25-14 ■) in the pediatric patient include:

- Altered mental status, from anxiety to unresponsiveness
- Apathy or lack of vitality (This may present as the child's inability to recognize a parent—an ominous sign.)
- Delayed capillary refill
- Rapid or weak pulse
- Pale, cool, and clammy skin
- Rapid breathing
- Falling or low blood pressure (a late sign)
- Absence of tears when crying
- In infants, a dry diaper that should be wet

Hypothermia can intensify shock in infants. They usually cannot shiver to warm themselves. Keep the infant warm and his head covered.

The care of pediatric patients in shock or at risk of going into shock is similar to care of the adult. If possible, lay the patient flat. It may be difficult to convince an agitated child to lie flat. Monitor the airway closely in case the child vomits. Provide oxygen and be prepared to assist ventilations if needed. Keep the patient warm and monitor closely, which includes taking frequent sets of vital signs.

Trauma

Injuries are a leading cause of death in infants and children. Blunt trauma is more common than penetrating injury. The basic life support care for a traumatized child is similar to that for an adult. As you assess the patient's airway, breathing, and circulation (ABCs), take care of any problem you find when you find it. Remember, children take longer to go into shock but deteriorate rapidly once the process starts. Do not let anything distract you from performing a rapid assessment and immediately providing treatment.

You should suspect trauma with certain mechanisms of injury such as in a motor vehicle collision. If the child was unrestrained, consider a head or neck injury. But if the child was wearing a seat belt, there is a possibility of an abdominal injury or lower spine injury.

Immobilizing very young children involved in a motor vehicle collision in a car seat should be done according to local protocols. If the integrity of the seat was compromised during the collision, it should not be used for immobilizing. Also, do not lean a child back in a car seat as it may impair breathing.

Any time a child has significant trauma, be concerned that the cervical spine, abdomen, and pelvic region might be injured. Your assessment should be thorough and repetitive. Pediatric patients are dynamic and can be difficult to assess. Check to make sure nothing was missed and to find problems that were initially undetected because the signs and symptoms were delayed.

Special Health Care Needs

Children who have certain types of physical or mental limitations have special health care needs. For example, a premature baby or a chronically ill child might be dependent on a mechanical device such as a ventilator. Many children with special health care needs receive care at home, attend school, and participate in activities throughout the community. In most cases, the parents or caregivers of these children have received some training on how to handle emergencies related to special health care needs. When EMS is called to provide care to one of these children, it may mean it is a true emergency beyond what the parent or caretaker feels comfortable handling or they may know that immediate hospital care is necessary.

When responding to a call for such a child, as always focus on the patient's ABCs. If a child is on a ventilator and is having trouble breathing, it is more important to assist ventilations than to determine what might be wrong with the device. In these situations, disconnect the device and ventilate using a bag-valve mask with an oxygen reservoir. If oxygen is not available, ventilate with a bag-valve mask until oxygen can be brought to the patient.

Keep in mind that parents and caretakers can be very good resources for information about the child's condition. They will probably know the child's baseline vital signs, medications, and how to operate the medical devices. In addition, they may have dealt with a similar problem previously and know what needs to be done. In many instances, the parents or caretakers may have initiated care before your arrival. Based on the circumstances, consider taking their lead and assist in providing care.

Sudden Infant Death Syndrome (SIDS)

sudden infant death syndrome (SIDS) the sudden death of an infant in the first year of life with no identifiable underlying cause.

Sudden infant death syndrome (SIDS) is defined as the sudden death of an infant in the first year of life with no identifiable underlying cause. In the past it was more commonly known as "crib death" or "cot death."

SIDS cannot be predicted or prevented. While placing a baby on his back to sleep and other recommendations may help reduce the chances of death, in fact, it is still not well understood. It almost always occurs while an infant is sleeping. The infant is typically healthy and was born prematurely. Between the ages of 4 weeks and 7 months, the infant suddenly dies without warning. No illness has been present, though there may have been recent cold symptoms. There is usually no indication of struggle.

Managing the SIDS Call

Unless the infant has *rigor mortis* (stiffness), immediately initiate basic life support, even if other signs make the effort appear hopeless. Begin CPR, and have someone activate the EMS system if it has not already been done.

The extreme emotional condition of the parents makes them victims as much as the baby. They will be in agony from emotional distress, remorse, and feelings of guilt. Avoid any comments that might suggest blame. Help them feel that everything possible is being done but do not offer false hope. Follow local protocols.

When you can, obtain a brief medical history of the infant. This should not delay or interfere with life support efforts in any way. Some of this information can be obtained from parents and some from observation. If necessary, have other medical personnel find out the following: When was the child put in the crib? What was the last time the parents looked in on the baby? What were the circumstances concerning the discovery of the infant? What was the position of the baby in the crib? What was the physical appearance of the infant in the crib? What else was in the crib? What was the appearance of the room and home? Is there medication present (even if it is for the adults)? What is the behavior of the people present? What is the general health of the infant (any recent illness, medications, or allergies)?

After ambulance personnel take over, encourage the parents to accompany their baby. Offer to make arrangements to stay with any other children until relatives or friends arrive. Support the parents in any way possible. While the resuscitation effort seems futile to them, parents may receive comfort from knowing that everything that can be done is being done.

It is very common for Emergency Medical Responders to experience emotions such as anxiety, guilt, or anger after a SIDS call. A debriefing or talking to a counselor, colleague, medical director, or spouse may be helpful. Ignoring feelings will not cause them to go away, and denying them can potentially be serious, resulting in a negative impact on your mental health.

Child Abuse and Neglect

The definition of **child abuse** is improper or excessive action so as to injure or cause harm. The term **child neglect** refers to giving insufficient attention or respect to a child who has a claim to that attention and respect.

Child abuse, or **nonaccidental trauma**, occurs in all parts of our society. The estimated number of children who are abused or neglected in the United States is staggering. Estimates range from 500,000 to over 4 million cases annually with thousands of abused children dying. These numbers are cause for alarm.

During an emergency call, the adult (often a parent) who abuses a child often behaves in an evasive manner. This person may volunteer little information or give contradictory information about what happened. However, a call for child abuse may be a call for help. Do not be judgmental. Focus on providing care for the child and transport to the hospital (a safe environment).

Signs and symptoms may include multiple bruises in various stages of healing; injury not consistent with the mechanism of injury described by the caregivers; patterns of injury that suggest abuse such as cigarette burns, whip marks, or hand prints; burns not consistent with the information provided by the caregivers; and untreated burns.

Also suspect possible abuse when there are repeated calls to the same address, when the caregivers seem inappropriately unconcerned or give conflicting stories, and when the child seems afraid to discuss how the injury occurred. If an infant or child presents with unresponsiveness, seizure, or signs of severe internal injuries but no external signs, suspect central nervous system injuries, or **shaken baby syndrome**.

child abuse improper or excessive action so as to injure or cause harm to an infant or child.

child neglect insufficient attention or respect given to a child who has a claim to that attention and respect.

nonaccidental trauma injuries caused by abuse.

shaken baby syndrome referring to an infant or child presenting with unresponsiveness, seizure, or signs of severe internal injuries but no external signs, causing suspicion of central nervous system injuries due to shaking of the child.

Signs and symptoms of possible neglect include lack of adult supervision; appearance of malnourishment; unsafe living conditions; untreated chronic illness, such as no medication for asthma; and delay in reporting injuries.

If you suspect abuse or neglect, first make sure that the environment is safe for you and the patient. Provide necessary emergency care. As time permits, observe the child and the caregivers. Observe for objects that might have been used to hurt the child. Look for signs of neglect in the child's general appearance. Remember, the responsibility of the EMR is to provide care and to facilitate getting the child to safety. Being a good observer is important, but do not investigate or get distracted away from giving treatment. Definitive determination of an abused or neglected child takes time and needs to be done by professionals such as law enforcement, social services, and physicians. The EMR must document thoroughly without being subjective or accusatory or drawing conclusions.

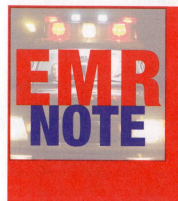

EMR NOTE

In cases of child abuse or neglect, a well-written prehospital care report that contains *objective* information can be a valuable tool in assisting officials who need to take action to protect a child through the legal or social services systems. Your observations from the field are vitally important to help physicians, social workers, or law enforcement officers to understand the events and circumstances that led up to a suspected abused or neglected child being brought to the hospital.

Sometimes what appears to be abuse or neglect may be the result of poor parenting or a result of actions that are acceptable in another culture. Jumping to conclusions is potentially counterproductive and distracts from the EMR's primary duty to the patient.

If you find yourself in a position of giving emergency care to a possible victim of child abuse or neglect, follow these guidelines:

- Only enter the home to access the child if it is safe. Don't assume the environment is safe even if the child made the call to 911. Be diligent to ensure you will not be in any danger. Do not put yourself at undue risk. Call for police assistance if there is any concern about safety for EMS personnel.

- Try to keep the parents calm and reassure them that the only reason you are there is to care for their child. Speak in a low, firm voice with the parents.

- Focus attention on the child while providing emergency care. When talking with the child, speak softly using the child's first name. Do not ask the child to re-create the situation that may have caused the injury while the parents are present. This can be done after the child is at the hospital.

- Do a full patient assessment as you would with any patient. Treat as you go. Note any suspicious abrasions, bruises, lacerations, and evidence of internal injury. Look for signs of head injury. Remember, you are there to provide emergency care, not to determine child abuse.

- Update the ambulance crew in the same way you would for any other child in need of care and treatment. You may need to be discreet.

- You are not expected to deal with child abuse issues on the spot unless the child is in immediate danger. In all suspected cases the child should be transported.

- Never confront parents with a charge of child abuse. Being supportive and nonjudgmental with parents will help them be more receptive to others providing emergency care.

- Accusations can delay transport and place the EMR at risk. Instead, report objective information to the transporting unit's crew. Focus on what you saw and what you heard. Be very cautious about providing subjective information (what you think). When transferring information, try to do it privately, away from the family and caretakers.

- Maintain total confidentiality regarding the incident. Do not discuss it with your family, friends, or anyone in your organization who is not authorized and does not have a specific need to know.

You must report your suspicions of child abuse to the proper authorities. It is critical to learn the reporting laws in your own state and reporting protocols and policies for your EMS system. Most states mandate EMS providers to report abuse and neglect. If you work in such a state, learn what abuse and neglect must be reported, to whom the report must be made, what information an EMR must give, what (if any) immunity is granted, and criminal penalties for failure to report.

Take Care of Yourself

The death of a child is emotionally wrenching, whether it occurs before you arrive, while you are giving care, or after you arrive at the hospital. For most EMRs this type of event is rare, but when it does occur you need to recognize when you are having a reaction to it. Feelings of fear, rage, helplessness, anxiety, sorrow, and grief are common, and in some cases there may be shame and guilt. These feelings may be more intense when a child dies. Unfortunately, how one reacts may not be related to the actions of the EMR. Even when the outcome occurs before EMS arrives or even if you do everything right while giving care, you may still have a reaction. Remember, some children will die despite your best efforts.

As an EMR, you need to control your emotions while you are treating a pediatric patient. In this way you can render the best assistance possible. After the call is over, however, you need to deal with your feelings. Talk them out. A critical incident stress debriefing (CISD) team may be helpful. But you can use other methods to discuss and deal with your feelings, for example, talking to a trusted friend, a colleague, the medical director, or a professional counselor. Don't deny your feelings or delay seeking help as it can potentially lead to serious and long-term problems.

✳ Stop, Review, Remember

Multiple Choice

Place a check next to the correct answer.

1. Which artery should be checked when assessing the pulse of an infant?

_____ a. Femoral

_____ b. Radial

_____ c. Carotid

_____ d. Brachial

2. Do not take a blood pressure in a child under what age?

_____ a. 5 years

_____ b. 3 years

_____ c. 7 years

_____ d. 9 years

3. An acute asthma attack occurs when:

_____ a. bronchioles spasm and contract.

_____ b. alveoli contract and some can rupture.

_____ c. the larynx swells and spasms.

_____ d. bronchi dilate, causing a choking sensation.

Emergency Medical Responder Practice

You arrive on the scene where a child has been injured. After determining the scene is safe, you enter and see an upset child on the couch with the mother by his side. You look around, observe the environment, and watch closely at how the child is interacting with his mother. You are thinking this call might involve child abuse.

1. What are seven indicators from this type of call that might alert you to suspect possible child abuse?

_____

_____

_____

_____

2. What action should you take when treating this child and following up on suspicions of possible child abuse?

_____

_____

_____

_____

You are dispatched to a call for a child who is having difficulty breathing. When you arrive, you see a child sitting up and leaning forward in what appears to be respiratory distress.

3. What are six signs you expect to see in a pediatric respiratory distress patient?

_____

_____

_____

_____

4. Which of the signs of respiratory distress are a serious finding that should alert you to be ready to support respiration with a bag-valve mask?

_____

_____

_____

_____

Identification

1. Place an X next to the signs and symptoms of shock that the EMR might find in a pediatric patient.

_____ Altered mental status   _____ Low blood pressure (late sign)

_____ Hyperactivity   _____ High blood pressure

_____ Inability to recognize parents   _____ Delayed capillary refill

_____ Rapid weak pulse   _____ Rapid capillary refill

_____ Slow strong pulse   _____ Absence of tears

_____ Rapid breathing   _____ Pale, cool, and clammy skin

_____ Slow breathing   _____ Warm, dry, and flushed skin

_____ Irregular respirations

2. What questions should you ask, as time and circumstances permit, during the resuscitation of a suspected sudden infant death syndrome baby?

1. _____

2. _____

3. _____

4. _____

5. _____

6. _____

7. _____

8. _____

9. _____

10. _____

THE LAST WORD

All anatomical structures in the infant's or child's airway, including the mouth and nose, are smaller than an adult's and are therefore more easily obstructed. The tongue takes up proportionally more space in the mouth than the tongue of an adult. As a result, it can block an infant's or child's airway more easily. The trachea is narrower, softer, and more flexible, so tipping the head too far back or allowing the head to fall forward can close the trachea.

Maintaining a good airway and ensuring quality breathing are the two most important concerns for an EMR when dealing with a pediatric emergency. Remember: If you do *not* have an airway, you will *not* have a patient. When assisting ventilations in a pediatric patient, be sure to watch for chest rise. This is a good indicator of whether your breaths are effective. Administer oxygen to the pediatric patient for any type of respiratory problem. If you do not have oxygen on scene, do not delay ventilations while you wait for it.

The primary cause of cardiac arrest in infants and children is an uncorrected respiratory problem. Because the chest wall is softer, they tend to rely more heavily on the diaphragm for breathing. Watch for excessive movement of the diaphragm. It can alert you to respiratory distress in these patients. With pediatric patients, all roads lead to the ABCs.

When performing a pediatric patient assessment, take what you can when you can get it. For example, if a child holds out a hand, it is a good time to check the pulse or capillary refill. Stop bleeding in a pediatric patient as quickly as possible. A comparatively small blood loss in an adult would be major for an infant or small child. In addition, they tend to compensate longer before going into shock. Be alert! They also decompensate very rapidly.

A child's skin surface is large compared to body mass. This makes children more susceptible to dehydration and hypothermia. Response to burns also can be more severe.

The interests of the infant and child must always be the foremost consideration when making patient care decisions. In cases of suspected abuse or neglect, EMS personnel may be the only advocates a child has. Report as objectively as you can what you have seen and heard. When you treat an ill or traumatized child, you are treating a family.

✳ Chapter Review

Multiple Choice

Place a check next to the correct answer.

1. Which of the following is *not* a sign of early respiratory problems?

    _____ a. Cyanosis

    _____ b. Noisy breathing

    _____ c. Normal mental status

    _____ d. Breathing with obvious effort

2. One sign of shock in children is:

    _____ a. warm and dry skin.

    _____ b. normal mental status.

    _____ c. slow respiratory rate.

    _____ d. weak and rapid pulse.

3. EMR care of childhood seizure includes:

    _____ a. administering oxygen after the seizure.

    _____ b. placing the patient in the supine position.

    _____ c. restraining the patient during the seizure.

    _____ d. placing a stick in the mouth to prevent biting.

4. Which of the following statements is *most* correct about an asthma emergency?

_____ a. It is not a serious medical emergency.

_____ b. You should gather a medical history.

_____ c. The patient will be awake and alert.

_____ d. Breathing will be slow and regular.

5. Which of the following may be the *best* solution to a situation in which parents are especially anxious?

_____ a. Raise your voice to distract them from their child's injuries.

_____ b. Keep them as far away as possible so they do not interfere with emergency care.

_____ c. Realize that they may be correct and could actually help you provide the proper care.

_____ d. Tell them that they are jeopardizing the life of their child and that you intend to report them.

6. Most cardiac arrests in infants and children result from:

_____ a. trauma-induced ventricular fibrillation.

_____ b. airway and respiratory problems.

_____ c. seizures.

_____ d. infection and dehydration.

7. Which of the following is a late sign of shock?

_____ a. Rapid breathing

_____ b. Pale, cool, and clammy skin

_____ c. Falling blood pressure

_____ d. Altered mental status

8. You are dispatched to a call at 11:00 p.m. for a child with breathing difficulty. Upon arrival you find a 4-year-old who is breathing with effort, flaring nostrils, restless, and making a "seal bark" noise. What do you think is the most likely problem of this child?

_____ a. Croup

_____ b. Asthma

_____ c. Epiglottitis

_____ d. Pneumonia

9. The prehospital report for a case involving suspected child abuse or neglect should contain what type of information?

_____ a. Judgmental

_____ b. Subjective

_____ c. Opinionated

_____ d. Objective

10. During the review of the circulatory status of a pediatric patient, you find that the skin is flushed. Of the following, what does this most likely indicate?

_____ a. Poor perfusion

_____ b. Fever

_____ c. Anxiety

_____ d. Trauma

Emergency Medical Responder Practice

You arrive on the scene of a 2-year-old who has been sick and vomiting. The mother, who appears frantic, is holding the sick child in her arms. The scene is safe.

1. As you approach the mother and the child, what should you be doing?

_____

_____

_____

_____

2. You observe the airway is open and breathing is rapid and shallow. Your young patient is lethargic and doesn't react to your presence or mind being touched. When you check capillary refill, it is delayed at 4 to 5 seconds. The child has a blanket covering him to keep him warm, but you also cover the head to ensure less body heat is lost. The mother is extremely anxious. What should you do next?

_____

_____

_____

_____

3. The physical examination has been completed and immediate emergency care provided. You turn your attention to obtaining a patient history. What questions should you ask?

_____

_____

_____

_____

4. The patient seems stable but you want to make sure the responding ambulance is updated. You give a brief radio report. What should this report contain?

_____

_____

_____

_____

5. Once you have assisted with packing the patient for transport and transitioned care to the transporting unit, you give a full patient update. As an EMR, what do you have left to do before you have completed this call?

_____

_____

_____

_____

Matching

Match the following descriptions with the appropriate term.

1. _____ Method of remembering the important components of pediatric assessment

2. _____ Injuries caused by abuse

3. _____ Insufficient attention or respect given to a child who has a claim to that attention or respect

4. _____ A high-pitched breathing sound usually heard during exhalation

5. _____ A bacterial infection that inflames the epiglottis

6. _____ Cornerstone of providing emergency care

7. _____ A sign of inadequate oxygenation

8. _____ A common viral infection of the upper airway, usually in a child 1 to 5 years of age

9. _____ Highest priority for the EMR when delivering care to a child

10. _____ Sucking in of the skin between the ribs, above the sternum, and above the clavicles

11. _____ A vital sign that does not have to be taken in children under 3 years of age

12. _____ A device that is only used in a patient without a gag reflex

13. _____ Occurs in children most often due to respiratory arrest

14. _____ A condition in which children compensate longer but decompensate quicker than an adult

15. _____ The type of information that should be contained in a prehospital care report for a suspected child abuse call

a. Wheezing
b. Cardiac arrest
c. Retractions
d. Nonaccidental trauma
e. Pediatric assessment triangle (PAT)
f. Oropharyngeal airway
g. Objective information
h. Open airway and breathing well
i. Croup
j. Assessment
k. Child neglect
l. Shock
m. Blood pressure
n. Cyanosis
o. Epiglottitis

Geriatric Patients

✳ **NAVIGATION GUIDE**

The following items provide an overview to the purpose and content of this chapter. The Education Standard and Competency are from the National EMS Education Standards.

Education Standard Special Patient Populations (Geriatrics)

Competency Recognizes and manages life threats based on simple assessment findings for a patient with special needs while awaiting additional emergency response.

Knowledge Area Geriatrics
- Impact of age-related changes on assessment and care

Objectives After reading this chapter, you should be able to:

1. Define key terms introduced in this chapter.
2. Describe the key differences in the anatomy and physiology of geriatric patients.
3. Discuss common age-related problems that must be considered in the assessment and management of elderly patients.
4. Relate the anatomical and physiological differences of geriatric patients to modifications in patient assessment and management.
5. Demonstrate effective techniques of approaching and communicating with geriatric patients.
6. Respond appropriately to the needs of the geriatric patient's caregivers.
7. Recognize the impact of psychosocial and economic issues, depression, substance abuse, and elder abuse and neglect on the health status of the elderly.
8. Adapt your index of suspicion of illness and injury in the elderly patient based on common mechanisms of injury, changes in pain sensation, and the potential for altered mentation.
9. Discuss the importance of determining the medications an elderly patient is taking.

Key Terms Page numbers indicate first major use in this chapter. The Margin Glossary in this chapter provides definitions as you read.

diaphoresis, p. 658

cataracts, p. 658

Alzheimer disease, p. 667

dementia, p. 667

NAVIGATION GUIDE *(continued)*

Media Resources Please go to **www.bradybooks.com** to access mykit for this text. You will find quizzes, critical thinking scenarios, weblinks, animations, and videos related to this chapter—and much more. Look for online information on seniors' health, aging hearts and arteries, and hypertension.

INTRODUCTION

As the population ages, you will respond to a larger number of geriatric patients. Many of these older patients have chronic conditions, take many medications, and have some kind of restricted mobility. Whether the elderly live on their own, in assisted-living facilities, or in nursing homes, many will need emergency medical assistance at some point.

You can expect to encounter geriatric patients in many different environments with various medical issues, such as a general medical emergency, a fall that was caused by low blood sugar, or a motor vehicle crash that precipitated a heart attack. Many calls can be challenging, requiring some of the most diligent care you will provide.

Prevention is always better than providing care to a patient who is injured when it could have been avoided. For example, if you encounter a patient who has fallen on a piece of loose carpet or whose home shows signs of a person who is unable to care for himself properly, try to alert someone who can correct the problem or assist the patient after he leaves the hospital.

Always treat older patients with respect and dignity, even when confronted with special challenges that you might encounter when assessing and treating geriatric patients. Be an advocate for your older patients and do not underestimate their abilities. Most will be able to understand what is happening and will expect an explanation of what you are doing. Although you may need to compensate for geriatric patients' impaired hearing or vision, or lack of mobility, they will have similar expectations as any patient you treat. If a patient is unable to answer questions needed for care and treatment, see if you have medical information easily accessible or consider asking a family member, neighbor, or caretaker.

CASE STUDY

THE CALL

You are dispatched to a residence of a 74-year-old male who is conscious and reported to be ill. No other information is available as the 911 call came from a neighbor. When you arrive, you find the patient sitting on a couch in the living room. He is unkempt with significant body odor and the smell of urine. Garbage and dirty dishes are scattered around. The scene is safe.

He snaps back that he did not want EMS; it was his nosy neighbor who called. You then ask how he feels. The patient replies that he has stomach pain. When you ask how long he has had the pain, he tells you his daughter is getting him some medicine and that she is going to be mad that someone called an ambulance.

It is obvious that more information is needed, and you begin your assessment.

■ Discussion: *What patient and environmental issues can you determine from your senses during the scene size-up?*

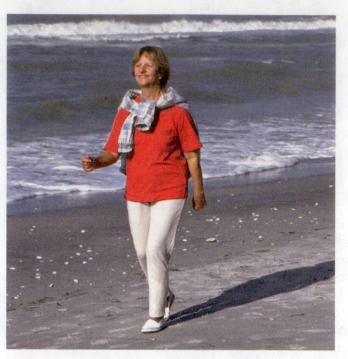

■ **Figure 26-1** Healthy, active geriatric adult.

ASK YOURSELF
- What are the key differences in the anatomy and physiology of geriatric patients?
- What common age-related problems must be considered in the assessment and management of elderly patients?
- How do you relate the anatomical and physiological differences of geriatric patients to modifications in patient assessment and management?
- Can you define key terms introduced in this chapter?

diaphoresis excessive perspiration.

cataracts opacity of the lens of the eye; among the common causes of blindness in adults.

Physical Changes and Challenges

The most common theories about aging relate to genetic makeup, the environment, and individual lifestyle (Figure 26-1 ■). Whatever the underlying cause, all body systems decline with age. This general decline in function includes changes in the skin, sensory organs, heart, blood vessels, and the respiratory, digestive, urinary, musculoskeletal, nervous, and immune systems. Basically every body system is affected and may be a factor when an older person is injured or becomes ill. The following review of these body systems will highlight important issues to consider when you provide care to a geriatric patient (Table 26-1).

The Skin

As people age, the skin can develop darkly pigmented areas which are most noticeable in lighter-skinned individuals. These areas are sometimes called "age spots" or "liver spots." The skin secretes less oil, making it drier and flakier. Skin secretions also contain substances that help protect against infection. However, as skin secretions decrease, so does the protection against infection.

Perspiration decreases, which is a contributing factor to heat-related emergencies in older adults. Some medications can further inhibit perspiration, so when an elderly patient is in shock you may not see the moisture on the skin from **diaphoresis** (excessive perspiration).

The skin of older adults tears quite easily as a result of loss of fat and weakening of the supportive structures within the skin. Patients who are confined to bed and do not receive proper care are prone to bedsores, which have serious and devastating consequences.

Sensory Organs

In general, aging leads to decreased sharpness of the senses. Visual changes include far-sightedness, **cataracts**, decreased night and peripheral vision, and less tolerance for glare. These changes can make it difficult to read directions on medication bottles or to tell the

TABLE 26-1 Physical and Functional Changes in the Older Adult

BODY SYSTEMS	CHANGES	COMPLICATIONS
Skin	Decreased perspiration Decreased oil secretion Loss of fat and weakening of supportive structures beneath the skin	Heat-related illness Masks signs of shock Decreased resistance to infection Skin is easily torn Bedsores
Sensory organs	Diminished vision Diminished hearing Diminished pain sensation Diminished taste and smell	Falls; vehicle crashes Unable to read directions for medication Unable to hear warnings such as smoke alarms or sirens May be unaware of injury or seriousness of injury Decreased appetite; malnutrition Unable to smell leaking gas or smoke
Respiratory system	Weakened chest muscles	Less able to compensate when the body needs more oxygen Less lung capacity
Heart and blood vessels	Decreased strength of heart contraction High blood pressure Blockage of blood vessels	Cannot meet higher demands for blood flow Heart attack, stroke, poor circulation to extremities Masks shock
Digestive system	Ulcers, tumors Dental problems	Gastrointestinal bleeding Malnutrition, choking on poorly chewed food
Urinary system	Incontinence	Catheterization may lead to infection
Musculoskeletal system	Diminished muscle strength Weakened bone structure	Minor falls or impacts can break bones
Nervous system	Fewer nerve fibers Alteration in chemical balance	Decreased sensory perception Depression Impaired sleep
Immune system	Less functional	Diminished ability to heal Infection Cancer

color of one pill from another. Visual changes may be a problem when driving and also contribute to many unintentional injuries such as falls and household injuries.

Hearing becomes less acute, especially in picking up high-pitched sounds. The senses of taste and smell are diminished, and there is less sensation in the skin. It is not difficult to imagine how older adults could fail to hear a siren while driving, fail to smell a gas leak or spoiled food, or be unaware when they sustain minor injuries. The diminished senses of taste and smell also contribute to a decreased appetite and nutritional problems that can endanger the overall health of an elderly patient. Be alert to these issues so you can tell the transporting unit for follow-up at the hospital.

Respiratory System

Aging results in weakening of the chest muscles and stiffening of the rib cage cartilage, making breathing less effective. In addition, the lungs lose some of their capacity to provide oxygen to the blood. As a result, the elderly are less able to compensate when they need more oxygen. It is not uncommon for elderly patients to have chronic obstructive

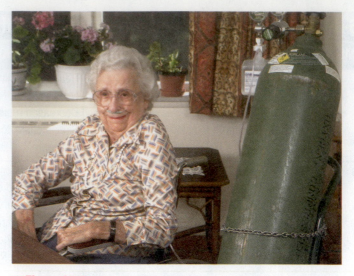

■ **Figure 26-2** Difficulty with breathing is a common emergency among the elderly.

pulmonary disease (COPD) from long-term smoking. Because of other changes in the lungs and the immune system, infections such as pneumonia are common (Figure 26-2 ■).

Heart and Blood Vessels

The ability of the heart to contract with force declines with age. When the body demands increased blood flow, the heart tries to compensate by contracting more often. If it contracts too often, the heart's chambers do not have enough time to completely fill with blood before the next contractions, so instead of increasing blood flow, a heart rate that is too rapid may result and actually worsen circulation.

Because of the effects of certain medications, the heart of a patient with heart disease or high blood pressure is unable to beat faster. This means that the pulse rate may be normal in patients with blood loss, even when you would expect it to be rapid.

Many older adults have high blood pressure; this can lead to a heart attack or stroke. Significant blood loss will lead to a drop in blood pressure. But in a person whose blood pressure is usually high, a blood pressure in the normal range may actually represent a drop. Shock due to blood loss may go unrecognized because of this. Decreased blood pressure is usually a late sign of shock so be alert for the usual signs and symptoms of shock. Consider the mechanism of injury and monitor the elderly trauma patient's mental status. In such cases a decrease in the level of responsiveness may be the first indication of shock.

In addition, genetic and lifestyle factors contribute to changes in the blood vessels over time, such as blockage or weakening of arteries that can affect the brain and the heart. Stroke and heart attack are common presentations that the Emergency Medical Responder may encounter.

Digestive System

With age, the digestive system slows, producing fewer secretions for the breakdown of food. This, along with other changes, may lead to indigestion or heartburn, gas production, and constipation. Since the stomach empties more slowly, vomiting may occur during illness and injury.

The elderly may also suffer from ulcers or disorders of the intestinal tract, which can lead to bleeding. Medications such as aspirin and some medications for arthritis are common causes of this bleeding. Such bleeding may be evident in vomit or from bloody or dark, tarry stools. Enough blood can be lost this way to result in shock.

Decreased taste and smell may lead to a decrease in appetite and dental problems. Fatigue may cause eating to be difficult. For these reasons—and others such as poverty and depression—the elderly may suffer from malnutrition. Malnutrition affects general health and makes existing medical problems worse. Be alert and pass this information along to the transporting EMS unit.

Urinary System

Elderly men may suffer from blockage of urine flow due to enlargement of the prostate gland, making bladder and kidney infection more likely. Elderly women are also more susceptible to infections of the urinary tract.

Elderly patients with urinary tract infections can be quite ill. Overwhelming infection may occur, causing changes in circulation that lead to shock. This type of shock, called septic shock, should be suspected when the patient has signs and symptoms of shock without blood loss. Also, expect to see fever, elevated heart rate, and decreased mental status in the elderly patient with septic shock. There may be pain, although painless urinary tract infection is fairly common in the elderly. As an EMR, you will treat this type of shock the same as shock due to blood loss.

Musculoskeletal System

Muscle strength and bone mass decrease with age. Older patients are less active and may tire more easily, contributing to falls and other injuries. In some cases, they may be too frail to do common chores such as fixing meals, bathing, or laundry due to this decline in the musculoskeletal system. Even minor falls commonly can result in broken bones in the elderly. When a hip is broken, the decrease in mobility often leads to a decline in the patient's overall health, such as bedsores and a decline in mental status. About one half of all geriatric patients who sustain a hip fracture die within one year of the injury.

Nervous System

Decreases in the number of nerve fibers and changes in the chemical balance of the brain may lead to decreased perception, changes in balance and coordination, and altered sleep patterns. These changes are factors that contribute to injuries among the elderly.

Many people believe that impairments in thinking and memory (often referred to as *dementia*) are normal processes of aging, but this is not the case. It may be a factor, but most of the geriatric patients you encounter probably do not suffer from dementia. When you are called for an elderly patient, consider the presence of an abnormal condition involving perception, balance, and coordination as being an underlying cause of an acute illness and not normal. Sometimes confusion and agitated behavior among the elderly are temporary, caused by illness or the effects of medication and not a stand-alone medical condition.

Immune System

Common illnesses, such as influenza, have a much higher fatality rate in the elderly. Though fever is often a sign of infection, it may *not* be present in the elderly. In addition, the increased risk of infection and decreased ability to heal after an injury or surgery may be serious and can be fatal.

Response to Medication

The body's ability to respond to and eliminate medications also changes with age. The liver, responsible for processing and detoxifying these medications, is not as efficient. This can result in patients having exaggerated responses to medications and more profound side effects compared to younger patients. Since older patients tend to be on several medications, life-threatening drug interactions can occur.

While asking a patient about medication during the history, information about starting on a new medication can be important. Make sure this information is included in the report to the transporting unit as it may be helpful to the physicians providing care at the hospital.

✴ Stop, Review, Remember

Multiple Choice

Place a check next to the correct answer.

1. Which of the following is a contributing factor for heat-related emergencies in an older patient?

   _____ a. Decreased perspiration

   _____ b. Hormonal changes

   _____ c. Loss of fat

   _____ d. Circulation changes

2. Which of the following is common in the elderly and makes breathing less effective?

   _____ a. Chronic lung congestion

   _____ b. Cartilage of rib cage becomes less rigid

   _____ c. Weakening of chest muscles

   _____ d. Widening of mediastinum

3. Which of the following is known to keep the heart from beating faster with blood loss in the elderly?

   _____ a. Effect of old age

   _____ b. Fluid intake

   _____ c. Depression of the nervous system

   _____ d. Medications

Emergency Medical Responder Practice

1. You respond to an assisted-living facility for a 72-year-old who tripped on a curb and fell. It is early evening and the sun is setting. What are five factors, due to age, that may have contributed to this patient falling?

   _____

   _____

   _____

   _____

   _____

2. What is emergency care for this patient?

   _____

   _____

   _____

   _____

3. What type of follow-up should be done?

_____

_____

_____

_____

Matching

Match the following conditions with the appropriate organ or system.

1. _____ Cataracts

2. _____ Bleeding evident by dark, tarry stools

3. _____ Age spots

4. _____ Forces of contractions decline with age

5. _____ Stiffening of cartilage

6. _____ Decreased perception

a. Skin

b. Sensory organs

c. Respiratory system

d. Heart

e. Digestive system

f. Nervous system

Psychosocial and Economic Factors

Many psychological, social, and economic factors impact the lives of the elderly. They include alcoholism, substance abuse, physical and psychological abuse, neglect, loneliness, and poverty. All of these factors have implications for the health of older adults. Being aware of these factors is a step toward developing empathy and compassion for your elderly patients. The clues to these issues can be helpful when providing care as well as follow-up treatment. Remember, the emergency department will not see what you see. Information about behavior, the environment in which the patient is found, and what the patient says may assist them in figuring out what is truly wrong with a patient. Make sure what you see and hear is communicated to the EMS providers who will be transporting.

Depression

Depression is not uncommon among older adults. This illness can lead to suicide or attempted suicide. A depressed patient may have poor hygiene, poor eating habits, and a disorderly living situation. In addition, frequent depression can lead to physical symptoms. Be alert to what the patient tells you about a significant life event such as the loss of a spouse or other family members or friends. Although depression often can be treated with therapy or medication, many depressed elderly do not get identified or diagnosed, and therefore are not getting treatment. As a result, it is still an underlying factor in suicide among the elderly.

Changes in the chemicals affecting the brain can cause depression, or the patient may be living alone and feeling isolated. Loss of independence and having to depend on others for help with daily activities may also be distressing. In some cases, the patient may feel shame, self-disgust, or embarrassment at the loss of a body function or changes in appearance.

ASK YOURSELF

■ What are some examples of the impact of psychosocial and economic issues, depression, substance abuse, and elder abuse and neglect on the health status of the elderly?

Substance Abuse

Health care providers often fail to suspect alcohol and other substance abuse as a factor in the medical condition of the elderly. This may include dependence on prescription drugs, as well as the abuse of illegal substances. It may seem shocking to think of an older adult as having a substance abuse problem, but a person who was in his 20s or 30s in the 1960s, a time when illicit drug use was popular, is now in his 60s or 70s.

Alcohol and substance abuse contributes to deterioration of physical health, may be a factor in altered mental status, and can contribute to injuries including those sustained in motor vehicle crashes.

Elder Abuse and Neglect

Physical and psychological abuse of the elderly and neglect of dependent elderly are often first detected by EMS providers. There are several risk factors for abuse, regardless of whether the older adult lives with a spouse, with his children, or in an extended-care facility. An older adult who requires assistance with daily activities, who has difficulty sleeping, who has lost bladder control, or who exhibits bizarre behavior due to altered mental status is more likely to be abused or neglected.

Abuse should be suspected when an injury seems inconsistent with the description of how it happened or when there are multiple injuries in various stages of healing (Figure 26-3 ■). The patient may be reluctant to discuss the nature of the injury in the presence of the abuser because of fear of punishment or because of feelings of shame or embarrassment. The neglected patient may be deprived of food and water, medications, and the assistance needed for activities such as bathing and changing clothing.

Do not confront the suspected abuser. Privately relate your suspicions to the arriving EMS crew. Follow local protocol.

ASK YOURSELF

■ How would you adapt your index of suspicion of illness and injury in the elderly patient based on common mechanisms of injury, changes in pain sensation, and the potential for altered mentation?

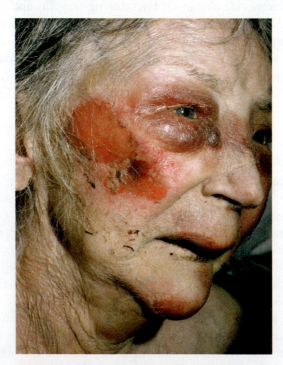

■ **Figure 26-3** Signs of elderly abuse or neglect.

Socioeconomic Concerns

Many older adults live on very limited incomes. As a result, they may not have adequate shelter, safety, food, or medications. The elderly may not be able to secure their homes against crime, make necessary repairs or upgrades to their homes, or otherwise maintain a safe environment. Lack of adequate heat or cooling can leave the older adult at risk of heat- and cold-related emergencies. Using alternative sources of heat, such as space heaters or an open oven, leads to burns, fires, and carbon monoxide poisoning.

The elderly with financial concerns also may not eat properly. They may take less medication than prescribed or may not take their medication at all in order to save money.

CASE STUDY

THE RESPONSE

As you start the assessment, you observe that the patient remains agitated. The airway is open and the patient is breathing adequately. You observe no signs of external bleeding and the patient denies falling or any other trauma. The vital signs show a slightly rapid pulse of 110, respirations of 26 and shallow, and blood pressure of 160/90. The skin is pale and very warm.

Next you take a SAMPLE history and find that the patient reports no allergies and he is taking atenolol, which is a beta-blocker. When you ask if he has been taking the medication on schedule, the patient tells you he does not remember the last time he took one. He is also vague about the last time he ate. You talk to the neighbor who called 911 to see if she has anything to add, but she does not.

While it has taken some time, the patient is warming up to you and lets you know he does not feel well and he has not eaten all day. The patient reports that he feels weak and is having trouble standing. You observe he has a persistent cough. He comments that his daughter must have forgotten to stop by with his medicine and food as she promised.

The patient allows you to apply a nonrebreather face mask at 15 lpm. You discuss going to the hospital because he isn't feeling well and appears to have a fever. He asks you to assist him with getting clean pants before going to the hospital and you do.

You take another set of vital signs, which are similar to the first set. You are concerned that not only is this patient sick but he may be neglected by his family.

■ Discussion: *What are other possible ways to obtain SAMPLE history information for this patient?*

Illness and Injury in the Older Adult

Common medical complaints in the elderly include chest pain, difficulty breathing, fainting, and an altered mental status (Figure 26-4 ■). Chest pain should always be considered serious. Difficulty breathing may occur due to lung or heart problems or because of airway obstruction. Fainting or near-fainting is common in the elderly. It may be due to a variety of causes such as side effects of medication, heart problems, internal bleeding, or changes in the blood vessels that supply the brain with oxygen. When an older adult has an altered mental status, such as a change in personality or behavior, a family member or caregiver usually summons help.

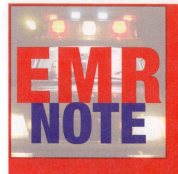

EMR NOTE

Decreased sensitivity to pain is a function of the aging process. Maintain a high index of suspicion and treat any complaint of pain in the elderly as a possible symptom of a serious illness or injury.

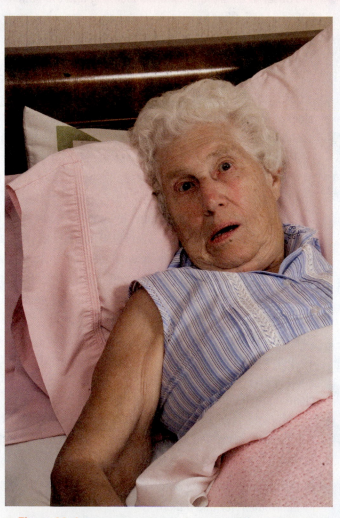

■ **Figure 26-4** Altered mental status, such as becoming confused or disoriented, is a common presentation of medical emergencies in the elderly.

The most common mechanisms of injury in the elderly are falls, burns, and motor vehicle crashes. These are usually due to effects of aging, such as diminished vision, hearing, and pain sensation, as well as loss of muscular strength, balance, and coordination. The physical changes associated with aging result in much less force needed to produce injury than in younger people. In addition, the effects of some medications can mask the seriousness of an older adult's injury. Therefore, injuries may be more serious than they appear.

Scene Size-Up

As with all calls, your first priority is your own safety and the safety of your crew. Size up the scene as you would for any emergency call. Keep in mind the following:

- An older adult with substance abuse problems, mental illness, or a condition such as **Alzheimer disease** (a form of **dementia**) may become violent. Be prepared.
- Stay alert for conditions that suggest abuse, neglect, or the patient's lack of self-care.
- Be careful of potential hazards, such as loose or missing handrails on porches and stairs, loose carpeting or throw rugs, and stairs and clutter in the house.
- Look for poorly functioning or alternative heat sources to warn you of possible carbon monoxide poisoning.
- Check for hygiene or environmental issues such as excessive garbage, pet excrement, or dirty clothes scattered around.

When approaching the elderly patient, focus on him rather than family members or caregivers who may be anxious to speak for him. This demonstrates respect for the patient, and it gives him more control over the situation. Make eye contact. Then, introduce yourself. Once you know the patient's full name, address the patient by that name—"Mr. Baker" or "Mrs. Smith" for example. Do not address the patient as "honey," "dear," "sweetheart," or similar terms.

Take a position at the patient's eye level (Figure 26-5 ■). It is less intimidating than towering over him. Offer a handshake to establish rapport and note the patient's skin temperature and ability to move and follow directions. Establish the chief complaint by asking for the reason why EMS was called today. Asking, "What is wrong?" is too vague and may only result in a lengthy recitation of both medical and nonmedical complaints. While this information is ultimately important, the

Alzheimer disease a progressive degenerative disease that attacks the brain and results in impaired memory, thinking, and behavior (the most common type of dementia in the elderly).

dementia the loss of brain function that results in a person having impaired memory, disorientation, decreased judgment, and lessening intellectual ability; usually a progressive process.

ASK YOURSELF

- How would you demonstrate effective techniques of approaching and communicating with geriatric patients?
- What is an example of an appropriate response to the needs of the geriatric patient's caregivers?

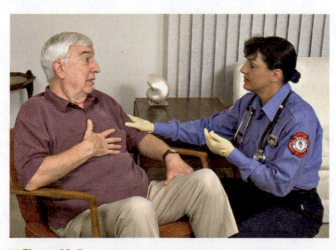

■ **Figure 26-5** Speak clearly and directly to the elderly patient.

immediate issue needs to be life threats. It is important to determine and treat these problems immediately. Information about medical complaints and other related problems should be identified when patient history is obtained.

Remember to be patient. Since the older patient may have poor vision, it's a good idea to position yourself right in front of him while you ask your questions. Do not raise your voice. Instead, face the patient and speak clearly. Position yourself where he has the best chance of seeing you. You might also put a hand on the patient to let him know where you are.

If your first attempt to communicate is unsuccessful, speak slightly louder but do not shout. Note that elderly people may find higher-pitched tones difficult to hear, so a person with a deeper voice may be more successful in communicating. If your patient has a hearing aid but is not wearing it, you may ask for it to be put in place. Another possible option is to write questions for the patient to read.

If your patient is not wearing his dentures (usually because they are uncomfortable), you may have a difficult time understanding what he is saying to you. If this is the case, you may ask him to put in his dentures.

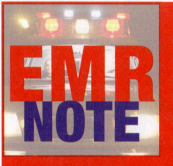

Don't forget about the possibility of a contagious disease in geriatric patients. Any patient, even an elderly one, could have a disease that can spread to you. Not only can older patients have human immunodeficiency virus (HIV) or hepatitis, they also may be at higher risk for tuberculosis (TB). *Remember:* Use Standard Precautions for all patients.

EMR Patient Assessment: The Primary Assessment

Perform a primary assessment as you would for any patient. However, keep the following in mind:

- For your general impression, be sure to note whether the patient appears clean, well groomed, and cared for. Lack of good hygiene could indicate the patient is not tending to his medical needs.

- To address mental status, find out from the patient's family or caregivers if a behavior related to the emergency is usual for the patient or if the changes have occurred suddenly. Specifically, what is different and how is it different?

- An elderly person who has had a stroke may have difficulty chewing, swallowing, or clearing the airway of secretions. In the unresponsive patient, dentures and other dental devices can cause airway obstruction.

- Pay attention to how the patient is posturing and working to breathe. Correct positioning of the head and neck for airway care may be a challenge due to a curvature of the spine that occurs with aging. If it is difficult for you to tilt the patient's head or position the airway properly, you may need to perform a jaw-thrust maneuver.

- For artificial ventilation, it may be easier to form a seal with the mask if you leave dentures in place. They can help to support the facial structure.

- Bleeding control in the elderly may be more difficult if the patient is taking aspirin or other blood-thinning medications. Expect it may take considerable time for clotting.

Physical Examination

Perform a physical exam, as you would for any patient who needs one (Figure 26-6 ■). If one is required, keep in mind that many elderly patients wear several layers of clothing, which may make the assessment more difficult to perform. Also, remember to look for any medical identification devices, such as bracelets or pendants.

Patient History

Gather a patient history as you would for any patient with a similar emergency. Only if it becomes apparent that your patient is not a reliable source of information should you go to others. Listen carefully to others who report a change in the patient's normal mental status as this is a critical piece of the history that the patient may be unable to self-express. Also, more seniors are now keeping medical data sheets so this information may be readily available to EMS. Some of the information on these sheets is the name of the physician, chronic medical conditions, medications, history of major illnesses and surgeries, and the patient's preference of hospital.

Some elderly patients may deny symptoms of illness or injury. There are many reasons. They may fear leaving home, going to a hospital, or losing independence or control. Some patients may even think that by going to the hospital they may not return home. They may have concerns about the cost of medical care, ambulance transport, and possible admission to a hospital. They also may be afraid to leave behind a spouse or sibling for whom they provide care. There may also be concern about a pet being left and who will care for it. If at all possible, assist in finding a solution. Sometimes this is as simple as asking if there is someone that could be called to help or finding a neighbor to assist.

Another issue in obtaining the history is that the patient may have only vaguely defined complaints, such as nausea or weakness. This can be true even with serious illness. Recent studies have shown that "weakness" is the most common chief symptom in older women with heart attacks. It is important to take all symptoms seriously, no matter how subtle.

Many elderly patients take several medications. Ask where the medications are and then read the labels yourself (Figure 26-7 ■). This is sometimes easier than asking the patient to remember and recite the name of each one. As time permits, ask if the patient is still taking all the medications you find. Just as important, ask if he is taking all his prescribed medications on schedule (Figure 26-8 ■).

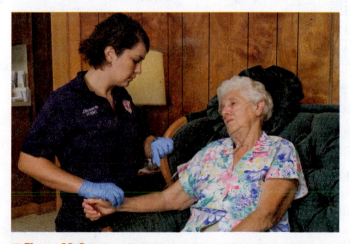

■ **Figure 26-6** Gather information from the geriatric patient while performing an assessment.

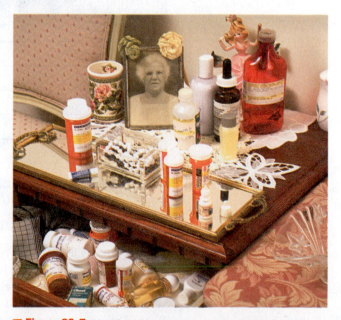

■ **Figure 26-7** Identify and record what medications the patient is taking.

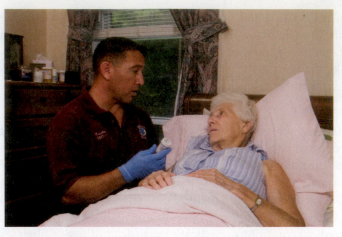

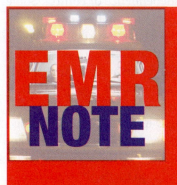

Figure 26-8 Ask the patient specifically about the medications that were taken.

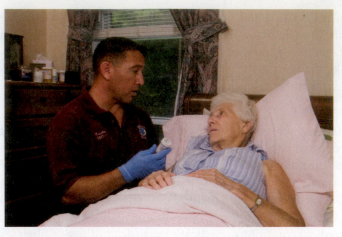

EMR NOTE

Many elderly patients take medications known as beta-blockers. This type of medication often is taken for high blood pressure or heart problems. One of the effects of this kind of drug is that it keeps the heart from beating too fast. The heart usually starts to beat faster in response to blood loss, but this medication keeps this from happening and this sign of shock may not be present. Be alert if a patient tells you he is taking a beta-blocker. Table 26-2 provides a list of some common beta-blockers.

TABLE 26-2 Common Beta-Blockers

GENERIC NAME	BRAND NAME
atenolol	Tenormin
metoprolol	Lopressor, Toprol XL
propranolol	Inderal, Inderal LA
carvedilol	Coreg
bisoprolol	Zebeta
sotalol	Betapace
labetalol	No brand name equivalent

EMR Patient Assessment: Secondary Assessment

The secondary assessment is the same as for any other patient. However, an ill or injured elderly patient is likely to show a slow, steady decline, not a sudden change that would alert you to a deteriorating condition. Do not be lulled into complacency because you observe little or no significant change from one set of vital signs to the next. Stay vigilant. Record all vitals and continually monitor them for any trends that may appear until care is transitioned to the EMS providers who will be transporting your patient.

Stop, Review, Remember

Multiple Choice

Place a check next to the correct answer.

1. Which of the following is a risk factor for abuse among the elderly?

   _____ a. Lives with a child

   _____ b. Loss of bladder control

   _____ c. Sleeps much of the day

   _____ d. Always acts in a composed manner

2. If an elderly person is on a limited income and can't pay the heating bill, which of the following might be a risk if an alternative device is being used to keep warm?

   _____ a. Fever

   _____ b. Open sores

   _____ c. Dementia

   _____ d. Burns

3. Which of the following is the most effective way to communicate with an elderly patient?

   _____ a. Tower over the patient.

   _____ b. Position yourself at the patient's eye level.

   _____ c. Call the patient by his first name.

   _____ d. Ask the patient, "What is wrong?"

Emergency Medical Responder Practice

1. You are called to a private residence for an unknown problem. When you arrive a police officer tells you it is safe and that the patient is a 78-year-old male who is conscious. The officer adds that the patient lives alone. List six psychosocial and economic factors that might be affecting this patient.

   _____

   _____

   _____

   _____

2. What should be done to assess this patient?

   _____

   _____

   _____

   _____

3. After seeing numerous bottles of alcohol in the garbage and scattered about, you talk to the patient about his drinking. He tells you he drinks at least half a bottle of hard liquor a day and sometimes more. The patient states he doesn't eat much and he appears quite agitated. What should you do for this patient?

   _____

   _____

   _____

   _____

4. Depression is not uncommon among older patients. List three findings that can be identified during the scene size-up that might alert you to the condition.

_____

_____

_____

_____

5. List three things that are important about medications and the elderly.

_____

_____

_____

_____

Matching

Match the following descriptions with the appropriate term.

1. _____ Deprived of food

2. _____ Feels shame

3. _____ Consuming large amount of alcohol

4. _____ Reluctant to discuss nature of injury

5. _____ Can't make needed repairs

a. Depression

b. Substance abuse

c. Abuse

d. Neglect

e. Socioeconomic problem

List

1. List three possible reasons why a patient may deny symptoms to avoid having to go to the hospital.

_____

_____

_____

2. What is one important point to remember about the ongoing assessment of an elderly patient?

_____

_____

_____

_____

TRANSITION

The ambulance radios they are on the scene and you get ready to transition care. Your report includes how you found the patient, including your survey of his house, his vital signs and that he seems to have a fever, information from the SAMPLE history, and the comment about the daughter not bringing in food and medicine as expected. You assist with packaging the patient for transport.

You return to quarters where you complete your prehospital care report and restock your supplies so you are ready for the next call.

■ Discussion: *Based on what you learned from the scene size-up and conversations with the patient, how would you ensure that information concerning the patient's living situation is provided to hospital personnel for follow-up by social services?*

THE LAST WORD

■ A misconception about the elderly is that they cannot live on their own. Despite the long list of possible problems discussed in this chapter, a majority of older adults experience good health, are independent and live active lives.

■ Functioning of the body's systems declines with age. The EMR's assessment and care should take the following changes into consideration:

  ■ *Skin.* A decrease in perspiration may be a contributing factor to heat-related emergencies. Diaphoresis, a sign of shock, may not occur.

  ■ *Sensory organs.* Changes in the senses contribute to many unintentional injuries, such as falls and burns. Vehicle crashes are the most common mechanism of injury in the elderly. Changes in sight, smell, and taste also contribute to decreased appetite and nutritional problems.

  ■ *Respiratory system.* Breathing becomes less effective in the elderly, causing a decreased ability to compensate when they need oxygen.

  ■ *Heart and blood vessels.* Changes due to age plus medication can cause ill or injured elderly patients to appear to have a normal pulse and blood pressure, causing shock and other conditions to go unrecognized.

  ■ *Musculoskeletal system.* Even minor falls commonly result in broken bones in the elderly.

  ■ *Immune system.* Common illnesses, such as influenza, have a higher fatality rate in the elderly. Also, an increased risk of infection and decreased ability to heal make injuries more serious and more often fatal.

  ■ *Response to medication.* Changes in the elderly patient's ability to respond to and eliminate medications can result in more profound side effects, as well as life-threatening drug interactions. The effects of some medications can mask the seriousness of an older adult's injury.

■ Patient assessment is the same for elderly patients as it is for any patient with a sudden illness or injury. However, there are differences in the general approach to the patient. Remember that the effects of aging and common medications can make the elderly less able to compensate for blood loss and less sensitive to pain. These factors can mask signs usually associated with serious injury or illness. Be sure to continually reassess your elderly patients for any change in mental status and physical condition.

✳ Chapter Review

Multiple Choice

Place a check next to the correct answer.

1. Elderly patients confined to bed are prone to bedsores because the skin has:

   _____ a. lost fat and the supportive structure has strengthened.

   _____ b. lost fat and the supportive structure has weakened.

   _____ c. built up fat and the supportive structure has strengthened.

   _____ d. built up fat and the supportive structure has weakened.

2. Which of the following are changes to vision expected in the elderly?

   _____ a. Farsightedness and improved peripheral vision

   _____ b. Nearsightedness and improved peripheral vision

   _____ c. Farsightedness and decreased peripheral vision

   _____ d. Nearsightedness and decreased peripheral vision

3. Which respiratory problem is the most common in the elderly?

   _____ a. Asthma

   _____ b. Fibrosis

   _____ c. Chronic obstructive pulmonary disease

   _____ d. Cancer

4. When a geriatric patient has a very rapid heartbeat, the end result will most likely be:

   _____ a. decreased blood flow.

   _____ b. increased blood flow.

   _____ c. no change in flow.

   _____ d. fluctuating flow.

5. Fewer secretions in the digestive system occur with the elderly, which may result in:

   _____ a. gallstones.

   _____ b. diarrhea.

   _____ c. celiac disease.

   _____ d. constipation.

6. Which of the following is *not* a sign or symptom of depression in the elderly?

   _____ a. Poor hygiene

   _____ b. Poor eating habits

   _____ c. Disorderly living situation

   _____ d. Rigid schedule for taking medication

7. Which of the following is a reason that a geriatric patient may be reluctant to share information about his abuser?

   _____ a. Feeling of shame

   _____ b. Lack of trusting EMS

   _____ c. Feeling of guilt

   _____ d. Confusion

8. Which of the following is a possible cause of fainting in the elderly?

   _____ a. Medications

   _____ b. Kidney disease

   _____ c. Overoxygenation of the brain

   _____ d. Good circulation

9. When coming into contact with a patient, a handshake can help the EMR identify:

   _____ a. bilateral strength.

   _____ b. interpersonal dynamics.

   _____ c. skin temperature.

   _____ d. reaction time.

10. When performing artificial ventilation on an elderly person who has dentures, which of the following is most likely to make this easier and more effective?

_____ a. Call for an EMT to use a nasal airway.

_____ b. Leave dentures in place.

_____ c. Remove dentures.

_____ d. Force dentures in place with a tongue depressor.

Matching

Match the following descriptions with the appropriate term.

1. _____ Effect that aging has on the rib cage cartilage
2. _____ Can cause the heart of the elderly patient not to beat faster
3. _____ Can affect urine flow in men
4. _____ May be caused by the decreased number of nerve fibers in the elderly
5. _____ Can be caused by the loss of independence
6. _____ Describes when an elderly patient is deprived of medication
7. _____ A common type of injury in the elderly
8. _____ May cause a patient to become violent
9. _____ A difficulty for some patients who have had a stroke
10. _____ Affects the ability of the blood to clot and may make controlling bleeding difficult
11. _____ A common cause of blindness in the geriatric adult
12. _____ Excessive perspiration
13. _____ Preferable to providing care to an injured patient
14. _____ Can easily be torn in elderly patients
15. _____ Has a much higher fatality rate in the elderly

a. Cataracts
b. Neglect
c. Stiffening
d. Skin
e. Swallowing
f. Change in coordination
g. Aspirin
h. Prevention
i. Influenza
j. Effect of certain medications
k. Enlarged prostate
l. Alzheimer disease
m. Depression
n. Burns
o. Diaphoresis

Emergency Medical Responder Practice

1. You arrive on the scene of a 74-year-old who appears not to have been well cared for. He has significant body odor and smells of urine. You notice garbage and dirty dishes scattered about. The patient is agitated and says in a loud voice, "Who called 911 and why are you here?" How would you respond?

_____

_____

_____

_____

2. You are now next to the patient and start the assessment. How should your initial assessment for the patient proceed, and what follows after that is done?

_____

_____

_____

_____

3. The SAMPLE history identifies that the patient is on beta-blockers and is taking aspirin. The vital signs are pulse 78 with an occasional irregular beat, respirations 20, and blood pressure 150/90. The skin is pale, cool, and mildly diaphoretic. The patient tells you his stomach hurts. Based on this information, do you think the patient may be bleeding internally and what may be the indicators you are observing?

_____

_____

_____

_____

4. What social and living conditions in the patient's home are a concern that should be included in your report to the transporting ambulance crew to pass on to the hospital?

_____

_____

_____

_____

CHAPTER 27

Special Populations and Situations

✱ NAVIGATION GUIDE

The following items provide an overview to the purpose and content of this chapter. The Education Standard and Competency are from the National EMS Education Standards.

Education Standard Special Patient Populations (Patients with Special Challenges)

Competency Recognizes and manages life threats based on simple assessment findings for a patient with special needs while awaiting additional emergency response.

Knowledge Area Patients with Special Challenges
  • Recognizing and reporting abuse and neglect

Objectives After reading this chapter, you should be able to:

1. Define key terms introduced in this chapter.
2. Describe the importance of interacting with the family and caregivers of patients with special challenges and considerations.
3. Give examples of common congenital and acquired diseases and conditions.
4. Discuss considerations in communicating with and caring for patients with sensory impairments and loss of mobility.
5. Explain the purpose, common problems, and emergency care of each of the following:
   a. Tracheostomies
   b. Ventilators
   c. Insulin pumps
   d. Implanted defibrillators
   e. Left ventricular assist devices
   f. Feeding tubes
   g. Indwelling catheters
   h. Urinary catheters
   i. Ostomy pouches
6. Describe the signs and management of the following:
   a. Physical abuse
   b. Sexual abuse
   c. Emotional abuse
   d. Financial abuse
   e. Neglect
7. Describe your roles and responsibilities as an EMR in situations involving abuse or neglect.

Key Terms Page numbers indicate first major use in this chapter. The Margin Glossary in this chapter provides definitions as you read.

palliative care, p. 680
hospice, p. 680

living will, p. 680
tracheostomy, p. 682

ventilator, p. 683
insulin pump, p. 683

Media Resources Please go to **www.bradybooks.com** to access mykit for this text. You will find quizzes, critical thinking scenarios, weblinks, animations, and videos related to this chapter—and much more. Look for online information on cerebral palsy and paraplegia. You will also find video clips on leukemia and cystic fibrosis.

INTRODUCTION

As an EMR, you will encounter a number of people who have special needs or who have advanced medical devices in their homes. These devices include machines that extend a person's ability to function and be comfortable, as well as machines that keep a patient alive. Special needs may be the result of medical, traumatic, emotional, behavioral, or developmental disorders. Responding to and caring for people with special needs is similar to any other call for service, in that it may be for such reasons as a fall, general illness, chest pain, seizures, or shortness of breath. What is different is that the preexisting conditions can complicate and quickly overwhelm your ability to assess and treat the patient. Although you are not expected to operate or diagnose problems with advanced medical devices, you should have some familiarity with various devices and their functions to ensure better care for a patient with special needs.

CASE STUDY

THE CALL ✳

As you are sitting at your desk writing a paper, you hear the tones go off on your radio. "St. Michael's College Rescue, respond to Cashman Hall for the report of a 4-year-old female with abdominal pain." Knowing that Cashman Hall has the college's day care center on its first floor, you respond to the building next to your dorm in record time.

■ Discussion: *What should you bring to this call if you are arriving independently?*

ASK YOURSELF

■ How would you describe the importance of interacting with the family and caregivers of patients with special challenges and considerations?

Technological Advances

In recent years, medical advances and insurance coverage changes have allowed the option for more people to have access to medical devices and care that was traditionally seen only in the hospital environment. Patients who may have previously been unable to survive at home are now able to live and work in a nonhospital environment. As a result of this increase in home-based care, prehospital providers are faced with an increasing number of calls for service to patients with devices and conditions that were previously not encountered by the EMR. These calls may be for a problem with the patient's medical device or may be entirely unrelated to the device.

You will encounter patients with special care needs that can occur in a variety of health care settings. You may respond to calls in personal residences, nursing homes, specialty rehabilitation centers, and specialized care facilities. You should familiarize yourself with any special health care settings in your community to better prepare for calls of this nature. Additionally, because many of these devices are portable, you may encounter patients with different devices and special care needs in almost any location.

EMR Patient Assessment: Special Patient Populations

Oftentimes, a patient with special needs will live with or be accompanied by a person who has training in the patient's condition and any devices that the patient uses. This person may be medically trained, such as a registered nurse (RN), certified nurse assistant (CNA), or home health aide, but more often will be a family member or friend. Although these family members may not have had formal medical training or certification, they are generally very familiar with the patient's special needs and comfortable with using the devices. The knowledge and techniques that family members have are taught to them by medical professionals before their family member (the patient) is discharged from a hospital. As they have a vested interest in being competent with the devices, family members are very thorough and deliberate with their understanding and application of the devices and their features. It is advisable to seek their input on any devices the patient has, and if they have been in a similar situation before. Some general questions should include:

- Has this problem ever occurred before? If so, what fixed it?
- Have you (or your family members/caregivers) been taught how to fix this problem?
- Have you tried to fix the problem? If so, what happened?

Asking questions such as "How do you normally move him?" or "Has she ever been transported by ambulance, and what worked well for the transfer?" will allow family members to be part of the solution and may ease the burden of the wide variety of medical devices. Assign a member of the EMS team to work with the family member regarding the medical device, while others on the team concentrate on assessment and treatment of the patient.

Congenital Diseases and Conditions

A congenital disease or condition is one that is present at birth. Some congenital diseases are genetic in nature, but others are not. An example is congenital heart disease where the heart or large blood vessels of the heart are malformed. Other examples include cleft palate; deafness; cerebral palsy, a neurological disorder that can cause developmental disabilities; and cystic fibrosis, a lung disorder that causes breathing difficulty as the patient ages.

Acquired Diseases and Conditions

An acquired disease or condition is one that occurs after birth. It may be the result of exposure to a virus or bacteria, or the result of trauma or a medical condition. Examples of acquired diseases and conditions include chronic obstructive pulmonary disease

ASK YOURSELF

- What are some examples of common congenital and acquired diseases and conditions?

ASK YOURSELF

■ Can you find and
define key terms
introduced in this
chapter?

(COPD), human immunodeficiency virus (HIV), acquired immune deficiency syndrome (AIDS), and traumatic brain and spinal cord injuries.

Some diseases may occur as a result of a congenital condition or may be acquired later in life. Examples include deafness and diabetes. A patient may be deaf from a congenital birth defect, or may become deaf from a loud explosion in a work environment. A patient may be born with diabetes, or may develop diabetes from lifestyle habits.

End of Life and Terminal Illness

As an EMR you will respond to patients suffering from terminal illness. Many of these patients have endured years of treatment and have reached a point where treatment will no longer provide relief from the pain of their disease process, or the disease has run its course and there is no further medical treatment available. You will find many of the patients receiving **palliative care**. Palliative care is also referred to as comfort care. These are measures aimed at making the last days of the patient's life more comfortable by providing pain management, intravenous fluids for dehydration, and oxygen to ease breathing. Many of these patients have do not resuscitate (DNR) orders or other palliative care orders.

palliative care a type of
medicine that is concerned
with providing comfort care
for patients with terminal
illnesses.

Palliative care is often provided by a **hospice** organization. Hospice is a community-based organization that provides palliative care to terminally ill cancer patients, although many hospices provide care to all terminally ill patients regardless of the disease. The goal of hospice is to provide care in the most comfortable environment possible for the terminally ill patient—usually the patient's home.

hospice a community-
based organization that
provides palliative care to
terminally ill patients.

When a patient dies under hospice care, many times the hospice nurse will deal with the death and 911 may not be called. However, if the hospice provider is unavailable or unable to respond the family may call 911. When you arrive on the scene, you may be confronted with the family and the patient's DNR. In most states an EMR can honor a valid DNR and withhold resuscitation efforts for a terminally ill patient. Laws governing DNRs and palliative care vary widely from state to state. In addition to a DNR, a patient may have a **living will** or other type of advance directive. Living wills provide direction to family members about a person's wishes if he becomes unable to make decisions about his care. In many states these documents do not allow the EMR to honor a request not to be resuscitated in the prehospital setting. Be sure to familiarize yourself with the laws and regulations in your state.

living will a document in
which a patient can make
known his will in regard to
advanced life support
measures in the case of
serious illness.

✸ Stop, Review, Remember

Multiple Choice

Place a check next to the correct answer.

1. You respond to a call for a 49-year-old female patient with terminal cancer in cardiac arrest. The patient's husband presents you with a DNR. You should:

   _____ a. begin care.

   _____ b. contact medical direction.

   _____ c. withhold CPR.

   _____ d. contact the patient's family physician.

2. COPD is a(n) _____ condition.

   _____ a. chronic

   _____ b. acute

   _____ c. treatable

   _____ d. acquired

3. One of the best sources of information on a patient with congenital illness is the patient's:

_____ a. chart.

_____ b. doctor.

_____ c. family member.

_____ d. nurse.

4. A person suffering from a terminal illness may have a _____ to guide family members about his wishes if he becomes unable to make decisions about his care.

_____ a. living will

_____ b. DNR

_____ c. palliative care

_____ d. doctor's order

5. While obtaining the history on your patient, you find out that he suffered a brain injury in a motor vehicle collision. This is an example of a(n) _____ chronic condition.

_____ a. acute

_____ b. acquired

_____ c. long-term

_____ d. short-term

Matching

Match the following description with the term.

1. _____ A community-based organization that provides palliative care to terminally ill patients

2. _____ A type of medicine that is concerned with providing comfort care for patients with terminal illnesses

3. _____ A document in which a patient can make known his will in regard to advanced life support measures in the case of serious illness

a. Palliative care

b. Hospice

c. Living will

EMR Emergency Care: Physical Impairments

ASK YOURSELF

■ What are some considerations in communicating with and caring for patients with sensory impairments and loss of mobility?

You may encounter patients who have some measure of physical impairment. These impairments range from those that affect the patient's senses (such as sight or hearing) to those that affect the patient's functioning (such as use of a wheelchair, or developmental disabilities).

Patients who call EMS may have a variety of impairments that affect their hearing, speech, or sight. When one of these senses has been removed, you must take extra care and time to help the patient adjust. It is, however, important to remember that these impairments do *not* necessarily affect the patient's ability to think for himself. Each limitation requires different approaches and considerations when treating the patient. Impairments to sight can be partial or complete (Figure 27-1 ■). Determine if the patient has poor vision, or no vision. The patient may know the layout of his home very well, so if anything is moved during the call be careful to return it to its original position. If the patient has a guide dog, federal law under the Americans with Disabilities Act (Section 36.104 of Title 3) allows for the patient to bring the dog with him in an ambulance, unless it is a direct threat to others (such as barking or growling).

Hearing Loss

Hearing loss is more common in the elderly, but it is not restricted to the older patient (Figure 27-2 ■). Not all patients with hearing loss can read lips, and in most cases, yelling

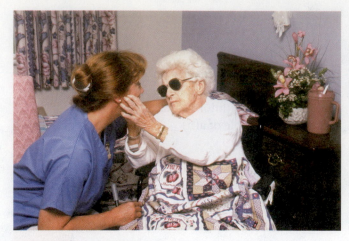

■ **Figure 27-1** Interacting with a visually impaired patient.

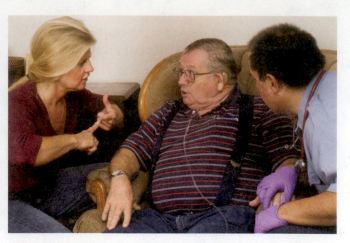

■ **Figure 27-2** Communicating with a deaf patient can be challenging.

ASK YOURSELF

■ What is the purpose, common problems, and emergency care of each of the following?
  ■ Tracheostomies
  ■ Ventilators
  ■ Insulin pumps
  ■ Implanted defibrillators
  ■ Left ventricular assist devices
  ■ Feeding tubes
  ■ Indwelling catheters
  ■ Urinary catheters
  ■ Ostomy pouches

or slowing down your speech will only make matters worse. One of the easiest ways to communicate with a patient who is deaf or hard of hearing is to write down your questions and actions on a piece of paper. Many dispatch centers and communities will also have a telecommunications device for the deaf/teletypewriter (TDD/TTY) phone, which is a user terminal with keyboard input and printer or display output used by the hearing and speech impaired.

A patient who is unable to speak may need to write answers to questions, or may use a TDD/TTY phone, or may type words into a computer that then speaks the words.

Mobility

Difficulty walking or standing is certainly a problem many of the elderly contend with, but problems with gait and balance can occur at any age. Carefully assess a person's abilities and if he uses any devices to help (canes, walkers, braces, or others). Patients who use wheelchairs may be difficult to completely assess, as they may be unable to stand. Carefully assess these patients in their position of comfort.

EMR Emergency Care: Medical Devices

Tracheostomy Tubes

tracheostomy a surgical opening placed in the front of the neck in the trachea where a tube can be placed to provide an airway for a patient who requires long-term mechanical ventilation.

Tracheostomy patients can range from infants to the very elderly. A tracheostomy is a surgical opening in the neck into the trachea, called a stoma. A short breathing tube and flange are inserted into the stoma. This allows the patient to breathe through it, instead of the nose and mouth (Figure 27-3 ■).

Patients with a tracheostomy may or may not be able to speak, depending on their condition. They may be able to speak by covering the tracheostomy tube briefly, with a speaker valve attached to the tube, or with an electronic box applied to their larynx. Do not assume that a patient with a tracheostomy can or cannot speak.

A frequent problem with tracheostomy tubes is a buildup of mucus in the tube. Suctioning of the tube may be needed quite regularly, often every few hours. This is especially common during times of distress, in the first few weeks after tube insertion, or if the patient has a respiratory infection.

A patient with a tracheostomy requires extensive care, and caregivers are provided with substantial training. Caregivers should be very familiar with the procedures used to suction the tube. Caregivers may also be familiar with how to change and replace the

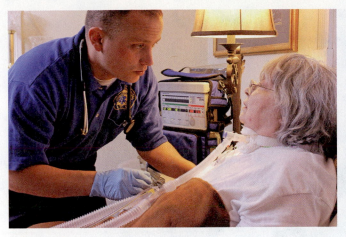

■ **Figure 27-3** EMS treats a patient with a tracheostomy at home. (© Ray Kemp/911 Imaging)

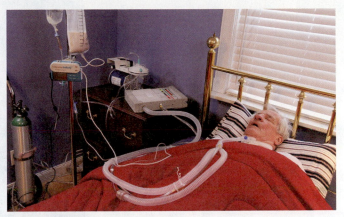

■ **Figure 27-4** Emergency medical assistance may be necessary for patients using medical equipment at home. (© Ray Kemp/911 Imaging)

inserted tracheostomy tube, as it generally needs to be cleaned on a regular basis. This is not a procedure for the EMR, but caregivers may have forgotten to do this and can be reminded of it.

Ventilators

A home **ventilator** is a device that breathes for a patient. It weighs anywhere from several pounds to over 20 pounds, and can range in size from a desktop computer to the size of a textbook. The ventilator is attached to a ribbed tube (called a ventilator circuit) of various lengths that enters the trachea. This tube may be attached to a tube in a stoma in the neck or may be attached through an endotracheal tube in the mouth (Figure 27-4 ■). Although the patient is dependent upon the ventilator for breathing, the patient may still lead an active lifestyle. One of the best examples of this was Christopher Reeve, who was paralyzed from the neck down in 1995. He lived until 2004, after acting in, narrating, and directing several movies and television shows; writing a book; winning a Grammy and an Emmy award; running a major charity foundation; and raising two children.

The patient on a home ventilator may call EMS for a variety of problems with the device. Similar to a tracheostomy tube, the patient may have mucous plugs and secretions develop that require suctioning. The patient may develop infections or respiratory distress. Additionally, the home ventilator depends on AC power, and power failures may be cause for concern. Ventilators do have backup batteries, generally lasting for an hour or more. In the event of power failure, the patient with a ventilator should have a bag-valve mask connected to his tracheostomy tube and you will assist with ventilations.

Insulin Pumps

People who have diabetes may have an **insulin pump** to help better regulate their blood glucose levels. These devices, often worn on a belt and about the size of a cell phone, have a small tube that is implanted into the abdomen (Figure 27-5 ■). The pump, at a predetermined rate, injects insulin into the patient and prevents the patient from having to perform injections.

Implanted Defibrillators

A patient may also have an **automatic implanted cardiac defibrillator (AICD)**. Implanted cardiac defibrillators are placed under the skin with wires inserted into the heart. The AICD varies in size from slightly larger than a 9-volt battery to the size of a wallet. It is

ventilator   a mechanical device that provides positive pressure ventilation to patients who are unable to breathe on their own due to disease or spinal cord injury; in the home setting, usually used on patients who have a tracheostomy.

insulin pump   a small device about the size of a cell phone or pager that provides a constant flow of insulin to an insulin-dependent diabetic, allowing the person to live a more normal life.

automatic implanted cardiac defibrillator (AICD)   a small device that is implanted in the patient's left chest to monitor the electrical rhythm of the heart and provide a shock to reset the heart into a normal rhythm if needed.

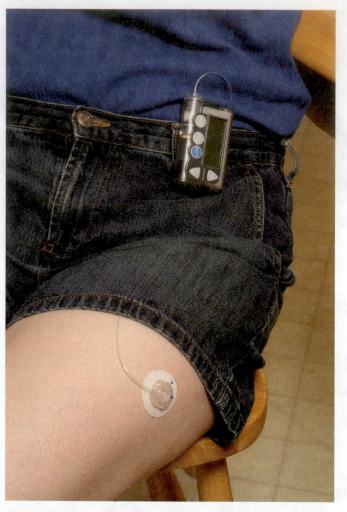

■ **Figure 27-5** An insulin pump automatically regulates the amount of insulin that the patient needs.

generally implanted in the upper left chest area, although occasionally it may be implanted in the area of the left upper quadrant of the abdomen. It is generally palpable through the skin (Figure 27-6 ■).

The implanted defibrillator is designed to detect life-threatening cardiac rhythms. The AICD delivers a single high-energy shock when a life-threatening rhythm is detected. This

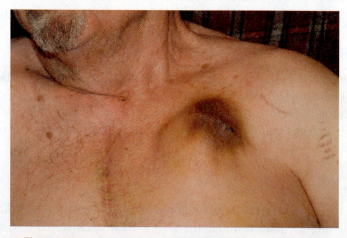

■ **Figure 27-6** Patient with an implanted defibrillator. (© Michal Heron)

shock is often very painful to the patient, generally rated as a 6 out of 10 on a pain scale. If the single shock does not correct the rhythm, or the rhythm returns, other shocks will be delivered, one at a time, until the problem is resolved or the machine is turned off. The machine can only be turned off by a special magnet, and generally only in a hospital setting. Although muscle twitches may be seen in the patient, providers and caregivers will not be harmed or shocked if the AICD shocks while they are touching the patient. The AICD is not dangerous if it shocks when the patient is wet. Patients are generally instructed to call their doctor if they feel fine after a shock; however, they should go to the hospital or call EMS if they are not feeling well, if they are shocked more than twice in any 24-hour period, or if they have any symptoms of dizziness, chest pain, or shortness of breath.

Most patients who have one or both of these devices have had a significant cardiac medical history. They may be on multiple medications, and may carry wallet cards or wear bracelets that identify that they use one of these devices.

Left Ventricular Assist Device

One of the more recent advances is the advent of the **left ventricular assist device (LVAD)**. In cases of severe left-sided heart failure, a heart transplant may be required. While the patient is waiting for a suitable donor, the LVAD serves as a "bridge to transplant." The LVAD takes blood from the left ventricle through an inserted tube, sends the blood to a pump implanted in the abdomen, which pressurizes the blood, and then sends the blood to the aorta for transport to the body. An external tube from the abdomen is connected to an external pump battery and control panel (Figure 27-7a ■).

left ventricular assist device (LVAD) a temporary external device that can assist a weak or failing heart to pump blood until a donor heart can be found.

Feeding Tubes

A feeding tube is used on patients who are unable to feed themselves and can't swallow. They may be used short term, during a recovery from surgery, or long term for chronic conditions. A feeding tube is commonly seen in two forms—a nasogastric tube (NG tube), which is inserted through the nose into the stomach, and a gastric feeding tube (G tube), which is surgically implanted through the skin of the abdomen into the stomach (Figure 27-7b ■).

Indwelling Catheters

You may encounter some patients who have a central IV catheter. A patient who receives frequent IV therapy, such as with chemotherapy, may have one of a variety of these catheters. Inserted in a hospital with surgery, they prevent patients from having to suffer from multiple needlesticks. The **indwelling catheter** may be found in the chest wall or in either arm, or implanted under the skin.

indwelling catheter a surgically implanted IV catheter for patients receiving long-term IV medications like chemotherapy.

Urinary Catheters

A **urinary catheter** is used for patients who have lost the ability to urinate or have lost the ability to regulate when they urinate. Most catheters are inserted into the bladder through the penis or urethral opening, and use a balloon to hold the tubing in place. The external tubing is connected to a collection bag, which may be a bag strapped to a leg, or a larger drainage bag, called a down drain, that hangs on the side of a patient's bed.

urinary catheter a tube placed in the bladder to drain the urine.

Ostomy Pouches

You may also encounter patients who have an **ostomy** pouch or bag. Ostomy bags are connected to a section of bowel that is surgically pulled up through, and attached to, the abdominal wall to allow for fecal drainage. An ostomy pouch, or bag, is usually attached to a patient's leg or to the abdominal wall and often will not be visible under clothing.

ostomy surgically created hole where urine or feces can be eliminated from the body.

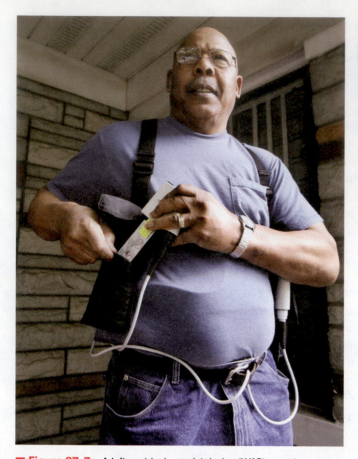

■ **Figure 27-7a** A left ventricular assist device (LVAD) uses two battery packs. (© AP Photo/M. Spencer Green)

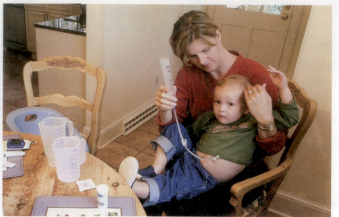

■ **Figure 27-7b** Most parents are very familiar with how to operate the devices helping their children. (© AP Photo/The Charlotte Observer, David T. Foster III)

✳ Stop, Review, Remember

Multiple Choice

Place a check next to the correct answer.

1. A device that allows a patient with hearing loss to communicate with the 911 call center is the:

   _____ a. AICD.

   _____ b. TDD/TTY.

   _____ c. ventilator.

   _____ d. LVAD.

2. A patient with diabetes may have a(n) _____ to help regulate his blood glucose level.

   _____ a. insulin pump

   _____ b. ventilator

   _____ c. IV catheter

   _____ d. feeding tube

3. You are assessing a patient with a complaint of abdominal pain. On inspection of the abdomen, you note a bag attached over a surgical opening in the abdominal wall. This is known as a(n):

   _____ a. urinary catheter.

   _____ b. indwelling catheter.

   _____ c. ostomy.

   _____ d. ectomy.

4. You are assessing a patient who has a small implanted device in his left chest. He states that it was put in to treat his irregular heartbeat. You know that he most likely has a(n):

_____ a. LVAD.

_____ b. defibrillator.

_____ c. AICD.

_____ d. ACID.

5. Your patient suffered a spinal cord injury and now has a surgical opening in his neck through which a breathing tube was placed. You know this to be a:

_____ a. tracheostomy.

_____ b. urineostomy.

_____ c. colonostomy.

_____ d. cricothyrotomy.

True/False

Mark whether each of the following statements is true (T) or false (F).

1. _____ Most catheters are inserted into the bladder through the penis or vaginal opening, and use tape to hold the tubing in place.

2. _____ The AICD varies in size from slightly larger than a 9-volt battery to the size of a wallet, and is generally implanted in the upper left chest area.

3. _____ The insulin pump injects insulin into the patient at a predetermined rate and prevents the patient from having to perform injections.

CASE STUDY

THE RESPONSE

When you arrive at the day care center, the director, Nancy Stevens, tells you that Savannah, a 4-year-old female, came in this morning looking very tired and like she had been crying. She did not want to have a midmorning snack and within an hour was holding her belly and complaining of "a real bad pain" in her stomach. You sit down next to Savannah, and she smiles at the funny faces you make at her. She points to her stomach and says it hurts really bad. She reluctantly lifts her shirt to show you her abdomen, and you notice multiple bruises, in colors of brown, yellow, and black. You ask her what happened, and she quickly covers up and will not answer any more questions.

■ Discussion: *What are your first suspicions from Savannah's reaction?*

Abuse

The EMR may encounter abuse, or suspect that a patient is being abused. Abuse can take many forms, including financial and neglect (Figures 27-8a through 27-8c ■). Abuse can also be performed against any age or sex.

EMR Patient Assessment: Abuse

During care and assessment of patients, you may become suspicious that a form of abuse has occurred.

ASK YOURSELF

■ What are the signs of the following?
- Physical abuse
- Sexual abuse
- Emotional abuse
- Financial abuse
- Neglect

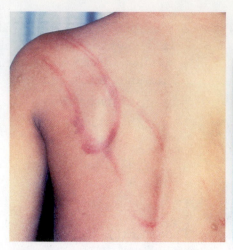

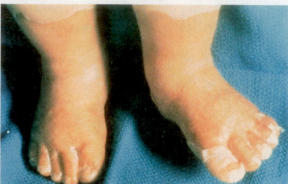

Figure 27-8a Child abuse: Cord bruises to the back. *(© Robert A. Felter, MD)*

Figure 27-8b Child abuse: Stocking burns to the feet. *(© Robert A. Felter, MD)*

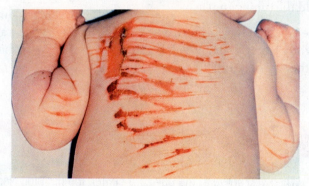

Figure 27-8c Child abuse: Cigarette lighter burns to the back. *(© Robert A. Felter, MD)*

physical abuse unexplained bruises (especially in various stages of healing), broken bones, welts, burn marks, bruises in the shape of objects (such as irons or cigarettes), hitting, shaking.

sexual abuse rape or inappropriate/nonconsensual sexual touching; signs include bruising or trauma around the genitalia or anus, and torn, stained, or bloody undergarments.

emotional abuse threatening, bullying, insults, harassment.

financial abuse monetary exploitation, theft, abuse of access to the patient's finances.

neglect malnutrition, dehydration, inappropriate clothing, soiled diapers, unsafe living conditions, soiled bedding, poor personal hygiene.

Forms of abuse include:

- **Physical abuse**
- **Sexual abuse**
- **Emotional abuse**
- **Financial abuse**
- **Neglect**

The EMR should observe for both the suspected physical findings as well as the actions of the patient and caregivers/family members. The patient may seem frightened to answer questions about the cause of injuries, have vague or conflicting stories of how they happened, or not answer questions at all. The patient may attempt to discuss financial abuse. Caregivers may prevent the patient from being interviewed or assessed without them present, or attempt to prevent the patient from answering questions by answering for him.

Although you may suspect child abuse, you should *never* confront or accuse the caregiver, guardian, or family member. Some medical disorders and cultural beliefs may mimic abuse, but are not considered abuse. Physicians and abuse specialists are best qualified to evaluate abuse in a neutral, nonconfrontational environment.

EMR Emergency Care: Abuse

The EMR is legally obligated in all 50 states to report suspicions of abuse—be it to a child or an adult—to specific agencies. In some states, it may be a department of child welfare or elder abuse, and in others it may be a law enforcement department. Generally, reporting your suspicions to a higher medical authority (EMT, paramedic, RN, physician, or other) is not enough, so you should check your local protocols and legal reporting requirements. In all 50 states, the provider is protected from criminal and civil litigation for reporting suspicions of abuse.

In addition to individual state reporting requirements, you should document findings and suspicions of abuse by carefully and factually describing what was seen, said, or heard during assessment and treatment of the patient. This documentation should be included with the prehospital care report. You may be required to submit your documentation to the local or state agency you initially reported your concerns to.

ASK YOURSELF

■ What are your roles and responsibilities as an EMR in situations involving abuse or neglect?

CASE STUDY

TRANSITION

As the ambulance arrives, the day care director says she has called Savannah's mother, who will meet you at the hospital. Mike, an EMT, arrives from the ambulance, and you tell him of your findings. Savannah decides that an ambulance ride would be fun. She goes with you to the ambulance, where you and Mike play a game of taking pulses and blood pressures and palpating her abdomen. You find that her heart rate is 108, her blood pressure is 92/58, and her abdomen is very tender. You arrive at the hospital, and Savannah's mother rushes to the stretcher and holds Savannah's hand. Privately, you give your report to the emergency physician, and tell her of your concerns of abuse. After saying good-bye to Savannah, you go the EMT room, call the local number for the state office of child welfare, and tell of your concerns about bruises of various stages, Savannah's complaints, and her unwillingness to tell what happened. Together, you and Mike then write a prehospital care report, ensuring you do not make any false accusations and that you accurately report the events during the call. Two weeks later, you learn that Savannah's uncle has been arrested for child abuse.

■ Discussion: *Are you required to report suspected abuse? Would you report it if it is not required?*

THE LAST WORD

When assessing patients with a medical or traumatic problem, the EMR may find patients that have special needs or devices. When confronted with a medical device, you should attempt to determine what type of device it is and what it is used for. Often the patient or caregivers will be well informed and can provide a wealth of information on the device. You should not attempt to alter, stop, or start the function of this device, but rather, assess the problems and provide any care necessary, using knowledgeable caregivers to control the device. You may also encounter patients with special needs due to impairments of their senses or physical abilities. Being sensitive to their needs, you should assess and care for any problems discovered, using alternative means of communication and assessment to best help the patient. If you suspect abuse in any patient, do not accuse anyone of the abuse. Follow your specific jurisdiction's reporting requirements. Appropriately document and relay concerns to the next member of the health care team.

✴ Chapter Review

Multiple Choice

Place a check next to the correct answer.

1. A common problem for people who have a tracheostomy tube is:
   - _____ a. mental impairment.
   - _____ b. chest pain.
   - _____ c. inability to eat.
   - _____ d. mucus in the tube.

2. True or False: Speaking louder to a patient with hearing impairment is helpful.
   - _____ a. True
   - _____ b. False

3. Patients with vision impairment will:
   - _____ a. have a guide dog.
   - _____ b. have a white cane.
   - _____ c. wear dark glasses.
   - _____ d. not always be apparent.

4. Patients who have a terminal illness may have a _____ to prevent EMS providers from performing CPR in the event of their death.
   - _____ a. DNR
   - _____ b. living will
   - _____ c. power of attorney
   - _____ d. hospice

5. _____ is an organization that provides end-of-life comfort care to patients with terminal illnesses.
   - _____ a. Home health care
   - _____ b. Hospice
   - _____ c. Hospital
   - _____ d. Living will

6. A tube that drains urine from the bladder is a(n):
   - _____ a. ostomy.
   - _____ b. IV catheter.
   - _____ c. urinary catheter.
   - _____ d. Hickman catheter.

7. True or False: Providing comfort measures for terminally ill patients at the end of life is known as palliative care.
   - _____ a. True
   - _____ b. False

8. A mechanical device that provides positive pressure ventilations via a tracheostomy tube is a(n):
   - _____ a. bag-valve mask.
   - _____ b. respirator.
   - _____ c. ventilator.
   - _____ d. iron lung.

9. When preparing a patient for transport who complains of weakness and uses a cane to assist in his mobility, you should:
   - _____ a. leave the cane at home so it won't be lost.
   - _____ b. have the family bring the cane to the hospital later.
   - _____ c. transport the cane to the hospital.
   - _____ d. not concern yourself with the cane.

Matching

Match the following descriptions with the appropriate term.

1. _____ Breathing tube inserted into a stoma
2. _____ Helps control blood sugar levels
3. _____ An implanted defibrillator
4. _____ Inserted into the bladder
5. _____ Used for frequent IV therapy
6. _____ Provides advance directives
7. _____ Assists a weak heart
8. _____ Provides nutrition via a tube in the stomach

a. AICD
b. Urinary catheter
c. Insulin pump
d. Indwelling catheter
e. Tracheostomy tube
f. Living will
g. Feeding tube
h. LVAD

Critical Thinking

1. Where in your response area would you be likely to find a high number of patients with medical devices?

_____

_____

_____

_____

2. What methods or items might help you assess and ask questions of a person with developmental disabilities?

_____

_____

_____

_____

EXPLORE **mybradykit**™

PEARSON

Please go to **www.bradybooks.com** to access mykit for this text. You will find quizzes, critical thinking scenarios, weblinks, animations, and videos related to this chapter—and much more. Look for online information on cerebral palsy and paraplegia as well as video clips on leukemia and cystic fibrosis.

Register your access code from the front of your book by going to **www.bradybooks.com** and selecting the mykit links.

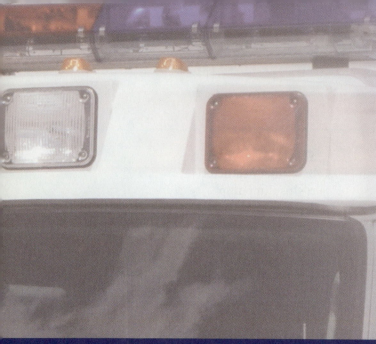

Review and Practice Examination

Assess what you have learned in this section by checking the best answer for each multiple-choice question. When you are done, check your answers against the key provided in Appendix B.

1. The lower end of the uterus that opens during labor to allow childbirth is called the:
   a. _____ fallopian tube.
   b. _____ endometrium.
   c. _____ cervix.
   d. _____ vagina.

2. The temporary organ of pregnancy that provides nourishment and oxygen to the fetus is the:
   a. _____ amniotic sac.
   b. _____ cervix.
   c. _____ placenta.
   d. _____ birth canal.

3. Which of the following occurs during stage one of labor?
   a. _____ The cervix dilates.
   b. _____ The baby moves through the birth canal.
   c. _____ Crowning.
   d. _____ The placenta is delivered.

4. There is generally time to transport a woman in labor if her contractions are at least _____ minute(s) apart.
   a. _____ 1
   b. _____ 3
   c. _____ 5
   d. _____ 10

5. A 30-year-old pregnant patient is having contractions 3 minutes apart. Which of the following indicates that you should prepare to deliver the baby on the scene?
   a. _____ The due date is in 3 weeks.
   b. _____ The mother says she feels as though she needs to have a bowel movement.
   c. _____ The mother previously had a cesarean section.
   d. _____ This is the mother's first pregnancy.

6. When assisting with delivery of an infant, you see the infant's scalp at the vaginal opening, and the vaginal area is bulging. You should:
   a. _____ attempt to suction the mouth and nose before the head is delivered.
   b. _____ place several pillows under the mother's hips to slow the progress of delivery.
   c. _____ insert your fingers on either side of the infant's head and pull gently.
   d. _____ place the palm of your hand gently over the infant's head.

7. Which of the following is the most critical piece of information to communicate to incoming EMS units following a delivery?
   a. _____ The contractions were 30 seconds to 1 minute apart at the time of delivery.
   b. _____ This is the mother's third delivery.

c. _____ The amniotic fluid was greenish brown.

d. _____ The baby had a bowel movement after delivery.

8. During labor, which of the following is normal prior to delivery of the infant?

a. _____ The umbilical cord appears in the birth canal.

b. _____ Clear fluid gushes from the vagina during contractions.

c. _____ The infant's feet appear at the vaginal opening.

d. _____ The placenta is delivered.

9. Which of the following is part of the ideal care of a normal newborn immediately after delivery?

a. _____ Keeping him at the level of the vagina until the umbilical cord is clamped

b. _____ Holding him by the heels and lightly slapping the buttocks

c. _____ Rinsing him off with saline or water

d. _____ Clamping the umbilical cord before it stops pulsating

10. Following a normal delivery, you have clamped and cut the umbilical cord. The mother states she is having contractions again, and the protruding part of the umbilical cord becomes longer. You should:

a. _____ firmly massage the lower abdomen in a downward motion.

b. _____ gently pull the cord to deliver the placenta.

c. _____ place an additional clamp on the umbilical cord and cut it again.

d. _____ encourage the mother to bear down like she did when she delivered the baby.

11. Following delivery, you notice about 250 mL (1 cup) of blood loss from the mother's vagina. You should:

a. _____ cover the vaginal area with sanitary napkins.

b. _____ place absorbent dressings in the vaginal opening.

c. _____ turn the mother on her left side, administer high-flow oxygen, and elevate the legs.

d. _____ immediately notify the incoming EMS unit.

12. A woman who is 7 months pregnant complains of general swelling, headaches, vomiting, and blurred vision. Her blood pressure is 162/90. These signs and symptoms are most consistent with:

a. _____ spontaneous abortion.

b. _____ preeclampsia.

c. _____ eclampsia.

d. _____ ectopic pregnancy.

13. Which of the following indicates the need for CPR in a newborn?

a. _____ The body is pink, but the extremities are blue.

b. _____ Respirations are less than 50 per minute.

c. _____ The infant cries for 30 seconds, then stops.

d. _____ Heart rate is less than 60 per minute.

14. You are assessing a 4-year-old with a severe cough and suspected fever. She is crying and upset. Her mother is very anxious and has tears in her eyes. Which of the following is the best way to initially handle this situation?

a. _____ Firmly tell the mother she must stay calm.

b. _____ Allow the mother to hold or stay near the child.

c. _____ Ask the mother to leave the room.

d. _____ Wait to assess the child until someone else is present.

15. Which of the following is true of the differences between adults and children?

a. _____ Children have much less body surface area for their size, allowing them to conserve body heat.

b. _____ Sick children compensate for a longer period of time and deteriorate gradually.

c. _____ Infants' and small children's airways can be obstructed by hyperextending the neck when positioning the airway.

d. _____ Most adult equipment can easily be adapted to the care of infants and children.

16. You have responded for a report of a sick infant. Of the following, which is the most important aspect of forming an initial impression of the patient's condition?

a. _____ Assessing the level of responsiveness

b. _____ Checking for fever

c. _____ Palpating the abdomen

d. _____ Taking a blood pressure

17. The three components of the pediatric assessment triangle are:
    a. _____ heart rate, presence of fever, and pulse oximetry.
    b. _____ pupil reaction, skin color, and appearance.
    c. _____ work of breathing, pupil reaction, and presence of fever.
    d. _____ appearance, work of breathing, and skin assessment.

18. In the pediatric assessment triangle, *appearance* refers to:
    a. _____ approximate age, weight, and height.
    b. _____ muscle tone, interactiveness, and consolability.
    c. _____ pulse, respiration, and blood pressure.
    d. _____ skin color, behavior, and initial position.

19. Maintaining the airway of a pediatric patient is made easier by:
    a. _____ the use of a nasal airway rather than an oral airway.
    b. _____ placing a folded small towel under the shoulders.
    c. _____ padding under the head.
    d. _____ hyperextending the neck and head.

20. When checking the pulse of an infant with respiratory distress, you should check the _____ pulse.
    a. _____ brachial
    b. _____ radial
    c. _____ carotid
    d. _____ femoral

21. A 19-month-old toddler fell off a small riding toy and struck his chin on the sidewalk. He has a laceration under his chin. He is crying frantically and struggles to move away when you try to look at his injury. A good way to initially attempt to gain his cooperation would be to:
    a. _____ tell him if he doesn't stop crying that his mommy will have to leave the room.
    b. _____ ask the mother to hold his arms and head still to keep him from moving.
    c. _____ see if he has a favorite toy or stuffed animal that will help comfort him.
    d. _____ tell him he won't have to get stitches if he'll just let you look at his cut.

22. Which of the following is true concerning the technique for bag-valve-mask ventilations in infants and children?
    a. _____ It is better to use a bag-valve mask that is too small than one that is too large.
    b. _____ High pressures are needed to overcome the resistance to airflow of the smaller trachea.
    c. _____ The bag should be squeezed gently, just until the chest rises.
    d. _____ A rate of 40 ventilations per minute for infants and 30 ventilations per minute for children should be used.

23. True or False: 30 percent of pediatric trauma cases are related to inappropriate management of the patient's airway.
    a. _____ True
    b. _____ False

24. Which of the following statements concerning croup is true?
    a. _____ The classic presentation of croup is the onset of a "seal bark" at night.
    b. _____ The child with croup mostly has wheezing while he is active or playing during the day.
    c. _____ Croup is a bacterial infection that causes swelling of the epiglottis.
    d. _____ It is never an emergency, although first-time parents can become very alarmed by it.

25. True or False: You should assume that seizures in children are from a rapid increase in temperature due to fever.
    a. _____ True
    b. _____ False

26. A 2-year-old female had a seizure, prompting her mother to call 911. When you arrive, the patient is drowsy and hard to awaken, but responds to a light pinch of her trapezius muscle with brief eye-opening and crying. She is breathing 26 times per minute and has a pulse of 120. She has hot, moist, flushed skin. Which of the following is appropriate in the management of this patient?
    a. _____ Open the airway with a head-tilt, chin-lift, apply oxygen by nonrebreather mask, remove heavy clothing, and sponge the skin with rubbing alcohol.

b. _____ Insert an oral airway, administer oxygen by nonrebreather mask, and cover the patient with blankets.

c. _____ Place her on her left side, apply blow-by oxygen, remove heavy clothing, and wipe the skin with a tepid wet washcloth.

d. _____ Place the child in a bathtub of cold water and ask the mother to administer acetaminophen (Tylenol) or ibuprofen (Motrin) by mouth.

27. A 2-year-old patient is very drowsy and difficult to awaken. His father states he has had a fever and cough for 3 days and has not had an appetite or much interest in drinking juice or water. Which of the following would be most concerning?

a. _____ The patient's temperature has been between 100°F and 102°F.

b. _____ Capillary refill time is about 1 1/2 seconds.

c. _____ The parents have not given a dose of ibuprofen (Motrin) for 4 hours.

d. _____ The patient has not had a wet diaper for 6 to 8 hours.

28. Which of the following injuries should you most highly suspect in a 7-year-old female who was wearing a seat belt during a front-end motor vehicle collision?

a. _____ Skull fracture

b. _____ Femur fracture

c. _____ Lower spine injury

d. _____ Facial lacerations

29. You are called to the home of a 3-year-old child who has a tracheostomy and is dependent on a ventilator. The parents are panicked because the ventilator is not working properly and they have been unsuccessful in correcting the problem. Which of the following should you do?

a. _____ Use a bag-valve mask to ventilate the patient.

b. _____ Apply a nonrebreather mask with 12 liters per minute of oxygen.

c. _____ Ask what type of problems the parents are having with the ventilator.

d. _____ Call the patient's home health equipment company for instructions on how to troubleshoot the ventilator.

30. You have responded for a call of an infant not breathing. As you arrive, a woman runs to you with a 4-month-old infant in her arms. The infant is limp, gray in color, and not breathing, and you can't find a brachial pulse. Which of the following is the highest priority?

a. _____ Find out if the woman is the child's mother.

b. _____ Begin CPR.

c. _____ Ask when was the last time anyone saw the infant alive.

d. _____ Look for any signs of child abuse.

31. Which of the following expected signs is less likely to be present in the elderly patient in shock?

a. _____ Altered mental status

b. _____ Diaphoresis

c. _____ Pale skin

d. _____ Nausea and vomiting

32. Which of the following changes should you anticipate when assessing an elderly patient?

a. _____ Decreased ability to see objects that are near

b. _____ Thickening of the skin

c. _____ Hypersensitivity to sound

d. _____ Increased appetite

33. True or False: Substance abuse is almost never a problem in the elderly.

a. _____ True

b. _____ False

34. A 79-year-old woman reports that she fell and now has severe pain in her right hip. Which of the following questions will help you the most in determining the nature of the problem?

a. _____ Do you live here alone?

b. _____ Have you broken your hip before?

c. _____ Did you take your blood pressure medicine today?

d. _____ How were you feeling just before you fell?

35. Which of the following statements is true concerning responding to calls for elderly patients?

a. _____ Confusion and loss of memory are normal parts of aging.

b. _____ There is virtually no risk of violence when responding to calls for elderly patients.

c. _____ Assume that the elderly have normal hearing and mental status until it appears otherwise.

d. _____ Elderly patients rarely, if ever, make suicide attempts.

36. You have just asked an 89-year-old patient what happened that caused his wife to call 911. He does not answer immediately. The first thing you should do is:
    a. _____ raise your voice and repeat your question.
    b. _____ ask his wife what happened.
    c. _____ give the patient a little longer to answer.
    d. _____ ask the patient if he has a hearing aid.

37. A 76-year-old patient has a laceration on her shin from accidentally hitting her leg with a shovel while she was working in the garden. Although the laceration seems relatively minor, it continues to bleed. Which of the following questions may give you information about why the bleeding is continuing?
    a. _____ Do you take aspirin?
    b. _____ Have you had a fever?
    c. _____ Have you been depressed lately?
    d. _____ Do you know what day it is?

38. Your 68-year-old patient tells you he takes metoprolol. A logical follow-up question would be:
    a. _____ Do you have heart problems or high blood pressure?
    b. _____ Do you have diabetes?
    c. _____ Do you have a history of lung problems?
    d. _____ Do you smoke or drink alcohol?

39. A good way to establish rapport with an elderly patient is to:
    a. _____ use the patient's first name to address him.
    b. _____ call the patient "partner" or "hon."
    c. _____ speak in a loud voice when you approach the patient.
    d. _____ offer a handshake when you introduce yourself.

40. Your 84-year-old patient, who is cared for by his son and daughter-in-law, is wearing pants that are wet with urine and has bruises on his forearms. The room where he stays has several days of laundry on the floor and dirty glasses and dishes on the dresser. The patient's daughter-in-law called 911 because the patient seems confused today. Which of the following is an appropriate approach?

    a. _____ Call law enforcement and report your suspicions of abuse.
    b. _____ Tell the patient and family that it would be a good idea for him to let the ambulance take him to the hospital.
    c. _____ Tell the family you understand their frustration, but there is really nothing EMS can do about the situation.
    d. _____ Ask the son and daughter-in-law why the patient is wet and living in a dirty room.

41. An example of a congenital condition is:
    a. _____ AIDS.
    b. _____ paralysis due to spinal cord injury.
    c. _____ COPD.
    d. _____ a malformation of the heart.

42. A 27-year-old female who is paralyzed from the shoulders down has a service dog that assists her with her daily activities. The patient is sick today with a fever and believes she has a urinary tract infection. She tells you she has to take her dog, Nadia, with her. What is the best way to handle this situation?
    a. _____ Let the patient know that the dog is welcome as long as its behavior does not endanger anyone.
    b. _____ Tell the patient that animals are not allowed in ambulances or medical facilities under any circumstances.
    c. _____ Ask the patient to see the dog's official papers to verify that it is a service animal.
    d. _____ Tell the patient that it is up to the ambulance crew to make these decisions on a case-by-case basis, but bringing the animal is discouraged.

43. One of the easiest ways to communicate with a patient who has a hearing impairment is to:
    a. _____ mouth your words slowly and in a slightly exaggerated manner.
    b. _____ use pen and paper.
    c. _____ call dispatch for an American Sign Language interpreter.
    d. _____ speak only when necessary, and use a loud voice when doing so.

44. Which of the following statements is true regarding patients with tracheostomies?
    a. _____ It is not possible to speak with a tracheostomy.
    b. _____ No one but a physician or respiratory therapist is permitted to care for tracheostomies.
    c. _____ A common problem is that mucus accumulates in the tube.
    d. _____ A patient with a tracheostomy must be on a ventilator.

45. Your patient has a device implanted under the skin of his upper left chest. His wife states that it is an AICD. This device is used to:
    a. _____ deliver insulin to diabetic patients in precise dosages.
    b. _____ provide tube feedings to patients who cannot swallow.
    c. _____ assist in pumping blood for patients with severe heart failure.
    d. _____ detect and shock life-threatening heart rhythms.

46. An indwelling catheter is used to:
    a. _____ access the venous system to deliver drugs without the need for frequent IV sticks.
    b. _____ drain urine from the bladder.
    c. _____ collect fecal matter after surgery on the intestine.
    d. _____ deliver food directly to the stomach of a patient who cannot swallow.

47. The tube that attaches a ventilator to a patient's tracheostomy is called a(n):
    a. _____ ventilator circuit.
    b. _____ endotracheal tube.
    c. _____ ostomy pouch.
    d. _____ LVAD.

48. A patient has a tube inserted directly through the abdominal wall into the stomach so he can receive feedings. This is called a(n):
    a. _____ NG tube.
    b. _____ indwelling catheter.
    c. _____ ostomy pouch.
    d. _____ G tube.

49. A patient states he has an AICD. This tells you that the patient has a history of:
    a. _____ diabetes.
    b. _____ heart disease.
    c. _____ stomach problems.
    d. _____ lung problems.

50. Which of the following is true concerning EMRs reporting suspicions of abuse?
    a. _____ EMRs can only report child physical and sexual abuse.
    b. _____ The EMR's obligation to report is usually satisfied by reporting suspicions to incoming EMS units.
    c. _____ EMRs in all 50 states have legal protections when reporting suspicions of abuse.
    d. _____ EMRs must verbally report abuse, but are not expected to prepare written documentation.

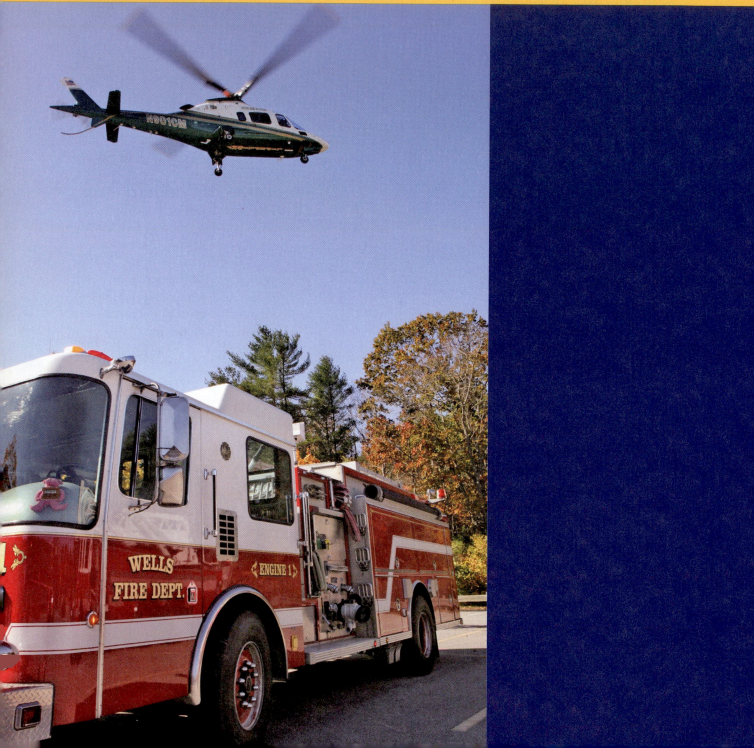

SECTION 7
Operations

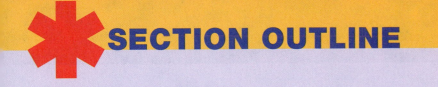

SECTION OUTLINE

In this section you will cover the following EMS Education Standards:
- EMS Operations

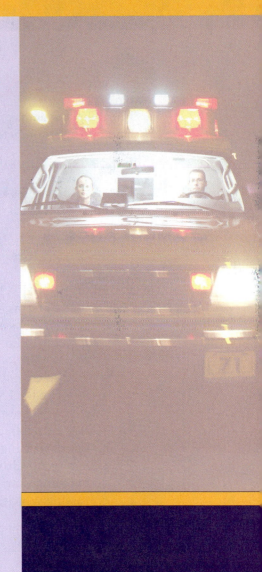

Operations

✳ NAVIGATION GUIDE

The following items provide an overview to the purpose and content of this chapter. The Education Standard and Competency are from the National EMS Education Standards.

Education Standard EMS Operations (Principles of Safely Operating a Ground Ambulance)

Competency Uses knowledge of operational roles and responsibilities to ensure patient, public, and personnel safety.

Knowledge Area Principles of Safely Operating a Ground Ambulance
- Risks and responsibilities of emergency response

Objectives After reading this chapter, you should be able to:

1. Define key terms introduced in this chapter.
2. Explain the steps of ensuring apparatus and equipment readiness.
3. Explain the EMR's considerations in responding to emergency calls, including:
   a. Safety of the EMR, partners, other emergency responders, EMS personnel, and the public
   b. Use of warning lights and siren
   c. Emergency driving in traffic
   d. Avoiding distractions
   e. Passing vehicles
   f. Approaching intersections
   g. Parking
4. Select the appropriate personal protective equipment for a call.
5. Describe the EMR's responsibilities in managing the scenes of a variety of types of emergency calls, including:
   a. Residential and non-highway scenes
   b. Transferring care to the EMS crew
   c. Interacting with other emergency responders

Key Terms Page numbers indicate first major use in this chapter. The Margin Glossary in this chapter provides definitions as you read.

360-degree survey, p. 706   *National Institute for Occupational Safety and Health (NIOSH), p. 707*

Media Resources Please go to **www.bradybooks.com** to access mykit for this text. You will find quizzes, critical thinking scenarios, weblinks, animations, and videos related to this chapter—and much more. Look for online information on roadside vehicle safety, emergency vehicle safety, and ambulance cleaning and disinfection.

INTRODUCTION

As an EMR, you must conduct the daily operations of arriving for your shift, getting a report from the off-going crew, checking your apparatus, and making sure that the vehicle is stocked and safe to operate. When dispatched to a call, you must confirm the address and plan your route. You must operate the apparatus in a safe manner with due regard for the safety of others. When you arrive you must take appropriate Standard Precautions and use personal protective equipment. You must interact with other responders, including law enforcement, fire service, and EMS on the scene (Figure 28-1 ■). Finally, you will provide patient care and transfer care to EMS for transport to the hospital.

CASE STUDY

THE CALL

You arrive at your station for duty 15 minutes before shift change as usual. You check the assignment board and see that you and your partner, Eddie King, are assigned to the Quick Response Vehicle brush truck. This vehicle serves as a first response unit for medical emergencies in your district.

You receive a report from the off-going crew. They inform you that they ran seven calls during the last shift. They restocked the supplies used but noted that the fuel level is below three-fourths of a tank.

You and your partner get the checklist and start checking your apparatus. You first raise the hood and check the oil, transmission fluid, and power steering fluid. Next you check the batteries, belts, and hoses. Your partner starts the truck and sounds the horn and siren. Then he turns on the emergency warning lights as you walk around the apparatus and check each light. All are working correctly.

Now you move on and check the medical equipment while your partner checks the apparatus's firefighting equipment. You check the oxygen bottles, automatic external defibrillator (AED), airway equipment, and bandage supplies. The portable oxygen tank is low and you are missing two trauma dressings. You replace the dressings and change the oxygen tank. You file the apparatus checklists while your partner fuels the truck.

With the truck checked and fueled, you and your partner are ready to begin your shift. Soon after you finish filing your vehicle checklist, the tones go off. You are dispatched to 137 Williams Street for breathing problems.

You write down the address, and your partner checks the map and plans your route of travel. You get in your unit and put on your seat belts. Your partner starts the engine and raises the bay door. As soon as you clear the bay, you notify the dispatch center that you are en route. The dispatch center informs you that you are responding to a 27-year-old female who is having difficulty breathing due to an asthma attack.

■ Discussion: *What is the purpose of following this protocol?*

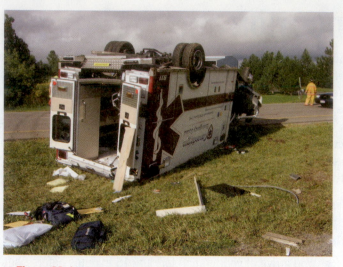

ASK YOURSELF

■ What are the steps of ensuring apparatus and equipment readiness?

Apparatus and Equipment Readiness

As an EMR you are responsible for ensuring that your apparatus and equipment are ready to respond to a call at a moment's notice. Whether you are a volunteer or paid EMR, you must check your apparatus and equipment at the beginning of each shift. Most often you will begin this process by receiving a report from the off-going crew.

All emergency vehicles should receive a daily safety inspection to ensure that they are safe to respond to an emergency. This inspection should check the following basic components:

■ Tire inflation pressure

■ Engine oil, power steering fluid, and transmission fluid (Figure 28-2 ■)

■ Fuel level

■ Headlights, turn signals, backup lights, and scene lights

■ Emergency warning lights

■ Siren, horn

■ Communications equipment

■ Medical equipment (Figure 28-3 ■)

■ Safety equipment

If you find that the fluids are low, only refill with the manufacturer's approved products. Adding an unapproved product could void any manufacturer's warranty. Refer to your department's procedures for vehicle maintenance. Any vehicle that is found to be unsafe to operate should be taken out of service until repairs by a qualified service technician can be made.

If you find a malfunction in the vehicle's radio system and there is no backup system, take the vehicle out of service and notify your supervisor.

Fire apparatus, ambulances, and other types of emergency vehicles require routine maintenance to ensure their continued safety. Refer to the manufacturer's specific recommendations for service intervals.

Additionally the vehicle must be stocked with the necessary Standard Precautions and personal protective equipment. Your apparatus should have latex-free gloves in various sizes (small, medium, large, and extra large) and masks that meet the standards for respiratory precautions (for example, N95 or P100 masks). Finally, you must have safety vests with reflective striping that meet ANSI standards for being a rip-away type.

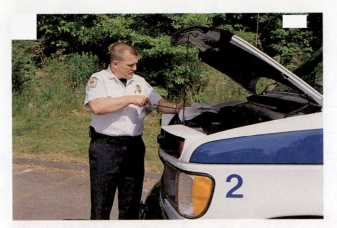
Figure 28-2 Check and prepare the emergency vehicle.

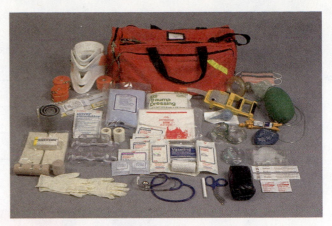
Figure 28-3 Basic emergency responder's medical kit.

Stop, Review, Remember

Multiple Choice

Place a check next to the correct answer.

1. Which of the following fluids on an emergency vehicle should be checked daily?

   _____ a. Engine oil

   _____ b. Power steering fluid

   _____ c. Transmission fluid

   _____ d. All of the above

2. You have just checked the engine oil in your emergency vehicle and see that it is at the add mark. You should:

   _____ a. notify the chief and take the vehicle out of service.

   _____ b. make a note in the log and run the vehicle anyway.

   _____ c. add the appropriate grade of oil to the vehicle's engine and recheck the engine oil level to make sure it is full.

   _____ d. make a note to add the appropriate grade of oil upon return.

3. During the vehicle inspection, you find that your radio is not working. You should:

   _____ a. keep the vehicle in service and just use a portable handheld radio for your vehicle's communications.

   _____ b. take the vehicle out of service.

   _____ c. take the vehicle out of service and notify your supervisor.

   _____ d. keep the vehicle in service and notify your supervisor.

4. When fueling your emergency vehicle, you find that the fuel cap is missing. You should:

   _____ a. take the vehicle out of service and get a replacement cap; then the vehicle should be put back in service.

   _____ b. keep the vehicle in service and report the missing fuel cap.

   _____ c. report the missing fuel cap.

   _____ d. tell the person who fueled the vehicle that the cap is missing and let him get it back without the chief knowing.

5. You are inspecting your oxygen equipment and see that the oxygen tank's pressure is under 500 psi. You should:

   _____ a. make note of the pressure and make sure the spare is full.

   _____ b. change the tank out immediately.

   _____ c. change the tank out after you finish checking off the vehicle and filing your report.

   _____ d. let the next crew change out the tank.

List

1. List six basic elements of an ambulance daily inspection.

_____

_____

_____

_____

CASE STUDY

THE RESPONSE ✳

Traffic is heavy as your partner maneuvers the vehicle in and out of traffic. As you approach the intersection the light turns red. Your partner steers the vehicle to the left turn lane and stops. He sounds the air horn as you both begin scanning the intersection. You make eye contact with the drivers on the right and see that they are all stopped while your partner checks the intersection to the left. Then you tell your partner, "clear right." He takes a quick look and proceeds through the intersection.

You travel another six blocks and turn onto Williams Street. You slow down and begin to scan for the number 137 on the houses. You arrive on scene. Your partner parks the unit above the entrance to the driveway, leaving the ambulance room to use the driveway. You call dispatch and inform them that you have arrived. You exit the vehicle and get your equipment from the side compartment.

As you enter the home, you hear the patient wheezing from across the room. She looks at you and in a gasping sentence says, "I… can't… breathe!" You can see she has an inhaler in her hand. Your partner begins to take a SAMPLE history from your patient's husband while you begin helping your patient. You introduce yourself and she says her name is "Mary" in a gasping breath.

The patient is sitting in a tripod position. You can see that she is using accessory muscles to breathe. You can hear her wheezing without placing your stethoscope on her chest. You count her respirations, 38 and labored.

■ Discussion: *What decisions regarding her breathing will you make?*

ASK YOURSELF

■ What are an EMR's considerations in responding to emergency calls, including:
  ■ Safety of the EMR, partners, other emergency responders, EMS personnel, and the public
  ■ Use of warning lights and siren
  ■ Emergency driving in traffic
  ■ Avoiding distractions
  ■ Passing vehicles
  ■ Approaching intersections
  ■ Parking

Responding to an Emergency Call

When the call for help comes in, you have a responsibility to answer that call. You must make every effort to ensure your safety, your partner's safety, and the safety of other emergency responders (law enforcement officers, EMTs, and paramedics) and the public at large (Figure 28-4 ■).

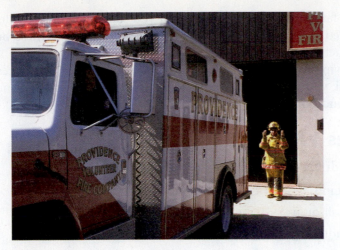

Figure 28-4 Whenever possible, travel in pairs to ensure the safety of your patient and the vehicle.

Safety is the first consideration of every 911 response. That consideration begins with making sure the apparatus is safe to respond and continues at the time of dispatch. The type or nature of call (for example, a domestic violence call) may reference the need to stage and wait for law enforcement to arrive and secure the scene. Next you will need to get the address and plan a safe route to the scene. You should take into account traffic patterns, construction, and other things that might delay your response.

Once you are in the vehicle, be sure to wear the safety belt. Supplemental restraint systems work best when combined with the use of a seat belt. The best practice for radio communication is for the driver to concentrate on vehicle operations and for the passenger to handle radio communications.

Warning Lights and Sirens

Turn on all the vehicle's warning lights and use the siren and air horn to alert other drivers of your presence. Emergency warning lights make your vehicle more visible but distracted drivers may not see you. Remember that the siren uses sound but it has a limited range. It is possible to "outrun" the siren sound. That means you are traveling faster than the effectiveness of the siren. Emergency lights and sirens do not give you the right-of-way. In most states you are merely asking for the right-of-way. The legal standard for emergency vehicle operations is "with due regard for the safety of others." This means you must operate the vehicle taking into account the safety of the public, not just the emergency you are responding to. If you are involved in a motor vehicle collision (MVC) and ruled at fault, you can be held both civilly and criminally liable.

Driving to an Emergency in Traffic

When driving to an emergency in traffic you may exceed the posted speed limit. When responding remember that speed is a factor in well over half of all collisions involving emergency vehicles. Having lights and siren on your vehicle does not give you the right to drive recklessly. Many states limit the speed that emergency vehicles can travel over the posted speed limit. Others simply require you to consider the safety of others when operating an emergency vehicle.

In some systems you may respond as a lone responder. You should take extra precautions when driving and operating the radio. Be sure that you do not become distracted. Remember, fatigue can cause delayed reaction time and poor decision making, increasing the risk to all personnel. If you become fatigued, take a short nap. The best strategy for combating fatigue is to get as much rest as you can and maintain a normal sleep pattern. Caffeinated drinks may provide a short-term increase in alertness, but does not help perception, reaction time, or decision making.

While driving to an emergency with lights and sirens or while responding to an emergency call, you should consider turning off the lights and siren and notifying dispatch of the conditions.

Distractions

The following driver distractions can be a danger to driving safely:

- mobile computer
- global positioning systems
- mobile radio
- cell phone
- vehicle stereo
- wireless devices
- eating/drinking

Minimize distractions when driving. You must not talk on the cell phone, read or send text messages when driving at any time. With the advent of the electronic age, emergency services also have advanced systems. New technologies like mobile data terminals send and receive data from a central system located in the 911 area. This new technology incorporates global positioning system (GPS) mapping software. It is easy to become distracted, which increases your risks of being involved in a motor vehicle collision.

Passing a Vehicle

When approaching a vehicle from behind while driving in traffic, slow down, and don't tailgate. Give the driver time to see you and react. Let the driver find a safe place to pull off the road to allow you to pass. When passing, remember to check the road ahead and only proceed if it is safe. You may come across an aggressive driver, someone who may tailgate you, fail to yield the right of way to you, or pass you unlawfully. You should slow down and back off and allow them to get away from you. If someone is tailgating you, turn off the lights and siren and notify dispatch to have law enforcement respond to your location, as you continue to your destination.

Intersections

Intersections are one of the most frequent places for emergency vehicles to become involved in a motor vehicle collision. When you approach an intersection slow down, even if the light is green in your lane of travel. Come to a complete stop if the light is red in your lane of travel. Check both sides of the intersection. When you have verified that it is safe, proceed slowly through the intersection until you have cleared the other side.

Parking

When approaching the scene, you should do a **360-degree survey** in all directions and look for hazards like downed utility lines or fluids leaking from damaged vehicles involved in a collision. Never drive through fluids leaking from a vehicle. The heat from your catalytic converter could ignite gasoline vapors from a leaking fuel tank. Choose a location that is uphill and upwind from the scene. If the incident is still in the roadway

ASK YOURSELF

- Can you define key terms introduced in this chapter?
- How do you select the appropriate personal protective equipment for a call?

360-degree survey a safety measure where you survey the scene in all directions as you approach, looking for hazards.

If operating fire apparatus, police cruiser or similar emergency vehicle, park vehicle with emergency lights activated to protect personnel at scene.

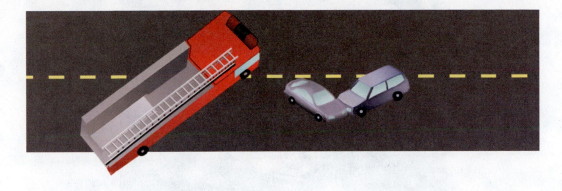

If responding in a personal vehicle or vehicle without appropriate emergency warning devices, park past the scene out of the flow of traffic.

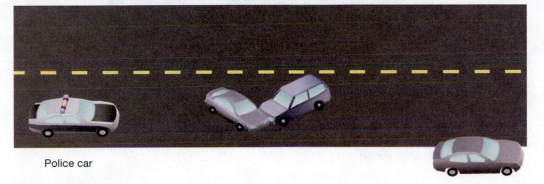

Police car

Personal vehicle

■ **Figure 28-5** Park the vehicle in a defensive manner at an emergency scene.

when you survey the scene, it may be necessary to park your vehicle in a defensive manner. In other words, place your vehicle between yourself and oncoming traffic and the scene (Figure 28-5 ■).

Personal Protective Equipment

The last thing you need to do before approaching the scene is don appropriate personal protective equipment (PPE) and take Standard Precautions. When you respond to a motor vehicle collision, you should wear protective clothing approved for auto extrication like firefighter turnout gear. Also you must don a traffic safety vest with reflective striping to improve your visibility to other drivers on the road (Figure 28-6 ■).

When responding to medical calls, you must take appropriate Standard Precautions. This will depend on your patient's condition and the likelihood of you coming in contact with infectious substances. Wear gloves when you may come in contact with these substances. Protect your face and clothes from splashing substances. You should wear a **NIOSH**-approved N95 respirator if you suspect your patient might have tuberculosis (TB). The symptoms of TB are cough with bloody sputum, fever, and night sweats.

National Institute for Occupational Safety and Health (NIOSH) As part of the Centers for Disease Control and Prevention, the *NIOSH* is responsible for conducting research and making recommendations for the prevention of work-related illnesses and injuries.

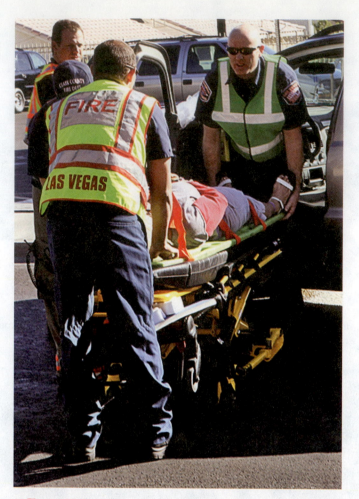

■ **Figure 28-6** Wearing the reflective safety vest improves visibility of the EMS provider.

✳ Stop, Review, Remember

Multiple Choice

Place a check next to the correct answer.

1. Safety is the responsibility of:

    _____ a. law enforcement.

    _____ b. EMRs.

    _____ c. firefighters.

    _____ d. all of the above.

2. The most dangerous place to be while driving emergency traffic is:

    _____ a. passing a vehicle in oncoming traffic.

    _____ b. driving at night.

    _____ c. passing through an intersection.

    _____ d. leaving the station.

3. When passing a vehicle on a two-lane road where the driver cannot pull off the road easily, you should:

    _____ a. pass immediately as soon as you get within passing distance.

    _____ b. slow down and allow time for the driver to see you and pull over.

    _____ c. slow down, allow time for the driver to see you, and pass only when it is safe to do so.

    _____ d. drive close behind the driver, pressing the air horn to cause the driver to stop and pull over so you can pass.

4. While responding to an emergency call, you approach an intersection and the traffic light turns yellow. You should:

_____ a. accelerate through the intersection while changing the tone on the siren.

_____ b. slow down, change the tone on the siren, look both ways, and then proceed through the intersection.

_____ c. maintain your speed, change the tone on the siren, look both ways, and then proceed through the intersection.

_____ d. slow down, come to a complete stop, change the tone on the siren, look both ways, and when all traffic has stopped proceed through the intersection.

True/False

Mark whether each of the following statements is true (T) or false (F).

1. _____ When driving an emergency vehicle, you do not have to wear a seat belt.

2. _____ Caffeinated drinks like coffee restore your alertness as well as a nap.

3. _____ By using lights and sirens, you are asking for the right-of-way from other drivers.

4. _____ When being tailgated by an aggressive driver while responding to an emergency, you should shut off the lights and siren and continue on to your destination.

5. _____ When parking on the scene of a motor vehicle collision, you should park your vehicle between yourself and the lane of travel.

6. _____ When involved in a scene where auto extrication is being done, you do not need to worry about blood or body fluids.

7. _____ If you are involved in a motor vehicle collision while operating an emergency vehicle, you are immune from criminal or civil liability.

Scene Management

As you've learned throughout this text, managing the scene is a priority for all emergency personnel. The first duty of all emergency personnel is safety (Figure 28-7 ■). As an EMR you must be alert for safety concerns at all times. Be aware of your surroundings. Remember that the scene of an emergency call is a dynamic environment and subject to change at any moment. You should be prepared to react to that changing environment. If the scene becomes unsafe, you may need to leave for your safety. Be sure to notify dispatch of the changing conditions and any time you have to evacuate the scene.

Residential Scenes

When dispatched to a call where the scene is a residence, pay particular attention to the dispatch information. Trauma-related dispatch codes are often related to assaults, shootings, stabbings, or domestic violence. Be sure that the scene is secured by law enforcement before you arrive. If law enforcement has not secured the scene, it may be necessary to stage or wait at a secure location close by. Once law enforcement has secured the scene, you may proceed on in. Remember, just because the scene is secure does not mean it cannot become unsafe at any moment.

Approaching the Scene: Residence/Non-Highway

As you learned in the early chapters of this book, when you arrive on scene you must do a 360-degree survey to look for any dangers such as loose pets in the area. If a dangerous dog confronts you, return to the safety of your vehicle, then radio dispatch and see if

ASK YOURSELF

- How would you describe an EMR's responsibilities in managing the scenes of a variety of emergency calls, including:
  - Residential and non-highway scenes
  - Transferring care to the EMS crew
  - Interacting with other emergency responders

Place warning devices several hundred feet from the accident scene back to oncoming traffic.

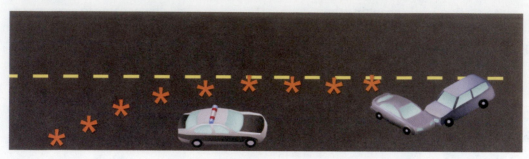

Police car

Place warning devices before the curve or at the crest of a hill to warn oncoming traffic.

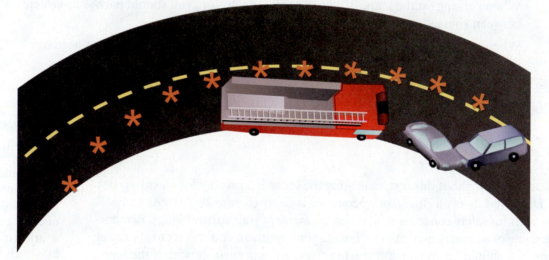

■ **Figure 28-7** When necessary, place warning devices at an emergency scene.

someone from the residence can secure the pet. If no one from the residence is available, have law enforcement respond and secure the pet.

Take note of suspicious individuals, or anyone who causes you to have an uneasy feeling. One thing that cannot be taught from a textbook is something referred to as "gut instincts." These feelings that something is not quite right have served many emergency responders over the years. Listen to your instincts.

Once you have surveyed the scene and are sure it is safe, and you have your Standard Precautions in place, you may enter the residence. As you enter the residence, survey your surroundings and be aware of the exits. Never allow yourself to be cut off from the exit.

Once you have entered the residence, introduce yourself to the patient and begin your assessment and treatment. As an EMR, you will often act as a first responder for the EMS system you are affiliated with. In many systems you will gather information for the responding EMS crew. Many EMS systems have patient information forms that you will need to fill out. Additionally you should have family members gather the patient's medications for the EMS crew to take with the patient to the hospital.

When treating patients, you will frequently interact with their family members. Many times these people are great sources of information and are genuinely concerned about their family member who you are treating. On rare occasions you will encounter a family member who is noncooperative and may even become disruptive to your efforts to care for the patient. You can handle these family members by assigning someone to talk to them. These family members are motivated by concern for their loved one and may not realize that they are inhibiting the patient's care. Sometimes family members can become irrational and could pose a threat to you or your crew. Again try to communicate with the family member and explain the situation and what you are doing to care for their loved one. If this does not work and you feel you are in danger, call for law enforcement and be ready to leave the scene.

Transferring Care

While you are on the scene, you will care for the patient until the EMS crew arrives. Then you will transfer care of the patient to the EMTs or Paramedics on the ambulance. You should give a report to the EMS crew including the SAMPLE history and any treatment that you provided for the patient. Then step back and let the EMS crew take over care of the patient. The EMTs or Paramedics will often re-interview the patient and obtain another SAMPLE history as they take over the care. Do not be offended by this. During the heat of the moment, a patient may leave out important details of the event or may forget that he is allergic to a particular medication. After they have obtained their history and stabilized the patient, you may assist them in packaging and moving the patient to the ambulance for transport to the hospital. Once this is completed, you should check the scene for your equipment and return to your vehicle to return to service. Be sure to restock your supplies after each call.

Interaction with Other Emergency Responders

In addition to EMTs and Paramedics, you will interact with the patient's family members, bystanders, firefighters, law enforcement officers, nurses, and physicians. The interactions may become stressful at times. Remember to be professional and courteous. As an EMR you are a representative of your department to the public. In today's world of mass media, you can never tell when you are being recorded.

✳ Stop, Review, Remember

Multiple Choice

Place a check next to the correct answer.

1. You are responding to an assault call where domestic violence is suspected to be the cause of the call. You should:

_____ a. enter the scene and apprise law enforcement if domestic violence was the cause of the assault.

_____ b. wait at the staging area until law enforcement officers arrive and secure the scene.

_____ c. wait in a staging area until you see the law enforcement vehicle pass; then follow them on to the residence.

_____ d. call dispatch and have them call the residence to see if the assailant is still there; if he is not there, you can proceed to the residence.

2. You are responding to a motor vehicle collision. When you approach the scene, you see that a tanker truck has collided with a small freight truck. You should perform a:

_____ a. 360-degree scene survey and park downhill and downwind.

_____ b. 360-degree scene survey and park downhill and upwind.

_____ c. 360-degree scene survey and park uphill and downwind.

_____ d. 360-degree scene survey and park uphill and upwind.

3. You are on the scene of a 56-year-old male with chest pain; the ambulance is 5 minutes away. The patient's irate son arrives on scene and starts screaming at his father that he is going to die waiting on the ambulance. The son insists that he should drive his father to the hospital. It is evening rush hour and the hospital is 25 minutes away. You should:

_____ a. let the son drive the father to the hospital, and use your emergency vehicle to clear a path for him.

_____ b. tell the patient that he should not go with his son because the ambulance will be there in 5 minutes and his son is stupid for suggesting that he drive him to the hospital.

_____ c. tell the irate son that you have called the police and he will be arrested if he remains on scene.

_____ d. calmly explain to both the patient and the son that the ambulance is only 5 minutes away and that the trip in the car would take 25 minutes in normal conditions and may take even longer since it is rush hour.

4. After transferring care of an elderly female patient complaining of abdominal pain and dementia, you remember that you forgot to write that the patient has an allergy to penicillin on your data sheet that you gave the EMTs. You should:

_____ a. call the EMTs en route to the hospital and notify them of the patient's medication allergy.

_____ b. call the EMTs after they arrive at the hospital and notify them of the patient's medication allergy.

_____ c. call the EMTs after they have cleared the hospital and notify them of the patient's medication allergy.

_____ d. tell no one about your mistake and just pretend that you don't know about the patient's medication allergy.

5. You overhear two police officers discussing the details of the call you are on where a patient was killed by an apparent drunk driver. They are unaware that a TV news crew has arrived on scene and is filming their conversation. You should:

_____ a. finish what you are doing and clear the scene and let the police officers deal with the media on their own.

_____ b. wait until they are done talking, call them over, and let them know that their conversation was recorded by the TV news crew.

_____ c. walk over to the two police officers and without drawing attention to yourself point out that they are secretly being recorded.

_____ d. go tell the TV news crew that they should not be taping the police officers while they are conducting their investigation.

Case Study

A 73-year-old woman playing at a slot machine in a gambling establishment is experiencing nausea and shortness of breath. Her husband becomes alarmed and asks for aid. Because of the patient's age, the establishment calls 911 for EMS help rather than evaluate her in their first-aid suite. You arrive on scene as an EMR. The patient's respirations are 50 and her blood pressure is 100/65. She tells you that she vomited about 2 minutes before you arrived, and she has pain in her arm.

1. Do you agree with this decision to call 911?

_____

_____

_____

2. What items from the ambulance did you bring into the gambling establishment to evaluate the patient?

_____

_____

_____

3. What are your first steps?

_____

_____

_____

TRANSITION

You immediately place the patient on oxygen via a nonrebreather mask. Next you take her pulse, which is 120 and weak. You notice that her nail beds have a bluish discoloration to them, indicating cyanosis. You place the oxygen saturation monitor on her fingertip; it reads 82 percent. As she begins to breathe the oxygen, her oxygen saturation slowly begins to rise. You check her blood pressure and find that it is 136/84.

Your partner reports the results of the SAMPLE history. She began having problems with her asthma last night. She has used her metered-dose inhaler eight times between last night and this morning. She has a history of asthma, she is allergic to peanuts, and she did not eat breakfast due to her breathing problems. She takes albuterol by inhaler and Singulair for her asthma.

You take the portable radio and call Medic 11, the paramedic ambulance, to respond to the scene. You give them a quick report on the patient's condition. They advise they have an estimated time of arrival of 4 to 5 minutes.

You reassess your patient. She is still alert, but only able to talk in one-word gasps. She is breathing 34 times a minute, her oxygen saturation has come up to 91 percent, she has a pulse of 120, and her blood pressure is 134/78.

You hear the ambulance approaching, and your partner goes out to help the paramedics bring in their equipment. You reassure your patient that the paramedics are here.

You give the paramedics a quick update on the patient. One sets up a nebulizer treatment while you finish a quick reassessment. After starting the nebulizer treatment, they begin to set up an IV. You assist in getting Mary on the stretcher. Once the IV is started, Mary is moved to the ambulance and is on the way to the hospital for further treatment.

■ Discussion: *What will you do to get ready for the next call?*

THE LAST WORD

You will respond to many calls for help over your career as an EMR. Remember your first priority is your safety and the safety of other emergency personnel, the patient, and bystanders on the scene. You can never be too safety conscious.

Every response to a call for help begins with preparation. As an EMR you must be diligent and check your vehicle and its equipment daily. Once the call comes, you are required to respond. When operating an emergency vehicle, you must take into account the traffic conditions and safety of the public.

When you arrive, survey the scene and park your vehicle in a defensive manner. Be aware of traffic and possible scene hazards. Provide care to the patient and work with other emergency responders to ensure the patient's smooth transition to the hospital for further care.

✳ Chapter Review

Multiple Choice

Place a check next to the correct answer.

1. The primary objective of responding to any 911 call is:

   _____ a. speed.

   _____ b. safety.

   _____ c. good public image.

   _____ d. patient care.

2. Engine oil, transmission fluid, and other vital fluids in an emergency vehicle should be checked:

   _____ a. daily.

   _____ b. weekly.

   _____ c. bi-weekly.

   _____ d. monthly.

3. While performing your vehicle's daily inspection, you notice that the left front tire has a nail embedded in the tread. You should:

   _____ a. make a note of the nail and operate the vehicle as usual.

   _____ b. change the tire yourself.

   _____ c. take the vehicle out of service and have the nail hole repaired.

   _____ d. pull the nail out yourself to save the department some money.

4. You are inspecting your vehicle's oxygen equipment and find a regulator that is leaking when you open the valve on the tank despite your attempts to tighten the regulator's locking pin down. You should:

   _____ a. make a note of the leak on the checklist and use the regulator anyway.

   _____ b. not worry about the leak.

   _____ c. worry that the leak could cause an explosion.

   _____ d. take the leaking regulator out of service and replace it with a new one.

5. While responding to a 911 call during rush hour, you observe a driver following on your bumper through two intersections. You should:

   _____ a. shut off your emergency lights, notify dispatch, and continue on to the call.

   _____ b. notify dispatch and have law enforcement intercept the driver.

   _____ c. stop your vehicle, tell the driver to stop following you, and lecture him on the dangers of following an emergency vehicle.

   _____ d. continue on to your call but slow down as you go through the intersections to allow other drivers to see the car following you.

6. You are approaching the scene of a motor vehicle collision. You should:

_____ a. look for a place to park out of the way of traffic uphill and upwind.

_____ b. park blocking traffic for your safety.

_____ c. perform a 360-degree survey of the scene, and park uphill and upwind.

_____ d. drive past the scene and park out of the way of traffic.

7. You respond to an assault call at a single-family home. Law enforcement is on scene. They advise the scene is secure; however, as you approach the house you notice a suspicious person hiding in the bushes. You should:

_____ a. use your vehicle's spotlight and public address system to warn law enforcement of the suspicious person.

_____ b. stop and notify dispatch via radio of the suspicious person and have law enforcement check on the person before entering the scene.

_____ c. proceed on into the house because the person is probably a neighbor who is curious about the emergency vehicles.

_____ d. sound the air horn as you approach to frighten the suspicious person away.

8. You are responding to a call for breathing problems. When you assess your patient, she states that she has been running a fever and started coughing up blood tonight. You should put a:

_____ a. surgical mask on both yourself and the patient.

_____ b. NIOSH-approved N95 or P100 respirator mask on the patient.

_____ c. NIOSH-approved N95 or P100 respirator mask on yourself.

_____ d. NIOSH-approved N95 or P100 respirator on yourself and a surgical mask on the patient.

9. You are responding to a motor vehicle collision at night during the winter. The temperature has dropped and you have just run through a patch of black ice where you temporarily lost control of your vehicle. You should:

_____ a. slow down and notify dispatch that black ice is forming on the road.

_____ b. slow down, turn off your emergency warning lights and siren, and notify dispatch that road conditions are becoming treacherous.

_____ c. continue on to the call as if nothing has happened, being thankful that you did not wreck your vehicle.

_____ d. slow down, leave your emergency warning lights on, and notify dispatch that road conditions are becoming treacherous.

10. You and your partner have responded to several 911 calls after midnight. It is now 3:00 a.m. and you notice that your partner has just nodded off at a stoplight while returning to the station after your last call. You should:

_____ a. offer to drive back to the station and tell him to get a cup of coffee when you get back to the station.

_____ b. offer to drive back to the station and tell him to take a nap as soon as you get back to the station.

_____ c. let him drive back to the station but have him roll the windows down and turn up the radio.

_____ d. let him drive back to the station but keep him awake by talking to him as he drives.

CHAPTER 29

Incident Management

NAVIGATION GUIDE

The following items provide an overview to the purpose and content of this chapter. The Education Standard and Competency are from the National EMS Education Standards.

Education Standard EMS Operations (Incident Management)

Competency Uses knowledge of operational roles and responsibilities to ensure patient, public, and personnel safety.

Knowledge Area Incident Management
- Establish and work within the incident

Objectives After reading this chapter, you should be able to:

1. Define key terms introduced in this chapter.
2. Describe the purpose of the National Incident Management System (NIMS).
3. Discuss each of the six major components of NIMS.
4. Describe each of the five key elements of an incident command system (ICS).
5. Operate within an ICS in a given scenario.

Key Terms Page numbers indicate first major use in this chapter. The Margin Glossary in this chapter provides definitions as you read.

incident command system (ICS), p. 717

National Incident Management System (NIMS), p. 717

unified command, p. 720

incident commander (IC), p. 721

Media Resources Please go to **www.bradybooks.com** to access mykit for this text. You will find quizzes, critical thinking scenarios, weblinks, animations, and videos related to this chapter—and much more. Look for online information on START and resources for emergency workers. You will also find a video clip on responding to children during a disaster.

INTRODUCTION

One of the more dynamic aspects of emergency care is that a responder never knows when the next call will come or what it will bring. Providers sometimes talk about going to "the big one"—an incident that taxes the abilities of the responder and the EMS system, and may receive local, state, or even national attention. Regardless of the cause—a natural disaster, a wildfire, a terrorist event, or a bus crash—many resources will be needed, and an organized, systematic method of managing these resources will be required. Providing and operating an incident management system is critical for the EMR during a large-scale incident.

One of the biggest challenges with large-scale incidents is that they occur relatively infrequently. The EMR can quickly become overwhelmed when faced with multiple injuries; numerous responders from EMS, police, and fire agencies; as well as governmental officials, reporters, and investigators. What happens if you are first on the scene? What happens if you respond once the system has been established? Working within the framework of an **incident command system (ICS)** and the **National Incident Management System (NIMS)**, the EMR can hold a variety of roles and functions. It is important to have a basic grasp of how each works.

ASK YOURSELF

- Can you define key terms introduced in this chapter?

incident command system (ICS) an expandable or collapsible system that focuses on goals and objectives and uses common terms to refer to its officers.

National Incident Management System (NIMS) a unified structure for public and private entities to work together to respond in all types of domestic incidents.

CASE STUDY

THE CALL

It is a bright and sunny afternoon. You and your partner, Ron, are enjoying some ice cream. The radio crackles to life: "Squad 16, respond to Highway 10 eastbound for the report of a vehicle crash in the breakdown lane. State police will be responding. Call came from a passerby on a cell phone, and we are receiving multiple calls that there may be several patients." You both throw your ice cream into the trash and start responding. You arrive first, and you find a large passenger van that has rolled over multiple times. It seems like there are people everywhere—patients, bystanders, and others trying to help those injured. As you pick up the radio to tell dispatch that you are on scene, you see several cars crash into each other on the westbound side of the highway, driven by people who were rubbernecking at the van accident (Figure 29-1 ■). You think to yourself, "This afternoon sure did change quickly!"

- Discussion: *Where and how do you and your partner begin?*

National Incident Management System

The National Incident Management System (NIMS) was federally mandated in 2003 by President George W. Bush. In *Homeland Security Presidential Directive (HSPD)-5, Management of Domestic Incidents*, President Bush directed the Secretary of Homeland Security to develop and administer the system. The NIMS forms a unified structure for public and private entities to work together to respond in all types of domestic incidents. The NIMS is centered on the concepts of preparing for, responding to, and recovering from a major incident. All federal agencies, and any agency receiving federal preparedness support, must implement and

ASK YOURSELF

- What is the purpose of the National Incident Management System (NIMS)?

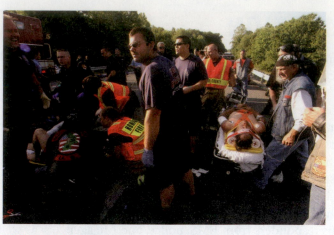

■ Figure 29-1 Multiple motor vehicle collision.

ASK YOURSELF

■ What are the six major components of NIMS?

use the NIMS. Any agency not using the NIMS incident command system may not be eligible for federal funding or reimbursement when responding to a domestic incident.

The NIMS has six major components:

- Command and management
- Preparedness
- Resource management
- Communications and information management
- Supporting technologies
- Ongoing management and maintenance

These components work in conjunction with one another to ensure an overall successful operation.

Command and Management

The command of NIMS is based on three systems:

- *Incident command system.* Defining an operation's structure, operation, and direction during an incident
- *Multiagency coordination system.* Defining the interaction and organization of supporting groups and agencies
- *Public information system.* Communicating systems and procedures to the public

Preparedness

The preparedness component is generally undertaken prior to an incident and involves:

- *Planning.* Analyzing what equipment and personnel are available, where hazards are, or what potential incidents may occur
- *Training.* Providing education on incident command, incident management, and multiagency cooperation and interaction
- *Exercises.* Conducting multijurisdictional drills to test the systems in place
- *Personnel qualification and certification.* Ensuring management and responding personnel meet national standards and are officially certified

- *Equipment acquisition and certification.* Ensuring responding personnel have the necessary equipment and that it is interoperable with other jurisdictions
- *Mutual aid.* Ensuring the means to assist other jurisdictions with resources, services, and support during an incident
- *Publications management.* Developing and publishing standardized forms for use during incidents

Resource Management

This component creates the methods to inventory, disperse, track, and return resources during and after an incident. This may range from personnel assisting from federal task forces and other states, to the use of helicopters and generators.

Communications and Information Management

This component sets up processes for collecting, interpreting, and disseminating information to incident managers and those impacted by the incident.

Supporting Technologies

This component is designed to ensure that communications systems (both voice and data) are functional and interoperable. It is also responsible for record keeping, and obtaining any specialized technologies that may be required during an incident.

Ongoing Management and Maintenance

This aspect was designed for long-term organization, and to review and refine the NIMS.

✳ Stop, Review, Remember

Multiple Choice

Place a check next to the correct answer.

1. The National Incident Management System (NIMS) was instituted in:

    _____ a. 2001.

    _____ b. 2002.

    _____ c. 2003.

    _____ d. 2004.

2. In order to receive federal funding for response to a domestic incident, you must use the NIMS.

    _____ a. True

    _____ b. False

3. Who is responsible for ensuring that all agencies, both public and private, adopt and utilize the NIMS ICS guidelines?

    _____ a. The President of the United States

    _____ b. The Federal Emergency Management Agency

    _____ c. The Secretary of Health and Human Services

    _____ d. The Secretary of Homeland Security

4. The three major elements of command and management are the incident command system, _____, and public information systems.

    _____ a. multijurisdictional drills

    _____ b. publications management

    _____ c. multiagency coordination systems

    _____ d. interagency cooperation agreements

5. The function of resource management is to:

_____ a. inventory, disperse, track, and return resources during and after an incident.

_____ b. track personnel during and after an incident.

_____ c. track equipment during and after an incident.

_____ d. disperse equipment and personnel to an incident.

CASE STUDY

THE RESPONSE ✴

As you stare in disbelief at the six heavily damaged cars with multiple occupants involved in the crash on the opposite side of the highway, a state police cruiser, a fire engine, and ambulances begin arriving on the scene. You call in to dispatch, "Squad 16 is on scene with two separate crashes. Squad 16 will be incident command and Ambulance 5 will be EMS command. We will need an additional ten ambulances and an EMS supervisor to be west side EMS." Upon their arrival, a state police sergeant, a fire deputy chief, and an EMS chief form a unified command, while you maintain east side EMS command.

■ Discussion: *Why do you think this EMR chose the need for 10, not fewer, additional ambulances? What is the next step in setting up an incident command?*

ASK YOURSELF

■ What are the five key elements of the incident command system (ICS)?

Incident Command System

The incident command system (ICS), used in the command and management portion of the NIMS, is an organizational method that is designed to be the same in any region, and in any type of response (hazardous materials, terrorism, fires, multiple-casualty incidents, or others). It focuses on achieving goals or objectives through safety of its responders, as well as effective and efficient use of resources available. The ICS is easily expandable and retractable, meaning that it can be used on any size incident, from a single car crash to a hurricane of immense proportions. The ICS can be set up in advance (such as for a large community event) or for an unplanned disaster. Some advantages of the ICS are:

■ Common terminology—Position titles and resource descriptions are defined regardless of department rank or status. For example, the incident commander might be the fire chief or the police captain. However, during the incident this person would be the incident commander. Other ICS titles can be section chief, team leader, or staging officer (Figure 29-2 ■).

■ Clear chain of command—This clarifies who is in charge of making overall decisions.

■ **Unified command**—All agencies work together to establish goals and make decisions (for example, fire chief, EMS chief, and police chief).

■ Unity of command—Each element reports to one supervisor only.

■ Manageable span of control—Each supervisor is responsible for no more than three to seven elements (with no more than five being the recommendation).

unified command all agencies working together to establish goals and make decisions.

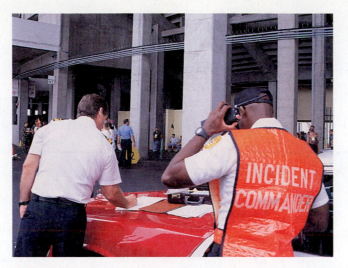

■ **Figure 29-2** Incident commander. *(© Mark C. Ide)*

There are five common elements found in an ICS structure:

- ■ **Incident commander (IC)**—the person who bears overall responsibility for the incident
- ■ Operations—carries out all incident objectives, such as directing a team to search a specific area to find a lost child
- ■ Planning—plans incident objectives in cooperation with the incident commander
- ■ Logistics—provides resources to carry out incident objectives, such as requesting a helicopter to perform roof rescues of stranded civilians during a major flood
- ■ Finance/administration—tracks resources from mobilization to demobilization, and provides an accounting of the cost of the incident

The ICS framework is easily modified, but the general structure would appear as in Figure 29-3 ■.

If you are first on the scene as an EMR, you may take the role of incident commander, requesting more equipment and resources.

As more of the resources you have requested arrive, you may exceed your span of control, perhaps making someone else in charge of requesting equipment (logistics), and another person in charge of the specific steps needed (operations). The ICS chart might look like Figure 29-4 ■.

As the incident continues, the operations section may determine that different areas are involved in the incident (for example, two floors of a building, or both sides of a highway) and may establish divisions to be in charge of each area. A division is a level that divides an incident geographically. The ICS chart might look like Figure 29-5 ■.

With this method, you can see that the incident commander only has to interact with the operations section and the logistics section, while the operations section is in charge

incident commander the person who bears overall responsibility for the incident.

ASK YOURSELF

■ How does an EMR operate within the ICS?

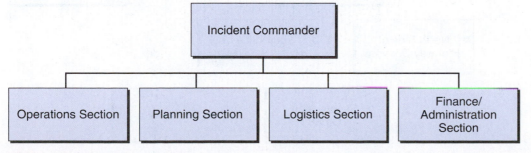

■ **Figure 29-3** Incident command system.

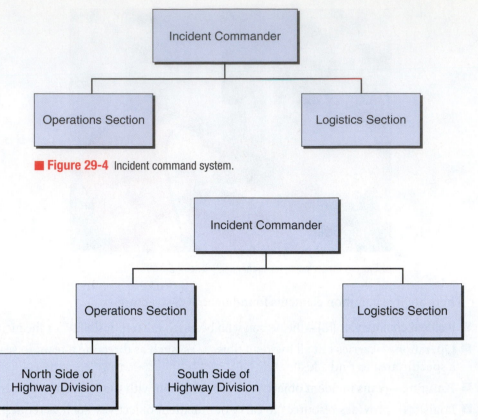

■ **Figure 29-4** Incident command system.

■ **Figure 29-5** Expanded ICS to include specific locations of the incident.

of the north side and south side divisions. As needs grow, the particular resource can be requested from logistics and assigned to a particular branch. For example, the north side division finds it needs an extrication team and a fire suppression team to cut open a car. The south side has no need of this resource, but does require two more EMRs to help carry a large patient. As these requests are made, they can be assigned to the correct branch to perform the needed function. These specific resources are known as groups. The ICS chart would now look like Figure 29-6 ■.

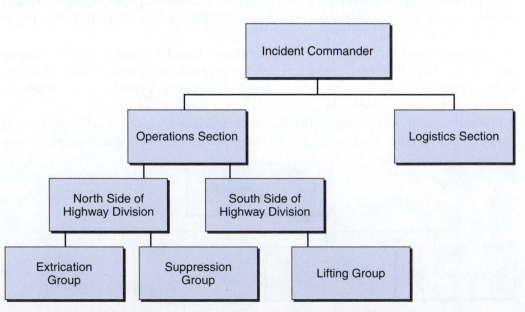

■ **Figure 29-6** Expanded ICS to include additional groups to address specific issues.

In most instances, you will be working in a group once the incident is established, but you should be familiar with all aspects of the incident command system, as the EMR may be needed to fill any role during an incident. To gain a better understanding, the EMR should take Federal Emergency Management Agency (FEMA) ICS-100 (An Introduction to Incident Command System) or equivalent, as well as FEMA's IS-700 (NIMS, An Introduction).

✳ Stop, Review, Remember

Multiple Choice

Place a check next to the correct answer.

1. What is considered the best range for a span of control?
   _____ a. one to three elements
   _____ b. three to five elements
   _____ c. five to seven elements
   _____ d. three to seven elements

2. This branch of the ICS provides the objectives for the incident.
   _____ a. Logistics
   _____ b. Planning
   _____ c. Finance/administration
   _____ d. Operations

3. This branch of the ICS carries out the objectives for the incident.
   _____ a. Logistics
   _____ b. Planning
   _____ c. Finance/administration
   _____ d. Operations

4. In the ICS, when different agencies work together on a single incident this is known as:
   _____ a. unity of command.
   _____ b. unified command.
   _____ c. chain of command.
   _____ d. incident command.

5. The person who bears overall responsibility for the incident is the:
   _____ a. incident commander.
   _____ b. police chief.
   _____ c. fire chief.
   _____ d. planning section chief.

CASE STUDY

TRANSITION ✳

Over the next hour, a total of 17 people are transported to local hospitals. Four are flown by helicopter to a regional trauma center. The EMS chief congratulates you on establishing ICS early and setting the tone for the incident. Your partner Ron, returning from assisting with one of the patients who was flown, looks at you and says, "Definitely time for that ice cream now!"

■ Discussion: *Were the 10 ambulances you originally called for enough? What happens when you find out you need additional resources as the call progresses? How would you determine the need for you to call for air transport?*

When you are faced with a large-scale incident, the demands of patient care, resource management, and multiple agencies attempting to gain information and accomplish their specific goals can become quickly overwhelming. By using the National Incident Management System (NIMS) and the incident command system (ICS), the EMR will be able to provide an adaptable and efficient framework to better handle major incidents.

✳ Chapter Review

Multiple Choice

Place a check next to the correct answer.

1. The use of clear titles such as incident commander or planning section chief is an example of:

    _____ a. chain of command.

    _____ b. unity of command.

    _____ c. common terminology.

    _____ d. command structure.

2. The command of the NIMS is based on three systems. Which of the following is *not* one of them?

    _____ a. The incident command system

    _____ b. Supporting technologies

    _____ c. Multiagency coordination

    _____ d. Public information

3. Training and exercises are considered part of what NIMS component?

    _____ a. Preparedness

    _____ b. Resource management

    _____ c. Command and management

    _____ d. Ongoing maintenance and management

4. The part of the NIMS command and management that passes information to the public during an incident is the:

    _____ a. public information system.

    _____ b. publications information.

    _____ c. joint information center.

    _____ d. liaison officer.

5. A mutual aid agreement between two jurisdictions is an example of _____ in the NIMS for incident management.

    _____ a. planning

    _____ b. preparation

    _____ c. partnership

    _____ d. preparedness

6. When a state or local government develops a system of interoperable communications so that police, fire, and EMS can all communicate with each other, this is an example of the _____ function of the NIMS.

    _____ a. voice over IP

    _____ b. resource management

    _____ c. supporting technology

    _____ d. planning

7. The incident command system is an adaptable system that can be used to respond to which of the following types of incidents?

    _____ a. Hurricane, forest fire, or flood

    _____ b. The Super Bowl

    _____ c. A single-car motor vehicle collision

    _____ d. All of the above

8. The role of incident commander on a major event should be assumed by:

    _____ a. the senior fire officer.

    _____ b. the senior EMS officer.

    _____ c. the senior person on the first-in unit.

    _____ d. the senior police officer.

Matching

Match the following descriptions with the appropriate term.

1. _____ Only one supervisor
2. _____ Carries out incident objectives
3. _____ Bears overall responsibility for the incident
4. _____ Provides incident resources
5. _____ All organizations in command
6. _____ Multijurisdictional drills to test the systems in place
7. _____ Develops the incident objectives
8. _____ Tracks all resources in and out of the incident

a. Operations
b. Incident commander
c. Logistics
d. Unity of command
e. Unified command
f. Finance/administration
g. Planning
h. Exercises

Critical Thinking

1. What might an ICS look like in your community?

_____

_____

_____

_____

2. How do you think the organizations in your community (fire, police, EMS, local and state governmental officials) could learn and practice NIMS?

_____

_____

_____

_____

Special Operations

✳ NAVIGATION GUIDE

The following items provide an overview to the purpose and content of this chapter. The Education Standard and Competency are from the National EMS Education Standards.

Education Standard EMS Operations (Hazardous Materials, Multiple Casualty Incidents, Air Medical, Vehicle Extrication)

Competency Uses knowledge of operational roles and responsibilities to ensure patient, public, and personnel safety.

Knowledge Areas Hazardous Materials
- Risks and responsibilities of operating in a cold zone at a hazardous material or other special incident

Multiple Casualty Incidents
- Triage principles
- Resource management

Air Medical
- Safe air medical operations
- Criteria for utilizing air medical response

Vehicle Extrication
- Safe vehicle extrication
- Use of simple hand tools

Objectives After reading this chapter, you should be able to:

1. Define key terms introduced in this chapter.
2. Describe common locations and situations in which hazardous materials are encountered.
3. Recognize the U.S. Department of Transportation (DOT) and National Fire Protection Association (NFPA) 704 systems of placards to identify hazardous materials.
4. Use the DOT Emergency Response Guidebook to find information about hazardous materials.
5. Discuss other sources of information on hazardous materials.
6. Describe the hot, warm, and cold zones of hazardous materials incidents.
7. Explain the EMR's role at a hazardous materials incident.
8. Discuss the goals of managing multiple casualty incidents (MCIs).
9. Given several descriptions of patients in an MCI, use the START and JumpSTART triage systems to categorize patients.

NAVIGATION GUIDE *(continued)*

10. Describe the EMR's role in vehicle extrication.
11. Explain the key components of vehicle extrication.
12. Recognize indications for aeromedical transport.
13. Discuss the considerations of setting up an appropriate landing zone.
14. Explain the safety considerations associated with approaching a medical aircraft.

Key Terms Page numbers indicate first major use in this chapter. The Margin Glossary in this chapter provides definitions as you read.

placard, p. 727
material safety data sheet, p. 732
mass casualty incident, p. 735

simple triage and rapid treatment (START) system, p. 735
extrication, p. 739

pinned, p. 740
entrapment, p. 740
aeromedical transport, p. 743

Media Resources Please go to **www.bradybooks.com** to access mykit for this text. You will find quizzes, critical thinking scenarios, weblinks, animations, and videos related to this chapter—and much more. Look for online information on traffic safety and air medical services. You will also find a video clip on rapid extrication.

INTRODUCTION

A special operations situation is any incident where you may encounter hazardous materials, mass casualties, or critical patients who will require aeromedical evacuation to a trauma center for treatment. A severe motor vehicle collision may have all of these elements in one single event.

Hazardous Materials

The U.S. Department of Transportation (DOT) defines a hazardous material as "any substance or material incident in a form which poses an unreasonable risk to health, safety, and property when transported in commerce."

Every day we encounter hazardous materials. They are found in the buildings we enter. Many are shipped in trucks and trailers of all shapes and sizes, in railroad cars, and by air or pipeline. Even though there are many regulations and safety procedures in place, exposures to hazardous materials do occur. The DOT and other agencies have developed warning systems in an attempt to assist emergency personnel responding to events involving hazardous materials (Figure 30-1 ■).

U.S. Department of Transportation Placard System

The DOT requires a diamond-shaped sign called a **placard** to be placed on certain containers when hazardous materials are being transported (Figure 30-2 ■).

The DOT classifies hazardous materials into nine classes. Additionally there may be numbers that show a division of the class of hazardous material that is being transported (Figure 30-3 ■).

A four-digit ID number may be shown on the placard, or it may be on an adjacent orange panel displayed next to the placard on the ends and sides of a cargo tank, vehicle, or rail car. You can reference the placard along with the ID number in the DOT Emergency

ASK YOURSELF

- Can you define key terms introduced in this chapter?
- How would you describe common locations and situations in which hazardous materials are encountered?
- How would you recognize the U.S. Department of Transportation (DOT) and National Fire Protection Association (NFPA) 704 systems of placards to identify hazardous materials?

placard diamond-shaped sign placed on certain containers when hazardous materials are being transported.

THE CALL

You are dispatched to a busy intersection for a motor vehicle collision involving an 18-wheeler truck and a minivan. You and your partner get in the quick response vehicle (QRV) and drive toward the scene.

As you approach the scene at the intersection, you note that the 18-wheeler is in fact a tanker truck that has struck the side of a minivan, and there is heavy damage to the minivan.

Your partner stops the QRV, and you take out the binoculars and survey the scene. You read the placard on the tanker with the binoculars. It is a white diamond with a red flame and the numbers 1293 inside of it. The tanker is intact and there is no damage or leaks to the tank.

Your partner looks up the placard and finds that the truck is carrying gasoline. You radio dispatch and have additional fire units dispatched to the scene to assist with a possible hazardous materials event.

Your partner maneuvers the unit to an uphill-upwind position to park the vehicle on the scene.

■ Discussion: *What should you do if there is gas leaking from the truck?*

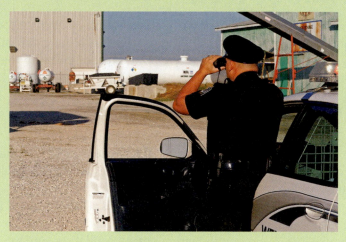

A police officer identifying a hazardous situation from a distance.

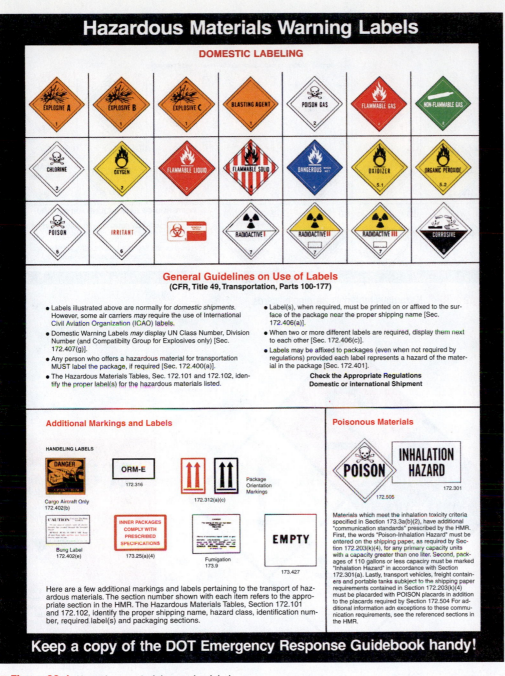

Figure 30-1 Hazardous materials warning labels.

Response Guidebook for information on what material is in the container and what initial safety measures you may need to take in the event of a spill (Figure 30-4 ■).

Additional sources of information include invoices, shipping papers (barges and trains), and bills of lading (trucks). These documents identify the type, quantity, origin, and destination of the hazardous materials. Often these documents are kept in the wheelhouse of a water-going vessel, in the cab of a truck, or with the engineer.

Remember that placards are required either by the weight of the material or by the class of the hazardous material being shipped. A hazardous material may not have a placard if it does not meet the requirements for having a placard on the vehicle, so always err on the side of caution when approaching any scene.

ASK YOURSELF

■ How would you use the DOT Emergency Response Guidebook to find information about hazardous materials?

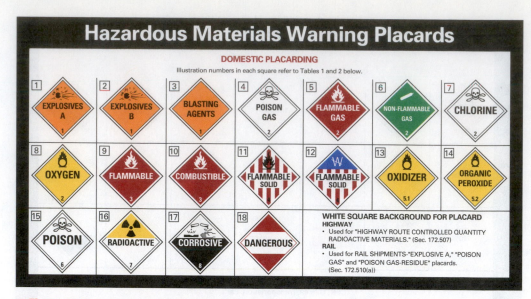

Figure 30-2 Hazardous materials warning placards.

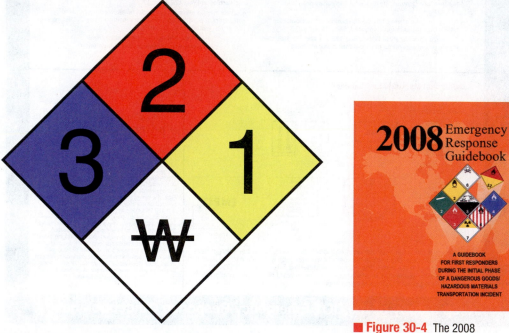

Figure 30-3 NFPA 704 placard for a building.

Figure 30-4 The 2008 Emergency Response Guidebook.

ASK YOURSELF

■ What are some other sources of information on hazardous materials?

NFPA 704 Placard System for Buildings

When you respond to a building, be aware of the possibility of encountering hazardous materials. The National Fire Protection Association (NFPA) has developed a voluntary marking system to alert emergency responders to the characteristics of hazardous materials stored in stationary tanks and facilities. This standardized system, known as NFPA 704, uses numbers and colors on a sign to indicate the basic hazards of a specific material being stored in large containers or at a manufacturing site. The NFPA 704 label is diamond shaped and is divided into four parts, or quadrants (Figure 30-5 ■).

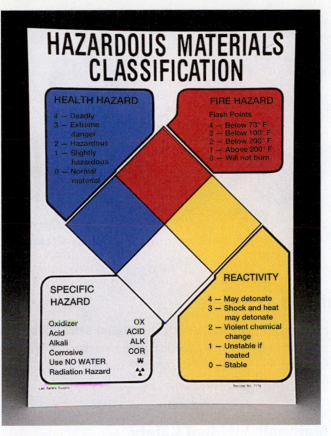

Figure 30-5 NFPA 704 classification system.

- The top left quadrant is *blue*, and contains a numerical rating of the substance's health hazard. Ratings are made on a scale of 0 to 4. A zero, or no code at all in this quadrant, means that no unusual hazard would result from the exposure. A rating of 4 indicates a severe hazard and that a very short exposure could cause serious injury or death.

- The top right quadrant of the NFPA symbol contains the substance's fire hazard rating. As you might expect, this quadrant is *red*. Again, number codes in this quadrant range from 0 to 4, with 3 representing a serious fire hazard.

- The bottom right quadrant, colored *yellow*, indicates the substance's likelihood to explode or react. As with the health and fire hazard quadrants, ratings from 0 to 4 are used to indicate the degree of hazard. If a 2 appears in this section, the chemical is moderately unstable, and even under *normal* conditions may explode or react violently. A zero in this quadrant indicates that the material is considered to be stable even in the event of a fire.

- The bottom left quadrant is *white* and contains information about any special hazards that may apply. There are three possible codes for the bottom quadrant of the NFPA symbol. OX means this material is an oxidizer. It can easily release oxygen to create or worsen a fire or explosion hazard. The symbol W̶ indicates a material that reacts with water to release a gas that is either flammable or hazardous to health. If the material is radioactive, the usual tri-blade "propeller" symbol for radioactivity will appear.

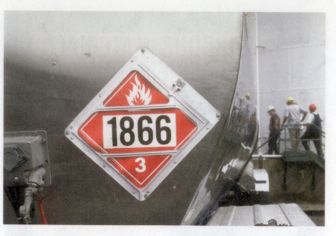

■ **Figure 30-6** A vehicle carrying hazardous materials will carry this warning placard.

Material Safety Data Sheets

material safety data sheet the manufacturer's information about the chemicals contained in the product.

Employers are required to maintain a current **material safety data sheet** (MSDS) from the manufacturer for each hazardous chemical in the workplace. You should only attempt to retrieve the MSDS if it is safe to do so. Be sure to give the MSDS to the EMTs transporting the patient to the hospital.

Hazardous Materials Incident Safety

ASK YOURSELF

■ How would you describe the hot, warm, and cold zones of hazardous materials incidents?

An incident where hazardous materials have escaped or may escape their containers is referred to as a hazmat incident (Figure 30-6 ■). To operate safely in a hazmat incident, you need to understand how an incident response will be conducted.

The hazmat incident is divided into special areas called zones:

■ The hot zone is the area directly around the incident where hazardous materials have breached their container. This area is contaminated with hazardous materials. Entering this zone without proper protective equipment or training will cause you to become contaminated.

■ The warm zone is the area surrounding the hot zone where hazmat technicians dress in their level A or B suits to prepare to enter the hot zone. Level A and B suits are specially designed to be resistant to chemicals. They also incorporate a self-contained breathing apparatus (SCBA) to provide breathable air to the hazmat technician. Patient decontamination occurs in the warm zone also. Decontamination is the process of cleaning contaminants from the patients who were in the hot zone.

■ The cold zone is the area that surrounds the warm zone. There are no contaminants in the cold zone, and no special equipment is needed to be in the cold zone. Patients who have been decontaminated are brought to the cold zone for triage and transport (Figure 30-7 ■).

ASK YOURSELF

■ What is the EMR's role at a hazardous materials incident?

Incidents involving hazardous materials should be handled by specially trained hazmat technicians. You should never enter the hot zone of a hazmat incident. Be sure to contain patients who are contaminated in the hot zone. Remember that patients who leave the hot zone can spread contaminants to others and increase the size of the hot zone (Figure 30-8 ■).

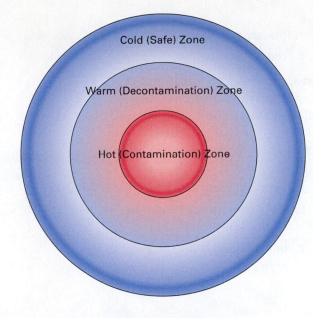

Hot (Contamination) Zone

Contamination is actually present.
Personnel must wear appropriate protective gear.
Number of rescuers limited to those absolutely necessary.
Bystanders never allowed.

Warm (Decontamination) Zone

Area surrounding the contamination zone.
Vital to preventing spread of contamination.
Personnel must wear appropriate protective gear.
Life-saving emergency care is performed.

Cold (Safe) Zone

Normal triage, stabilization, and treatment are performed.
Rescuers must shed contaminated gear before entering
the cold zone.

■ **Figure 30-7** Three control zones.

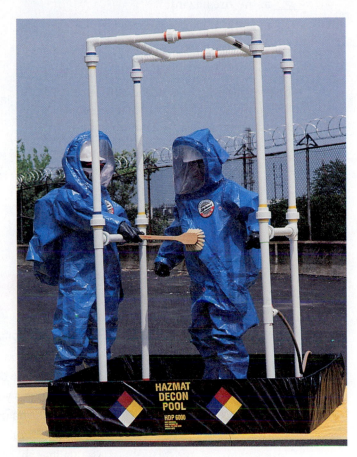

■ **Figure 30-8** Rescuers in the decontamination process.

✳ Stop, Review, Remember

Multiple Choice

Place a check next to the correct answer.

1. The U.S. Department of Transportation (DOT) defines a *hazardous material* as:

   _____ a. a poison or chemical that could harm you.

   _____ b. any substance or material in a form that poses an unreasonable risk to health.

   _____ c. a substance that must be marked with a placard to be shipped or stored.

   _____ d. a poison or chemical that is not harmful to you.

2. The National Fire Protection Association 704 system is used to mark buildings for _____ with a multicolored diamond sign.

   _____ a. occupancy

   _____ b. hazards

   _____ c. flammable materials

   _____ d. chemical materials

3. You arrive at a building for a medical call. The red quadrant of the NFPA symbol contains the number 3. This means there is:

_____ a. no fire hazard.

_____ b. a minimal fire hazard.

_____ c. a serious fire hazard.

_____ d. a moderate fire hazard.

4. When responding to a motor vehicle collision involving a vehicle that transports hazardous materials, you should look for _____ during your scene size-up.

_____ a. material safety data sheets

_____ b. invoices, shipping papers, and bills of lading

_____ c. placards

_____ d. red diamonds

5. When approaching an incident scene involving hazardous materials with a vehicle containing visible placards, you can use the _____ to gather initial information on the material inside the vehicle.

_____ a. material safety data sheet (MSDS)

_____ b. DOT Emergency Response Guidebook

_____ c. bill of lading

_____ d. NFPA 704 placard system

CASE STUDY

THE RESPONSE

Two additional fire companies arrive on scene and lay hoses. The scene is now secure, making it safe for you to approach. The chief of the first fire company on scene calls incident command and designates you as the triage officer.

As you get out of your vehicle, you meet the driver of the tanker truck carrying his bill of lading and other papers about the gasoline in the tanker. He tells you that the minivan ran a red light, and he could not stop in time and hit them. He tells you there are several people in the minivan and they all look real bad. You have your partner stay with the driver and you go to check on the patients in the minivan.

You approach the minivan with your turnout gear on. You are able to open the passenger's side sliding door with little effort. You count six patients total. The driver appears to be pinned in by the damage to the vehicle. You realize that you have a multiple casualty incident. You call for three additional ambulances to help with the patients and have the heavy rescue unit proceed on to your location. Next you begin to use the START triage system to sort the patients according to the severity of their injuries.

■ Discussion: *Read on to understand the START triage system. How will you determine which patients are a priority for immediate care?*

Mass Casualty Incidents

Mass casualty incidents (MCIs) bring to mind terrorist attacks, severe storms, and large-scale disasters. However, a mass casualty incident or multiple casualty incident is any event that overwhelms the resources of the responders on scene. A simple motor vehicle collision involving a school bus full of children can quickly tax the resources of any EMS system. Effective management of an MCI is achieved by using the incident command system (ICS) model (for more information on the ICS model, refer to Chapter 29, "Incident Management).

No matter the role you are assigned on an MCI, you must work as a team to deliver the most care to the largest number of patients. Remember the goal of managing an MCI is to quickly and effectively triage, treat, and transport all patients to the most appropriate medical facility.

mass casualty incident an event that overwhelms the resources of the responders on scene.

Triage

As an EMR you may serve as the triage officer on the scene of an MCI.

Triage is the process of sorting patients by the severity of their injuries so that the most severely injured patients get treated first. The idea was first practiced in Europe by Napoleon's chief surgeon, Dominique Jean Larrey, who would sort the wounded from the battlefield according to the severity of their wounds.

In modern times there have been many effective systems of triage developed. In an effort to establish a uniform system, the Department of Homeland Security has chosen the **Simple Triage and Rapid Treatment (START) system** to be the national model and it is incorporated into the National Incident Management System (NIMS). The START system guides you in using your resources to do the most good for the greatest number of patients. It can be accomplished with no equipment and minimal training.

The START system was designed for use on adult patients. A modified system called JumpSTART was designed for use on pediatric patients. Tags are placed on the patient after being seen by the triage officer (Figure 30-9a ■).

All triage can begin with sorting the walking wounded to secondary triage by simply asking all patients who can walk to come to an area that you designate. Be sure that another EMR is there to provide care.

The START system differs from the initial assessment you have been taught in this book in that you begin with an assessment of breathing and then move on to assessment of perfusion and finally mental status.

Simple Triage and Rapid Treatment (START) system a simplified system using respirations, circulation, and mental status as the basis for triage.

Example of the Use of START Triage

To assess an adult patient in an MCI, first assess for breathing. If the patient is not breathing, you should open the airway and reassess. If the patient is still not breathing, you will classify the patient as nonsalvageable, or unable to be saved, and move on to the next patient. Although it seems contradictory to your training to not begin CPR, in an MCI you have limited resources and you are trying to help the most patients with the resources you have.

The JumpSTART System

The JumpSTART triage system is designed for use on pediatric patients (ages 1–8) and differs slightly from the triage system for adult patients. Airway problems are the primary cause of cardiac arrest in pediatric patients (refer to Chapter 25). The JumpSTART system

ASK YOURSELF
- What are the goals of managing mass casualty incidents (MCIs)?
- Given several descriptions of patients in a mass casualty incident, how would you use the START and JumpSTART systems to categorize patients?

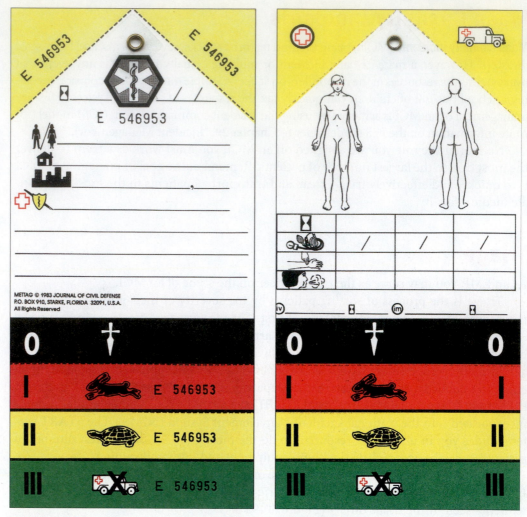

Figure 30-9a Example of a commonly used triage tag (front and back).

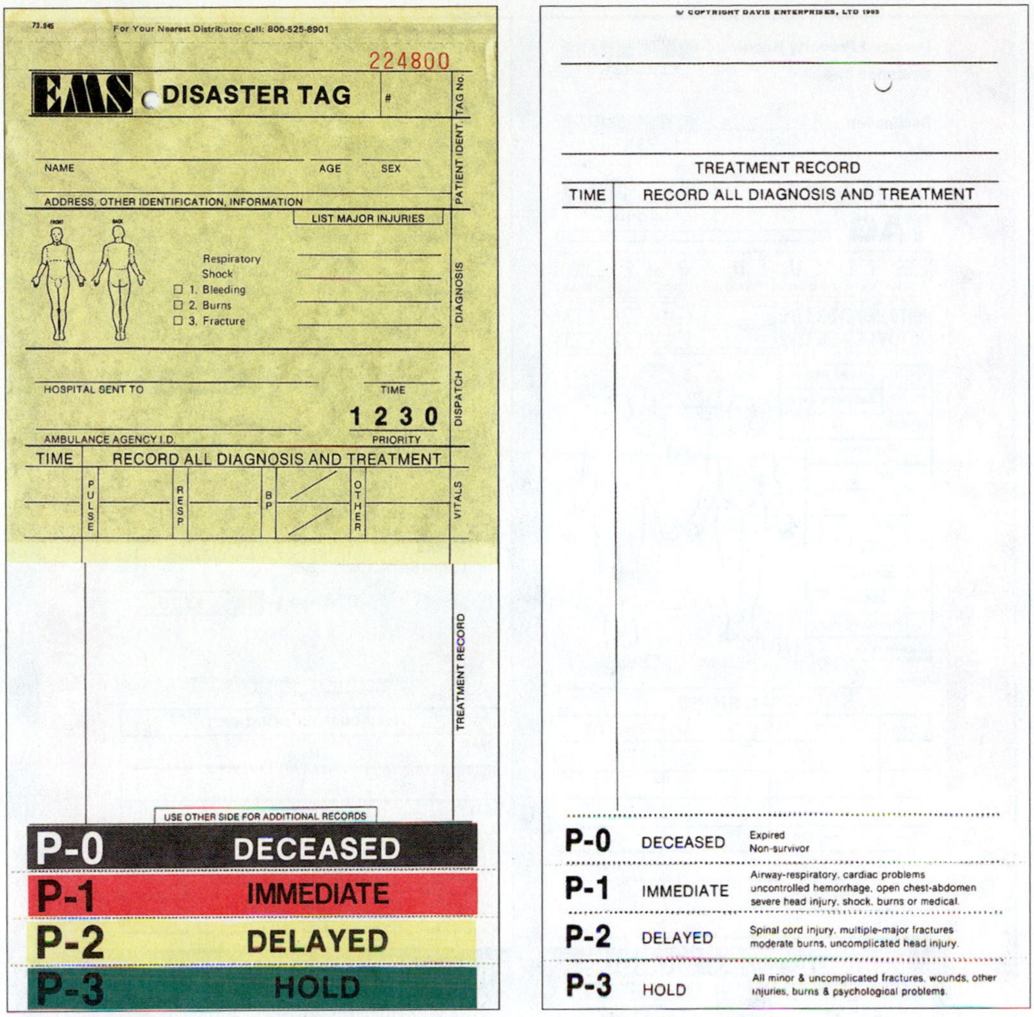

■ Figure 30-9b Example of a commonly used EMS disaster tag (front and back).

addresses that difference by allowing for the provider to give rescue breaths to "jump start" breathing in the pediatric MCI patient (Figure 30-9b ■).

- ■ If the patient is not breathing after airway opening, check for a peripheral pulse. If there is no pulse, tag the patient deceased/nonsalvageable and move on.
- ■ If there is a peripheral pulse, give five mouth-to-barrier ventilations. If apnea persists, tag the patient as deceased/nonsalvageable and move on.

If breathing resumes after the "jump start," tag the patient as immediate (highest priority) and move on (Figure 30-9c ■ and Figure 30-10 ■).

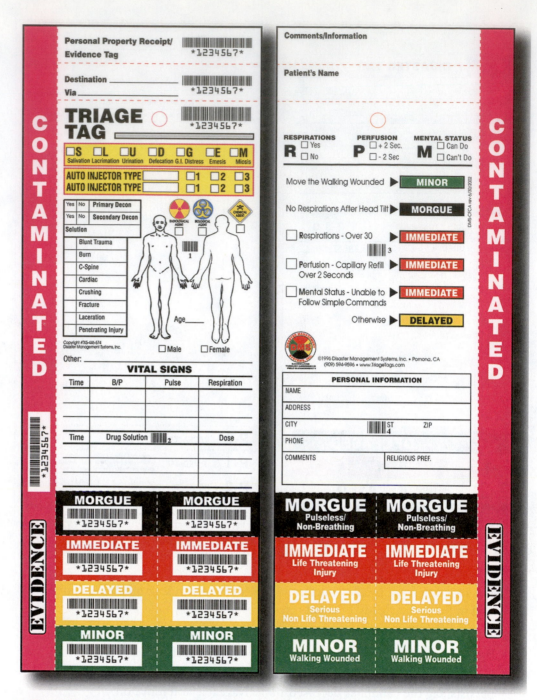

Figure 30-9c Example of a contaminated patient tag (front and back).

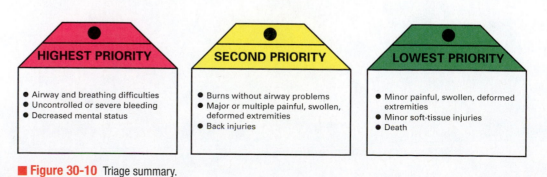

Figure 30-10 Triage summary.

Multiple Choice

Place a check next to the correct answer.

1. Which of the following is a mass casualty incident (MCI)?

    _____ a. A single vehicle is involved in a collision. There is one minor trauma and one patient ambulatory on scene.

    _____ b. A school bus rolls over. The driver is pinned in, and there are no other passengers.

    _____ c. A car has brake failure and strikes a crowded storefront with many shoppers.

    _____ d. A large tanker truck is struck by a freight train at a crossing. The driver is nonsalvageable.

2. Only a large-scale MCI will require use of the incident command system.

    _____ a. True

    _____ b. False

3. The term *triage* means to:

    _____ a. separate.

    _____ b. sort.

    _____ c. categorize.

    _____ d. divide.

4. The START triage system begins with an assessment of:

    _____ a. level of consciousness.

    _____ b. airway.

    _____ c. breathing.

    _____ d. pulse.

5. The JumpSTART triage is used in pediatric patients because:

    _____ a. children are more likely to survive a trauma.

    _____ b. children need assisted ventilations in all trauma emergencies.

    _____ c. the primary cause of cardiac arrest in children is a heart problem.

    _____ d. the primary cause of cardiac arrest in children is a respiratory problem.

Extrication

Extrication is the process of disentangling a patient from wreckage or debris that prevents access to render care and transport (Figure 30-11 ■).

Over the years the equipment has changed but the principle remains the same, to safely and quickly extricate the patient from the wreckage of a motor vehicle collision. You will

extrication the process of disentangling a patient from wreckage or debris that prevents access to render care and transport.

ASK YOURSELF

- What is the EMR's role in vehicle extrication?
- What are the key components of vehicle extrication?

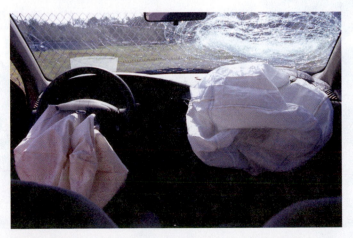

■ **Figure 30-11** Discharged air bag. (© Stephen Bell Photographic Productions)

need to wear appropriate personal protective equipment (PPE) including a helmet, gloves, NFPA-approved coveralls or firefighter's coat and pants (often called bunker gear), and steel-toed boots before you enter the scene to assist with patient care or begin extrication.

First you need to determine if the patient is truly pinned in the vehicle or just entrapped.

■ To be **pinned** in means that a part of the patient's body is entangled in the wreckage. The wreckage must be removed before the patient can be safely removed from the vehicle.

■ **Entrapment** means that the patient is free inside the vehicle, but due to damage to the vehicle the patient cannot be accessed or safely removed from the wreckage.

Vehicle Stabilization

The process of extrication begins with scene safety. Ensure that you are not in danger from traffic or unsafe scene conditions. Next the vehicle must be assessed for stability. A vehicle that has been involved in a motor vehicle collision may lose its stability due to the position it came to rest in or damage suffered during the collision (Figures 30-12a and 30-12b ■).

Unstable vehicles must be stabilized using cribbing. Cribbing material is often made from blocks of treated lumber cut in various shapes or lengths, although there are various commercial devices available. The cribbing is placed under the vehicle between the frame and the ground to provide stability. Once the vehicle is stabilized the true work of extrication can begin (Figures 30-13a through 30-13c ■).

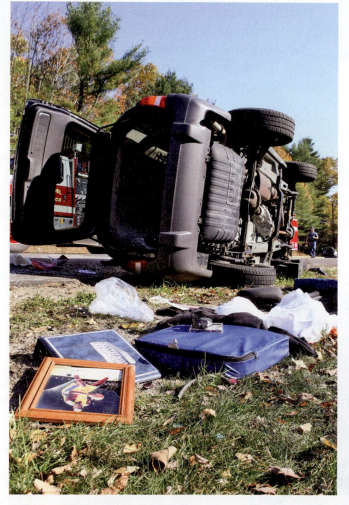

■ **Figure 30-12a** Unstable vehicle.

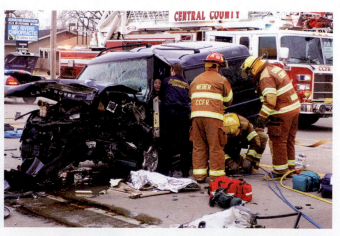

■ **Figure 30-12b** Entrapped patient receiving EMS care. (© Ray Kemp/911 Imaging)

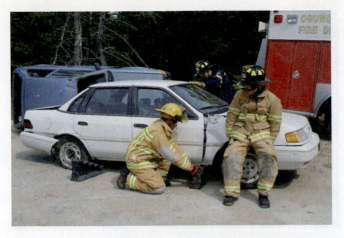

■ **Figure 30-13a** Stabilizing a car on its wheels with cribbing.

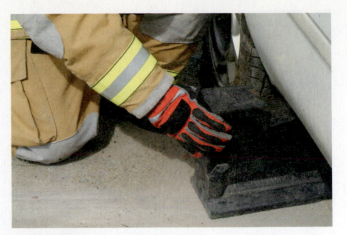

■ **Figure 30-13b** Placing a step chock.

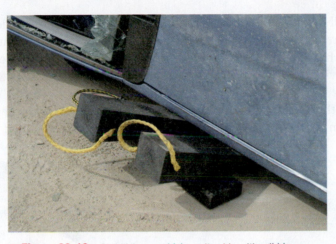

■ **Figure 30-13c** Stabilizing a vehicle on its side with cribbing.

Gaining Access

Gaining access is the process of entering the vehicle to care for the patient. It may be as simple as opening an undamaged door on the other side of the vehicle, or it may require the use of hydraulic extrication tools. There is an old saying that you should always remember: "Try before you pry." This means to check all the doors and windows to see if they open. Sometimes gaining access may be as simple as unlocking the door. If the door is locked and the patient can unlock the door without moving around or twisting his body or neck, you can ask him to unlock the door for you.

If it is unsafe for the patient to unlock the door or the patient is unresponsive, you can break a window using a spring-loaded center punch. If you use a center punch, break the glass on the opposite side of the car from the patient to prevent glass from covering the patient. If you can safely open a door after breaking the glass and unlocking it, you can enter the vehicle and begin to assess and treat your patient. A center punch will not work on laminated glass like the front windshield (Figure 30-14 ■).

Occasionally damage to the vehicle will be too great for you to open the doors without using simple or hydraulic tools. Simple tools like the pry bar or the Halligan tool are used to force doors open and allow for removal of the patient from the vehicle (Figure 30-15 ■).

Hydraulic extrication tools like the Hurst Jaws of Life are used in place of manual extrication tools. Hydraulic tools can easily cut most metal found in today's cars, and they give the rescuer the advantage of both speed and power when it comes to patient extrication (Figure 30-16 ■).

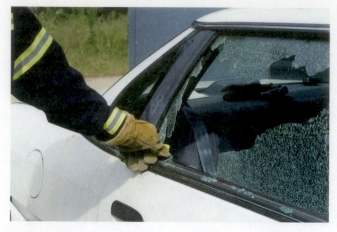

■ **Figure 30-14** Spring-loaded center punch.

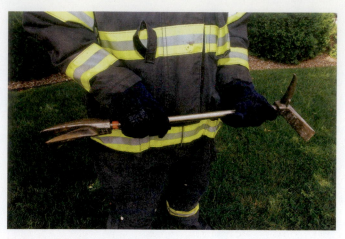

■ **Figure 30-15** EMR holding a pry bar.

Occasionally damage to a vehicle is so great that to extricate the patient the roof has to be partially removed. This is known as flapping the roof. In order to accomplish this, the windshield has to be removed. Removing the windshield can be done with an ax or a commercial device like a glass saw or a reciprocating saw (Figure 30-17 ■).

Patient extrication is a time-sensitive matter. As you may recall, the "golden hour" is one hour from the time of injury to arrival at the trauma center for the best outcome. Vehicle extrication is dangerous and should only be attempted by qualified personnel.

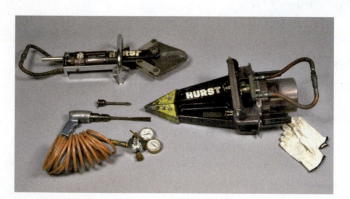

■ **Figure 30-16** Heavy rescue equipment.

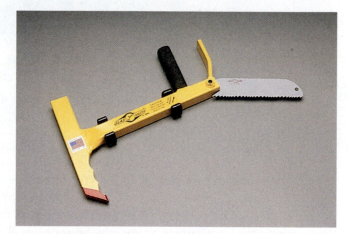

■ **Figure 30-17** Glas-Master saw.

✳ Stop, Review, Remember

Multiple Choice

Place a check next to the correct answer.

1. You respond to a motor vehicle collision where the driver is free from mechanical obstructions but you are unable to gain access due to damage to the doors on both the passenger and driver sides. You would radio into dispatch and state that the driver is:

   _____ a. pinned.

   _____ b. stuck.

   _____ c. free.

   _____ d. entrapped.

2. Before extrication can begin, you must stabilize the vehicle. To stabilize a vehicle with damage to the right front passenger side, you would most likely place _____ under the frame of the vehicle before you begin extrication.

_____ a. cribbing

_____ b. wheel chocks

_____ c. air bags

_____ d. nothing (you don't need to stabilize the vehicle)

3. When providing care to a patient in a motor vehicle collision who is entrapped in the vehicle, you should have appropriate personal protective equipment on. This would include:

_____ a. firefighting gloves and a helmet.

_____ b. non-latex gloves and a firefighting coat.

_____ c. non-latex gloves, helmet, and firefighting coat, pants, and boots.

_____ d. non-latex gloves, helmet, eye protection, and firefighting coat, pants, and boots.

4. The time from when the incident occurs to when the patient should be at the trauma center in order to have the best chance of survival is the:

_____ a. platinum ten.

_____ b. golden hour.

_____ c. titanium ten.

_____ d. silver hour.

5. You are preparing to use a center punch to gain access to a vehicle. The mother of an infant accidentally locked her keys in the car. The temperature is over 100 degrees and the infant is in a center-mounted rear-facing car seat. You should use the center punch on the:

_____ a. rear window.

_____ b. rear driver's or passenger's side window.

_____ c. front windshield.

_____ d. front driver's or passenger's side window.

Aeromedical Rescue

The use of helicopters to transport critical patients from the scene of an injury to a hospital began during the Korean War. Injured soldiers were flown to a mobile army surgical hospital (MASH) unit to receive surgical care for their wounds. This use of rapid **aeromedical transport** to a hospital greatly decreased the casualty rates compared to World War II. This led to the development of helicopter transport for civilian use, improving the outcome of trauma patients in modern times (Figure 30-18 ■).

aeromedical transport the use of a helicopter to provide quick transport of a critically ill or injured patient to a trauma center.

ASK YOURSELF

■ What are the indications for aeromedical transport?

■ What are the considerations of setting up an appropriate landing zone?

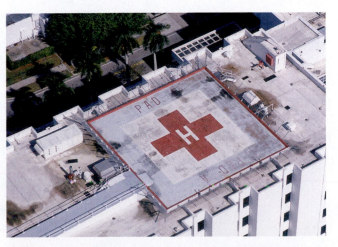

■ **Figure 30-18** Aeromedical transport—a hospital landing pad.

ASK YOURSELF

■ What are the safety considerations associated with approaching a medical aircraft?

Indications for Aeromedical Transport

Using a helicopter to transport a patient to a trauma center does have risks to the patient and the flight crew. It is therefore necessary to weigh the risks and benefits to the patient.

A patient who may require immediate surgical intervention in order to save his life should be considered a candidate for aeromedical transport. The following are reasons to consider the patient a candidate:

■ Head trauma

■ Spinal trauma

■ Chest trauma

■ Abdominal trauma

■ Heart attack

■ Acute stroke with symptom onset less than 3 hours ago

Calling for the Helicopter

You should call for the helicopter anytime you find a patient who will benefit from helicopter transport. Be sure to defer to your local protocols on helicopter transport. In general, however, most EMS systems allow for the initiation of helicopter transport by any law enforcement, EMS, or fire department personnel.

The Landing Zone

Choosing a site for a landing zone (LZ) is a task that you may assist with. The site should be a flat area at least 100 by 100 feet (Figure 30-19a ■). The best choices are a large flat field or a parking lot that has no lampposts. The slope of the landing zone should not be greater than 8 degrees. The area should be free of utility lines (Figure 30-19b ■). If utility lines are present, be sure to mark their location with lighting or even with a piece of fire apparatus. Radio the exact location and a good description of the landing zone to the pilot. Your description should include the following items:

■ Terrain—For example, "Your LZ is a large field with several large oak trees south of the field."

■ Landmarks—"There is a large water tower to the west of the LZ. The LZ is marked with fire apparatus to either side of the LZ."

■ Major hazards—"There are utility lines marked with a tanker at the north side of the LZ. Three police cars with blue light bars mark the LZ."

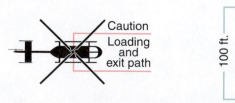

■ **Figure 30-19a** Setting up a landing zone.

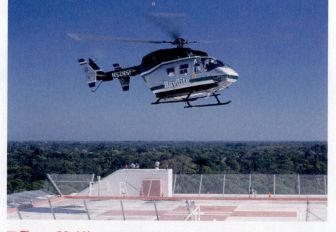

■ **Figure 30-19b** Helicopter coming in for a landing.

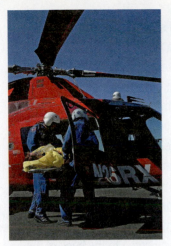

■ **Figure 30-20a** Flight crew loading a patient for transport by helicopter.

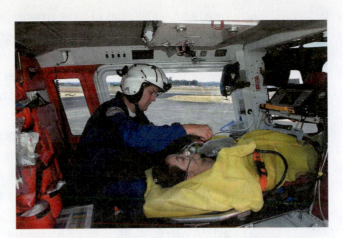

■ **Figure 30-20b** Flight crew treating a patient on board a helicopter.

Approaching the Aircraft

Allow the aircraft to land. If you are assisting with the landing zone or loading or unloading the helicopter, you must always approach from the front of the aircraft in full view of the pilot. *Never approach the aircraft from the rear around the tail rotor* (Figures 30-20a and 30-20b ■).

CASE STUDY

TRANSITION (VIA HELICOPTER)

With the help of your team, you have triaged and extricated all of the passengers from the minivan except for the driver, who remains pinned in the vehicle by the heavy damage from the truck striking the driver's side. You take over holding manual cervical spine stabilization for the patient as the team prepares for extrication.

The heavy rescue unit arrives on scene and begins the process of extricating the driver. They place blocks under the frame of the vehicle to stabilize it. Then they use the hydraulic cutting tool commonly known as the Jaws of Life to begin to cut the minivan apart. The team quickly begins to disassemble the minivan from around the patient. The passenger's side door is removed. The windshield is then cut out and the posts connecting the roof to the front of the minivan are cut. Then, the roof is flapped open. At almost the same time the dashboard is rolled back and the patient is free.

As the last of the vehicle is removed from around the patient, she is quickly moved to a backboard with your help. She is secured to the backboard and taken to a waiting ambulance to be transported to the landing zone where a helicopter will transport her to the local trauma center for surgeons to treat her injuries. The patient is loaded into the ambulance and the 2-mile trip to the landing zone begins. The patient's breathing has become shallow and slow. The paramedics ask to begin positive pressure ventilations with a bag-valve-mask resuscitator as they start an IV and prepare to place an advanced airway. The paramedic at the head places an endotracheal tube in the patient's airway and confirms placement of the tube by listening over the lungs and the stomach as you squeeze the bag-valve mask.

The short ride to the parking lot designated as the landing zone ends quickly. The paramedic begins to give his report to the helicopter crew. You continue to ventilate the patient. As you gaze out the back window of the ambulance, you watch as the helicopter lands about 200 feet from the rear of the ambulance. The flight crew exits the aircraft with their stretcher and equipment. They come to the back of the ambulance. The flight crew enters the ambulance and a quick report is given to the flight paramedic. He does a quick assessment of the patient and confirms the placement of the endotracheal tube. The flight paramedic confirms the possibility of a head injury. The patient is then transferred to the helicopter crew's stretcher for a hot load. The flight paramedic explains that the blades of the helicopter will be spinning and that you have to keep your head low to avoid injury. You approach the side of the helicopter, keeping your head low as you assist the flight crew in loading the patient. You back away and the pilot signals the firefighter in charge of the landing zone that he is ready to lift off. The last patient is now on her way to the trauma center.

■ Discussion: *Why would you choose to have this patient flown to a trauma center? What are the advantages and disadvantages of aeromedical evacuation?*

THE LAST WORD

As an EMR, you will have the potential to respond to a special operations situation at any time. Any incident where you encounter hazardous materials, mass casualties, or critical patients who require aeromedical evacuation to a trauma center for treatment will require you to call on your knowledge of special operations. Remember that you will face many additional hazards in special operations situations. Your personal safety is the most important part of any special operation.

When you are faced with hazardous materials, remember to use all the resources available such as the 704 placarding system, DOT vehicle placards, and the DOT Emergency Response Guidebook. This will help to ensure your personal safety and the safety of those around you.

A multiple or mass casualty incident is any situation where the number of patients overwhelms the resources that you have. Use the triage system to prioritize who you treat and to treat as many patients as possible.

Finally when requesting aeromedical transport, time and the patient's condition must be weighed against the risks of flying the patient. While helicopter transport provides a quick way to the hospital, it may not be the fastest, safest, or most economical way to get the patient to the trauma center.

Chapter Review

Multiple Choice

Place a check next to the correct answer.

1. A possible reason that you might consider using a helicopter to transport a patient to the hospital is:

    _____ a. head injury.

    _____ b. heart attack.

    _____ c. spinal injury.

    _____ d. all of the above.

2. Which of the following would make the best landing zone for a helicopter?

    _____ a. A hillside with a slope of 25 degrees

    _____ b. A parking lot with numerous utility lines overhead

    _____ c. An interstate highway closed to all traffic

    _____ d. A small gravel parking lot close to a store with glass windows

3. You should approach a helicopter from the rear of the aircraft.

    _____ a. True

    _____ b. False

4. Your patient has a gunshot wound to the abdomen. The patient's heart rate is 124, blood pressure is 84/55, and respirations are 24. It is 29 minutes by ground to the closest trauma center. Is this patient a good candidate for aeromedical evacuation?

    _____ a. Yes

    _____ b. No

5. Helicopters were first routinely used to transport soldiers during:

    _____ a. World War II.

    _____ b. the Vietnam War.

    _____ c. the Korean War.

    _____ d. World War I.

6. You arrive at a building for a medical call. The blue quadrant of the NFPA symbol contains the number 2. This means there is:

    _____ a. no health hazard.

    _____ b. a minimal health hazard.

    _____ c. a serious health hazard.

    _____ d. a moderate health hazard.

7. Patient decontamination occurs in the:

    _____ a. hot zone.

    _____ b. warm zone.

    _____ c. cold zone.

    _____ d. decontamination zone.

8. You are assigned to triage at a motor vehicle collision. The first patient you assess is a male who appears to be about 30 years old. He is not breathing after opening the airway. You should tag him as:

    _____ a. green.

    _____ b. yellow.

    _____ c. red.

    _____ d. black.

9. Your patient has a stab wound to the arm and the bleeding is controlled with a pressure dressing. The patient's heart rate is 90, blood pressure is 118/64, and respirations are 18. It is 50 minutes by ground to the closest trauma center. Is this patient a good candidate for aeromedical evacuation?

    _____ a. Yes

    _____ b. No

10. You respond to a motor vehicle collision where the driver of a vehicle is trapped. The dash is collapsed on his legs, preventing him from moving. You would radio dispatch and state that the driver is:

    _____ a. pinned.

    _____ b. stuck.

    _____ c. free.

    _____ d. entrapped.

11. You are observing a motor vehicle collision that involves a tanker truck with hazardous materials from a safe distance. The area directly around the incident is known as the:

    _____ a. hot zone.

    _____ b. warm zone.

    _____ c. cold zone.

    _____ d. terminal zone.

12. You respond to a call at a manufacturing facility. The patient had a chemical splashed in his eyes. The facility's response team has already begun to flush the patient's eyes at the eye wash station. You can consult the _____ for information on the chemical that the patient was exposed to.

_____ a. material safety data sheet

_____ b. DOT Emergency Response Guidebook

_____ c. bill of lading

_____ d. NFPA 704 placard system

13. An incident where patients outnumber resources is known as a:

_____ a. minor casualty incident.

_____ b. major casualty incident.

_____ c. mass casualty incident.

_____ d. heavy casualty incident.

Matching

Match the following descriptions with the appropriate term.

1. _____ The patient is free inside the vehicle but cannot be accessed due to damage to the vehicle

2. _____ Manufacturers' information about the chemicals contained in their products

3. _____ The process of disentangling a patient from wreckage or debris that prevents access to render care and transport

4. _____ The first 60 minutes after a traumatic injury

5. _____ Any substance or material in a form that poses an unreasonable risk to health

6. _____ Area where patients who have been decontaminated are brought for triage and transport

7. _____ Area where hazmat technicians dress in their level A or B suits

8. _____ Diamond-shaped sign placed on certain containers when hazardous materials are being transported

9. _____ The area directly around the incident where hazardous materials have breached their container

10. _____ A part of the patient's body is entangled in the wreckage and will require removal of the wreckage before the patient can be removed

a. Hazardous material
b. Placard
c. Material safety data sheet
d. Extrication
e. Pinned
f. Entrapment
g. Golden hour
h. Hot zone
i. Warm zone
j. Cold zone

Terrorism and Natural Disasters

✦ NAVIGATION GUIDE

The following items provide an overview to the purpose and content of this chapter. The Education Standard and Competency are from the National EMS Education Standards.

Education Standard EMS Operations (Multiple Casualty Incidents, Terrorism and Disaster)*

Competency Uses knowledge of operational roles and responsibilities to ensure patient, public, and personnel safety.

Knowledge Areas Multiple Casualty Incidents, Terrorism and Disaster
- Risks and responsibilities of operating on the scene of a natural or man-made disaster

Objectives After reading this chapter, you should be able to:

1. Define key terms introduced in this chapter.
2. Explain the EMR's considerations in personnel safety when responding to natural disasters or acts of terrorism.
3. Explain how the concepts of time, distance, and shielding apply to the approach to emergencies.
4. Recognize the possibility that responders may be targets of terrorist attacks.
5. Discuss the EMR's responsibilities in the response to terrorist acts and natural disasters.
6. Describe the considerations of the 360-degree assessment and scene size-up in terrorist attacks and natural disasters.
7. Relate each of the following steps to the response to a terrorist attack or natural disaster:
   a. Ensuring your safety
   b. Keeping distance from an unsecured scene
   c. Denying entry to the scene to those not authorized
   d. Remaining vigilant for secondary events
   e. Communicating
   f. Using the incident command system (ICS)
   g. Establishing a perimeter
   h. Having an escape plan

Key Terms Page numbers indicate first major use in this chapter. The Margin Glossary in this chapter provides definitions as you read.

personal protective equipment, p. 752

time, distance, and shielding, p. 752

protect from harm, p. 753

greater good, p. 753

360-degree assessment, p. 756

*This section of the National EMS Education Standards is currently subject to ongoing collective and cooperative review and input from all stakeholders, including the Department of Transportation, Department of Homeland Security, and Department of Health and Human Services.

NAVIGATION GUIDE (continued)

Media Resources Please go to www.bradybooks.com to access mykit for this text. You will find quizzes, critical thinking scenarios, weblinks, animations, and videos related to this chapter—and much more. Look for online information on smallpox, anthrax, and blast injuries.

ASK YOURSELF

■ Can you define key terms introduced in this chapter?

INTRODUCTION

Although very different in their nature and cause, terrorist incidents and natural disasters hold much in common for the Emergency Medical Responder (EMR). Both types of incidents can create panic and confusion. Both affect the health and safety of many patients in a relatively short period of time.

These incidents can result in hundreds of trauma patients at once due to mechanisms ranging from explosive devices in terrorist events to flying debris from a hurricane or tornado. Many patients may also suffer from medical problems from an extreme heat wave, or the release of a toxic chemical. These events can create new problems for a patient, such as heatstroke or respiratory distress, as well as worsen existing problems, such as asthma or cardiac problems (Figures 31-1a through 31–1c ■).

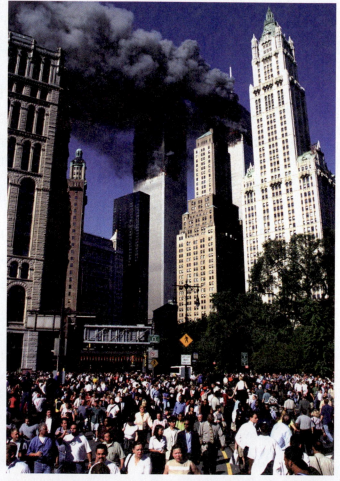

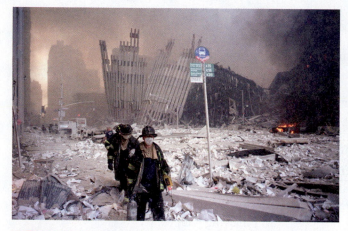

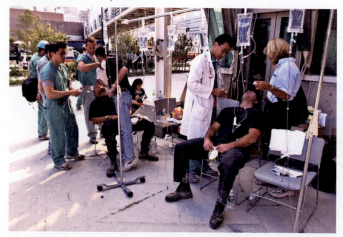

■ **Figure 31-1a** Firefighters at the destroyed World Trade Center. (© Neville Elder/Corbis)

■ **Figure 31-1b** A medical treatment center at the World Trade Center 2001 bombing. (© Orjan F. Ellingvag/Dagbladet/Corbis)

■ **Figure 31-1c** People fleeing lower Manhattan after the September 11, 2001, terrorist attack on the World Trade Center. (© Richard Cohen/Corbis)

THE CALL ✳

You have just been assigned to ride on an engine company that is stationed near an industrial complex. You and the rest of the engine company are sitting around the table just as lunch is being served when you hear the rumble of an explosion and feel the building begin to shake. Simultaneously everyone rushes outside to see a large column of smoke arise from a chemical plant about 5 miles away. Just then two more explosions rock two nearby buildings, each about a mile away from the initial incident.

A long string of dispatch tones begin to sound, and the dispatcher begins to speak: "Stations 1, 2, 3, 5, 6, and 7, Battalion Chief 1, Hazmat 1 respond to an explosion at Omni Chemical Manufacturing. Possible terrorist event. Witnesses on scene report a tanker truck crashed through the main gate, drove into the processing building, and then exploded." You feel a lump in your throat. While you are donning your turnout gear, dispatch diverts some of the responding stations to the other two explosions at two different manufacturing facilities. In both cases, witnesses report similar stories that a truck crashed into the building and then exploded.

You take your seat on the engine as it pulls out of the station. The captain calls out over the intercom to be on the lookout for secondary devices. You learned about responding to a mass casualty event while you were in class, and now it is happening.

■ Discussion: *Remember what you learned in Chapter 30. What triage equipment will be necessary?*

Personal Safety

Even with the best intentions, you and other EMRs must resist the urge to rush in and provide care too quickly during a terrorist or natural disaster. Your ability to respond, provide care, and organize during a chaotic incident will be lost if you are injured or killed. You must take certain steps to help protect yourself.

Mind-Set

The EMR must adopt the mind-set of safety first. During an incident such as a natural disaster or terrorist event, the landscape of your response area may change dramatically. Picture a terrorists' bomb exploding in or near a building. Debris, jagged metal, severed electrical wires, and ruptured gas, water, and sewer lines will lead to new and unexpected hazardous conditions. As an EMR, you must consider these obstacles when responding to such an incident, and ask yourself, "What here can hurt me?"

In the event of a natural disaster, streets, hospitals, and familiar landmarks may be flooded, demolished, or simply nonexistent. Structures, bridges, and overpasses may be unstable, and many of the same problems as in a terrorist event (such as debris and broken gas lines) can occur.

ASK YOURSELF

■ What are an EMR's considerations in personnel safety when responding to natural disasters or acts of terrorism?

Personal Protective Equipment (PPE)

EMRs can take the steps of protecting themselves with the proper use of **personal protective equipment** (PPE). The PPE selected will vary by conditions faced, but should include an approved helmet, work gloves, steel-toed safety boots, and medical exam gloves. Other PPE that may be required includes respiratory protection, such as a dust mask, particulate filter (N95 or P100), or self-contained breathing apparatus (SCBA); protective jacket and pants (such as NFPA-approved structural firefighting coat and pants); gowns and face masks; and attire for local weather conditions (such as a raincoat or winter coat).

Time, Distance, and Shielding

The EMR must balance the need for rapid response with the need to avoid becoming part of the incident. Using the concepts of **time, distance, and shielding**, EMRs can position themselves to respond as quickly and safely as possible. These concepts generally refer to radioactive materials. *Time* refers to limiting how long you handle or are exposed to the material. *Distance* is the concept of putting a minimum recommended distance between yourself and the material. *Shielding* is using a protective barrier between yourself and the material. In the case of terrorist incidents, EMRs should use the same concepts, regardless of whether radioactive materials are involved:

■ Time: Responders must have time to evaluate the safety and stability of the scene. An injured or killed responder will not help resolve the incident.

■ Distance: Incidents of this magnitude can quickly overrun a responder (for example, a fire station is not necessarily protection from a tornado or hurricane). Maintaining a safe distance will allow the EMR to carefully evaluate the whole incident, rather than just a small portion of it.

■ Shielding: In the event of a natural disaster or terrorist attack, the EMR should have preplanned protection. The EMR should know where to stage to remain safe and then respond quickly, but not become part of the incident.

Responders as Targets/Secondary Attack

Unfortunately, terrorism incidents may be nonselective and injure or kill many people, including emergency responders. Terrorist incidents have also been known to have secondary incidents that are aimed at injuring or killing emergency caregivers after the initial incident in order to disrupt the emergency services response. Figure 31-2 ■ shows several weapons that may be used by terrorists.

With natural disasters, additional events such as earthquake aftershocks, building collapses, and multiple tornadoes may occur. These events may also inflict heavy damage to responders who are attempting to provide care. It is important for EMRs to consider these possibilities and be alert for any indications of secondary events.

Patient Care Priorities

Patient care during a terrorist event is focused on providing care for a large group of patients with limited resources.

Inform the Patient of Your Actions

Emergency responders have an obligation to inform a patient of the care they are administering and to ensure the patient has given informed consent. A person who has been

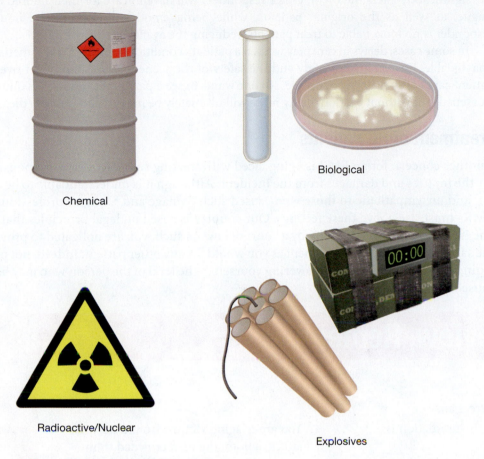

Chemical

Biological

Radioactive/Nuclear

Explosives

■ Figure 31-2 Types of terrorist weapons.

injured in a natural disaster or terrorism event will most likely be frightened, confused, and disoriented. You will provide considerable help to the patient with calm and clear information about what you are going to do to help treat him and how you will bring him to safety. Some patients may be difficult to access or be trapped by debris. One of the important aspects of care that an EMR can provide is reassurance and explanation of the activities around the patient (for example, extrication).

Protect from Harm

As emergency caregivers, we have an obligation to our patients to **protect from harm**. This skill is best determined by common sense. For example, although you may be worried about a possible neck injury, if the patient is near a burning building and in danger, it would be best to move him quickly away from that danger. Simple tasks, such as covering a cold patient with a blanket or providing shade for those in the sun, can help prevent further medical problems from developing.

Greater Good

One of the concerns many EMRs have is the delay in care that may result when responders stay clear of a scene until it is determined to be safe. You will need to make a decision that provides for the **greater good**. You might think, "I could just run and get one or two people to safety." Although this may be seen in television shows and movies, the reality is that many

protect from harm the EMR's responsibility to protect patients from further harm in certain situations, such as removing a patient from a burning building.

greater good the need to assess the scene, request adequate resources, and enter the scene when it is reasonably safe to do so to help as many patients as possible.

emergency care providers have been killed doing just that. The injury or death of a responder significantly alters the event. Other responders will have to care for their injured colleague, as well as the original patients, while being emotionally upset. The injured responder is no longer able to treat patients, reducing the available pool of EMRs.

In some cases, delays in care may worsen a patient's condition. However, it is sometimes unavoidable. Ensuring your safety and the safety of the scene will result in better overall patient care to the majority of people. No one wants to see a patient die or have his injuries worsened, but without caution, many more will ultimately be injured and possibly die.

Treatment of All Patients

Another concern for an EMR is being faced with treating someone who is responsible for the injuries and damages from the incident. Although it is understandable to be angry and unsympathetic to those who caused such damage and harm, as professionals, EMRs must rise above these feelings. Our country is based on legal principles that no one is guilty until proven guilty by a court of law. As such, you are obligated to provide the same level of care and treatment as you would for any other patient. Indeed, not providing this care would only be lowering yourself to the level of the person who may have caused the incident.

✳ ⬧ Stop, Review, Remember

Multiple Choice

Place a check next to the correct answer.

1. The best protection against radiation is:
   - _____ a. time.
   - _____ b. distance.
   - _____ c. shielding.
   - _____ d. all of the above.

2. When confronted with a mass casualty situation, utilizing your resources to treat the most patients and protect as many people as possible from injury is known as:
   - _____ a. the greater good.
   - _____ b. the most good.
   - _____ c. treating all patients.
   - _____ d. treating all serious patients.

3. Which of the following is your best respiratory protection on the scene of a structural collapse or other high dust environment?
   - _____ a. N100 mask
   - _____ b. P95 mask
   - _____ c. SCBA
   - _____ d. None of the above (You do not need respiratory protection.)

4. You are triaging victims from a terrorist attack, a bombing on a crowded train station. You find a possible suspect in the group of victims you are assessing. You should:
   - _____ a. let him die; after all he just killed over 50 people.
   - _____ b. triage him last; after all he caused his own injuries.
   - _____ c. triage him as normal, but notify a law enforcement officer quietly about him.
   - _____ d. point him out to the crowd and let them deal with him.

5. In every mass casualty event, the overall responsibility of the event is given to the:
   - _____ a. police chief.
   - _____ b. highest ranking fire officer on scene.
   - _____ c. highest ranking EMS officer on scene.
   - _____ d. incident commander.

True/False

Mark whether each of the following statements is true (T) or false (F).

1. _____ As an EMR, you should be concerned about secondary devices at any suspected terrorist attack.

2. _____ When responding to a mass casualty event, you do not have to inform your patient of what you are doing because you will have to move quickly from patient to patient.

3. _____ A tornado has just come through an open air music festival where there are between 2,000 and 3,000 people in attendance. This is an example of a domestic terrorist event.

4. _____ As an EMR, your first priority in any terrorist event or natural disaster is your personal safety.

5. _____ You are assigned to do triage on a motor vehicle collision where a tour bus has overturned. There are numerous patients. The first patient you find, an approximately 60-year-old male, does not begin breathing after you open his airway. You should black tag him.

ASK YOURSELF

■ What are the considerations of the 360-degree assessment and scene size-up in terrorist attacks and natural disasters?

■ How do you relate each of the following steps to the response to a terrorist attack or natural disaster?
  ■ Ensuring your safety
  ■ Keeping distance from an unsecured scene
  ■ Denying entry to the scene to those not authorized
  ■ Remaining vigilant for secondary events
  ■ Communicating with other responders
  ■ Using the ICS
  ■ Establishing a perimeter
  ■ Having an escape plan

Scene Size-Up

As an EMR, understanding the size and components of the scene is a key undertaking. Upon arrival at an incident, you should perform a primary assessment by deliberately walking around the scene and carefully, yet quickly, observing its features. If the scene is too large to

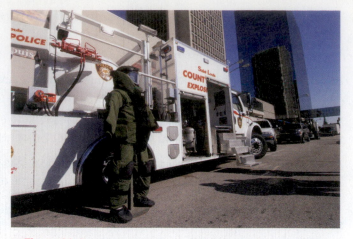

■ **Figure 31-3** A bomb technician by the bomb squad truck. (© Ray Kemp/911 Imaging)

360-degree assessment
a careful and deliberate walk around the scene scanning for dangers or hazards to all responders.

accomplish this, perform the **360-degree assessment** on the designated section you are working in, and perform a new assessment at every new area you work in. Think of it like purchasing a new home—you would not buy a new home without walking all the way around it, inspecting it for hidden problems or concerns. In much the same way, an arcing power line may be behind a pile of debris. A building may look stable on one side, but treacherous on another. Taking the time to evaluate the depth and breadth of the event is the scene size-up and can help the EMR determine the following:

- Scene hazards
- Routes of access/egress
- Number of patients
- Anticipated equipment needs

Keeping an open mind-set, coupled with a 360-degree assessment, can prevent you from having tunnel vision and attempting to access patients from a treacherous route. During the assessment, you may find a safer, and possibly easier, access route. Additionally, you may notice several ways out, should an unforeseen problem develop on the scene. These escape routes may never be needed, but will help protect responders' lives if known beforehand.

In much the same way a hazard can be hidden by obstructions, so too can the existence of ill and injured patients. During an incident that has dramatically altered the landscape (be it through an explosion or natural disaster), you may find downed trees, rubble, and strewn vehicles that obscure your ability to accurately determine the number of patients that require care. Use the 360-degree assessment to help determine the number of patients that will require care, but resist the urge to begin treating these patients; your goal is to understand the scene more completely before rushing in.

A 360-degree assessment will also give you insight into the potential equipment needed at the incident. If a hissing broken gas pipe is found, fire and utility companies will be required; a car down an embankment after a hurricane or earthquake may require a rope rescue team.

Determine Number of Patients

You will estimate the approximate number of patients. Although this will not be 100 percent accurate, a rough idea is the most important (2 versus 20, for example). As noted in Chapter 30, a multiple casualty incident (MCI) protocol should be implemented anytime the number of patients exceeds the abilities of the system to assess, treat, and transport those patients. Thus, an MCI can vary in the number of patients and is based on system resources being overwhelmed.

Evaluate Need for Additional Resources

The EMR may be tempted to dive in to patient care too quickly during a large-scale emergency. After ensuring their own safety, EMRs must make a quick, initial determination of any additional resources needed—additional EMS providers, police and fire department response, or utility company response (such as gas, water, and electric companies). The EMR is not expected to be an expert in knowing all of the specific resources required for an incident, but rather someone who knows when to ask for an expert. Generally, the sooner into an incident this assistance is requested, the sooner these experts will be able to offer assistance and positively impact the EMS operations on scene (Figure 31-3 ■). Although there may be many patients in need of medical care, you must take a moment to evaluate any needs the scene has. As an EMR, you may very well be the first on the scene of an incident. Taking the extra minute to call for help and being as specific as possible will substantially increase the success and effectiveness of the emergency response as a whole. A radio report of "EMR 1 is on scene with a lot of people hurt and I need help" is not nearly as helpful as "EMR 1 is on scene with a school bus that has crashed into a house and there are approximately 20 people injured." If your dispatch center is prepared, it should be able to dispatch ambulances, fire equipment, and police units from this report. If it requires more specific information, you may need to follow up with "Please dispatch ten ambulances, an extrication unit, a fire engine, and the police department to the scene." Make sure you know what information a dispatcher will need from your initial radio report and requests.

Initial Actions—The "No Approach" Method

The EMS team should adopt the "no approach" method during the initial response to a terrorist or other disaster incident. In most cases, the EMR will not be equipped to determine the overall safety of incidents that involve such problems as hazardous materials, weapons of mass destruction, building collapse, and nuclear incidents. The EMR should initially stop short of the scene, so as not to become a part of the problem. The distance that the EMR should stay away from the scene varies with the type of incident. A cloud of toxic gas will require a greater distance away from its release point as compared to a house that has collapsed from an earthquake.

Along with maintaining a safe distance, the EMR should prevent those unauthorized and untrained from entering the scene. Although these people's intentions may be good, the potential is far too high for injury to allow them into a situation they are unprepared for. Establishing a perimeter around an incident can help prevent the entry of people who may otherwise be injured and become part of the problem. Perimeters should be set far enough away from the incident to allow emergency responders space to work, and to protect the public.

On a large-scale incident, the police department or the military may handle perimeter control, as the size may easily overwhelm one or two people. Barrier tape works well as an initial method to define a barrier, but may eventually be ignored, fall, or be knocked down by inclement weather. The best perimeter control is vigilance and the human eye. Denying entry may be as simple as telling someone not to enter an area because of safety concerns. For those who continue to enter a scene, law enforcement is sometimes required and should be available. By these actions, the EMR is preventing further injuries and complications to an incident. The EMR should wait until the scene is secured by appropriately trained teams. Only after the area is deemed safe, the EMR can enter and begin providing medical care to any patients.

The sooner an incident command system (ICS) is put into place, the better organized the incident will be. Review the information in Chapter 30 on ICS and the National Incident Management System (NIMS).

Secondary Events

As mentioned earlier in this chapter, secondary terrorist actions have been aimed at emergency caregivers to further create panic. Natural disasters, and even terrorism incidents that do not target emergency responders, may have secondary events that can kill or injure more patients or care providers. The collapse of buildings after tornadoes; roadway collapse from flooding; and fire, electrical, and gas hazards are just some of the problems that will at best complicate operations, and at worst will injure or kill many emergency responders.

As an EMR, you should look for suspicious objects, vehicles, devices, odd-colored smoke, and unauthorized personnel at all times. Use your common sense and listen for noises of cracking, hissing, or collapsing. Watch for visible hazards, shifting buildings, and suspicious activities. Also watch for outward signs of biological, nuclear, incendiary, chemical, and explosive (B-NICE) weapons. You may help self-administer or administer to other EMS providers a biological weapon or nerve agent antidote such as DuoDote (Figures 31-4a and 31-4b ■). The administration is similar to that of an Epi-Pen and should be disposed in the same manner.

Communicate with Other Responders

A terrorism incident or natural disaster will almost always bring a large response from a variety of services. Initial responders will generally include local EMS, fire, and police agencies. As an incident progresses, more agencies will need to become involved, such as federal and

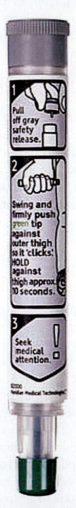

■ Figure 31-4a Example of a DuoDote kit—front, used to treat patients affected by a biological weapon, *(DuoDote™ is a trademark of Meridian Medical Technologies™, Inc.)*

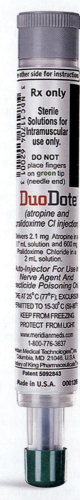

■ Figure 31-4b DuoDote kit—back. *(DuoDote™ is a trademark of Meridian Medical Technologies™, Inc.)*

state law enforcement agencies, the Federal Emergency Management Agency (FEMA), and military response teams (National Guard, bomb disposal teams, and others). These services will respond with their own specific goals and tasks, all of which will relate to the overall incident. Proper communication between these agencies can benefit the overall operation. For example, one of law enforcement's tasks is to gather evidence at a terrorism event. If a law enforcement officer knows of a piece of evidence he does not want disturbed, communication with the EMR can help prevent the EMR from inadvertently altering that evidence. Additionally, if the EMR needs to move a piece of evidence to provide patient care, communication with the police agency will also serve to resolve the incident. In a large-scale incident, many organizations will be involved, and communication without a plan would be chaotic and ineffective. Remember federal law enforcement agencies will lead the investigation, but they will utilize state and local agencies to help gather evidence and investigate the scene.

Stop, Review, Remember

Multiple Choice

Place a check next to the correct answer.

1. You have just responded to a motor vehicle collision and you are performing your 360-degree scene size-up. What are you looking for?

   _____ a. Scene hazards

   _____ b. Number of patients

   _____ c. Anticipated equipment needs

   _____ d. All of the above

2. The best way to manage a terrorist attack, disaster, or any mass casualty event is to utilize the:

   _____ a. START triage system.

   _____ b. National Incident Management System (NIMS).

   _____ c. incident command system (ICS).

   _____ d. Federal Emergency Management Agency (FEMA).

3. In the event of a terrorist attack you should adopt the "no approach" method, which is to:

   _____ a. wait for law enforcement to secure the scene and check for secondary devices.

   _____ b. wait for the hazmat team to assess the scene for the presence of hazardous materials.

   _____ c. stop short of the scene so as not to become part of the problem, relay a detailed scene size-up, and secure the scene.

   _____ d. immediately enter the scene and begin to help the victims.

4. You are completing a 360-degree scene assessment of a motor vehicle collision. Which of the following scenes would require additional resources?

   _____ a. A loaded 15-passenger van has collided with a dump truck.

   _____ b. A delivery truck has struck a large oak tree and the driver is pinned in.

   _____ c. A minivan with seven passengers has struck a pickup truck at 50 mph.

   _____ d. All of the above are scenes where additional resources could be required.

5. _____ is the key for overall effective management of any type of mass casualty event by all agencies involved.

   _____ a. Communication

   _____ b. Control

   _____ c. Command

   _____ d. Cooperation

True/False

Mark whether each of the following statements is true (T) or false (F).

1. _____ When you arrive on the scene of a mass casualty event, one of the first actions you should take is to deny entry to the scene to all but trained essential personnel.

2. _____ The incident command system spreads responsibility for the incident to all personnel represented at the scene.

3. _____ When responding to any incident, the most experienced responder usually assumes the role of initial incident commander.

4. _____ When arriving on any scene where the number of patients exceeds your ability to treat and transport them, you should implement the MCI protocol.

5. _____ Triage of patients in an MCI should begin after scene safety has been ensured.

CASE STUDY

TRANSITION

As the sun begins to set, you survey the scene. The main processing building at Omni Chemical is a pile of rubble. You look over the triage areas as you review the counts from the day: 44 green-tagged patients, 16 yellow-tagged patients, and 9 red-tagged patients were transported from the scene. In total, you triaged, decontaminated, and transported 69 patients from the scene. In the black triage zone, 22 body bags line the area taped off by the black scene tape. You believe that number will grow. There are 11 personnel unaccounted for who were working in the main processing building.

Feelings of frustration and anger arise in you. You just don't understand why someone would do this. What did these people do to deserve this kind of senseless attack? They just make chemicals used in health and beauty aids here. As the futility of the incident sets in, you notice a line of four black sedans with government plates being let through the police barricade. The FBI has arrived.

You have just spent the last 9 hours helping to manage chaos that ensued. Now you must spend the next few hours helping the FBI begin to piece together the evidence to try to determine who did this and why.

■ Discussion: *How will you deal emotionally with the aftermath of this scene?*

THE LAST WORD

Your response to a natural disaster or terrorist incident will be critical to the care and treatment of many injured people. Always keep in mind the following steps:

1. Ensure your safety and wear proper protective equipment.
2. Remain a safe distance away from an unsecure scene.

3. Deny entry to the scene to those who are untrained/unauthorized.
4. Remain vigilant for secondary events.
5. Communicate with other emergency responders.
6. Use the incident command system as soon as possible.
7. Establish a perimeter.
8. Establish an escape plan.

Chapter Review

Multiple Choice

Place a check next to the correct answer.

1. During a structural collapse where there are multiple patients, you may need to evacuate patients from an area where more debris could fall. Is it OK to do this with minimal or no spinal immobilization precautions?

_____ a. Yes, you do not have to follow treatment protocols during an MCI.

_____ b. No, you should never enter an area where debris may fall.

_____ c. Yes, you are protecting the patients from further harm.

_____ d. No, you should never move a patient who may be injured without spinal immobilization precautions.

2. Triage at an MCI begins by finding all the patients who can be _____ tagged.

_____ a. green

_____ b. yellow

_____ c. red

_____ d. black

3. The investigation of a possible terrorist attack would fall under the auspices of:

_____ a. local law enforcement.

_____ b. federal law enforcement.

_____ c. state law enforcement.

_____ d. military law enforcement.

4. You are responding to an explosion at a large manufacturing facility that covers several hundred acres. Due to the size of the event, you are unable to complete a full 360-degree assessment of the entire facility. What should you do?

_____ a. Stop and wait until a battalion chief arrives.

_____ b. Enter the scene and report to all other arriving units what you find.

_____ c. Do not enter the scene. Instead begin a 360-degree assessment of the entire facility.

_____ d. Perform the 360-degree assessment on the section you are going to be working in and notify dispatch to inform other responding units to assess their own sections.

5. When competing a 360-degree assessment of the scene, what should you do after estimating the number of patients as close as possible?

_____ a. Radio the hospital and have off-duty staff called in.

_____ b. Radio dispatch, initiate the MCI plan, and request an appropriate number of transport ambulances.

_____ c. You do not need to estimate the number of patients. Just have dispatch send you all of the ambulances they have.

_____ d. Radio all of the surrounding counties and request mutual aid.

Fill in the Blank

1. Using scarce resources to help the most people in the event of a mass casualty incident is an example of benefiting the _____ _____.

2. In the event of an incident where you are unsure it is safe to approach or radioactive or nuclear materials are involved, _____, _____, and _____ are your best protection.

3. When responding to a structural collapse where there is a lot of debris, the minimal level of PPE should include helmet, gloves, goggles or safety glasses, _____, and approved structural firefighting gear.

4. The _____ _____ _____ is a system to provide a flexible framework for organizing the chaos of running an incident and putting all of the responders on the same page.

5. _____ _____ is a careful and deliberate walk around the scene of an event and is the first step in beginning to manage any type of natural disaster or terrorist event.

Critical Thinking

1. What are some hazards that could be detected on a 360-degree assessment of a tornado that demolished a strip mall?

   _____

   _____

   _____

2. What are some feelings that you might experience if you had to respond to a natural disaster (such as a tornado or flood) that devastated your community?

   _____

   _____

   _____

3. What are some feelings that you might experience if you had to respond to a terrorist attack in your community?

   _____

   _____

   _____

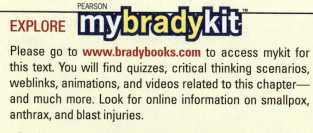

EXPLORE PEARSON mybradykit™

Please go to www.bradybooks.com to access mykit for this text. You will find quizzes, critical thinking scenarios, weblinks, animations, and videos related to this chapter— and much more. Look for online information on smallpox, anthrax, and blast injuries.

Register your access code from the front of your book by going to www.bradybooks.com and selecting the mykit links.

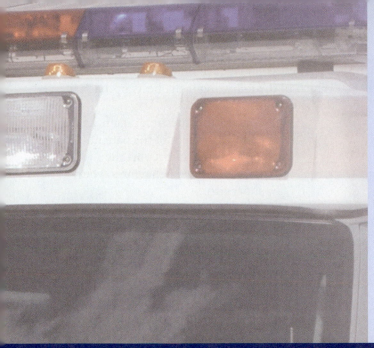

SECTION 7

Review and Practice Examination

Assess what you have learned in this section by checking the best answer for each multiple-choice question. When you are done, check your answers against the key provided in Appendix B.

1. While doing your routine vehicle check at the beginning of your shift, you notice that the engine oil level is slightly low. You should:
   _____ a. notify dispatch that you are out of service.
   _____ b. consult with your supervisor.
   _____ c. go out of service until maintenance can be performed.
   _____ d. add an approved engine oil.

2. Vehicle tire pressure, emergency lights and siren, and brake lights should all be checked at least:
   _____ a. on every call.
   _____ b. daily.
   _____ c. weekly.
   _____ d. monthly.

3. The best way to manage radio communications while driving is to:
   _____ a. steer with the left hand and hold the radio microphone with the right hand.
   _____ b. have your partner use the radio while you drive.
   _____ c. clip the portable radio microphone to your right shoulder.
   _____ d. keep the microphone in your right hand and keep both hands on the steering wheel.

4. While responding to an emergency call with your lights and siren on, you collide with a vehicle that does not yield the right-of-way to you at an intersection. The driver of the other vehicle is injured. Which of the following statements regarding this situation is most accurate?
   _____ a. You could face both civil and criminal liability.
   _____ b. The driver may sue for his injuries, but you cannot receive a traffic citation.
   _____ c. You are protected from both criminal and civil liability.
   _____ d. You can be ticketed, but you are protected from lawsuits.

5. Which of the following is the best example of failure to exercise due regard for others while operating an emergency vehicle?
   _____ a. Proceeding through a red light after checking that the intersection is clear
   _____ b. Sending a text message while driving
   _____ c. Driving 10 miles per hour over the posted speed limit
   _____ d. Passing other vehicles on their left

6. When approaching the scene of a motor vehicle collision, it is best to park your vehicle:
   _____ a. upwind from the damaged vehicles.
   _____ b. downhill from the damaged vehicles.
   _____ c. across lanes of oncoming traffic.
   _____ d. immediately next to the most seriously damaged vehicle.

7. You are responding to a motor vehicle collision. As you select your personal protective equipment, which of the following will you give the *lowest* priority?
   _____ a. Standard Precautions
   _____ b. Turnout gear
   _____ c. An N95 respirator
   _____ d. A reflective safety vest

8. You are responding to a residence on a call for a sick child with a fever. As you prepare to enter the scene, which of the following will you give the *highest* priority?
   _____ a. Gloves
   _____ b. Turnout gear
   _____ c. Reflective safety vest
   _____ d. N95 respirator

9. Upon approaching a house on a medical call, you are disturbed by the behavior of the person greeting you at the door, but you can't quite put your finger on what is bothering you. There are no weapons visible and no obvious signs of danger. The person tells you his "buddy" is down in the basement and he doesn't know what is wrong with him. Which of the following would be the best course of action?
   _____ a. Tell the person that you forgot something in your vehicle. Return to the vehicle and request law enforcement.
   _____ b. Proceed to the basement, but make sure the person is in front of you, instead of behind you.
   _____ c. Tell the person that you will need to wait with him on the porch until the ambulance arrives.
   _____ d. Tell the person you will need him to wait on the porch for the ambulance and ask him to direct you to the basement stairs.

10. After assessing a 79-year-old man with chest pain and administering oxygen to him, you give a report to the incoming ambulance crew. The EMT approaches the patient and asks the same questions you just gave him information about. Which of the following is the best approach in this situation?
    _____ a. Answer the questions again, as the EMT asks them of the patient.
    _____ b. Say nothing, but report the unprofessional behavior to your supervisor.
    _____ c. Recognize that patients may add or change information when asked the same question a second time.
    _____ d. Assume that you left out some important questions and apologize for not getting a better history.

11. Which of the following best explains the purpose of the National Incident Management System (NIMS)?
    _____ a. Its use is reserved for incidents in which terrorism is suspected.
    _____ b. It provides an organized, systematic method of managing resources and operations at large-scale incidents.
    _____ c. It provides a federal-level response to all large-scale incidents.
    _____ d. It allows for an identical response to every large-scale incident.

12. The defined interaction and organization of multiple groups and agencies who may respond to a large-scale incident is part of the _____ component of NIMS.
    _____ a. command and management
    _____ b. communications and information management
    _____ c. supporting technologies
    _____ d. ongoing management and maintenance

13. The person who has overall responsibility for the management of an incident is called the:
    _____ a. unified command.
    _____ b. operations sector.
    _____ c. incident commander.
    _____ d. logistics chief.

14. Which of the following is part of a typical element of the incident command system (ICS) structure?
    _____ a. Continuous quality improvement
    _____ b. Logistics section
    _____ c. Medical control
    _____ d. Air medical support

15. Which of the following best describes the role of the EMR in NIMS and ICS?
   _____ a. The EMR must be able to perform in any group or section assigned.
   _____ b. The EMR must be able to take incident command at any kind of incident.
   _____ c. The EMR must know the terms used in association with NIMS and ICS, but is not expected to work within the system.
   _____ d. The EMR must understand the structure and how to work within it.

16. Which of the following statements is true regarding public safety agencies' use of NIMS/ICS?
   _____ a. It is federally mandated that all agencies use NIMS/ICS.
   _____ b. Systems that do not use NIMS/ICS are not eligible for federal funding for the response to domestic incidents.
   _____ c. The only reason to use NIMS/ICS is to obtain federal funding.
   _____ d. Only supervisory personnel must be trained in NIMS/ICS.

17. When setting up an ICS, a manageable span of control is ideally no more than _____ elements.
   _____ a. three
   _____ b. five
   _____ c. seven
   _____ d. nine

18. Which of the following best explains the concept of unity of command in the ICS?
   _____ a. Each person reports to only one supervisor.
   _____ b. All agencies work together.
   _____ c. Each supervisor has no more than three to seven elements of responsibility.
   _____ d. It promotes the use of common terminology.

19. A hazardous material can be defined as:
   _____ a. any substance that is poisonous to human beings.
   _____ b. any substance transported by rail or highway in large quantities.
   _____ c. dangerous chemicals.
   _____ d. substances that pose an unreasonable risk to health, safety, and property.

20. A system of placards to identify hazardous substances being moved from one location to another has been developed by the:
   _____ a. Department of Homeland Security.
   _____ b. Department of Health and Human Services.
   _____ c. Department of Transportation.
   _____ d. National Fire Protection Association.

21. Identification numbers on hazardous material placards used in the transportation industry can be referenced to important information in the:
   _____ a. Emergency Response Guidebook.
   _____ b. material safety data sheet.
   _____ c. NFPA 704 system.
   _____ d. shipping papers.

22. An NFPA 704 placard would most likely be found on which of the following?
   _____ a. A tanker truck hauling gasoline
   _____ b. A liquid oxygen storage tank at a hospital
   _____ c. A railroad tank car full of ammonia
   _____ d. A cargo container of bleach on a ship

23. The blue area of an NFPA placard contains information about the _____ risk posed by the substance.
   _____ a. fire
   _____ b. explosion
   _____ c. water reactivity
   _____ d. health

24. In which of the following areas of an NFPA 704 placard would you find information on the potential for a substance to react or explode?
   _____ a. Top
   _____ b. Bottom
   _____ c. Right side
   _____ d. Left side

25. The highest level of risk posed by a substance is represented in the NFPA placard system by the number:
   _____ a. 0.
   _____ b. 1.
   _____ c. 3.
   _____ d. 4.

26. Material safety data sheets apply to hazardous materials when they:
   _____ a. pose minimal risk to health.
   _____ b. are transported by air.
   _____ c. are stored on military bases.
   _____ d. are used in the workplace.

27. You have responded to a report of a person who got a chemical in his eyes at work. Your first action should be to:
_____ a. irrigate the eyes with copious amounts of water.
_____ b. find the MSDS.
_____ c. ensure there is no risk of additional exposure to the chemical.
_____ d. call the fire department.

28. The EMR without additional training in the handling of hazardous materials operates in the _____ zone of a hazardous materials incident.
_____ a. cold
_____ b. cool
_____ c. warm
_____ d. hot

29. The process of removing a hazardous material from a patient's body is called:
_____ a. neutralization.
_____ b. decontamination.
_____ c. detoxification.
_____ d. lavage.

30. You are an EMR in a rural county of 450 square miles that has two centrally located transporting ambulances. Which of the following would be an MCI in this setting?
_____ a. A head-on crash between a van and a motorcycle with seven patients
_____ b. A carbon monoxide exposure involving three critical and two stable patients
_____ c. A nursing home fire with 15 minor injuries
_____ d. All of the above

31. The National Incident Management System uses the _____ system of triage.
_____ a. START
_____ b. OPQRST
_____ c. SAMPLE
_____ d. I-STAT

32. JumpSTART is a modified approach to triage used for _____ patients.
_____ a. medical
_____ b. pediatric
_____ c. burned
_____ d. unresponsive

33. You have responded to the scene of a restaurant/nightclub fire with at least two dozen seriously injured patients. Upon assessing the first adult patient you come to, you discover that he is not breathing and does not have a pulse. You should immediately:
_____ a. give two breaths, perform CPR for one minute, and recheck the breathing and pulse.
_____ b. apply the AED.
_____ c. move on to the next patient.
_____ d. request a paramedic to your location.

34. You have responded to a day care center struck by a tornado. You have at least 30 injured patients, mostly children. Your first patient is about 12 months old. You open the airway and find that he is not breathing. You should immediately:
_____ a. move on to the next patient.
_____ b. check a pulse.
_____ c. start rescue breathing.
_____ d. tag the patient as *immediate*.

35. In an MCI, which of the following patients would have the *lowest* priority for treatment and transport?
_____ a. A 33-year-old male has an open fracture of his right femur. He is awake and bleeding is controlled. He is anxious and complaining of pain, demanding that he be transported next.
_____ b. A 23-year-old female is approximately 8 months pregnant. She is not breathing and does not have a pulse.
_____ c. A 60-year-old male is unresponsive, but is breathing 12 times per minute and has a heart rate of 68.
_____ d. A 40-year-old female does not appear to have any physical injuries, but she is badly disturbed by the incident and is wandering around and crying hysterically.

36. You will be in the back seat of a vehicle, maintaining the patient's cervical spine alignment and airway during extrication. Which of the following must you be wearing to safely accomplish this task?
_____ a. Latex gloves
_____ b. N95 respirator
_____ c. Helmet
_____ d. Reflective safety vest

37. Upon arriving at the scene of a motor vehicle collision, you find that an unrestrained patient has his head caught between the floorboard and the clutch pedal. You should notify dispatch and the incoming units that the patient is:
_____ a. pinned.
_____ b. entrapped.
_____ c. extricated.
_____ d. disentangled.

38. Which of the following would be used to stop a vehicle on its wheels from rolling?
_____ a. Cribbing
_____ b. Stop chock
_____ c. Halligan bar
_____ d. Hurst tool

39. You have just arrived at the scene of a motor vehicle collision. There are two vehicles involved. A man is standing next to a vehicle on its wheels, holding a towel to a cut on his forehead. He says he was alone. The second vehicle, a small SUV, is on its side, and you can see movement inside. There is no obvious fire, no leaking fluids, no downed power lines, and no other immediately obvious dangers. Other units are already en route. The next thing you should do is:
_____ a. try to open the rear hatch of the second vehicle.
_____ b. notify dispatch that the patient is pinned.
_____ c. check the stability of the second vehicle.
_____ d. break the windshield glass by using a spring-loaded punch in a lower corner.

40. The best way to remove a windshield during extrication is to use a:
_____ a. spring-loaded center punch.
_____ b. Hurst tool.
_____ c. reciprocating saw.
_____ d. Halligan bar.

41. You have determined that there are no initial dangers at the scene of a motor vehicle collision involving a new BMW. The female driver of the vehicle is still sitting in the driver's seat. She is awake, but seems to be confused. You attempt to open the driver's door, but it seems to be locked. Which of the following would be safest, most efficient, and most likely to be successful?

_____ a. Ask if the patient can unlock the door.
_____ b. Open the back door behind the driver.
_____ c. Use a spring-loaded punch to break the driver's window so you can unlock the door.
_____ d. Use a pry bar to open the driver's door.

42. True or False: Air medical transport is always the best way to transport critically injured patients to a trauma center.
_____ a. True
_____ b. False

43. Which of the following is the best direction from which to approach a helicopter when assisting with air medical transport?
_____ a. From the high side of a slope
_____ b. From the rear
_____ c. In full view of the pilot
_____ d. From the downwind side

44. For which of the following patients would air medical resources be best used?
_____ a. A 7-year-old terminally ill cancer patient with difficulty breathing
_____ b. A 50-year-old motorcyclist who crashed without a helmet and seems to have a severe head injury
_____ c. A 14-year-old skateboarder who has an open fracture of his right forearm
_____ d. A 25-year-old unresponsive diabetic

45. Which of the following can create difficulties for EMRs responding to natural disasters or incidents of terrorism?
_____ a. Roads and streets may be impassable.
_____ b. Scene hazards are harder to predict than on routine calls.
_____ c. The resources needed, such as hospitals, may not be accessible.
_____ d. All of the above.

46. The most important considerations in protecting oneself from radiation hazards are:
_____ a. time, distance, and shielding.
_____ b. amount, type, and area.
_____ c. stability, wind direction, and dose.
_____ d. recognition, decontamination, and follow-up care.

47. You have responded to a report of an explosion at a coffee shop. When considering how to approach the scene, the first concern is:

_____ a. how many potential patients there are.

_____ b. the possibility of a second explosion.

_____ c. the types of injuries patients receive in explosions.

_____ d. getting everyone out of the structure as quickly as possible.

48. A small tornado has torn the roof off a grocery store. Several injured patients are in the parking lot and indicate to you that there are two seriously injured patients inside. Your next step should be to:

_____ a. communicate the need for additional resources, such as utility company response or the need for heavy rescue equipment.

_____ b. assess the seriously injured patients in the building.

_____ c. triage the patients who are out of the building.

_____ d. search the building for potential additional patients.

49. A small earthquake has damaged several houses in a neighborhood. As you are surveying the scene, an anxious man tells you his neighbor is trapped inside his home and he needs your help getting him out. Which of the following is the best way to handle this situation?

_____ a. Notify dispatch that you are entering a residence for search and rescue.

_____ b. Tell the man you must wait outside but encourage him to attempt a rescue.

_____ c. Try to calm the man and tell him you will need the additional resources that are on their way to safely rescue his neighbor.

_____ d. Use your public address (PA) system to instruct the trapped man to try to free himself.

50. You are responding to a report of a woman in labor during a heavy rainstorm. The road to the patient's home is along a river and is badly flooded. You are driving a large 4-wheel drive vehicle. You should:

_____ a. travel the road slowly and carefully.

_____ b. notify dispatch to have the woman meet you at the end of the road.

_____ c. use 4-wheel drive when entering the water.

_____ d. notify dispatch that the road is inaccessible by road due to flooding.

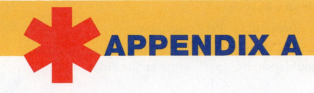

GLOSSARY

360-degree assessment a careful and deliberate walk around the scene scanning for dangers or hazards to all responders.

360-degree survey a safety measure where you survey the scene in all directions as you approach, looking for hazards.

A

abandonment leaving a patient after beginning the provision of care.

abdominal cavity the cavity that contains the stomach, intestines, liver, gallbladder, pancreas, spleen, appendix, and kidneys.

abdominal distention enlargement of the patient's abdomen due to pressure from within; typically a result of internal bleeding.

abrasion a rubbing or scraping force that penetrates and destroys the outermost layers of skin.

accessory muscle use the use of muscles in the neck, shoulder, and abdomen to assist in breathing.

acute abdomen a sudden onset of severe abdominal pain.

adolescence stage of life from 13–18 years.

advance directives legal documents giving a person's instructions on medical decisions.

Advanced EMT (AEMT) level of advanced training to start IVs and intubate.

aeromedical transport the use of a helicopter to provide quick transport of a critically ill or injured patient to a trauma center.

afterbirth the placenta, after it separates from the uterine wall and delivers.

agonal breathing infrequent, irregular gasping respirations, usually associated with respiratory/cardiac arrest.

agonal occasional and gasping, when referring to respiration.

air embolism air bubble in the bloodstream.

airborne droplets particulate matter suspended in respiratory secretions.

allergen any substance that causes an abnormal immune response or hypersensitivity.

allergic reaction an exaggerated immune response.

altered mental status condition of decreased alertness and responsiveness.

alveoli small sacs at the end of the respiratory tree where gas exchange takes place.

Alzheimer disease a progressive degenerative disease that attacks the brain and results in impaired memory, thinking, and behavior (the most common type of dementia in the elderly).

amniotic sac the sac of fluid in which the developing fetus floats; also called bag of waters.

amputation complete detachment of a body part from the rest of the body.

anaphylactic shock   another term for anaphylaxis.

anaphylaxis   a severe, potentially life-threatening allergic reaction.

anatomical position   the standard for the orientation of terms; the patient is standing and facing forward, with legs shoulder-width apart, arms at the sides, and palms turned forward.

anatomy   the study of structure.

angulated fracture   a normally straight bone that is bent due to a fracture.

anterior/ventral   toward the front.

antibodies   protein molecules produced by B cells as a primary immune defense.

apnea   no breathing.

appendicular skeleton   the arms and legs (upper and lower extremities).

arrhythmia   an abnormal electrical heart rhythm.

arteries   vessels that carry blood away from the heart.

arterioles   small arteries connected to the capillaries.

articulation   two bones moving together (as in a joint).

assault   the threat or act of physical harm.

asthma   respiratory condition causes airway narrowing/constriction.

asymmetry   unevenness.

atria   the two upper chambers of the heart.

auscultating   listening with your ears or with a stethoscope.

automated external defibrillator (AED)   a device designed to recognize fatal heart rhythms and send an electrical current through the chest to correct the problem.

automatic implanted cardiac defibrillator (AICD)   a small device that is implanted in the patient's left chest to monitor the electrical rhythm of the heart and provide a shock to reset the heart into a normal rhythm if needed.

autonomic nervous system   involuntary nervous system.

avulsion   an injury in which the force completely tears away large pieces of soft tissue.

axial skeleton   the skull, spinal column, and rib cage.

B

bacteria   organisms causing infection.

bandage compress   a dressing with a bandage attached.

barriers to communication   distractions or physical objects that impede one's assessment and care.

base station radio   mounted in a building.

battery   unlawful touching of a person.

battle sign   bruising behind the ears typically denoting an open head injury.

behavior   the manner in which we act.

behavioral emergency   any situation in which a patient's behavior is unacceptable or intolerable to the patient, the family, or the community.

birth canal   an anatomical passage made up of the cervix and the vagina.

bloody show   the plug of mucus that is discharged during labor.

blunt trauma   trauma (force) applied over a large area.

body fluids   blood, saliva, urine, and other substances produced by the body.

body mechanics   proper use of the body to lift.

boil line   point where the water below a low-head dam divides; part of the water continues downstream and part recirculates back into the boil.

bonding   the sense that needs will be met.

breach of duty   failure to perform or incorrectly performing an action.

bronchi   part of the airway branching off the trachea

burn center   hospital specializing in burn care.

C

capillaries   thin blood vessels where exchange of gases, nutrients, and wastes occurs.

capillary refill   the length of time it takes to refill the capillary beds of the skin after pressure forces the blood out of them; normal is less than 2 seconds.

carbon dioxide   a waste product of metabolism.

carbon monoxide (CO)   an odorless, colorless, tasteless poisonous gas that can be especially lethal.

cardiac arrest   the failure of the heartbeat; loss of all pumping action of the heart.

cardiac muscle   muscle type found only in the heart.

cardiopulmonary resuscitation (CPR)   timed artificial ventilations and chest compressions designed to maintain minimal circulation in a patient with cardiac arrest.

cardiovascular care center   hospital specializing in advanced cardiac care.

cataracts   opacity of the lens of the eye; among the common causes of blindness in adults.

central nervous system   brain and spinal cord.

cerebrospinal fluid   the protective liquid that surrounds the brain and spinal cord.

cervical spine   seven vertebrae forming the neck.

cervix   the neck of the uterus that connects to the uterus.

chief complaint   the main problem the patient is experiencing; why the patient has called you today.

child abuse   improper or excessive action so as to injure or cause harm to an infant or child.

child neglect   insufficient attention or respect given to a child who has a claim to that attention and respect.

chronic bronchitis   medical condition marked by a long-term accumulation of excess mucous in the lower airway.

chronic obstructive pulmonary disease (COPD)   term describing diseases which are long term in nature and cause an partial occlusion of the airway.

circulatory system   body system that delivers oxygen and nutrients to the cells, removes waste products, and consists of the heart, blood, and blood vessels.

clavicle   collarbone.

closed injury (fracture)   a broken bone that has intact skin overlying the injury.

closed wound   a wound in which the skin has not been broken.

closed-ended question or direct question   one that asks specific details or can be answered with a single word.

coccyx   four vertebrae forming the tailbone.

cognitive disabilities   impairment of thinking.

compensated shock   the early stages of shock where minimum perfusion is maintained through compensatory actions of the body such as increased heart rate and constriction of blood vessels.

concealment   a defensive position that hides your body but offers no protection.

concussion   a blow to the head that temporarily interrupts the function of the brain.

conduction   heat loss through direct contact with an object.

congestive heart failure   medical condition caused by backup of fluid in to the lungs from the heart's inability to properly pump.

continuity of care   ensuring a thorough transfer of a patient's progress and condition.

contusion   a bruise often caused by blunt force trauma; typically seen as a discolored and swollen area of soft tissue.

convection   heat loss through moving air or water passing over the body.

coronary arteries   arteries supplying the heart muscle with blood.

cover   a defensive position that hides your body, offering protection.

cranial cavity   the cavity that contains the brain.

cranium   part of the skull containing the brain.

crepitus   the grating sound made when broken bone ends rub together.

croup   a common viral infection of the upper airway, most common in children between the ages of 1 and 5 years.

crowning   the appearance of the baby's head or other body part at the opening of the birth canal.

Cushing triad   the three trends in vital signs denoting increasing intracranial pressure: decreasing pulse rate, increasing blood pressure, and abnormal respiratory patterns.

cyanosis   a bluish tint to skin, especially around lips and fingernail beds, resulting from hypoxia.

D

decapitation   injury causing separation of the head and neck.

decay   degrading of the skin and organ systems.

decompensated shock   the later stages of shock where compensation methods begin to fail due to the increasing lack of oxygen being delivered to vital organs.

decompensation   the failure of the body's steps to compensate for insult or injury.

deep   farther from the surface.

defibrillation   an electrical shock applied to the heart to correct lethal heart arrhythmias.

dementia   the loss of brain function that results in a person having impaired memory, disorientation, decreased judgment, and lessening intellectual ability; usually a progressive process.

dependent lividity   the pooling of blood in the lower areas of the body after death.

dependent   the lowest point in the body.

dermis   middle layer of the skin.

diabetes mellitus   commonly referred to as diabetes, a condition that prevents individuals from producing enough insulin or from using insulin effectively.

diabetes   common term for diabetes mellitus.

diaphoresis   excessive perspiration.

diaphragm   the large muscle that separates the chest from the abdomen and plays a major role in the mechanical function of breathing.

diastolic pressure   the pressure of the relaxation of the heart.

direct pressure   pressure placed directly onto a wound to slow or stop bleeding.

dislocation   an injury that occurs when a joint is disrupted; when a bone (or bones) that makes up part of a joint is forced out of place.

disposition   destination of a patient following your care.

distal   farther from the point of attachment (torso or trunk of the body).

distended   appearance of being expanded or swollen.

distracting injury   injury to one area that masks a more serious injury due to increased pain.

distraction   utilizing items to block or disorient an aggressor.

do not resuscitate order   written document of a patient requesting cardiac resuscitation not be performed.

dressing   a covering for a wound designed to absorb blood and wound drainage, control bleeding, and protect and cover the wound to prevent infection.

drowning   death from suffocation due to submersion.

drug abuse   the self-administration of one or more drugs in a way that differs from the approved medical or social practice.

durable power of attorney   document designating a legal decision maker.

duty to act   legal requirement to perform care.

E

early adulthood   stage of life from 20–40 years.

ecchymosis   bleeding beneath the skin; typically seen as "black and blue" discoloration as in a bruise.

eclampsia   a severe complication of pregnancy that produces seizure and possibly coma.

ejection   result of an unrestrained passenger leaving (or partially leaving) the confines of the vehicle during a collision.

emancipated minor   a minor who may receive the rights of an adult.

emergency medical dispatcher   person who is trained to answer and prioritize emergency calls.

Emergency Medical Responder (EMR)   training level to be a first responder to most calls.

emergency medical services (EMS) system   grouping of medical providers from 911 to the emergency department.

Emergency Medical Technician (EMT)   minimum training level to staff an ambulance.

emergency moves   moves done in extreme, life-threatening conditions.

emotional abuse   threatening, bullying, insults, harassment.

emphysema   respiratory disease often caused by smoking, resulting in a breakdown of the alveoli prohibiting gas exchange.

entrapment   the patient is free inside the vehicle but cannot be accessed due to damage to the vehicle.

epidermis   outermost layer of the skin.

epiglottitis   a bacterial infection that inflames the epiglottis; often resembles croup but is more serious.

ethics   moral judgments.

evaporation   the process by which sweat changes to vapor and has a cooling effect on the body.

evisceration   an open wound of the abdomen where abdominal organs, such as intestine, protrude.

exhalation   the process of air moving out of the chest cavity as the muscles used during inhalation relax.

expiration   movement of air out of the lungs.

exposure   contact with a substance.

expressed consent   when a patient gives permission for care.

exsanguinating hemorrhage   uncontrolled severe bleeding in massive volume that quickly leads to loss of total circulating blood volume.

external   outside.

extrication   the process of disentangling a patient from wreckage or debris that prevents access to render care and transport.

F

fallopian tube   one of the two tubes or ducts that extend up from the uterus to a position near an ovary.

febrile seizures   seizures caused by a rapid rise in body temperature usually resulting in a high fever.

femur   bone of the leg; largest bone in the body.

fetal position   position where the patient lies on his side with his legs drawn up and his arms across his abdomen.

fibula   smaller, lateral bone of the lower leg.

financial abuse   monetary exploitation, theft, abuse of access to the patient's finances.

flail segment or flail chest   two or more adjacent ribs that are broken in two or more places, creating a free-floating section.

fontanel   the soft spot between the cranial bones of the skull of an infant.

foramen magnum   the hole at the base of the skull where the spinal cord connects to the brainstem.

fracture   an injury that occurs when a bone is cracked or actually broken.

freely movable joints   bone joints that have a great range of motion.

frostbite   injury caused by extreme cold exposure.

G

gangrene   localized tissue death.

gastrointestinal (GI) bleeding   bleeding that occurs within the gastrointestinal tract (as in the stomach and/or intestines).

general impression   how the patient looks to you as you approach.

Glasgow Coma Scale assessment tool used to determine a person's level of consciousness based upon certain factors.

glucose a form of simple sugar that is the main source of fuel for the body's cells.

greater good the need to assess the scene, request adequate resources, and enter the scene when it is reasonably safe to do so to help as many patients as possible.

gross anatomy anatomy that looks at the structures visible to the naked eye.

H

hazardous materials substances that are harmful to health.

head-on collision vehicle struck from/at the front.

health care proxy document designating a legal decision maker for medical decisions.

Health Insurance Portability and Accountability Act (HIPAA) law regarding confidentiality of protected health information.

hematoma a large amount of bleeding beneath the skin; typically enough to raise a bluish discolored lump.

hemodialysis treatment where a patient's blood passes through a dialysis machine which filters out excess water and waste products; commonly called dialysis.

hemoglobin red blood cells.

hemostatic agent a drying agent applied to a wound to help control life-threatening bleeding.

hemothorax blood in the pleural space; can collapse the lung in the same manner as a pneumothorax.

herniation pressure forcing the upper portions of the brain downward and through the foramen magnum.

high-efficiency particulate air (HEPA) respirator or mask that filters ultrafine particles in the air.

homeostasis the body's state of balance between all the body processes.

hormones chemicals that help regulate various body systems and processes.

hospice a community-based organization that provides palliative care to terminally ill patients.

humerus bone of the arm.

hyperglycemia high blood glucose.

hyperthermia condition of higher than normal body temperature.

hypoglycemia low blood glucose.

hypotension low blood pressure.

hypothermia condition of lower than normal body temperature.

hypoxia low levels of oxygen in the body's tissues.

I

ilium major bone of the pelvic girdle; contains the iliac crests.

immovable joints bone joints that are fused together.

implied consent assuming permission of an unresponsive patient requiring care.

inadequate breathing respiration pattern not consistent with life.

incident command system (ICS)   an expandable or collapsible system that focuses on goals and objectives and uses common terms to refer to its officers.

incident command system   structure to allow for unified control of an incident.

incident commander   the person who bears overall responsibility for the incident.

index of suspicion   a general idea of how bad a person's injuries may be based upon the mechanism of injury.

indwelling catheter   a surgically implanted IV catheter for patients receiving long-term IV medications like chemotherapy.

infancy   stage of life from birth to 1 year of age.

infection   organisms invading the immune system, causing illness.

inferior   toward the feet.

inhalation   the process of bringing air into the chest cavity.

inspiration   movement of air into the lungs.

insulin   hormone that allows glucose to enter the body's cells.

insulin pump   a small device about the size of a cell phone or pager that provides a constant flow of insulin to an insulin-dependent diabetic, allowing the person to live a more normal life.

internal   inside.

internal bleeding   bleeding that occurs under the skin and is not visible externally; often occurs into the cavities of the body such as the abdominal cavity.

involuntary muscle   muscle type not under conscious control.

ischium   bone that forms the loops on the inferior pelvis.

K

kidney   organ of the urinary system that filters blood.

L

labor   the term used to describe the process of childbirth.

laceration   a cut to the skin and/or to the layers of soft tissue beneath the skin caused by a sharp object.

larynx   the voice box.

late adulthood   stage of life from 61 years and older.

lateral   away from the midline.

laterally recumbent   lying on one's side.

left   the patient's left.

left lateral recumbent   lying on left side.

left ventricular assist device (LVAD)   a temporary external device that can assist a weak or failing heart to pump blood until a donor heart can be found.

level of consciousness   a patient's responsiveness.

ligaments   structures that attach bone to bone.

liters per minute   the measure of oxygen delivery to a patient.

living will   a document in which a patient can make known his will in regard to advanced life support measures in the case of serious illness.

long axis   moving the patient while preserving the spine in-line position.

lumbar spine   five vertebrae forming the lower back.

lymph node   organ of the lymphatic system where white blood cells filter the blood.

M

mandible   movable bone of the lower jaw.

manual stabilization   using your hands to prevent movement of the head and neck.

mass casualty incident   an event that overwhelms the resources of the responders on scene.

material safety data sheet   the manufacturer's information about the chemicals contained in the product.

mechanism of injury (MOI)   the force that was applied to the patient to cause trauma.

meconium staining   greenish or brownish color to the amniotic fluid, which means the unborn infant had a bowel movement.

medial   toward the midline.

metabolism   all the physical and chemical changes that occur in the body, including digestion.

microscopic anatomy   anatomy that looks at the structures only visible through a microscope.

middle adulthood   stage of life from 41–60 years.

miscarriage   the natural loss of pregnancy before the 20th week; also called spontaneous abortion.

mobile radio   mounted in a vehicle.

modified chin lift   the chin lift used without the head tilt designed to minimize spinal movement while opening the airway.

Moro reflex   when startled, an infant throws his arms out, spreads his fingers, then grabs with his fingers and arms.

motorcycle collision   crash that involves a motorcycle and is especially dangerous due to lack of protection.

myocardial infarction   medical condition felt when a coronary artery becomes occluded or blocked.

N

narrative   the details of a provider's care of a patient.

National Incident Management System (NIMS)   a unified structure for public and private entities to work together to respond in all types of domestic incidents.

National Institute for Occupational Safety and Health (NIOSH)   as part of the Centers for Disease Control and Prevention, the NIOSH is responsible for conducting research and making recommendations for the prevention of work-related illnesses and injuries.

needlestick   accidental penetration of a needle.

neglect   malnutrition, dehydration, inappropriate clothing, soiled diapers, unsafe living conditions, soiled bedding, poor personal hygiene.

negligence   failure to follow a standard of care.

neutral position   the head is neither flexed forward nor extended back.

nonaccidental trauma   injuries caused by abuse.

nonrebreather mask   an oxygen delivery device that consists of a reservoir and a mask; designed to provide up to 90 percent concentration of oxygen to the patient.

O

O ring   a circular ring placed between an oxygen cylinder and a regulator to maintain a firm seal.

objective   factual documentation of events or conditions.

observation   assessment findings found by direct visualization.

occlusive dressing   a dressing that is made of material that is airtight and is designed to create a seal over certain types of wounds.

off-line medical direction   written physician orders directing care and assessment based on a general set of signs and symptoms.

on-line medical direction   physician orders received specific to an active patient's signs and symptoms.

one-way valve   a device that inserts into the ventilation port of a pocket face mask to prevent air and secretions from the patient from coming in contact with a rescuer.

open injury (fracture)   a broken bone that has perforated the skin overlying the injury.

open wound   a wound in which the skin has been broken.

open-ended question   one that can't be answered with a one-word answer.

orbit   the bony structure that houses the eye.

oropharyngeal airway   an airway adjunct inserted through the mouth to assist in maintaining an open airway.

orthopedic injury   an injury to the skeletal system and/or associated muscles, joints, tendons, and ligaments.

ostomy   surgically created hole where urine or feces can be eliminated from the body.

ovaries   glands storing ovum.

ovary   one of two almond-shaped glands in the female that produce the reproductive cell (the ovum).

overdose   an emergency that involves poisoning by drugs or alcohol.

ovum   the reproductive cell, or "egg."

oxygen saturation   the percentage of hemoglobin in the red blood cells that are saturated with oxygen.

oxygen supply tube   tubing that runs between a regulator and a device such as a pocket face mask to supply oxygen.

oxygenation   the levels of oxygen in the blood that will be carried to the body.

P

palliative care   a type of medicine that is concerned with providing comfort care for patients with terminal illnesses.

palmar reflex   when you place your finger in an infant's palm, he will grasp it.

palpating assessment findings found by pressing on body areas.

paradoxical breathing one side or section of the chest rising while the other side falls (as in a flail chest).

paradoxical motion movement opposite of the normal; in the chest, a section of ribs moving in the opposite direction of the majority of ribs.

Paramedic highest level of nationally recognized training.

patent an airway that is open and clear.

pathogens disease-causing agents.

patient data clinical information concerning a patient.

patient refusal see refusal of care.

pediatric assessment triangle (PAT) a method of remembering the important components of pediatric assessment: appearance, breathing, and circulation.

pediatric center hospital specializing in pediatric care.

pediatric patients patients who are infants or children.

pelvic cavity the cavity that contains the bladder, rectum, and internal female reproductive organs.

perfusion the consistent delivery of blood to adequately oxygenated cells.

peripheral nervous system nerves that transmit impulses to and from the central nervous system.

personal protective equipment may vary by conditions, but should include an approved helmet, work gloves, steel-toed safety boots, medical exam gloves, respiratory precautions for the environment, and NFPA-approved structural firefighting coat and pants. Also refers to equipment used to prevent the spread of disease.

personal space an area of approximately 3 feet around a patient where he feels comfortable.

pharynx throat.

physical abuse unexplained bruises (especially in various stages of healing), broken bones, welts, burn marks, bruises in the shape of objects (such as irons or cigarettes), hitting, shaking.

physiology the study of function.

pinned a part of the patient's body is entangled in the wreckage and will require removal of the wreckage before the patient can be removed.

placard diamond-shaped sign placed on certain containers when hazardous materials are being transported.

placenta a disk-shaped organ on the inner lining of the uterus that provides nourishment and oxygen to a developing fetus.

plasma yellowish liquid component of the blood.

platelets blood components that help with clotting.

pneumonia infection of the lungs.

pneumothorax a leak or tear in the lung causing air to fill in to the thoracic cavity.

poison any substance that can be harmful to the body.

portable radio carried on one's person.

posterior/dorsal toward the back.

posturing involuntary movement (flexion or extension) of the patient's limbs that occurs either spontaneously or in response to pain.

preeclampsia   a complication of pregnancy where the woman retains large amounts of fluid and has high blood pressure.

prehospital care report   paperwork for documenting your assessment and care of a patient.

preschool age   stage of life from 3–5 years.

professionalism   treating others as you would want to be treated.

prone   lying on stomach.

protect from harm   the EMR's responsibility to protect patients from further harm in certain situations, such as removing a patient from a burning building.

protocols   written guidelines or instructions describing assessment and care.

proximal   closer to the point of attachment (torso or trunk of the body).

proximate causation   harm caused by the action or inaction of a provider.

pubis   anterior portion of the pelvis.

public access defibrillation (PAD)   a program to distribute AEDs to lay rescuers especially in areas of high public use such as malls and airports.

public safety answering point   location where emergency calls are answered.

pulmonary ventilation   the process of moving air in and out of the lungs.

pulse oximeter   a device to measure the amount (percentage) of oxygen saturation in the blood.

pulse   the sensation of a change in pressure (a beat) in the arteries created by contraction of the heart.

puncture   a penetration of the skin that damages the soft tissue in the path of the penetrating object.

R

raccoon eyes   bruising around the eyes (similar to black eyes) typically denoting an open head injury.

radiation   heat loss involving the transfer of heat to an object without physical contact.

radius   lateral bone of the lower arm.

rear-end collision   vehicle struck from/at the rear.

reassessment   strategic ongoing assessments of the patient's condition and your interventions until the arrival of EMS.

recovery position   lying on left side to prevent inhalation of secretions.

red blood cells   blood cells that carry oxygen.

reflex   emergency nervous system response.

refusal of care   patient not permitting care.

regulator   a device that is attached to an oxygen cylinder to provide a measured flow of oxygen from the cylinder to the patient.

respiration   the process of using oxygen throughout the body and transporting the gas waste product carbon dioxide in and out of the body's cells, through the lungs, and out of the body.

respirations   heat loss through breathing.

retractions   the appearance of skin being "sucked in" between the ribs, over the clavicle, and above the sternum; indicates difficulty breathing.

retreat   moving away from danger.

right lateral recumbent   lying on right side.

right   the patient's right.

rigid eye shield   a special cup designed to protect the eye.

rigor mortis   stiffening of the muscles and joints after death.

roller bandage   a type of bandage commonly made from nonelastic material and packed in rolls; tends to cling together when rolled out onto itself.

rollover collision   vehicle that rolls causing multiple points of impact.

rooting reflex   when you touch a hungry infant's cheek, he will turn his head toward the side touched.

rotational collision   vehicle struck in a corner and/or caused to turn.

run data   administrative information such as agency and unit.

S

sacrum   five fused vertebrae forming the posterior pelvic girdle.

scaffolding   building on what one already knows.

scapula   shoulder blade.

scene size-up   the responder's impression of the overall scene.

school age   stage of life from 6–12 years.

scope of practice   rules, regulations, and laws that designate how you legally function.

secondary assessment   a second investigation to systematically assess the patient to determine what else may be wrong.

secondary injury   an injury that occurs as a result of movement after the original injury.

seizure   a sudden change in behavior or movement caused by irregular electrical activity in the brain.

Sellick maneuver   pressure applied to the cricoid cartilage that may prevent regurgitation and assist in the placement of advanced airway devices.

sexual abuse   rape or inappropriate/nonconsensual sexual touching; signs include bruising or trauma around the genitalia or anus, and torn, stained, or bloody undergarments.

shaken baby syndrome   referring to an infant or child presenting with unresponsiveness, seizure, or signs of severe internal injuries but no external signs, causing suspicion of central nervous system injuries due to shaking of the child.

shock   inadequate perfusion of the body.

side impact collision   vehicle struck from the side.

sign   a finding that is an objective or specific indication of a disease that can be observed.

Simple Triage and Rapid Treatment (START) system   a simplified system using respirations, circulation, and mental status as the basis for triage.

slightly movable joints   bone joints that have a limited range of motion.

sling and swathe   an immobilization technique formed by the combination of a sling (triangle bandage) around the affected arm and triangle bandages securing the arm to the rest of the body.

somatic nervous system   voluntary nervous system.

sphygmomanometer   a blood pressure cuff.

spontaneous pneumothorax   a pneumothorax that occurs without trauma; typically caused by a hole in the lung that occurs due to weakened tissue, typically caused by COPD and other congenital lung diseases.

sprain   an injury that occurs when ligaments that connect bone to bone are overextended and stretched beyond their normal range of motion.

Standard Precautions   use of protective equipment to prevent spread of disease.

sternum   the breastbone.

stethoscope   medical device used to auscultate or listen to noises not readily heard outside the body.

stoma   breathing hole in the neck directly into the trachea.

stomach   organ in the digestive system where material is churned with digestive chemicals.

strain   an injury that occurs when muscles and tendons are overworked or stretched and extended beyond their normal range of motion.

stroke   a condition that interrupts the blood supply to the brain.

stroke center   hospital specializing in advanced stroke care.

subcutaneous layer   innermost layer of the skin.

subjective   impressions relayed from the patient.

sucking chest wound   an open wound in the chest where air is pulled in and pushed out as the patient breathes.

sucking reflex   when you stroke a hungry infant's lips, he will start sucking.

suction catheters   devices that attach to a suction unit and are inserted into the pharynx to remove solids and liquids from the airway.

sudden cardiac death   phenomenon marked by cardiac arrest being the first cardiac symptom or arising soon after initial down time.

sudden infant death syndrome (SIDS)   the sudden death of an infant in the first year of life with no identifiable underlying cause.

suffocation   the deprivation of air exchange.

superficial   toward the surface.

superior   toward the head.

supine   lying on back, facing up.

symptom   a finding relayed to you from the patient; cannot be observed or measured.

systolic pressure   the pressure of the contraction of the heart.

T

temperament   the infant's reaction to his environment.

tendons   cords of tissue that connect muscles to bones.

tension pneumothorax   accumulated air in the pleural space that collapses the lung and puts pressure on the heart and great vessels, causing profound shock.

testicles   glands producing sperm.

therapeutic communication   conversing with a patient in a comforting and empathetic nature.

thoracic (chest) cavity   the cavity that contains the heart, lungs, great vessels, and esophagus.

thoracic spine   12 vertebrae forming the upper back.

tibia   larger, medial bone of the lower leg.

tiered response   system where EMTs and Paramedics respond separately.

time, distance, and shielding   concepts that the EMR must use to respond quickly and safely, while avoiding becoming part of the incident.

toddler phase   stage of life from 12–36 months.

tonsils   lymph nodes in the posterior oral cavity.

topographic anatomy   anatomy that looks at the external surfaces and the shapes given by underlying structures.

tort   a legal wrongdoing.

trachea   the windpipe.

tracheostomy   a surgical opening placed in the front of the neck in the trachea where a tube can be placed to provide an airway for a patient who requires long-term mechanical ventilation.

traction splint   a mechanical device that, when attached to an extremity, provides gentle pulling (traction) to help decrease pain and prevent muscle spasm.

transcient ischemic attack   signs and symptoms of a stroke that only last a short period of time. These temporary signs and symptoms may indicate a "mini-stroke." TIAs are often a warning sign of an impending stroke.

trauma center   facility capable of advanced trauma and specialty care on a 24-hour basis as governed by the American College of Surgeons.

trauma dressing   a large and absorbent dressing designed for major wounds.

traumatic asphyxia   massive blunt trauma applied over a large portion of the chest forcing blood out of the heart and in an opposite direction.

trending   charting of upward or downward patterns in vital signs.

triangle bandage   a bandage made from a large piece of unbleached cotton cut to form a triangle.

tripod position   sitting position used to assist the patient's respiration. This allows maximum chest capacity/maximum inspiration.

trust vs. mistrust   concept developed from an orderly, predictable environment versus a disorderly, irregular environment.

U

ulna   medial bone of the lower arm.

umbilical cord   an extension of the placenta through which the developing fetus receives nourishment while in the uterus.

unified command   all agencies working together to establish goals and make decisions.

unstable fracture   broken bones that are loose and uncontrolled.

ureter   tube that carries urine from the kidney to the urinary bladder.

urethra   canal that carries urine from the urinary bladder for elimination.

urgent moves   moves done quickly but providing protection.

urinary bladder   organ that stores urine.

urinary catheter   a tube placed in the bladder to drain the urine.

uterus   organ where fetus develops.

V

vaccination   injection to help prevent disease and illness.

veins   vessels that carry blood back to the heart.

velocity   speed of an object.

ventilation   the mechanical process of moving air in and out of the body.

ventilation port   the portion of the pocket face mask that protrudes up from the mask away from the patient; the site where the one-way valve is connected.

ventilator   a mechanical device that provides positive pressure ventilation to patients who are unable to breathe on their own due to disease or spinal cord injury; in the home setting, usually used on patients who have a tracheostomy.

ventricles   the two lower chambers of the heart.

Venturi mask   a mask that mixes room air with oxygen to create specific oxygen concentration percentages; often used in patients with chronic obstructive pulmonary disease (COPD) or on long-term oxygen therapy.

venules   small veins connected to the capillaries.

vertebrae   the individual bones of the spinal column.

voluntary muscle   muscle under conscious control.

W

wheezing   audible high-pitched breath sound heard when air passes through a constricted air opening.

white blood cells   blood cells that fight infection.

withdrawal   the effects on the body that occur after a period of abstinence from the drug or alcohol to which the body has become accustomed.

X

xiphoid process   the small protrusion at the inferior end of the sternum.

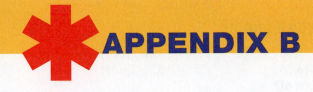

ANSWER KEY

CHAPTER 1

STOP, REVIEW, REMEMBER   (PP. 11–12)
MULTIPLE CHOICE

1. b (p. 9)
2. a (p. 8)
3. c (p. 10)
4. b (p. 9)

MATCHING

1. b (p. 9)
2. a (p. 9)
3. d (p. 9)
4. d (p. 9)
5. c (p. 9)

CRITICAL THINKING

1. It is a system where EMTs and Paramedics respond separately. (p. 10)
2. Patients most often come in contact with several components in the EMS system: personnel in human resources, transportation, and facilities. (pp. 6, 8)
3. The EMR is the first point of contact for assessment and beginning of treatment. The EMR's training is not as in-depth as the other levels, but the EMR is the important first responder to begin the assessment and lifesaving measures. (pp. 6–10)

CHAPTER REVIEW   (PP. 18–20)
MULTIPLE CHOICE

1. d (p. 8)
2. c (p. 9)
3. a (p. 9)
4. c (p. 10)
5. b (p. 10)
6. a (p. 9)
7. c (p. 11)
8. d (p. 15)
9. b (p. 16)
10. a (p. 10)

MATCHING

1. h (p. 9)
2. d (p. 10)
3. a (p. 10)
4. l (p. 9)
5. j (p. 8)
6. b (p. 10)
7. c (p. 10)
8. g (p. 9)
9. e (p. 10)
10. k (p. 8)
11. f (p. 10)
12. i (p. 9)

CRITICAL THINKING

1. Scene safety (p. 13)
2. Tiered response (p. 10)
3. Trauma center (p. 10)

CHAPTER 2

STOP, REVIEW, REMEMBER   (PP. 34–35)
MULTIPLE CHOICE

1. c (p. 24)
2. d (p. 24)
3. a (p. 24)
4. a (p. 25)
5. b (p. 26)

EMERGENCY MEDICAL RESPONDER PRACTICE

1. Not an exposure (pp. 26–27)
2. Exposure (pp. 26–27)
3. Exposure (pp. 26–27)
4. Not an exposure (pp. 26–27)

SHORT ANSWER

a. Airborne (pp. 27–28)
b. Bloodborne (pp. 27–28)
c. Bloodborne (pp. 27–28)
d. Bloodborne (pp. 27–28)
e. Airborne (pp. 27–28)
f. Airborne (pp. 27–28)

STOP, REVIEW, REMEMBER   (PP. 45–46)
MULTIPLE CHOICE

1. b (p. 35)
2. a (p. 35)
3. d (p. 36)
4. c (p. 37)
5. c (p. 44)

EMERGENCY MEDICAL RESPONDER PRACTICE

1. Do not move.
2. Move the driver to access the passenger.
3. Move the patient to the floor for airway care and CPR.
4. Move the patient to protect him from traffic.
5. Move the patient to protect him from hypothermia.

MATCHING

1. c (p. 38)
2. c (p. 38)
3. a (p. 38)
4. b (p. 38)
5. e (p. 38)
6. a (p. 38)

CHAPTER REVIEW   (PP. 48–50)

MULTIPLE CHOICE

1. c (p. 38)	6. d (p. 28)
2. d (p. 38)	7. a (p. 38)
3. c (p. 28)	8. d (p. 38)
4. b (p. 28)	9. a (p. 32)
5. a (p. 32)	10. c (pp. 38–44)

EMERGENCY MEDICAL RESPONDER PRACTICE

1. Emergency move
2. Urgent move
3. Emergency move
4. No move
5. Urgent move
6. Urgent move

SHORT ANSWER

1. The patient's weight, your abilities and limitations, the help available to you, the patient's condition, the patient's location, and the need for movement (choose three)
2. Precautions that are taken to prevent transmission of disease to the EMR. They are the same for all patients based on the potential for exposure to blood, body fluids, or airborne droplets.
3. Denial, anger, bargaining, depression, acceptance
4. Moving the patient (usually from the head) so that the spine stays in a straight line

CHAPTER 3

STOP, REVIEW, REMEMBER   (PP. 58–59)

MULTIPLE CHOICE

1. d (p. 53)	4. d (p. 57)
2. c (p. 53)	5. d (p. 62)
3. b (p. 54)	

MATCHING

1. d (p. 54)	5. b (p. 53)
2. f (p. 54)	6. e (p. 54)
3. h (p. 53)	7. g (p. 54)
4. a (p. 57)	8. b (p. 53)

CASE STUDY

1. She is able to consent for her treatment. Being a mother herself, she is most likely considered an emancipated minor. (p. 54)
2. She is able to consent for the treatment of her son. She is his legal next of kin and responsible for his care. (p. 54)
3. a. Fire chief (p. 54)

STOP, REVIEW, REMEMBER   (PP. 63–64)

MULTIPLE CHOICE

1. c (p. 60)	4. b (p. 62)
2. a (p. 59)	5. b (p. 62)
3. c (p. 61)	

TRUE/FALSE

1. T (p. 62)	4. T (p. 61)
2. F (p. 62)	5. T (p. 59)
3. F (p. 62)	

CASE STUDY

1. Breach of duty—He is required to respond to the call and therefore required to treat the patient on that call. (p. 62)
2. Proximate causation—He is required to treat the patient in a fair and ethical manner and do no further harm to the patient. (p. 62)
3. Abandonment—Once he has begun care, he must follow through until the care is passed to another medical provider or the patient withdraws his consent for treatment. (p. 62)

CHAPTER REVIEW   (PP. 67–69)

MULTIPLE CHOICE

1. a (p. 53)	6. d (p. 57)
2. b (p. 53)	7. b (p. 62)
3. d (p. 53)	8. a (p. 64)
4. b (p. 54)	9. d (p. 66)
5. a (p. 54)	10. c (p. 62)

CASE STUDY

1. Scene safety (p. 22)
2. Implied consent (p. 54)
3. No. (p. 61)
4. Request the police to remove the dangerous objects from the patient's surroundings. (p. 22)
5. Preserve any entry/exit wounds and note in detail any bruising or other findings on the physical examination. (p. 53)

CHAPTER 4

STOP, REVIEW, REMEMBER   (P. 75)

TRUE/FALSE

1. F (p. 72)	5. F (p. 74)
2. T (p. 73)	6. F (p. 74)
3. T (p. 74)	7. F (p. 74)
4. T (p. 72)	8. T (p. 74)

STOP, REVIEW, REMEMBER   (P. 79)
MATCHING

1. d (p. 78)
2. c (p. 75)
3. a (p. 75)
4. b (p. 75)
5. b (p. 75)
6. d (p. 78)
7. c (p. 75)
8. c (p. 75)

CHAPTER REVIEW   (PP. 79–81)
MULTIPLE CHOICE

1. c (p. 72)
2. c (p. 72)
3. c (p. 75)
4. a (p. 74)
5. b (p. 72)
6. a (p. 74)
7. d (p. 74)
8. d (p. 75)
9. c (p. 72)
10. b (p. 78)

MATCHING

1. b (p. 72)
2. o (p. 74)
3. c (p. 72)
4. e (p. 72)
5. f (p. 72)
6. a (p. 72)
7. g (p. 72)
8. h (p. 73)
9. i (p. 74)
10. s (p. 74)
11. j (p. 74)
12. d (p. 72)
13. k (p. 74)
14. l (p. 74)
15. n (p. 74)
16. p (p. 74)
17. m (p. 74)
18. q (p. 74)
19. r (p. 74)

EMERGENCY MEDICAL RESPONDER PRACTICE

1. Right lateral recumbent (p. 72)
2. Distal (p. 75)
3. Proximal (p. 74)

CHAPTER 5

STOP, REVIEW, REMEMBER   (PP. 90–91)
MULTIPLE CHOICE

1. c (p. 84)
2. c (p. 86)
3. b (p. 87)

EMERGENCY MEDICAL RESPONDER PRACTICE

1. Cervical
   Thoracic
   Lumbar
   Sacral
   Coccyx (p. 86)
2. Freely movable joint (p. 87)
3. Ligaments (p. 84)
4. Tendons (p. 87)

MATCHING

1. a (p. 84)
2. b (p. 84)
3. o (p. 86)
4. d (p. 84)
5. h (p. 86)
6. l (p. 86)
7. g (p. 86)
8. m (p. 86)
9. e (p. 84)
10. k (p. 86)
11. n (p. 86)
12. c (p. 84)
13. p (p. 86)
14. q (p. 86)
15. r (p. 87)
16. j (p. 86)
17. s (p. 87)
18. i (p. 86)
19. f (p. 86)
20. t (p. 89)

STOP, REVIEW, REMEMBER   (PP. 99–100)
MULTIPLE CHOICE

1. a (p. 93)
2. b (p. 95)
3. d (p. 96)

EMERGENCY MEDICAL RESPONDER PRACTICE

1. Red blood cells carry oxygen to the cells.
   White blood cells fight infection.
   Platelets help blood clot.
   Plasma transports components in the blood. (p. 96)

MATCHING

1. a (p. 84)
2. d (p. 92)
3. o (p. 96)
4. f (p. 93)
5. h (p. 93)
6. i (p. 93)
7. j (p. 95)
8. l (p. 95)
9. g (p. 93)
10. m (p. 95)
11. c (p. 92)
12. n (p. 96)
13. b (p. 91)
14. p (p. 96)
15. k (p. 95)
16. q (p. 96)
17. r (p. 96)
18. e (p. 93)
19. s (p. 96)
20. t (p. 99)

STOP, REVIEW, REMEMBER   (PP. 103–104)
MULTIPLE CHOICE

1. c (p. 100)
2. c (p. 101)
3. a (p. 101)

EMERGENCY MEDICAL RESPONDER PRACTICE

1. Epidermis
   Dermis (p. 100)

MATCHING

1. h (p. 101)
2. a (p. 100)
3. c (p. 100)
4. e (p. 101)
5. b (p. 100)
6. f (p. 101)
7. d (p. 101)
8. g (p. 101)

CHAPTER REVIEW   (PP. 108–112)

MULTIPLE CHOICE

1. b (p. 84)
2. b (p. 104)
3. d (p. 87)
4. a (p. 92)
5. b (p. 95)
6. d (p. 96)
7. c (p. 96)
8. b (p. 100)
9. a (p. 100)
10. b (p. 101)

EMERGENCY MEDICAL RESPONDER PRACTICE

1. composition of ambient air; condition of respiratory system, circulatory system, tissues and cells. Chemicals in the air may decrease available oxygen; airway obstruction, infection, and allergic reaction may impair the breathing process; blood flow diminishes if the heart pumps ineffectively; damaged tissues and cells impair ability to exchange gases, nutrients, and wastes. (p. 107)

LABEL (PP. 85, 97)

1. (A) Cervical
2. (B) Thoracic
3. (C) Lumbar
4. (D) Sacral
5. (E) Coccyx

1. (A) Clavicle
2. (B) Scapula
3. (C) Ribs
4. (D) Humerus
5. (E) Elbow
6. (F) Ulna
7. (G) Radius

MATCHING

1. j (p. 104)
2. a (p. 84)
3. f (p. 100)
4. c (p. 91)
5. d (p. 93)
6. g (p. 101)
7. b (p. 87)
8. e (p. 96)
9. h (p. 101)
10. i (p. 104)

MATCHING

1. b (p. 84)
2. f (p. 86)
3. g (p. 86)
4. i (p. 86)
5. j (p. 86)
6. l (p. 86)
7. w (p. 104)
8. n (p. 87)
9. a (p. 84)
10. p (p. 91)
11. q (p. 92)
12. m (p. 87)
13. c (p. 84)
14. r (p. 86)
15. k (p. 95)
16. s (p. 95)
17. d (p. 86)
18. t (p. 96)
19. o (p. 87)
20. u (p. 104)

21. v (p. 104)
22. x (p. 104)
23. e (p. 86)
24. y (p. 104)
25. z (p. 104)
26. h (p. 86)

TRUE/FALSE

1. T (p. 84)
2. F (p. 87)
3. T (p. 93)
4. F (p. 93)
5. T (p. 97)
6. F (p. 100)
7. T (p. 92)
8. F (p. 104)
9. T (p. 104)
10. T (p. 104)
11. F (p. 104)

CHAPTER 6

STOP, REVIEW, REMEMBER   (PP. 122–123)

MULTIPLE CHOICE

1. d (p. 117)
2. c (p. 119)

EMERGENCY MEDICAL RESPONDER PRACTICE

1. Answers may vary, but should include these points:
   - Adolescents try to achieve more independence and develop their own identity.
   - This is a time when self-destructive behaviors begin, such as use of tobacco, alcohol, illicit drugs, and unsafe driving. (p. 121)

MATCHING

1. c (p. 115)
2. b (p. 115)
3. a (p. 115)
4. d (p. 115)

CHAPTER REVIEW   (PP. 127–129)

MULTIPLE CHOICE

1. b (pp. 124–125)
2. c (p. 116)
3. c (p. 118)
4. c (p. 118)
5. c (p. 120)
6. a (p. 121)
7. b (p. 123)
8. a (pp. 124–125)
9. a (p. 125)
10. b (p. 125)

EMERGENCY MEDICAL RESPONDER PRACTICE

Living environment: Answers will vary. Can be used for class discussion on community resources.

Self-worth: Answers will vary. Can be used for class discussion on community resources.

Financial burdens: Answers will vary. Can be used for class discussion on community resources.

Death and dying: Answers will vary. Can be used for class discussion on community resources.

MATCHING

1. d (p. 119)
2. a (p. 114)
3. h (p. 125)
4. c (p. 118)
5. e (p. 120)

6. f (p. 123)
7. b (p. 117)
8. g (p. 124)

SECTION ONE REVIEW

1. d (p. 7)

   Rationale: EMRs may be volunteer or paid, and may work in a variety of settings, but patient transportation is not in the EMR's scope of practice. Regardless of the type of service or setting, the EMR's role is to provide lifesaving care in the first few minutes of patient contact while awaiting arrival of additional EMS personnel.

2. a (p. 9)

   Rationale: In order from least training to most training, EMS provider levels are EMR, EMT, AEMT, and Paramedic.

3. b (p. 10)

   Rationale: Of the many types of resources that may be available in a community, a trauma center is the specialized resource that provides critically injured patients with the best chance of survival.

4. a (p. 11)

   Rationale: Evaluation is the process of collecting data to see how the EMS system is performing and determining from the data any changes that need to be made. The medical director has a role in system evaluation, and system evaluation may be written in EMS regulations and policies.

5. d (p. 14)

   Rationale: Patient advocacy means to promote the rights of patients and let other health care providers know what the patient's needs and concerns are. Basically, advocacy is looking out for the patient's needs and rights.

6. a (p. 15)

   Rationale: Any method of double–checking or confirming information is an important means of reducing the risk of errors in patient care. There is a vast number of medications, making it difficult for any health care provider to be familiar with all medications. All levels of health care providers, including physicians, use a variety of quick reference guides to check information.

7. b (p. 16)

   Rationale: The data collected and reported by EMRs are very important in finding evidence to support practices in EMS. Evidence may also indicate that a skill that was once thought effective really is not.

8. a (p. 24)

   Rationale: The EMR should be observant to detect potential hazards, including violence, at any scene, but a large group of people is a situation that has a greater potential than the other situations described of leading to violence against EMS personnel, and if it does, you are outnumbered.

9. c (p. 24)

   Rationale: The bush might allow you to conceal yourself from sight, and retreating may be an option, but a tree would be more likely to stop the shotgun pellets.

10. c (p. 25)

    Rationale: Hazardous materials, such as chemicals and radioactive materials, are often transported in large enough quantities to pose a hazard by tractor trailer, trains, and cargo ships. Although nitroglycerin can be used in explosives, the form and amount in patient medications does not pose a hazardous materials risk.

11. c (p. 26)

    Rationale: It is not always possible to know which patients may have a communicable illness, and patients who do not immediately pose a risk of contact with body fluids may vomit unexpectedly. Therefore, a "standard" approach to patient care is emphasized for health care worker safety.

12. a (p. 28)

    Rationale: Of the various types of hepatitis, only vaccination against hepatitis B is both available and recommended for health care providers. The tuberculosis vaccine is rarely given. Instead, health care providers are usually tested for exposure to tuberculosis on an annual basis. Pneumonia vaccine is not routinely recommended for EMS personnel, but injury on the job can pose a risk of exposure to tetanus.

13. d (p. 28)

    Rationale: Patients may not know whether they have particular infectious diseases, and contact between the patient's blood and your intact skin does not constitute an exposure. The risk of infection is low, and is best prevented by thorough hand washing at the earliest opportunity. If hand-washing facilities are not immediately available, the next best step would be to clean the hands with an alcohol-based gel hand cleanser and change gloves.

14. a (p. 31)

    Rationale: You should wear eye and face protection when there is a risk of blood or body fluids coming into contact with your eyes, nose, or mouth. Of the options given, only suctioning and caring for a patient who is coughing blood would pose such a risk.

15. b (p. 32)

    Rationale: Remember, there is a difference between contact with body fluids and an exposure to body fluids. Contact with intact skin is not an exposure, but needlesticks, contamination of open skin, or contact with mucous membranes are exposures.

16. b (p. 35)

    Rationale: Like everyone else, different EMS providers can find different situations stressful. However, one of the situations listed as very stressful by many EMS personnel is calls dealing with ill and injured children.

17. d (p. 36)

Rationale: Family members can often become outwardly emotional when their loved ones are sick. This is a normal reaction, and there is nothing in the daughter's response at this point that indicates potential violence, although you should always continue to observe and evaluate the situation. The best way to handle such situations is to be calm and display empathy and compassion toward the patient and family.

18. c (p. 37)

Rationale: The symptoms described are common reactions to stress. Things that will definitely not help you cope with stress are alcohol, drugs, caffeine, and ignoring the situation. Physical activity, a healthy diet, and talking to someone—perhaps a professional counselor—are all effective ways of coping with stress.

19. a (p. 37)

Rationale: In most cases, EMS personnel are not required to begin resuscitative efforts if there are signs of obvious death, such as decomposition, rigor mortis, or decapitation. In the absence of these signs, the family's wishes usually cannot be honored unless there is a valid DNR order present for EMS personnel to inspect.

20. a (p. 38)

Rationale: Given the time elapsed since the patient and family found out that she was terminally ill, her refusal of treatment, and the husband's demeanor, it is most likely that he has reached the acceptance stage of grief, and it is unlikely that he would experience a sudden burst of anger after reaching this stage.

21. d (p. 41)

Rationale: Many back injuries in EMS personnel are due to improper lifting techniques, which include twisting or bending at the waist, and not having the feet about shoulder-width apart. Keeping your back straight and using your leg muscles are proper lifting techniques.

22. b (p. 41)

Rationale: The driver has a life threat to the airway and you must reach him without delay. An emergency move is indicated when you must move a less seriously injured patient to reach a patient with immediate threats to life.

23. a (p. 53)

Rationale: On-line medical direction means you are in voice contact with a physician by telephone or radio. This is sometimes called direct medical direction. Protocols are an example of off-line medical direction.

24. d (p. 54)

Rationale: In order to give medical consent, a patient must be 18 years of age or older and mentally competent. To truly consent to medical care, the patient must understand the risks, benefits, and options. Only in unusual circumstances are minors legally emancipated and able to give consent. In most cases, you must get consent from the parent or guardian of a patient under 18 years old.

25. b (p. 55)

Rationale: There are many situations in EMS where there is not a perfect solution, but we must make the best decisions we can, given the information we have and the time frame we must work in. Sometimes, we are making the "least bad" decision. In this case, we see the presence of alcohol and a possible indication that the patient has consumed alcohol, but we don't know enough to say that the patient is mentally incompetent and implied consent applies. Restraining the patient in these circumstances could very well lead to claims of battery and false imprisonment. Ethically, letting the patient walk away when he may be injured or have impaired judgment could be risky. Under no circumstances should an EMR transport a patient—it is not in the scope of practice. The best answer in this case is to first attempt to talk to the patient and remain nonjudgmental about the legalities and morals of his possible intoxication.

26. a (p. 59)

Rationale: In most cases, EMS personnel can honor valid DNR orders, but they must actually see the DNR and, in many cases, must then contact medical direction. If there was a delay in producing the DNR, or the nurse could not find it, then the EMR should start resuscitation.

27. b (p. 64)

Rationale: The patient is in immediate need of emergency medical care and, if possible, you must go to the patient, rather than having law enforcement move the patient. When entering a crime scene, though, take every precaution possible to avoid disturbing evidence while caring for the patient. In most cases, it is possible to provide good patient care while disturbing the crime scene as little as possible.

28. b (p. 72)

Rationale: The prefix "tachy" means rapid, and the root word or stem "card(ia)" refers to the heart.

29. b (p. 74)

Rationale: Anterior (and also the term ventral) refers to the front of the patient's body.

30. d (p. 74)

Rationale: Proximal means something is closer to the body with respect to the point of reference, while distal means something is farther away from the body with respect to the point of reference. Example: The elbow is distal to the shoulder, but proximal to the wrist. An injury between the elbow and wrist would be distal to the elbow, but proximal to the wrist.

31. c (p. 75)

Rationale: The thoracic cavity is the chest cavity, which contains the heart.

32. d (p. 75)

Rationale: Of the organs listed, only the liver lies in the upper right abdominal quadrant.

33. c (p. 84)

Rationale: Anatomy refers to the body's structure, rather than its function. Physiology refers to the body's functions, and the goal of physiology is to maintain homeostasis—a steady state of healthy conditions that the body maintains within narrow boundaries.

34. a (p. 86)

Rationale: The uppermost portion of the spine is known as the cervical spine. The term cervix means "neck."

35. b (p. 86)

Rationale: The ilia (iliac bones) make up the winglike lateral aspects of the pelvis.

36. c (p. 86)

Rationale: Anatomically speaking, the term leg refers to the thigh, which contains the femur, the largest, heaviest bone in the body. The bones of the lower leg are the tibia and fibula.

37. a (p. 87)

Rationale: A joint that allows movement in all directions, such as the ball-and-socket joint of the hip, is called a freely movable joint.

38. c (p. 87)

Rationale: Involuntary and smooth muscle refer to the muscles found in hollow organs. These muscle cells have a smooth appearance under the microscope, and we do not have to consciously think about the control of these muscles. Cardiac muscle is found only in the heart. Skeletal muscle, which appears striated (striped) under a microscope and functions under conscious control, allows movement of the extremities.

39. c (p. 91)

Rationale: The normal respiratory rate for adults is 12 to 20 breaths per minute.

40. a (p. 92)

Rationale: The larynx is the voice box.

41. a (p. 93)

Rationale: Air must pass through the nose or mouth, pharynx, larynx, trachea, bronchi, and bronchioles, before reaching the thin-walled alveoli, which are in close contact with capillaries returning blood from the body and capillaries that will return oxygenated blood to the heart to be pumped throughout the body.

42. c (p. 93)

Rationale: When the diaphragm contracts, it flattens, moving down toward the abdomen. This makes the chest cavity larger in volume. To equalize the air pressure between the atmosphere and the now-larger thoracic cavity, air flows inward through the nose or mouth.

43. c (p. 93)

Rationale: The term "cor-" refers to the heart. In this case, these are the arteries that arise directly from the aorta as it leaves the left ventricle of the heart, supplying the cardiac muscle with oxygenated blood.

44. d (p. 93)

Rationale: The left ventricle is the chamber of the heart that pumps blood throughout the entire body, requiring more forceful contraction than any other chamber of the heart.

45. c (p. 96)

Rationale: Platelets clump together when the lining of a blood vessel is damaged, forming a plug that stops bleeding.

46. a (p. 100)

Rationale: The subcutaneous layer (sub = beneath; cut(aneous) = skin) lies beneath the dermis and contains fat that provides the body with protection and gives it contours.

47. d (p. 101)

Rationale: Urine flows from the kidneys through the ureters to the urinary bladder, and out of the body through the urethra.

48. a (p. 102)

Rationale: Bladder is a general term that means "balloon." The urinary bladder is a hollow organ that expands to collect urine, while the gallbladder is a hollow structure that expands to store the bile that is produced by the liver.

49. c (p. 104)

Rationale: The lymph nodes throughout the body, including those in the neck, are part of the immune system and become swollen when they are working to fight an infection.

50. a (p. 104)

Rationale: The ovaries produce eggs, which are collected by the fallopian tubes, where, if sperm are present, the egg is fertilized and then travels to the uterus, where implantation occurs. The cervix is the lower part of the uterus, which opens during labor to allow childbirth.

51. c (p. 107)

Rationale: Perfusion, the delivery of oxygenated blood to the tissues, is necessary to cellular respiration, which provides the gas exchange needed to maximize metabolism, which, in turn, provides the energy needed to maintain homeostasis.

52. b (p. 114)

Rationale: A newborn is an infant in the first month of life, but infancy extends from birth to 1 year of age.

53. c (p. 114)

Rationale: An infant's heart rate is normally between 140 and 160 beats per minute.

54. c (p. 115)

Rationale: The startle reflex is normal in young infants.

55. a (p. 116)

Rationale: Infants have both an anterior and a posterior fontanelle that allows the head to be compressed as it passes through the birth canal and for rapid growth of the brain after birth.

56. c (p. 121)

Rationale: Adolescents are very concerned with body image, and an injury to the face can be very upsetting to patients in this age group. Her blood pressure is normal for her age, and magical thinking occurs in toddlers and preschoolers. Whether or not the patient has started menstruating is not relevant to her immediate prehospital care and will possibly embarrass the patient, especially if asked by a male EMS provider.

CHAPTER 7

STOP, REVIEW, REMEMBER   (PP. 148–149)
MULTIPLE CHOICE

1. a (p. 142)
2. c (p. 143)
3. d (p. 146)
4. a (p. 149)

TRUE/FALSE

1. T (p. 146)
2. T (p. 147)
3. F (p. 146)
4. F (p. 147)

CRITICAL THINKING

1. In jeopardy—He is gurgling on each breath. (pp. 144–148)
2. Log-roll him into a supine position. (pp. 144–148)
3. Late (pp. 144–148)

STOP, REVIEW, REMEMBER   (PP. 158–159)
MULTIPLE CHOICE

1. c (p. 149)
2. a (p. 149)
3. b (p. 152)
4. c (p. 155)
5. a (p. 158)

MATCHING

1. c (p. 150)
2. e (p. 152)
3. a (p. 149)
4. b (p. 150)
5. d (p. 154)

CRITICAL THINKING

1. Suction. (pp. 150–155)
2. Insert an oral airway. (pp. 150–155)

CHAPTER REVIEW   (PP. 178–180)
MULTIPLE CHOICE

1. b (p. 160)
2. a (p. 146)
3. b (p. 149)
4. b (p. 142)
5. c (p. 164)
6. c (pp. 171–172)
7. b (p. 158)
8. a (p. 147)
9. d (p. 170)
10. b (p. 148)

TRUE/FALSE

1. T (p. 162)
2. F (pp. 163–164)
3. F (p. 172)
4. F (p. 152)
5. T (p. 149)

CRITICAL THINKING

1. No (pp. 149–178)
2. No (pp. 149–178)
3. Nonrebreather mask (pp. 149–178)
4. Remove the nonrebreather mask, suction, resecure the airway by whatever means necessary (pp. 149–178)

CHAPTER 8

STOP, REVIEW, REMEMBER   (PP. 188–189)
MULTIPLE CHOICE

1. b (p. 184)
2. a (p. 184)
3. d (p. 184)
4. d (pp. 183, 185)
5. a (p. 185)

EMERGENCY MEDICAL RESPONDER PRACTICE

1. List any four of the following:
   a. Unresponsive mental status
   b. Airway compromise
   c. No breathing;
   d. cyanosis; No pulse (p. 185)
2. a. Immediate recognition and activation
   b. Early CPR
   c. Rapid defibrillation
   d. Effective advanced life support (pp. 187–188)
   e. Integrated post-cardiac arrest care

SHORT ANSWER

1. Answers will vary by student.

STOP, REVIEW, REMEMBER   (PP. 195–196)
MULTIPLE CHOICE

1. c (p. 190)
2. a (p. 191)
3. d (p. 191)
4. a (p. 191)
5. b (p. 191)

EMERGENCY MEDICAL RESPONDER PRACTICE

1. a. Check for responsiveness and scan the chest for breathing.
   b. Activate the EMS system. Request advanced assistance.
   c. Move the patient to a firm surface and position yourself.
   d. Check the pulse. (p. 191)
2. a. Two of the following: Pulse with compressions, chest rise with ventilations, skin
   b. color improvement (p. 194)

SHORT ANSWER

1. The compressor calls for the switch. After 30 compressions, the ventilator will administer two breaths, quickly move to

the patient's side, locate his hand position, and begin the next round of 30 compressions. The compressor simultaneously moves to the airway position and prepares to ventilate at the cycle's end. (pp. 192–193)

2. Be sure the EMS system has been activated; obtain an AED if one is nearby. (pp. 191–193)
3. Two of the following: Activate the EMS system early; push hard and fast; switch often to avoid fatigue; limit interruptions in compressions. (pp. 190–193)

CRITICAL THINKING

Ideally you would direct others in the park to call for help while you provide care. It is advisable to send more than one person to make sure help is called. If you are alone with no others in sight when faced with an adult patient who has collapsed you should go and call for help before beginning care. (pp. 190–193)

STOP, REVIEW, REMEMBER   (PP. 202–203)

MULTIPLE CHOICE

1. d (p. 197)
2. c (p. 200)
3. a (p. 201)

4. c (p. 201)
5. c (p. 201)

SHORT ANSWER

1. If there is any chance of a successful resuscitation in a pediatric patient, it will most likely be the result of the basic airway and ventilation management you will perform immediately. (p. 197)
2. Infants and newborns may need padding behind their shoulders to prevent airway occlusion when lying flat. (pp. 198–201)
3. Hypothermia (p. 201)

CRITICAL THINKING

1. Calls involving children are often difficult—and those for cardiac arrest may be the toughest. You may have profound effects of stress and overwhelming feelings after a call these calls. Follow the guidelines in the well-being chapter and remember that these emotions are normal. Unfortunately even your best efforts can't save every patient. (See Chapter 2)

CHAPTER REVIEW   (PP. 210–211)

MULTIPLE CHOICE

1. a (p. 185)
2. a (p. 191)
3. d (p. 193)

4. d (p. 193)
5. d (p. 206)

SHORT ANSWER

1. a. Excessively hairy chest
   b. Medication patches
   c. Pacemaker. (pp. 205–206)

2. a. Shave or replace original pads
   b. Remove patches and wipe away medication
   c. Offset pads away from pacemaker. (pp. 205–206)
3. a. V-tach
   b. V-fib (pp. 205–206)
4. a. Rescuer is exhausted or the patient is turned over to provider of equal or higher level.
   b. The patient is resuscitated.
   c. The patient has been declared dead by a proper authority. (pp. 190, 194)

CRITICAL THINKING

1. When two rescuers are present, tasks can be performed simultaneously. If the patient is pulseless, one EMR will begin CPR while the other prepares and applies the AED. Because the patient appears lifeless you will take the C-A-B approach to the primary assessment. (p. 205)
2. The DNR order reflects the patient's wishes. Many times the family is in denial and wants resuscitation initiated. Assure the order is current and valid. Do not begin resuscitation. Contact medical direction if you have questions or doubts. If there is a question about the validity of the DNR order or the order is not physically present, begin resuscitation. (p. 209)

CASE STUDY

1. Assess responsiveness, ensure the EMS system has been activated, call for ALS, open the airway, check breathing, and begin CPR. (pp. 183, 185)
2. This depends on whether you have an AED present or not. If the AED is immediately available your protocols will likely advise you to do this first. If the AED isn't available or no shock is advised, begin CPR. (p. 205)
3. Rigor mortis, dependent lividity (p. 209)

SECTION TWO REVIEW

1. a (p. 142)
   Rationale: Contraction of the chest muscles and lowering of the diaphragm cause the thoracic cavity to enlarge, which lowers the pressure inside of it with respect to the atmosphere, causing air to move into the lungs.
2. d (p. 142)
   Rationale: The anatomical location of the vocal cords is in the larynx, or voice box, which is below the pharynx and above the trachea and bronchi.
3. c (p. 143)
   Rationale: The alveoli are the thin, terminal air sacs of the lung, which are surrounded by capillaries, allowing gas to be exchanged between the thin walls of the alveoli and capillaries.
4. d (p. 146)
   Rationale: The body responds to hypoxia by trying to improve oxygenation through taking more breaths per minute and circulating oxygenated blood from the lungs more quickly throughout the body.

5. c (p. 149)

Rationale: The priorities of resuscitation, in order, are always airway, breathing, and circulation. An unresponsive patient who is snoring has a partial airway obstruction that must be relieved.

6. c (p. 146)

Rationale: The patient is unresponsive and must be adequately assessed and positioned for potential resuscitation, which cannot be accomplished with the patient in his recliner.

7. a (p. 158)

Rationale: The EMR must recognize that agitation, anxiety, and changes in mental status are indications of hypoxia, and that this particular patient is at high risk for hypoxia.

8. c (p. 149)

Rationale: With this patient's history of trauma to the head, he is at risk for spinal injury. The airway should not be opened with a head-tilt, chin-lift (unless all other measures prove inadequate). Suctioning must be performed immediately to prevent aspiration of blood into the lungs.

9. a (p. 158)

Rationale: The patient's airway must be cleared immediately and completely to prevent her from aspirating stomach contents into her lungs.

10. c (p. 158)

Rationale: The tongue is the most common cause of airway obstruction in the unresponsive patient, producing snoring sounds. Using a manual maneuver to pull the tongue away from the back of the pharynx relieves the obstruction.

11. d (p. 149)

Rationale: Despite the mechanism of injury that is consistent with a spinal injury, we must realize that the patient may have a spinal injury, which may be aggravated by moving, while he most definitely has an airway obstruction that will lead to hypoxia and death if not corrected.

12. a (p. 152)

Rationale: Suction alone, even with a large-bore, rigid suction catheter, is not likely to be an efficient and effective way of removing undigested food from the airway. The airway must be cleared as quickly and completely as possible before resuming ventilations.

13. c (p. 152)

Rationale: Forcing the suction catheter or inserting beyond the point where you can visualize it may result in damage to the soft tissue with swelling and bleeding that can further complicate airway management; however, the catheter must be inserted into the oropharynx, beyond the teeth, to be effective.

14. b (p. 154)

Rationale: An oral airway can help keep the tongue away from the back of the pharynx, but does not work on its own. Proper positioning of the airway must be maintained, and only a properly sized device is used. If used in patients who have a gag reflex, the device can stimulate gagging and vomiting.

15. a (p. 155)

Rationale: An oral airway is not used in patients who have a gag reflex.

16. c (p. 158)

Rationale: In early hypoxia the body compensates by increasing the heart and respiratory rates, but if hypoxia continues, the body's compensatory mechanisms fail and death will quickly follow.

17. c (p. 160)

Rationale: The term oximetry literally means oxygen measurement, which is the intent of pulse oximetry, although technically, oxygenation is measured indirectly by determining how saturated the molecules of hemoglobin in the red blood cells are.

18. c (p. 161)

Rationale: Pulse oximetry measures hemoglobin saturation. Normally, hemoglobin is saturated with oxygen, but carbon monoxide binds more readily with hemoglobin than oxygen and will provide a falsely high pulse oximetry reading, despite the fact that the patient is hypoxic.

19. b (p. 161)

Rationale: For safety, there are several mechanisms for identifying oxygen, one of which is its green cylinder or cylinder marking. Different gases have different colors associated with them.

20. a (p. 161)

Rationale: A regulator attaches to an oxygen cylinder to reduce the pressure in the tank to a safe level for patient administration.

21. a (p. 163)

Rationale: The bag of the BVM is squeezed to deliver positive pressure ventilation to patients with inadequate breathing. The other devices simply deliver oxygen under very low pressure, meaning that the oxygen will not be able to enter the lungs for ventilation.

22. d (p. 164)

Rationale: The reservoir bag of the nonrebreather mask stays inflated at all times to ensure that the patient receives oxygen with every breath. Typically, it takes a flow rate of 10 to 15 liters per minute to accomplish this goal.

23. c (p. 167)

Rationale: A flow rate in excess of 6 liters per minute, directly into the nostrils, will irritate and dry the mucous membranes.

24. b (p. 172)

Rationale: A breath delivered every 5 to 6 seconds will provide a ventilatory rate of 10 to 12 breaths per minute.

25. d (p. 172)

Rationale: Both pocket face masks and BVMs can be used with supplemental oxygen, and both can be used in a way that results in stomach distention. To deliver ventilations to the lungs, there must be an adequate seal with either device, to prevent air from escaping underneath the mask. A Venturi mask is used for precisely controlled oxygen delivery, not ventilation.

26. c (p. 184)
Rationale: Without a constant supply of oxygen supplied by adequate circulation, brain cells begin to die in as soon as 4 to 6 minutes, and irreversible damage begins in 8 to 10 minutes.

27. a (p. 185)
Rationale: As a rule, children have very healthy hearts but cannot compensate for respiratory problems for prolonged periods of time.

28. d (p. 185)
Rationale: Cardiac arrest means the heart has stopped pumping blood, which can only be confirmed by the absence of a pulse.

29. b (p. 194)
Rationale: It is reported that the child was choking, but laypersons can be mistaken about the presenting problem. As an EMR, you must proceed systematically. After establishing unresponsiveness and absence of breathing, the next step is to check a pulse, which is done at the carotid artery in the neck for children this age. Without checking the pulse, it would be premature to begin chest compressions.

30. c (p. 187)
Rationale: The first link in the chain of survival is recognizing the problem and notifying emergency personnel.

31. b (p. 188)
Rationale: In adults, the most common cause of cardiac arrest may be corrected by early defibrillation. It is critical to get EMS on the way without delay.

32. a (p. 190)
Rationale: CPR provides only about 1/4 to 1/3 of normal cardiac output, but may be able to provide enough perfusion to the vital organs to allow survival if the patient's heartbeat can be restored with defibrillation or medications.

33. c (p. 191)
Rationale: This is the current American Heart Association guideline for adult CPR.

34. c (p. 191)
Rationale: Although the chest wall must be allowed to recoil after each compression, the hands are not removed, so as not to lose the correct positioning. Ventilations are performed slowly and smoothly to prevent air from entering the stomach. The current American Heart Association guideline for adult CPR is 30 compressions to 2 ventilations.

35. a (p. 194)
Rationale: There are known complications of even properly performed CPR, including fractures of the ribs or sternum (especially in the elderly). The patient's best chance of survival is to perform CPR normally.

36. a (p. 198)
Rationale: CPR is started in infants with a heart rate less than 60. When CPR is indicated in children and infants, do not delay. If EMS has not been contacted, perform 2 minutes of CPR first, then contact 911.

37. d (p. 198)
Rationale: The airway of a small child is best maintained by placing padding under the shoulders to prevent flexion of the neck by the larger head. Chest compressions are not needed in this child.

38. c (p. 201)
Rationale: Although chest compressions can be performed in newborns and small infants by encircling the chest with the hands and placing the thumbs over the sternum, the chest must still be allowed to recoil fully following each compression.

39. d (p. 199)
Rationale: 30 compressions to 2 ventilations is the current American Heart Association guideline for one-rescuer child CPR.

40. c (p. 203)
Rationale: The two arrhythmias that can be terminated with defibrillation are ventricular tachycardia (without a pulse) and ventricular fibrillation.

41. b (p. 206)
Rationale: An AED is used after the EMR determines a patient is pulseless and delivers shocks to those patients in cardiac arrest who are in either ventricular tachycardia or ventricular fibrillation.

42. b (p. 208)
Rationale: The heart must be perfused for defibrillation to have the best chance of being successful. A patient who has been "down" for longer than 4 or 5 minutes should receive 2 minutes of CPR to perfuse the heart before attempting defibrillation.

43. d (p. 205)
Rationale: Most manufacturers recommend the placement described in choice "d" to allow electricity to pass through the heart as it travels between the pads.

44. a (p. 205)
Rationale: The patient's best chance for survival is following current American Heart Association guidelines for CPR and defibrillation without delay. However, the pads must not be placed directly over any implanted cardiac device.

45. c (p. 206)
Rationale: Not every patient in cardiac arrest is in a shockable rhythm. Properly maintained AEDs are unlikely to fail, and are not designed to determine whether conditions are dangerous.

46. a (p. 206)
Rationale: Cardiac arrest in children is rarely due to a shockable rhythm but an AED can be used on a patient of any age.

47. c (p. 208)
   Rationale: Return of spontaneous circulation does not automatically mean breathing will resume.
48. b (p. 209)
   Rationale: The patient is in cardiac arrest with obviously fatal wounds, making attempts at resuscitation futile.
49. c (p. 206)
   Rationale: It may take AEDs up to 15 seconds to analyze.
50. a (p. 206)
   Rationale: Anyone in contact, directly or indirectly, with a patient who is being defibrillated can be shocked by the electrical current.

CHAPTER 9

STOP, REVIEW, REMEMBER (PP. 228–229)

MULTIPLE CHOICE

1. c (p. 223)
2. a (p. 225)
3. c (pp. 226–227)

TRUE/FALSE

1. F (pp. 226–227)
2. T (p. 227)
3. T (p. 227)

CRITICAL THINKING

1. No. They may have more information concerning the scene that was not given to EMS on initial dispatch. (p. 224)
2. Retreat from the area in your ambulance and advise police of the location of the individual. (p. 224)
3. Step away from the patient and advise one of the police officers. (p. 224)

STOP, REVIEW, REMEMBER (PP. 236–237)

MULTIPLE CHOICE

1. b (p. 230)
2. a (p. 231)
3. c (p. 232)
4. d (p. 232)

TRUE/FALSE

1. F (p. 231)
2. T (p. 232)
3. T (pp. 234–235)

CRITICAL THINKING

1. Scene safety (p. 232)
2. Any—Multiple points of impact can create forces on all angles of the body. (p. 232)
3. Ejection—In the surrounding area of the crash scene (p. 232)

CHAPTER REVIEW (PP. 240–241)

MULTIPLE CHOICE

1. b (p. 224)
2. c (p. 224)
3. d (pp. 226–227)
4. b (p. 227)
5. b (p. 232)

SHORT ANSWER

1. People, pets, chemicals, unstable surfaces, fire, vehicles (pp. 223–227)
2. The height the patient fell from
   The part of the patient that struck the surface
   The surface the patient fell on
   Whether anything broke the fall or caused additional injuries during the fall (p. 234)
3. Mass- or multiple-casualty incident—determining the proper resources are available (p. 241)

CRITICAL THINKING

1. determining the number of patients (p. 232)
2. police, fire department, and/or traffic assistance (pp. 237–238)
3. Anyone in the collision should sign a refusal. Anyone under 18 or not able to make a legal consented decision must be transported. (See Chapter 3)

CHAPTER 10

STOP, REVIEW, REMEMBER (PP. 252–254)

MULTIPLE CHOICE

1. d (p. 248)
2. b (p. 248)
3. c (p. 248)
4. a (p. 246)
5. d (p. 247)

EMERGENCY MEDICAL RESPONDER PRACTICE

1. Head tilt, chin lift (p. 249)
2. Head tilt, chin lift (p. 249)
3. Jaw thrust (p. 249)
4. Head tilt, chin lift (p. 249)
5. Jaw thrust (p. 249)

SHORT ANSWER

1. A chief complaint is the patient's answer to the question "Why did you call EMS?" (p. 246)
2. Spinal precautions are steps you take to protect the spine, including holding the head and neck still and preventing the patient from moving. Do this if the patient has a mechanism of injury that causes you to believe the spine may be injured. (p. 247)
3. No. Once you have identified a response at a higher level, you will stop checking. A patient who responds verbally will respond to pain. (p. 248)

MULTIPLE CHOICE

1. c (p. 254)
2. b (p. 254)
3. a (p. 254)
4. c (p. 256)
5. d (p. 256)

EMERGENCY MEDICAL RESPONDER PRACTICE

1. The patient appears to be breathing adequately but is breathing somewhat rapidly and may have experienced trauma. Anxiety may indicate hypoxia. This patient would be given oxygen by nonrebreather mask or nasal cannula. (p. 254)
2. Inadequate breathing. Assist ventilations with pocket face mask or bag-valve-mask ventilation while maintaining spinal stabilization and the jaw thrust if necessary. (p. 254)
3. Breathing adequately. Apply oxygen by nonrebreather mask or nasal cannula. (p. 254)
4. Inadequate breathing. Assist ventilations with pocket face mask or bag-valve mask while maintaining spinal stabilization. (p. 254)

CRITICAL THINKING QUESTIONS

1. Adequate breathing is normal in rate and depth. Inadequate breathing has a diminished depth, a rate above or below normal, or both rate and depth problems. Patients who are breathing inadequately not only have diminished breathing but also look sick. They have poor skin color and usually an altered mental status. (p. 254)
2. This is a potentially serious condition and most likely means that there is a spinal cord injury. You should take great care to treat the patient without moving the spine except when the patient is in physical danger. (p. 256)
3. It means the patient has hypotension. The body can't put out enough pressure for the pulse wave to reach the wrist. The pulse is palpable at the carotid artery in the neck because it is close to the heart. (p. 254)

CHAPTER REVIEW   (PP. 259–261)

MULTIPLE CHOICE

1. b (p. 246)
2. b (p. 252)
3. d (p. 254)
4. c (p. 258)
5. c (p. 249)

SHORT ANSWER

1. The scene size-up is done before you reach the patient. It ensures safety and checks other factors you should know before you reach the patient. The primary assessment deals with life threats and is the first assessment you do upon reaching the patient. (p. 243)
2. No. If a patient looks good and is breathing adequately, he has a pulse. When the heart stops, responsiveness is lost almost immediately. Breathing ceases quickly thereafter. Although there may be some agonal breathing during this time, there is no true breathing. (p. 254)
3. So you can see any potentially serious injuries to vital areas such as the chest and abdomen. You should find this out as quickly as possible in your assessment. In medical and trauma patients, you will be able to assess for breathing more efficiently. (p. 258)

CRITICAL THINKING

1. Most Emergency Medical Responders would agree with this statement. This is where the most lifesaving treatments are performed—the ABCs. Without these your patient will die. (p. 244)
2. Keep ventilating. The leg can wait. It may look bad but won't kill the patient. If you stop ventilating the patient will die. (p. 254)
3. These tell you about circulation perfusion status. If the skin doesn't receive good blood flow, it reacts by becoming cool, pale, and moist. The pulse increases to improve cardiac output in cases of shock. (p. 254)

CASE STUDY

1. You should position the patient on his side and suction out his mouth. If there is a lot of vomitus, you could sweep it out with your fingers and a gauze pad. Be careful the patient doesn't bite. (p. 252)
2. The patient's breathing should be assessed for both rate and depth. Both must be adequate for breathing to be adequate. This means breathing within normal rates—not very slow or very fast. It must also be deep. (p. 254)
3. You should have gloves and face protection (eyewear at a minimum). If spraying is likely, use a mask/face shield combination. (p. 247)
4. Roll the patient to his side and suction with a large-bore suction catheter. You may also sweep with your gloved fingers if you don't believe you will be bitten. (p. 252)
5. The patient is "U" (unresponsive). (p. 248)
6. Advise that the patient has a decreasing mental status with vomiting causing potential airway problems. Include that alcohol was suspected by school officials as well as any other vital signs or treatments you have given. This patient would be assigned a high priority. (p. 248)

CHAPTER 11

MULTIPLE CHOICE

1. c (p. 264)
2. a (p. 265)
3. a (p. 267)
4. d (p. 267)
5. a (p. 268)

EMERGENCY MEDICAL RESPONDER PRACTICE

1. S Signs and Symptoms (p. 267)
2. A Allergies (p. 267)
3. M Medications (p. 267)
4. P Past Medical History (p. 267)
5. L Last oral intake (p. 268)
6. E Events (p. 268)

SHORT ANSWER

1. The chief complaint is, in the patient's own words, what is bothering him today. (p. 264)
2. When the patient cannot communicate with you directly, look for clues from the scene in general. Family members and caregivers often are a great source of information. Use clues from the patient including medical alert jewelry, medications he is taking, and other physical findings. Consider also scene clues. (p. 265)
3. The MOI is the force that was applied to the patient to cause the trauma. (p. 267)

STOP, REVIEW, REMEMBER (PP. 278–279)
MULTIPLE CHOICE

1. b (p. 272)
2. b (p. 271)
3. b (p. 273)
4. a (p. 273)
5. c (p. 276)

SHORT ANSWER

1. The pulse is a wave of pressure created by contraction of the heart that can be felt in the arteries throughout the body. (p. 272)
2. Auscultation involves using a stethoscope and listening for the systolic and diastolic blood pressures. Palpation only obtains the systolic and is done by palpating and noting when the pulse distal to the cuff returns. (p. 274)
3. Gasping respirations, also called agonal respirations are not adequate and require the EMR to ventilate the patient using a pocket face mask or BVM. (p. 271)

CRITICAL THINKING

1. A pulse oximeter may report near 100% saturation in cases of trauma and shock. In cases of internal bleeding, blood may be saturated at 100% but blood volume is seriously low. Carbon monoxide poisoning saturates the hemoglobin in the blood with carbon monoxide rather than oxygen giving a false reading. (p. 276)
2. In this case the sun is likely causing the patient's constricted pupils. Shade the patient's eyes and look for dilation of the pupils as a sign of reactivity. (p. 277)

CHAPTER REVIEW (PP. 280–281)
MULTIPLE CHOICE

1. d (p. 265)
2. c (p. 267)
3. a (p. 270)
4. d (p. 271)
5. b (p. 273)

SHORT ANSWER

1. Carbon monoxide (CO) poisoning can give you a false normal reading on a pulse oximeter. The CO molecule occupies the same space on the hemoglobin as oxygen would and may be read by a pulse oximeter. Because the hemoglobin is fully saturated, your oximetry may be normal or even high even though your patient is profoundly hypoxic. (p. 276)
2. Squeeze the fingernail of an adult or the forearm of a child. This gentle squeeze should turn the skin white. When the squeeze is released, blood and a pink color should return to that area. In a healthy person this return should take no more than 2 seconds. (p. 273)
3. Abnormal pupil findings: No reaction—hypoxia, brain injury; Dilation—hypoxia, shock; Constricted—narcotic overdose, stroke; Unequal—brain injury, stroke (Note: Unequal pupils are a normal finding in some healthy people). (p. 277)

CRITICAL THINKING

1. Trending can help you see progress or failure of your interventions. It can also help you predict potential downturns in your patient. (p. 270)
2. Blood pressure looks only at pressure in the system and not at where the blood is going. Although pressure may be normal, blood may be shunted away from vital organs. (p. 273)

CASE STUDY

1. When a patient cannot communicate with you directly, look for clues from the scene in general. Family members and caregivers often are a great source of information. Use clues from the patient including medical alert jewelry, medications he is taking, and other physical findings. (p. 265)
2. SAMPLE (p. 267)
3. wrap cuff around patient's upper arm; find the radial pulse; inflate cuff; palpate radial pulse; inflate cuff 30 mmHg more once pulse is lost; deflate cuff slowly; palpate the radial pulse. Record systolic pressure upon return of radial pulse, do not record a diastolic pressure when palpating. (p. 275)

CHAPTER 12

STOP, REVIEW, REMEMBER   (PP. 288–289)

MULTIPLE CHOICE

1. d (p. 286)
2. b (p. 287)
3. a (p. 287)
4. c (p. 292)

MATCHING

1. b (p. 288)
2. d (p. 292)
3. c (p. 292)
4. a (p. 287)

CRITICAL THINKING

1. Seriously ill; trauma patient. (pp. 283–288)
2. Not at first glance. No, the lacerations would not cause him to be in shock. The EMR must assume further injury. (pp. 283–288)
3. Yes. When the medics arrive, they tell you that he is having a heart attack. It appears as though the heart attack happened first and that he went off the road as a result of it. (pp. 283–288)

STOP, REVIEW, REMEMBER   (PP. 297–298)

MULTIPLE CHOICE

1. a (p. 292)
2. c (p. 295)
3. b (p. 296)
4. a (p. 297)

TRUE/FALSE

1. F (pp. 292–293)
2. T (p. 295)
3. F (p. 288)
4. T (p. 297)

CRITICAL THINKING

1. Torso (pp. 286–297)
2. Blood pressure; heart rate; respirations (pp. 286–297)
3. Not necessarily; transport the patient immediately. (pp. 286–297)

CHAPTER REVIEW   (PP. 301–303)

MULTIPLE CHOICE

1. b (p. 298)
2. b (p. 299)
3. a (p. 300)
4. c (p. 287)
5. b (p. 292)
6. c (p. 296)
7. a (p. 297)
8. b (p. 297)

TRUE/FALSE

1. T (p. 299)
2. F (p. 288)
3. F (pp. 291–292)
4. T (p. 292)
5. T (p. 298)
6. T (p. 300)
7. F (p. 287)
8. F (pp. 292–293)

CRITICAL THINKING

1. Abnormal vital signs (pp. 283–301)
2. Pain on palpation to the abdomen (pp. 283–301)
3. Unexplained pain to the head (pp. 283–301)
4. Unstable bones/joints in the pelvis (pp. 283–301)

CHAPTER 13

STOP, REVIEW, REMEMBER   (PP. 311–312)

MULTIPLE CHOICE

1. a (p. 306)
2. c (p. 307)
3. b (p. 307)
4. a (p. 310)

TRUE/FALSE

1. T (p. 310)
2. T (p. 306)
3. F (p. 307)
4. T (p. 307)

CRITICAL THINKING

1. In patients that have severe distress your primary assessment is the first priority. You will perform interventions for life-threatening conditions (applying oxygen for respiratory distress, controlling severe bleeding) before asking detailed history questions (pp. 306–311)
2. Questions that help to immediately establish the nature of the problem such as "Your wife tells me you were having chest pain." Or "Did you take these pills?" are relevant and won't delay your primary assessment. (pp. 306–311)
3. Hypoxia may cause anxiety or confusion. He will likely not be able to remember some of his significant medical history. He may also appear agitated. Anxiety or distress from family members can worsen this. (pp. 306–311)

STOP, REVIEW, REMEMBER   (PP. 315–316)

MULTIPLE CHOICE

1. d (p. 312)
2. a (p. 313)
3. b (p. 314)
4. b (p. 314)

TRUE/FALSE

1. T (p. 312)
2. F (p. 314)
3. T (p. 313)
4. F (p. 314)

CRITICAL THINKING

1. Determine how the patient's current mental status compares to his normal status at the facility. Determine if there have been sudden or gradual changes. (pp. 306–315)
2. No. Elderly patients should never be assumed to have Alzheimer's or disabilities. Many lead very vibrant lives

but simply need assistance with daily activities. Some facilities have special units or specialize in Alzheimer's patients. Ask about each patient's specific medical history. (pp. 306–315)

3. In this case the staff will. If he is living with his wife (couples often move into these facilities) she may also have information. Even if the patient appears to have an altered mental status be sure to talk with him and reassure him as you provide care. (pp. 306–315)

CHAPTER REVIEW (PP. 321–322)

MULTIPLE CHOICE

1. c (p. 306)
2. b (p. 307)
3. a (pp. 307–308)
4. c (p. 313)
5. a (p. 314)
6. b (pp. 317–318)
7. d (pp. 318–319)
8. b (p. 319)

TRUE/FALSE

1. T (p. 307)
2. F (p. 307)
3. F (p. 310)
4. T (p. 310)
5. F (p. 314)
6. F (p. 319)
7. T (p. 319)
8. F (pp. 318–319)

CRITICAL THINKING

1. Every effort should be made to convince the patient to accept your care and the care and transportation of the ambulance personnel. (pp. 306–321)

2. It is a common tenet of mechanism of injury that if there is a death of an occupant in the vehicle, other occupants in the same vehicle are considered seriously injured until proven otherwise. If the crash killed one person the others could be seriously injured. (pp. 306–321)

3. Your approach depends on your patient and your relationship with them. Since you have no authority to force him to go, the best course of action is to provide facts and rationale for your insistence they go to the hospital. Enlist the help of the police if this is not successful. (pp. 306–321)

SECTION THREE REVIEW

1. a (p. 225)
   Rationale: A shrub may hide, or conceal, you from view, but does not provide substantial protection from a violent person or any weapons he has.
2. b (p. 226)
   Rationale: The safest course of action is to first stop and use binoculars to gain additional information before getting closer or assuming that hazardous materials are involved.
3. d (p. 226)
   Rationale: The Department of Transportation Emergency Response Guidebook contains essential information about hazardous materials, including the initial isolation distance for specific hazardous materials.

4. b (p. 235)
   Rationale: A building collapse requires special rescue techniques to prevent injury to responders, and further injury to survivors.
5. b (p. 230)
   Rationale: Mechanism of injury is used to develop an index of suspicion for what types of injuries are likely, and their severity, but cannot give information about whether the injuries actually exist.
6. b (p. 231)
   Rationale: Occupants in frontal impact collisions continue to move forward, in the direction the vehicle was traveling. The patient who takes the down-and-under pathway will receive the first impact to the lower extremities, which will absorb some of the injury, decreasing impact to other parts of the body. (However, these additional impacts are still capable of producing severe injury.)
7. d (p. 232)
   Rationale: Whiplash occurs in rear impact collisions when the body is propelled forward, but the head lags behind. A properly positioned headrest will prevent the head from lagging behind and injuring the neck.
8. c (p. 232)
   Rationale: Injuries are most likely on the side of impact (the left, in this case). In lateral collisions, as the body accelerates away from the point of impact, the head lags behind and exceeds the normal range of motion of the neck.
9. d (p. 234)
   Rationale: A fall 2 to 3 times the patient's height (average 11 to 12 feet or higher) is considered significant.
10. b (p. 243)
    Rationale: The primary assessment is focused on finding and correcting problems that can immediately result in death—that is, problems with the airway, breathing, or circulation.
11. a (p. 246)
    Rationale: Although you've gained valuable information, several steps are still required to complete the primary assessment.
12. d (p. 246)
    Rationale: The chief complaint is what the patient tells you in his own words is the reason why he needs emergency medical care.
13. c (p. 247)
    Rationale: A patient reported to have trouble breathing is at risk for hypoxia, which can manifest as combative behavior as the brain is deprived of oxygen.
14. b (p. 248)
    Rationale: The patient is awake, but because he is confused, cannot be said to be alert, according to the AVPU mnemonic. He does, however, respond verbally.

15. b (p. 248)

Rationale: The appropriate next step is to lightly shake the patient, before applying a painful stimulus or assuming that the patient is unresponsive.

16. a (p. 250)

Rationale: Following the steps of the primary assessment, you have determined that the airway is open and the patient is breathing well enough to speak normally and maintain alertness. Although we know the patient has a pulse, it is still necessary to determine more information about her circulation by assessing the radial pulse.

17. b (p. 256)

Rationale: The EMR does a gross check of the central nervous system by assessing level of consciousness and testing the patient's ability to move and detect touch in all four extremities.

18. d (p. 258)

Rationale: It is not acceptable to state the patient's name or other confidential information over the radio. The most immediately useful information to the incoming EMS unit is the patient's level of consciousness.

19. a (p. 264)

Rationale: The key to getting the patient's history is being able to talk to him and listen to him.

20. b (p. 265)

Rationale: A symptom is something the patient is experiencing, but that cannot be measured by the EMR. The chief complaint, in this case, is the chest pain.

21. d (p. 264)

Rationale: Past medical history can have an impact on medical and traumatic conditions, although the point in the assessment at which the history is obtained can vary depending on the nature of the problem.

22. c (p. 270)

Rationale: Whenever time and the patient's condition allow, the EMR obtains a complete set of vital signs initially, and takes follow-up vital signs to detect changes in the patient's condition.

23. d (p. 271)

Rationale: An infant's normal respiratory rate is from 25 to 50 breaths per minute.

24. c (p. 271)

Rationale: The normal adult respiratory rate is between 12 and 20 per minute.

25. b (p. 273)

Rationale: All of the patient's vital signs are within normal limits for his age, but the pale, cool skin suggests that he is compensating for shock and perfusion is not normal.

26. a (p. 275)

Rationale: For several reasons, a particular patient's blood pressure may be difficult to hear. It is important to use actual data, not estimates or guesses. However, proper procedures must be followed to obtain an accurate reading (not "c"). Palpation can give only the systolic reading, but is more accurate than an improperly taken auscultated blood pressure.

27. d (p. 277)

Rationale: The patient's mental status and vital signs are inconsistent with a brain injury or shock, and contact lenses do not interfere with pupil constriction.

28. c (p. 277)

Rationale: Hypoxia would be a cause of dilated, nonreacted pupils, and a brain injury can cause dilated or unequal pupils. However, narcotics are a cause of constricted pupils, and the patient's primary assessment findings are consistent with narcotic overdose.

29. b (p. 276)

Rationale: The lack of correlation between the pulse you obtained and the pulse reading on the pulse oximeter, along with the patient's lack of other signs of hypoxia point to an incorrect oximetry reading.

30. c (p. 273)

Rationale: Children tend to compensate well for shock (but not for long), leading to the vital signs within normal limits, but the delayed capillary refill and the 2-day history of vomiting indicate poor perfusion.

31. a (p. 284)

Rationale: More information will be obtained through the history of a medical patient than from any of the other choices.

32. a (p. 290)

Rationale: The 13-year-old male has a significant mechanism of injury that requires manual stabilization of the head and neck. The other patients lack a mechanism consistent with trauma to the spine.

33. b (p. 292)

Rationale: Asymmetry refers to unevenness.

34. d (p. 296)

Rationale: Tenderness is a sensation of pain that occurs when the affected area is palpated.

35. b (p. 287)

Rationale: A less serious injury that prevents the patient from noticing a more serious injury—that is, distracts the patient from the more serious injury—is called a distracting injury.

36. c (p. 297)

Rationale: Hypothermia will worsen the patient's condition, and she needs to be kept as warm as possible, but it is a mistake to avoid looking for a potentially life-threatening problem related to the patient's breathing. This patient has a serious mechanism of injury—especially for her age—and should not be moved. The best choice is to both assess the injury and keep the patient as warm as possible.

37. a (p. 291)

Rationale: The proper term for an abdomen that seems to be enlarged by gas or fluid is distended.

38. d (p. 296)

> **Rationale:** Once pain is elicited, avoid unnecessarily causing additional pain. In the case of the pelvis, a fracture can lead to serious bleeding, which can be aggravated by rocking or pressing on the pelvis.

39. b (p. 299)

> **Rationale:** Combined with the mechanism of injury, the vital signs are consistent with a serious closed head injury, not the increased heart rate and decreased blood pressure associated with shock or an injury to the heart or lungs.

40. c (pp. 306–307)

> **Rationale:** Remember, you are in someone else's home and owe them courtesy and professionalism. You are more likely to gain cooperation when treating others courteously.

41. a (p. 307)

> **Rationale:** In this case, the patient is stable and the EMS unit is nearby. The ambulance will provide a private location to obtain the patient's history, which, for a young female with abdominal pain, will include questions she will not feel comfortable answering in front of others.

42. c (p. 307)

> **Rationale:** This is the distance at which we are comfortable with others.

43. d (p. 310)

> **Rationale:** Starting with an introduction and an open-ended question will provide more information than asking closed-ended or leading questions, or focusing on what seems obvious to you.

44. c (p. 313)

> **Rationale:** Portable radios can be carried on the belt or in the hand. Mobile radios are installed in vehicles.

45. c (p. 313)

> **Rationale:** A closer distance makes the communication too loud or distorted, while a distance farther away will not be heard.

46. a (p. 314)

> **Rationale:** Your goal is accurate communication. The patient will be aware of his disability and will not likely be offended by being asked to write something down, although he may feel frustrated by his difficulty in making himself understood. Do not take control away from the patient by immediately turning to the family or disregarding his attempts to communicate with you. If the patient cannot communicate in writing, it may be necessary to then ask the family for information.

47. b (p. 318)

> **Rationale:** Of the choices listed, only b is directly considered patient data.

48. c (p. 319)

> **Rationale:** Except for c, the choices listed are factual and could be determined or observed by someone else. The patient's experience of pain is not something that could be seen or measured by another person.

49. a (p. 319)

> **Rationale:** Except for choice a, assumptions are being made about the cause of the patient's condition, which could have alternative explanations.

50. c (p. 319)

> **Rationale:** As much is communicated by the condition of the report as is communicated by what is actually recorded in the report.

CHAPTER 14

STOP, REVIEW, REMEMBER   (PP. 343–344)

MULTIPLE CHOICE

1. b (p. 335)
2. a (p. 336)
3. d (p. 338)
4. a (p. 340)

TRUE/FALSE

1. F. (p. 341)
2. T (p. 340)
3. T (p. 339)
4. F (p. 355)

CRITICAL THINKING

1. Assure the patient has a patent airway. (p. 341)
2. No, but his altered mental state may give you clues as a symptom and must be taken into consideration in handling or moving the patient. (p. 341)
3. As an EMR, your treatment will be the same and you must call for immediate transport. (p. 343)

STOP, REVIEW, REMEMBER   (PP. 347–348)

MULTIPLE CHOICE

1. a (p. 344)
2. b (p. 346)
3. a (p. 346)

TRUE/FALSE

1. T (p. 346)
2. F (p. 345)
3. T (p. 347)

CRITICAL THINKING

1. Altered mental status or is unresponsive, inability to speak more than a few words without catching his breath, minimal movement of the chest when breathing, difficulty breathing, using more muscles than usual to expand the chest, sitting in the tripod position, pale, cool, or moist skin. (p. 346)

CHAPTER REVIEW   (PP. 351–353)
MULTIPLE CHOICE

1. c (p. 345)
2. d (p. 345)
3. a (p. 348)
4. c (p. 349)
5. d (p. 340)
6. b (p. 339)
7. c (p. 336)
8. a (p. 339)
9. c (p. 337)
10. a (p. 337)

TRUE/FALSE

1. F (p. 337)
2. T (p. 335)
3. T (p. 335)
4. T (p. 336)
5. F (p. 345)

CRITICAL THINKING

1. It is cardiac in nature. (p. 337)
2. The symptom of the CHF is difficulty with breathing. (p. 337)
3. Call for immediate transport and assure he is breathing. Check his vital signs. (p. 350)
4. Document and communicate his breathing difficulty, chest pain, and the water bubbling sound. Communicate his vital signs. (p. 350)

CHAPTER 15

STOP, REVIEW, REMEMBER   (PP. 363–364)
MULTIPLE CHOICE

1. d (p. 358)
2. c (pp. 358–359)
3. a (p. 361)

EMERGENCY MEDICAL RESPONDER PRACTICE

1. altered mental status, sweet, fruity, or acetone-like breath, flushed, warm, dry skin, hunger and thirst, rapid weak pulse, intoxicated appearance, staggering, slurred speech, frequent urination, reports that the patient has not taken the prescribed diabetes medications
2. Hyperglycemia. The slow onset of signs and symptoms, consuming food (probably overeating due to the scenario), unknown when insulin was last taken, and unusual breath odor all lead toward hyperglycemia.
3. notify EMS; Standard Precautions; monitor airway, breathing, circulation; mental status, and vital signs frequently, position the patient; administer high-flow oxygen, and sugar, if allowed by your local protocol, provide emotional support; notify the responding EMS if you administered sugar and any changes

TRUE/FALSE

1. T (pp. 360–361)
2. F (p. 358)
3. T (p. 358)
4. T (p. 359)
5. F (p. 358)

STOP, REVIEW, REMEMBER   (PP. 369–370)
MULTIPLE CHOICE

1. c (p. 364)
2. c (p. 364)
3. a (p. 367)
4. b (p. 369)

EMERGENCY MEDICAL RESPONDER PRACTICE

1. Stroke
2. See page 367.
3. See pages 368–369.
4. See page 369.

LIST

1. See page 366.
2. See page 368.

STOP, REVIEW, REMEMBER   (PP. 382–383)
MULTIPLE CHOICE

1. b (p. 376)
2. d (p. 377)
3. a (p. 381)

EMERGENCY MEDICAL RESPONDER PRACTICE

1. See page 376.
2. See page 380.
3. See page 380–381.

MATCHING

1. c (p. 371)
2. a (p. 371)
3. b (p. 371)
4. d (p. 372)

CRITICAL THINKING

1. What was the substance involved? How much of the substance was involved? When did the poisoning occur? What is the patient's approximate weight? What has the patient or others done to relieve the signs and symptoms? (p. 374)

CHAPTER REVIEW   (PP. 388–390)
MULTIPLE CHOICE

1. b (pp. 357–358)
2. b (p. 359)
3. b (pp. 361–362)
4. b (p. 361)
5. c (p. 364)
6. d (pp. 368–369)
7. b (pp. 367–368)
8. a (p. 381)
9. c (p. 374)
10. c (pp. 385–387)

MATCHING

1. m (p. 377)
2. o (p. 379)
3. g (p. 359)
4. n (p. 377)
5. q (p. 384)
6. h (p. 364)
7. f (p. 358)
8. l (p. 377)
9. d (p. 358)
10. c (p. 358)
11. k (p. 371)
12. a (p. 356)
13. e (p. 358)
14. p (p. 384)
15. i (p. 364)
16. b (p. 358)
17. j (p. 367)

EMERGENCY MEDICAL RESPONDER PRACTICE

1. Immediately notify the responding EMS personnel, take appropriate Standard Precautions, closely monitor and maintain the patient's airway and breathing, position the patient, and administer high-flow oxygen.
2. No. The patient's level of responsiveness is only painful (on the AVPU scale) and, therefore, he may not be able to control his own airway.
3. Yes. Altered mental status changes in a patient, in this case his level of responsiveness with a history of diabetes, is enough to consider this patient as unstable.

CHAPTER 16

STOP, REVIEW, REMEMBER   (PP. 398–399)

MULTIPLE CHOICE

1. b (pp. 392–393)
2. c (pp. 394–395)

EMERGENCY MEDICAL RESPONDER PRACTICE

1. monitor and maintain the patient's airway, breathing, and circulation; place the patient in a position of comfort; administer high-flow oxygen; monitor the patient's mental status and vital signs frequently; provide emotional support to the patient; notify the responding EMS of any changes in the patient's condition
2. severe respiratory distress, wheezing, rapid pulse, low blood pressure, pale, red, cyanotic, hives, itching, swelling around eyes, mouth, tongue, altered mental status, nausea, vomiting
3. notify EMS; Standard Precautions; monitor and maintain airway, breathing, and circulation, mental status, and vital signs often, position patient; administer high-flow oxygen; remove allergen, if possible; ask if patient used his epinephrine auto-injector; provide emotional support notify responding EMS of changes in condition

CRITICAL THINKING

1. Answers will vary but should include professionalism and truthfulness. (pp. 393–394)

STOP, REVIEW, REMEMBER   (PP. 402–403)

MULTIPLE CHOICE

1. a (p. 399)
2. d (p. 400)

EMERGENCY MEDICAL RESPONDER PRACTICE

1. abdominal pain (local, diffuse, or crampy); abdominal tenderness, local or diffuse; rigid, tense, or distended abdomen; anxiety; reluctance to move; loss of appetite; nausea; vomiting; diarrhea (may be extensive); blood in the vomit (bright red or "coffee grounds") or blood in the stool (bright red or black, tarry); signs of shock; fever
2. notify the responding EMS; take Standard Precautions; monitor and maintain airway, breathing, and circulation; place the patient in a position of comfort; administer high-flow oxygen; monitor the patient's mental status and vital signs frequently; provide emotional support to the patient; notify the responding EMS of changes in the patient's condition

LIST

1. Answers may vary, but should include some ingested (food, pills), inhaled (carbon monoxide, chemicals), absorbed (poison ivy, chemicals), and injected (sting, bite, drugs).

CHAPTER REVIEW   (PP. 405–407)

MULTIPLE CHOICE

1. b (pp. 392–393)
2. b (p. 393)
3. a (p. 394)
4. c (pp. 394–395)
5. c (p. 396)
6. b (p. 399)
7. c (pp. 399–401)
8. a (pp. 399–401)
9. c (p. 403)
10. c (p. 404)

MATCHING

1. d (p. 394)
2. g (p. 400)
3. h (p. 403)
4. f (p. 400)
5. b (p. 394)
6. a (p. 394)
7. c (p. 394)
8. e (p. 399)

EMERGENCY MEDICAL RESPONDER PRACTICE

1. Size up the scene and take all necessary precautions.
2. abdominal pain (local, diffuse, or crampy); abdominal tenderness (local or diffuse); rigid, tense, or distended abdomen; anxiety; reluctance to move; loss of appetite;

nausea; vomiting; diarrhea (may be extensive); blood in the vomit (bright red or "coffee grounds") or in the stool (bright red or black, tarry); signs of shock; fever

3. notify the responding EMS; take Standard Precautions; monitor and maintain airway, breathing, and circulation; place the patient in a position of comfort; administer high-flow oxygen; monitor the patient's mental status and vital signs frequently; provide emotional support to the patient; notify the responding EMS of changes in the patient's condition

SECTION FOUR REVIEW

1. b (p. 336)
   Rationale: Deoxygenated blood from the body enters the right side of the heart, where it is pumped to the lungs for oxygenation. The oxygenated blood returns to the left atrium of the heart.

2. c (p. 337)
   Rationale: Arteries and arterioles distribute oxygenated blood to the capillary level, where gases can be exchanged through the thin walls of the capillaries, before blood returns to the heart through the venous system.

3. a (p. 337)
   Rationale: The heart muscle receives its blood supply from the coronary arteries, which branch directly from the aorta.

4. c (p. 337)
   Rationale: Asthma causes constriction of the small airways (bronchioles) through muscle contraction and inflammation. Air makes a whistling or wheezing sound as it tries to exit through the narrowed airways.

5. b (p. 337)
   Rationale: A myocardial infarction is a heart attack. The heart muscle is deprived of oxygenated blood, resulting in pain.

6. a (p. 338)
   Rationale: Narrowing of the blood vessels of the heart, often due to plaque, reduces blood flow to the muscle, causing pain—especially at times of increased oxygen demand, such as exercise or stress.

7. d (p. 338)
   Rationale: Angina pectoris is often brought on by stress or exercise, and relieved by rest.

8. b (p. 339)
   Rationale: Ventricular fibrillation is a cardiac electrical disturbance that results in the inability of the heart to pump blood and produce a pulse.

9. b (p. 339)
   Rationale: When pain is located in one place, but feels like it also goes to other areas, this is known as radiation.

10. a (p. 341)
    Rationale: A medical history is important, but the patient needs oxygen first. The patient should be allowed to assume a position of comfort, and AED pads are not indicated.

11. d (p. 341)
    Rationale: The patient is not in cardiac arrest, so AED pads are not indicated. Assisting with ventilations takes precedence over obtaining a blood pressure or performing an examination.

12. b (p. 343)
    Rationale: The patient's history is important, but he first needs oxygen, no matter what his pulse oximetry reading is.

13. c (p. 343)
    Rationale: Nitroglycerin and aspirin are two drugs that can benefit the patient having a myocardial infarction. Albuterol is an inhaled drug often used for asthma, and epinephrine would be used by the patient with an anaphylactic reaction.

14. b (p. 435)
    Rationale: Chronic bronchitis is a form of chronic obstructive pulmonary disease (COPD) characterized by episodes of inflammation, increased mucus production, and productive cough.

15. d (p. 435)
    Rationale: Either the right or left sides of the heart can fail. When the left side fails, pressure in the pulmonary circulation increases, forcing fluid into the lungs.

16. a (p. 431)
    Rationale: The patient with a severe asthma attack will not get better without medication. The patient's decreased chest movement and decreased level of consciousness are due to respiratory failure and hypoxia, not improvement in his condition.

17. b (p. 348)
    Rationale: Patients with congestive heart failure have difficulty breathing when they lie flat and often sleep with several pillows or in a recliner.

18. c (p. 349)
    Rationale: Rhonchi indicate fluid in the larger airways, such as might be heard with bronchitis, while crackles (rales) are fine sounds associated with fluid in the smaller airways, such as might be heard in the patient with pulmonary edema.

19. d (p. 341)
    Rationale: While there are many things to do when caring for a patient with difficulty breathing, providing oxygen is one of the EMR's highest priorities.

20. a (p. 349)
    Rationale: The body uses more energy, and requires more oxygen, during anxiety. Calming the patient will help reduce the amount of oxygen his body needs.

21. d (p. 349)

Rationale: No matter the cause, a patient who is not ventilating one lung is not receiving oxygen at the cellular level. The EMR plays an important role in the care of such patients by providing supplemental oxygen.

22. b (p. 350)

Rationale: Unresponsive patients are vulnerable and cannot protect their airways. They may need assistance with breathing and circulation.

23. a (p. 358)

Rationale: Although cells need oxygen as part of the energy production process, the fuel that is used for energy is glucose.

24. d (p. 360)

Rationale: A pulse of 64, respirations of 20, and warm skin are all within normal expectations for adult patients. A fruity odor to the breath can be a sign of a diabetic emergency, which could explain the patient's confusion.

25. c (p. 358)

Rationale: Insulin is a hormone secreted by the pancreas in response to increased blood glucose. It helps glucose gain entry into cells.

26. d (p. 358)

Rationale: Although there are many causes of altered mental status, the patient has the classic signs of untreated diabetes (increased thirst and urination) in addition to altered mental status that has occurred over a few days, rather than suddenly. This is most consistent with the hyperglycemia that accompanies untreated diabetes.

27. a (p. 361)

Rationale: The patient is confused, but there is no indication that he is combative or violent. First encourage the patient to consume some sugar before deciding if other actions are necessary.

28. c (p. 364)

Rationale: Strokes are sometimes called "brain attacks" because they result from an obstruction of blood flow to brain tissue, just like a heart attack results from obstruction of blood flow to cardiac tissue.

29. b (p. 364)

Rationale: Some types of strokes can be reversed with drugs that break up the blood clot obstructing blood flow to brain tissue, but these drugs must be given within a few hours of onset of the signs and symptoms.

30. b (p. 366)

Rationale: Although a more thorough neurological assessment may include things such as pupil reaction, the Cincinnati Prehospital Stroke Scale can identify many strokes by checking for ability to speak, arm drift, and facial droop.

31. c (p. 367)

Rationale: The patient's signs and symptoms are very typical of stroke. Oxygen would be a priority as part of the primary assessment over any of the other choices.

32. d (p. 369)

Rationale: Consecutive or prolonged seizures represent a life-threatening emergency known as status epilepticus.

33. b (p. 371)

Rationale: Ingestion is entry to the body by eating or drinking a substance.

34. a (p. 379)

Rationale: It is critical to care for the airway, breathing, and circulation once the scene is safe, but if the patient is still being exposed to fumes, he must be removed from the area before being treated, and you must avoid entering a scene in which you could be exposed to a hazardous material.

35. b (p. 394)

Rationale: An allergen is a type of antigen—a foreign protein—that produces an allergic (hypersensitivity) reaction when it reacts with antibodies in the body.

36. d (p. 394)

Rationale: An allergen does not directly cause signs and symptoms. In fact, these substances do not affect most people. Some people produce antibodies to these substances and when the allergen and antibody interact, their cells release substances, such as leukotrienes and histamine, that actually cause the signs and symptoms.

37. a (p. 394)

Rationale: Hives in a patient who is alert and in no distress are most likely due to an allergic reaction. Antibiotics are a common allergen, making an allergic reaction more likely in this patient.

38. a (p. 395)

Rationale: The patient needs oxygen, regardless of his pulse oximetry reading. Epinephrine is an important treatment for anaphylaxis, and the patient may still be receiving venom if the stinger is in place.

39. a (p. 396)

Rationale: Pale skin, chest pain, and anxiousness are side effects of epinephrine, indicating that the epinephrine is causing vasoconstriction and having an effect on the heart.

40. b (p. 399)

Rationale: The most important action for this patient is maintaining the airway and providing oxygen. Knowledge of the exact allergen will not change treatment at this point, and complete vital signs should be taken only after the airway and breathing are addressed.

41. d (p. 396)

Rationale: Because epinephrine is a short-acting drug, some auto-injectors come in packages of two.

42. c (p. 396)

Rationale: It is important to ensure the entire dose of epinephrine is delivered by holding the unit against the thigh for 10 seconds.

43. b (p. 400)

Rationale: This position seems to provide the most comfort for patients with abdominal pain by reducing tension on the abdominal wall.

44. a (p. 401)

Rationale: This position will provide the most protection for the patient's airway during continued vomiting.

45. b (p. 404)

Rationale: Taking steps to improve the patient's perfusion is the first priority.

46. c (p. 394)

Rationale: It is most important to reassess the patient to detect any changes in the vital signs.

47. b (p. 403)

Rationale: A heart rate of 124 is higher than normal, and is a sign of hypovolemia.

48. d (p. 400)

Rationale: The quadrant in which the patient complains of pain should always be palpated last.

49. a (p. 403)

Rationale: Dialysis is used to remove wastes from the blood of patients whose kidneys are not functioning.

50. c (p. 404)

Rationale: It is most important to first stop the bleeding using direct pressure. Do not take a blood pressure or use a tourniquet in an extremity with a shunt.

CHAPTER 17

STOP, REVIEW, REMEMBER (PP. 424–425)
MULTIPLE CHOICE

1. b (p. 419)
2. c (p. 420)
3. a (p. 421)
4. c (p. 423)

TRUE/FALSE

1. T (p. 419)
2. F (p. 419)
3. F (pp. 420–421)
4. T (pp. 420–421)

CRITICAL THINKING

1. You will size up and manage the scene initially including assuring safety and calling for additional EMS resources so the person can be removed from the vehicle. (pp. 420–421)
2. As in question one you will assure your safety and that of the patient. Your primary assessment will begin with assessing the patient's breathing and clear the airway, if possible. (p. 420)
3. Primary assessment revolves around the ABCs for all patients. You would still take spinal precautions because the patient was involved in what appears to be a significant MOI crash. (pp. 420–422)

CHAPTER REVIEW (PP. 428–430)
MULTIPLE CHOICE

1. a (p. 426)
2. d (p. 426)
3. c (p. 423)
4. a (p. 420)
5. b (p. 424)
6. c (p. 423)
7. b (p. 426)

TRUE/FALSE

1. T (p. 427)
2. T (pp. 420–421)
3. F (p. 423)
4. F (p. 421)
5. T (pp. 420–421)
6. T (p. 424)
7. F (p. 420)

CRITICAL THINKING

1. The scene size-up determines that it is unsafe for you and the patient due to the electrical wires. Appropriate resources should be called immediately and do not approach until it is safe. (pp. 420–421)
2. You should assess airway, breathing, and circulation. (p. 423)
3. The mechanism of the fall and the fact that his upper legs (femurs) are fractured indicate that internal blood loss and shock is possible. Prompt transport to a trauma center (where available) is appropriate here. (p. 418)

CHAPTER 18

STOP, REVIEW, REMEMBER (PP. 441–442)
MULTIPLE CHOICE

1. c (p. 439)
2. a (p. 434)
3. a (p. 434)
4. c (p. 438)
5. c (p. 437)

EMERGENCY MEDICAL RESPONDER PRACTICE

1. Capillary (p. 440)
2. Arterial (p. 439)
3. Venous (p. 439)

SHORT ANSWER

1. Not enough oxygen getting to the cell. Underperfused. (p. 434)
2. Small blood vessels in the skin constrict to shunt blood to the core of the body. This limits the amount of blood near the surface of the skin and thus creates a pale appearance. (p. 437)
3. In irreversible shock, organs and organ systems have died and cannot be returned to normal function. In decompensated shock, these systems are failing, but not necessarily dead yet. (p. 438)

STOP, REVIEW, REMEMBER   (PP. 446–447)
MULTIPLE CHOICE

1. c (p. 443)
2. a (p. 443)
3. d (p. 443)

4. d (p. 443)
5. c (p. 444)

EMERGENCY MEDICAL RESPONDER PRACTICE

1. Direct pressure (p. 443)
2. Hemostatic agent (p. 444)
3. Tourniquet (p. 444)

CRITICAL THINKING

1. High-flow O₂ maximizes the oxygen in the blood. It is important in a severe bleeding patient because that person has lost and is losing his oxygen transport system. Therefore he needs to maximize what he has left circulating. (p. 443)
2. Patients can lose blood due to fractures, and splinting helps minimize this blood loss. A person in shock cannot afford to lose any more blood than he has already lost. (p. 445)

CHAPTER REVIEW   (PP. 450–452)
MULTIPLE CHOICE

1. d (p. 449)
2. b (p. 447)
3. c (p. 438)

4. a (p. 434)
5. a (p. 448)

SHORT ANSWER

1. Seated upright and slightly forward to allow drainage of the nose without impairing breathing. This position also discourages the swallowing of blood. (p. 448)
2. Any blood loss adds to the total amount lost. A patient with internal bleeding cannot afford to lose additional blood from an external wound. (p. 448)
3. The body increases heart rate to compensate for the challenge of shock. What blood is left is pumped faster. (p. 437)

CRITICAL THINKING

1. Some experts say massive bleeding (exsanguinating hemorrhage) kills faster than even airway or breathing interruption. (p. 443)
2. This question addresses scene safety. Consider the threat of bloodborne pathogens vs. the need to treat this patient. (p. 443)
3. First signs of allergy: hives, itch, runny nose. Anaphylaxis would be seen if airway, breathing, or circulation problems occurred. (p. 449)

CASE STUDY

1. Ensure adequate airway and breathing. (p. 443)
2. If you find massive bleeding, take steps to control it immediately. (pp. 443–444)
3. Spurting blood indicates arterial bleeding. (p. 443)
4. Apply direct pressure, apply a pressure dressing, consider a hemostatic agent (if protocol allows), and consider a tourniquet if previous steps are unsuccessful. (p. 443)
5. Shock (p. 437)
6. Assist the patient to lie flat, preserve heat, apply high-flow oxygen, and arrange rapid transport. (p. 448)

CHAPTER 19

STOP, REVIEW, REMEMBER   (PP. 463–464)
MULTIPLE CHOICE

1. d (p. 455)
2. c (p. 458)
3. b (p. 455)

4. a (p. 456)
5. a (p. 461)

MATCHING

1. e (p. 458)
2. a (p. 458)
3. d (p. 458)

4. b (p. 458)
5. c (p. 459)

SHORT ANSWER

1. Air may be pulled in through the hole rather than through the trachea. (p. 455)
2. Sealing it completely may allow pressure to build up and cause a tension pneumothorax. Sealing only three sides allows air to escape if pressure begins to build. (p. 456)
3. A tension pneumothorax puts pressure on the heart and/or great vessels to cause shock. A simple pneumothorax does not. (p. 458)

STOP, REVIEW, REMEMBER   (PP. 469–470)
MULTIPLE CHOICE

1. c (p. 464)
2. a (p. 464)
3. d (p. 465)

4. a (p. 467)
5. b (p. 468)

EMERGENCY MEDICAL RESPONDER PRACTICE

1. ■ Clean away large debris. (p. 465)
   ■ Cover the organs with a moist sterile dressing and then an occlusive dressing. (p. 465)
   ■ Prevent heat loss. (p. 465)
   ■ Never push organs back into the cavity. (p. 465)

CRITICAL THINKING

1. Yes, this patient has the potential for damage to abdominal organs such as the liver and spleen, but in particular the great vessels with lower quadrant pain. (p. 467)
2. The object may be preventing blood loss. Removing the object may cause more bleeding. (p. 466)

CHAPTER REVIEW   (PP. 470–473)
MULTIPLE CHOICE

1. a (p. 455)
2. d (p. 455)
3. c (p. 465)
4. d (p. 465)
5. c (p. 466)

SHORT ANSWER

1. Crepitus refers to the grating sound of broken bone ends rubbing together. (p. 458)
2. Many abdominal injuries also involve lung tissue. An occlusive dressing protects against pneumothorax, "just in case." (p. 465)
3. "Closed abdominal injury" implies that the skin is intact over the wound. (p. 466)

CRITICAL THINKING

1. Shock can be caused by the actual blood loss of the hemothorax or by the creation of a tension hemothorax by creating enough pressure to put pressure on the heart and great vessels in the chest. (p. 458)
2. Assess and control the airway (consider bag-valve mask). Take appropriate steps to dress and bandage the evisceration. Arrange rapid transport. (p. 468)
3. Ensure the ABCs. Remove the branch from the tree if possible, secure, and protect in place (do not remove the impaled object). Arrange rapid transport. (p. 466)

CASE STUDY

1. Assess the airway. (p. 468)
2. Suction and secure the airway. Consider an airway adjunct. (p. 468)
3. Shock (p. 467)
4. Internal bleeding (p. 467)
5. Decompensated shock (p. 467)

CHAPTER 20
STOP, REVIEW, REMEMBER   (PP. 480–481)
MULTIPLE CHOICE

1. a (p. 477)
2. c (p. 476)
3. d (p. 478)
4. b (p. 479)
5. b (p. 478)

EMERGENCY MEDICAL RESPONDER PRACTICE

1. a. Abrasion b. Open (p. 477)
2. a. Contusion b. Closed (p. 476)
3. a. Hematoma b. Closed (p. 476)
4. a. Laceration b. Open (p. 478)
5. a. Puncture b. Open (p. 478)

SHORT ANSWER

1. Damage to the underlying internal abdominal organs and potentially internal bleeding. (p. 476)
2. Scene safety. Severe bleeding and shock, air entering the great veins of the neck. (p. 479)
3. Scene safety. Damage to the underlying internal organs of the chest; in particular lung, heart, and great vessel injury. Internal bleeding and shock, interruption of the mechanism of breathing. (p. 479)

STOP, REVIEW, REMEMBER   (PP. 490–491)
MULTIPLE CHOICE

1. a (p. 482)
2. d (p. 487)
3. c (p. 483)
4. d (p. 486)
5. d (p. 483)

EMERGENCY MEDICAL RESPONDER PRACTICE

1. ■ Do not remove. (p. 487)
   ■ Secure the pencil in place using bulky dressings, roller bandage, and tape. (p. 487)
   ■ Secure and protect the object during transport. (p. 487)

SHORT ANSWER

1. Bending may cause bandages to tighten and cut off blood flow to the extremity. (p. 486)
2. Leaving digits exposed allows for ongoing assessment of distal circulation, sensory function, and motor function. (p. 486)
3. An effective dressing is sterile or clean, bulky, absorbent, and large enough to cover the entire wound. (p. 484)

STOP, REVIEW, REMEMBER   (PP. 500–501)
MULTIPLE CHOICE

1. d (p. 491)
2. d (p. 491)
3. a (p. 491)
4. d (p. 494)
5. d (p. 498)

EMERGENCY MEDICAL RESPONDER PRACTICE

1. ■ Arrange transport (consider a burn center). (p. 495)
   ■ Consider other injuries (complete a primary assessment). (p. 496)
   ■ Bandage with clean dry dressing. (p. 497)

SHORT ANSWER

1. 18 percent (p. 494)
2. 18 percent (p. 494)
3. Actual burns to mouth, nose, or face; hair or eyebrows burnt; difficulty speaking; difficulty breathing; presence of soot in sputum (p. 497)

CHAPTER REVIEW (PP. 502–503)

MULTIPLE CHOICE

1. a (p. 491)
2. b (p. 478)
3. c (p. 497)
4. c (p. 477)
5. d (p. 483)

SHORT ANSWER

1. Remove loose debris, wrap in gauze moistened with sterile saline, place in a sealed plastic bag labeled with the patient's name, place bag in a container with ice (never use dry ice, place the part directly on the ice, or immerse the part in water), arrange transport (p. 489)
2. White, pale, and has a leathery feel; potentially little pain. (p. 493)

CRITICAL THINKING

1. Recovery of the knife will allow you to assess the size of the knife and therefore the potential size of the wound it created. (p. 479)
2. Do not approach until you are sure power has been cut to the dryer. Conduct the primary assessment. Treat airway, breathing, and circulation problems. Treat any burns related to the electrocution. Arrange transport. (p. 498)
3. Consider the emotional impact of a serious facial injury. Consider the need to transport to a facility with appropriate resources to repair such a wound. (p. 479)

CASE STUDY

1. In the primary assessment you would want to address the chest wound. The open wound to the chest (the back is the posterior border of the chest cavity) must be sealed. Administer oxygen by nonrebreather mask. You observe that bleeding is already controlled. (p. 479)
2. You must seal the open chest wound immediately. This can be done with a gloved hand if you don't have an occlusive dressing immediately available. (p. 479)
3. The open chest wound could cause pneumothorax or tension pneumothorax as well as internal bleeding leading to shock. This patient should be considered a high priority. Advise incoming EMS units of the information you find. (p. 479)

CHAPTER 21

STOP, REVIEW, REMEMBER (PP. 510–511)

MULTIPLE CHOICE

1. a (p. 505)
2. c (p. 505)
3. b (p. 506)
4. c (p. 507)
5. a (p. 509)

EMERGENCY MEDICAL RESPONDER PRACTICE

1. Any three of these: altered mental status, weakness, numbness, inability to move one side of the body, vision problems, posturing, pupil changes, loss of balance or difficulty walking, nausea and vomiting after the injury (p. 508)
2. Any three of these: obvious deformity, visible fracture; pain and/or tenderness at point of impact; cerebrospinal fluid (CSF) leaking from ears, nose, mouth, or the wound itself; pupil changes; Battle sign; bruising behind the ears; raccoon eyes (p. 509)

SHORT ANSWER

1. Pressure forcing the brain down through the foramen magnum. Signs include altered and decreasing mental status, Cushing triad, posturing, and changes to pupil response. (p. 508)
2. The brainstem controls airway and respiratory function. Damage to that area can impair function. (p. 508)
3. Constant reassessment will help identify patterns that will allow you to recognize ominous signs of pressure building in the skull. Mental status changes, raccoon eyes, Battle sign, and even some pupil changes can occur long after the initial injury and will require your ongoing attention to find. (p. 508)

STOP, REVIEW, REMEMBER (PP. 518–519)

MULTIPLE CHOICE

1. c (p. 514)
2. a (p. 513)
3. c (p. 514)
4. c (p. 514)
5. d (p. 516)

EMERGENCY MEDICAL RESPONDER PRACTICE

1. Any three of these: difficulty opening or closing the mouth, swallowing, speaking, or closing the jaw properly (teeth are misaligned on closing the mouth), pain, tenderness or deformity in the area around the ears, missing or dislodged teeth (p. 513)
2. Any three of these: obvious deformity of the bones surrounding the eye, difficulty moving the eye, double or impaired vision, numbness around the eye (p. 514)

SHORT ANSWER

1. Do not touch the roots, rinse off debris with tap water, and place the tooth in a glass of milk (if available). If milk is not available, wrap the tooth in gauze moistened with sterile saline. (p. 513)
2. Apply direct pressure (one side only). Consider an occlusive dressing. (p. 513)
3. Flush the eye with clean water (follow local protocol), visualize the foreign object (either under the lower lid or under the upper lid), and remove the object with the corner of a piece of sterile gauze. Turn the upper lid over a cotton swab to provide better access. (p. 515)

CHAPTER REVIEW   (PP. 532–534)

MULTIPLE CHOICE

1. b (p. 506)
2. c (p. 510)
3. a (p. 508)
4. c (p. 519)
5. d (p. 521)

SHORT ANSWER

1. Keeping the bones aligned as one unit in a natural, anatomical position (p. 521)
2. Brief loss of consciousness, temporary confusion or altered mental status, amnesia (especially of the moments before or immediately after the event), repetitive questioning, seizure, nausea and vomiting, incontinence (p. 509)
3. pain and/or tenderness over the area of the spinal column, pain with movement, numbness and/or tingling in the arms or legs, paralysis or difficulty moving any of the extremities, loss of sensation in the extremities, incontinence (loss of bowel or bladder control), priapism, deformity of the spine (p. 521)
4. Torso, pelvis, head. (p. 526)
5. One provider holds in-line stabilization of the head and directs movements to keep the head in line with the rest of the body. Two other providers position themselves on the same side of the patient and reach across the body. One grabs the patient's shoulder and hip, and the other grabs the patient's upper thigh and lower leg. Coordinated movement is critical. (p. 527)

CRITICAL THINKING

1. A closed head injury has no room for pressure to build. (p. 508)
2. Consider the emotional impact of a facial injury. (p. 512)
3. Life threat to the patient or to a patient blocked by your patient (p. 529)

CASE STUDY

1. Check airway, breathing, and circulation (ABCs). (p. 513)
2. Massive bleeding, air in great vessels, c-spine injury (p. 513)
3. Direct pressure, occlusive dressing. Do not compress both sides of the neck simultaneously. (p. 513)
4. Injury to the cervical spine is now more likely. (p. 519)
5. This patient would most likely keep you busy managing just the life threats. Be sure to suction the airway as needed and ventilate if required. You will probably be called to assist EMS with full spinal immobilization. (p. 522)

CHAPTER 22

STOP, REVIEW, REMEMBER   (PP. 540–541)

MULTIPLE CHOICE

1. a (p. 537)
2. d (p. 537)
3. a (p. 538)
4. c (p. 538)
5. d (p. 537)

EMERGENCY MEDICAL RESPONDER PRACTICE

1. Twisting force (p. 538)
2. Direct force (p. 537)
3. Indirect force (p. 538)
4. Indirect force (p. 538)
5. Direct force (p. 537)

SHORT ANSWER

1. Days lost at one's job (p. 536)
2. Simple tasks that would become much more difficult (p. 536)
3. Ability to get from one location to another (p. 536)

STOP, REVIEW, REMEMBER   (PP. 548–549)

MULTIPLE CHOICE

1. a (p. 542)
2. b (p. 544)
3. c (p. 543)
4. d (p. 544)
5. a (p. 547)

EMERGENCY MEDICAL RESPONDER PRACTICE

1. Four or more of the following: tenderness or pain on touching; deformity; open wounds and exposed bone; crepitus; loss of range of motion or being unable to move an extremity; swelling; bruising or discoloration; loss of sensation; loss of circulation; the patient may tell you he heard the sound of bone breaking. (p. 542)
2. Four or more of the following: communicate with the patient; maintain manual immobilization; expose injury before splinting; dress open wounds first;

straighten angulated injuries; assess circulation, sensation, and motor function before and after application; consider padding a splint; immobilize above and below the injury (p. 544)

CRITICAL THINKING

3. Answers will vary. Sample: Many household items could be used. Wood, broom handles, sporting equipment (shin guards), cardboard, rolled up magazines, and pillows could all be used. Consider patient comfort and pad appropriately. (p. 547)

CHAPTER REVIEW (PP. 553–555)

MULTIPLE CHOICE

1. d (p. 549)
2. a (p. 549)
3. d (p. 549)
4. c (p. 551)
5. c (p. 550)

SHORT ANSWER

1. Rotated foot or a shortening of one leg compared to the other (p. 551)
2. Some EMS systems allow for the use of the pneumatic antishock garment (PASG) to treat unstable pelvic fractures. (p. 551)
3. Pass the sling around affected arm with the point of the triangle to the elbow using a small knot to hold the elbow. Pass other sides of the sling around arm and tie. Try to keep the knot off the patient's neck. Secure arm to body with two to three cravats around chest. (p. 544)

CRITICAL THINKING

1. To ensure that circulation and blood flow are adequate (p. 543)
2. Splinting is a way to control both external and internal bleeding related to a fracture. (p. 551)
3. To maximize the possibility of reattachment to the patient (p. 552)

CASE STUDY

1. Answers are for discussion based on the students' answers. (p. 550)
2. Answers are for discussion based on the students' answers. (p. 550)
3. Answers are for discussion based on the students' answers. (p. 551)
4. Answers are for discussion based on the students' answers. (p. 551)

CHAPTER 23

STOP, REVIEW, REMEMBER (PP. 566–568)

MULTIPLE CHOICE

1. b (p. 558)
2. d (p. 559)
3. c (p. 565)

EMERGENCY MEDICAL RESPONDER PRACTICE

1. Answers should include four of the following: cool/cold skin temperature; shivering; impaired judgment; decreased mental status; initially rapid, then slow pulse; lack of coordination; complaints of joint/muscle stiffness; stiff/rigid posture. (p. 560)
2. Notify EMS; take Standard Precautions; scene size-up; make sure EMS system is activated; remove patient from cold and cover with blanket; administer oxygen; remove wet clothing; monitor vital signs; comfort, calm, and reassure patient. (p. 562)
3. When transportation is delayed 100°F to 105°F (p. 565)
4. Notify EMS; Standard Precautions; scene size-up; be sure EMS system is activated; remove patient from cold and from wet clothing; administer oxygen; protect, stabilize, and do not massage hands; comfort, calm, reassure patient; check for hypothermia (p. 564)

MATCHING

1. b (p. 558)
2. d (p. 558)
3. e (p. 558)
4. a (p. 558)
5. c (p. 558)
6. M (p. 563)
7. S (p. 563)
8. M (p. 563)
9. M (p. 563)
10. S (p. 563)
11. S (p. 563)
12. M (p. 563)
13. S (p. 563)
14. L (p. 564)
15. G (p. 560)
16. G (p. 560)
17. L (p. 564)

CRITICAL THINKING

1. Medical condition, trauma condition, use of drugs or alcohol, exposure to poisons, age of the patient (p. 559)
2. You're not dead until you're warm and dead. (p. 564)

STOP, REVIEW, REMEMBER (PP. 572–573)

MULTIPLE CHOICE

1. b (p. 568)
2. c (p. 570)
3. d (p. 570)
4. d (p. 569)
5. b (p. 568)

MATCHING

1. b (p. 568)
2. a (p. 568)
3. c (p. 568)

EMERGENCY MEDICAL RESPONDER PRACTICE

1. Answers can include: weakness; exhaustion; muscle cramps; dizziness, faintness; rapid pulse, strong at first, but weakens headache; seizures; loss of appetite; nausea; vomiting; altered mental status/unresponsiveness; skin that is moist, pale, and normal to cool in temperature or hot and moist or hot and dry (p. 569)
2. Notify EMS; take Standard Precautions; remove patient from heat; administer oxygen; loosen/remove clothing; fan moist, pale, and normal to cool skin, while applying a mist of water; for hot and dry/moist skin, apply cold packs to neck, armpits, and groin; keep skin wet/take vital signs often; advise incoming units of signs of shock (p. 570)
3. High heat; high humidity; exercise or strenuous activity; medical condition; use of drugs or alcohol; age of the patient (p. 568)

CHAPTER REVIEW   (PP. 579–581)

MULTIPLE CHOICE

1. c (p. 558)
2. b (p. 559)
3. b (p. 563)
4. c (p. 563)
5. a (p. 564)
6. c (p. 562)
7. b (p. 565)
8. c (p. 568)
9. c (p. 569)
10. d (p. 576)

EMERGENCY MEDICAL RESPONDER PRACTICE

1. Perform a scene size-up and assess for any dangers. (p. 578)
2. Answers can include: weakness; exhaustion; muscle cramps; dizziness, faintness; rapid pulse that is strong at first, but becomes weak as damage progresses; headache; seizures; loss of appetite; nausea; vomiting; altered mental status, possibly unresponsiveness; skin that is moist, pale, and normal to cool in temperature or hot and moist or hot and dry (p. 569)
3. Notify EMS; take Standard Precautions; remove patient from heat; administer oxygen; loosen/ remove clothing; fan surface of moist, pale, and normal to cool skin, while applying a mist of water; for hot and dry or moist skin, apply cold packs to neck, armpits, and groin; keep skin wet/take vital signs often; advise incoming units of signs of shock (p. 570)

MATCHING

1. m (p. 575)
2. f (p. 558)
3. a (p. 558)
4. i (p. 564)
5. e (p. 558)
6. k (p. 574)
7. d (p. 558)
8. c (p. 558)
9. b (p. 558)
10. g (p. 559)
11. h (p. 559)
12. j (p. 568)
13. l (p. 574)

SECTION FIVE REVIEW

1. a (p. 417)
   Rationale: Observations of improved trauma care in the Korean and Vietnam wars, and the 1966 white paper made better trauma care the focus of initial EMS system development.
2. d (p. 419)
   Rationale: The American College of Surgeons sets the criteria for four levels of trauma centers, depending on their capabilities for caring for trauma patients.
3. c (p. 420)
   Rationale: All of the responses are part of the scene size-up, but scene safety is always the highest priority.
4. a (p. 423)
   Rationale: A primary assessment is performed on all patients, even if it is as straightforward as observing that the patient is in no immediate distress as you approach him. This patient has an isolated injury, making a head-to-toe exam unnecessary. Vital signs are a routine part of care for every patient
5. b (p. 427)
   Rationale: Patients are considered higher risk for life-threatening injury if the Glasgow Coma Scale score is less than 12.
6. b (p. 426)
   Rationale: Although the patient has no eye-opening response, the lowest score possible in each section of the Glasgow Coma Scale is 1.
7. a (p. 426)
   Rationale: There are up to 6 points possible for motor response. In this case, the patient obeys commands, which warrants the highest score.
8. b (p. 423)
   Rationale: The patient's behavior could be due to any of several different reasons, but hypoxia is a life-threatening potential cause for his behavior and he must be treated for hypoxia.
9. c (p. 437)
   Rationale: One of the earliest signs of shock, along with pale skin and anxiety, is increased heart rate. The other responses represent late signs of shock.

10. b (p. 437)

Rationale: Although it is not unheard of for young female patients to have normal blood pressures similar to that of the patient, we must assume that the blood pressure is starting to drop, especially in the presence of a very weak rapid pulse, shallow rapid respirations, and pale, cool, sweaty skin. We cannot tell from signs and symptoms at what point a patient enters irreversible shock, because it is a cellular event.

11. b (p. 439)

Rationale: The blood pressure may be normal, but it is normal because of vasoconstriction in peripheral tissues and decreased perfusion to those areas.

12. c (p. 437)

Rationale: Not all shock is due to external bleeding. Signs of hypoperfusion include weakness and faintness (often described by patients as dizziness).

13. d (p. 443)

Rationale: The patient's airway must be opened and cleared of blood with suction, and he must receive bag-valve mask ventilations to ensure that his lungs are ventilated.

14. c (p. 443)

Rationale: Although any clean cloth will do in a pinch to control bleeding, sterile dressings are preferred. In addition, you should look at the laceration so you know what you are dealing with. In this case, the patient does not have signs of shock, so a quick peek at the wound while swapping the washcloth for a dressing will not endanger the patient.

15. d (p. 444)

Rationale: The patient's most immediate threat to life is ongoing hemorrhage. Having him lie down will increase perfusion to the brain and can be accomplished almost simultaneously with preparing a tourniquet. Oxygen is important, but the patient's airway is open and he is breathing. Allowing bleeding to continue while setting up oxygen for administration will result in continued significant blood loss.

16. a (p. 448)

Rationale: Although sitting up would allow gravity to assist in controlling bleeding from the nose, the patient is showing early signs of shock and complains of nausea. She should be placed on her side as you control the bleeding and ready yourself to suction her airway if she vomits.

17. d (p. 462)

Rationale: The patient's respiratory rate of 40 and his drowsiness indicate respiratory distress. He is in immediate need of assisted ventilations and oxygen. The blood pressure and exact nature of the allergy will not change the EMR's immediate treatment, and can be obtained once the patient is being ventilated. Although the parents must be contacted, care must not be delayed to do so in this case.

18. a (p. 456)

Rationale: This wound is large enough to allow air to enter the thoracic cavity with each breath, resulting in an accumulation of air outside the lung that will compress the lung and interfere with ventilation. Taping three sides prevents air from getting in, but creates a "relief valve" to prevent further accumulation of any air that may be escaping from an injured lung.

19. b (p. 456)

Rationale: Air under pressure inside the thoracic cavity can escape if the occlusive dressing is lifted as the patient exhales.

20. d (p. 458)

Rationale: The medical term hemothorax literally means blood in the chest cavity.

21. a (p. 458)

Rationale: Subcutaneous means beneath the skin, and emphysema refers to a condition of air being trapped—in this case, under the skin.

22. c (p. 459)

Rationale: The patient shows signs of good oxygenation, but this may change if it is painful for her to take a breath of normal depth. Splinting the injured area with a pillow can provide some relief without restricting movement of the chest wall.

23. d (p. 462)

Rationale: The mechanism of injury and physical signs are consistent with traumatic asphyxia, and a risk of spinal injury. The patient's respiratory rate and depth indicate respiratory depression. He needs assistance breathing.

24. c (p. 466)

Rationale: Exposed abdominal organs are protected from drying out and further contamination by placing a moist, sterile, occlusive dressing over them.

25. c (p. 466)

Rationale: The patient's fall puts him at risk for spinal injury. Placing him supine will move the stake, as will attempting to saw it off without help to stabilize the object. Any movement of the stake can result in additional injury and potentially uncontrollable bleeding. Additionally, the object should only be shortened if it is impossible to transport the patient without doing so.

26. d (p. 478)

Rationale: Soft tissue injuries can result in significant bleeding and, if they involve the face or neck, can obstruct the airway. However, most soft tissue injuries are not life threatening, though they may be the most obvious problem, distracting the patient and the EMR from other injuries.

27. a (p. 476)

Rationale: Hematomas under the skin (especially over bony areas such as the skull) are usually self-limiting since, as blood accumulates in a limited space, the pressure on the injured vessels controls bleeding.

Swelling of the scalp will not be life threatening, and a closed wound carries little chance of infection. However, the mechanism of injury puts the patient at risk for injury to the brain, which can be life threatening.

28. c (p. 478)
Rationale: A tearing away of the skin, which often results in a loose flap of skin attached by a narrow band of tissue, is called an avulsion.

29. b (p. 478)
Rationale: After the scene size-up, assessing and managing the airway is the first problem. Keep in mind that dramatic soft tissue injuries have the potential to distract you from your priorities in patient care.

30. a (p. 483)
Rationale: A dressing is placed over the wound and ideally is sterile, is able to absorb blood and fluids, and will not stick to the wound when removed. A dressing should be slightly larger than the area of the wound.

31. c (p. 487)
Rationale: Open or closed wounds of the neck can compromise the airway and be life threatening. An occlusive dressing is used to prevent air from entering the large blood vessels in the neck. A circumferential dressing is never used on the neck, as it may interfere with blood flow and obstruct the airway.

32. a (p. 489)
Rationale: Remember, an EMR is of little use to a patient if he is injured. Scene safety is a top priority, and there are hazards at this scene that must be controlled.

33. b (p. 490)
Rationale: As an EMR, your first priority is your own safety. Animal control officers are specifically trained and equipped to manage animals that may be dangerous. If animal control is not available in your area, it might be preferable to check with dispatch to see if someone in the residence is able to secure the animal before you approach.

34. b (p. 491)
Rationale: Partial-thickness burns (formerly referred to as second-degree burns) are characterized by blistering and pain.

35. c (p. 494)
Rationale: Of the choices given, burns of the face are most concerning because they may be an indication of airway burns or smoke inhalation, and carry the potential for scars that may impact the patient's subsequent quality of life. Therefore, patients with facial burns are best managed in a burn center.

36. a (p. 500)
Rationale: Electrical burns may have exit wounds and may produce long bone fractures, but finding them is not the first priority. Electrical burns usually are not associated with large areas of the body surface. But, electricity travels through the body internally and may cause damage to the heart, nerves, muscles, and blood vessels.

37. b (p. 508)
Rationale: Temporary loss of memory is typical of concussions, but not a specific indication of increased pressure within the skull. Increased pressure within the skull is associated with high blood pressure, a slowing pulse, unequal pupils, abnormal respirations, and a decreasing level of responsiveness.

38. c (p. 509)
Rationale: Of the choices given, the highest priority is airway management. Because of the mechanism of injury, protecting the spine from movement is important but will be challenging since the patient is having a seizure. Trying to restrain the head while the rest of the body is moving will result in movement of the neck.

39. a (p. 509)
Rationale: A fracture of the portion of the skull that connects to the ear can allow cerebrospinal fluid mixed with blood to leak from the ear.

40. d (p. 515)
Rationale: The eyes move together, so covering the uninjured eye to prevent it from moving in response to visual stimuli will help keep the injured eye from moving.

41. c (p. 524)
Rationale: Cervical collars are designed to limit motion, but cannot prevent movement by themselves. A collar that does not fit properly can force the neck out of neutral alignment, increasing the potential for injury.

42. a (p. 529)
Rationale: Because removing a helmet carries a risk of movement of the neck, they are typically only removed if they interfere with management of the airway.

43. b (p. 538)
Rationale: A strain is a tearing or stretching of muscle fibers.

44. c (p. 549)
Rationale: Although simple and time-tested, a sling and swathe is the best way to immobilize an injured shoulder.

45. b (p. 549)
Rationale: A traction splint may benefit the patient with a femur fracture by overcoming the contraction of the strong thigh muscles to allow gross alignment of the bone ends.

46. d (p. 552)
Rationale: The best way to preserve the exposed tissues, nerves, and blood vessels of the amputated part is by grossly decontaminating it with sterile saline, wrapping it in a sterile saline-moistened dressing, placing it in a plastic bag, and keeping it cool, but not putting it directly on ice.

47. a (p. 560)
Rationale: The shivering mechanism breaks down with progressive hypothermia. A lack of shivering in a cold patient is a sign of a progressively decreasing core temperature.

48. d (p. 562)

Rationale: Warming a severely hypothermic patient is complicated, and should only be carried out in a hospital setting. Removing wet clothing will help reduce further heat loss from the body.

49. a (p. 568)

Rationale: Heatstroke is a life-threatening emergency in which the body's cooling mechanisms are not working and the core temperature climbs dangerously high.

50. c (p. 570)

Rationale: A patient with decreased responsiveness should never be given anything by mouth. Cooling the patient is important, but cooling too quickly, such as by icing the patient, may result in shivering, which will produce more body heat.

CHAPTER 24

STOP, REVIEW, REMEMBER   (PP. 601–603)

MULTIPLE CHOICE

1. b (p. 593)
2. c (p. 593)
3. d (p. 596)

MATCHING

1. b (p. 593)
2. g (p. 591)
3. f (p. 591)
4. c (p. 593)
5. a (p. 591)
6. d (p. 593)
7. e (p. 593)

LIST

1.
   1. Dilation of the cervix (p. 593)
   2. Expulsion (p. 595)
   3. Placenta (p. 595)
2.
   1. Sheets and towels, sterile if possible and sterile gloves and gown
   2. One dozen 4-inch square gauze pads
   3. Two or three sanitary napkins
   4. Rubber suction syringe and baby receiving blanket
   5. Surgical scissors for cutting the umbilical cord and cord clamps or ties
   6. Foil-wrapped germicidal wipes
   7. Large plastic bags (p. 597)

EMERGENCY MEDICAL RESPONDER PRACTICE

1. Any five of the following:
   1. Have you had a baby before? What is your due date?
   2. Did you receive prenatal care? Did a doctor say you are having more than one
   3. baby or warn of complications? Are you having contractions? How far apart are they?
   4. Did your water break? When? What color was the fluid?
   5. Do you feel the sensation of a bowel movement? (p. 596)
2. Crowning (bulging in the vaginal area) (p. 596)

STOP, REVIEW, REMEMBER   (PP. 612–613)

MULTIPLE CHOICE

1. a (p. 604)
2. c (p. 608)
3. a (p. 611)

EMERGENCY MEDICAL RESPONDER PRACTICE

1.
   1. Dry the infant.
   2. Wrap in a clean, warm blanket.
   3. Place the baby on his side with head slightly lower than trunk.
   4. Clean the mouth and nose, and suction mouth and nose again if needed.
   5. Provide tactile stimulation, if the baby is not active or actively crying.
   6. Administer blow-by oxygen. (p. 603)
2. Provide artificial ventilation at 30–60 breaths per minute using a bag-valve mask. Check to make sure there is proper alignment of the airway. Place a towel under the infant's shoulders. Reassess every 30 seconds. (p. 604)
3. Start CPR with a compression rate of 120 per minute and a ratio of compressions to breaths of 3:1. (p. 604)

MATCHING

1. d (p. 611)
2. f (p. 612)
3. a (p. 610)
4. e (p. 611)
5. b (p. 610)
6. c (p. 611)

PLACE IN ORDER

1. 6, 2, 9, 4, 7, 5, 1, 8, 3 (p. 599)

CHAPTER REVIEW   (PP. 614–617)

MULTIPLE CHOICE

1. b (p. 591)
2. a (p. 593)
3. d (p. 596)
4. c (p. 600)
5. d (p. 601)
6. b (p. 604)
7. a (p. 606)
8. c (p. 605)
9. d (p. 593)
10. b (p. 612)

MATCHING

1. d (p. 595)
2. b (p. 591)
3. j (p. 600)
4. g (p. 611)
5. a (p. 596)

6. i (p. 611)
7. f (p. 599)
8. h (p. 611)
9. e (p. 593)
10. c (p. 611)

EMERGENCY MEDICAL RESPONDER PRACTICE

1. Do a check of the ABCs and determine if there are any immediate care issues that need to be provided. Then move on to taking patient vital signs, obtaining history information, and asking specific questions about the pregnancy in order to determine if delivery is imminent. (p. 595)

2. Transport the patient for delivery at the hospital. This is her first delivery and the contractions are longer than 5 minutes apart. She does not feel like she has to bear down, and she has no sensation like wanting to move her bowels. She has given no indication that she feels like the baby is about to be born. (p. 595)

3. This patient can develop eclampsia. Keep the patient calm and provide reassurance. If the patient is willing, have her lie down on her left side and provide oxygen. If the husband is calm, have him sit next to his wife and provide comfort. Avoid rough movement, try to maintain a low level of light and noise. Assess and be alert for the possibility of a seizure. (p. 610)

4. ALS Unit 10 this is EMR Unit 2. I am with a pregnant patient in her late 20s. Her water has broken and is 2 weeks from her due date. Delivery does NOT seem imminent as contractions are 10 to 15 minutes apart and this is her first delivery. Her pulse of 90, respirations 22, blood pressure is 190/110. She has pregnancy-induced hypertension. She is calm, on her left side, receiving oxygen. (p. 595)

5. Complete a prehospital care report and restock your vehicle so you are prepared for the next call. (p. 608)

CHAPTER 25

STOP, REVIEW, REMEMBER   (PP. 643–644)

MULTIPLE CHOICE

1. d (p. 625)
2. b (p. 621)
3. c (p. 627)

4. a (p. 632)

EMERGENCY MEDICAL RESPONDER PRACTICE

1. Five from this list: altered mental status, apathy/lack of vitality, pale, cool, clammy skin, rapid respiration rate, absence of tears when crying, rapid or weak and thready pulse, delayed capillary refill, falling blood pressure (p. 645)

2. Try to lay the child flat (make sure the position doesn't interfere with breathing).
Provide oxygen (be prepared to assist ventilations). Keep the patient warm and as calm as possible. Take vital signs often. Provide rapid transport. Make sure that the assessment and treatment you provide is given to the transporting unit. (p. 645)

3. Five from this list: rapid irregular breathing, exhaustion, changes in level of consciousness (or sleepiness), cyanosis, rapid pulse, dropping blood pressure, signs of dehydration, wheezing (usually when child exhales), respiratory distress (late sign), quiet or silent chest (with shallow respirations). (p. 639)

MATCHING

1. b (p. 622)
2. e (p. 622)
3. d (p. 622)

4. c (p. 622)
5. a (p. 622)

SHORT ANSWER

1. (p. 632)

Anatomical Difference	Impact on Assessment and Treatment
Larger tongue	Can block airway
Flat nose and face	Difficult to obtain good airway seal with face mask
Shorter neck	Difficult to stabilize and immobilize
Larger body surface	Prone to hypothermia
Faster respiratory rate	Muscles fatigue easily, can lead to respiratory distress
Heart can sustain faster rate for longer period of time	Can compensate longer before showing signs of shock

2. Possible answers: Has the child had seizures before? Is this seizure pattern normal? Do they always occur with fever? Did family members have seizures as children? How many seizures in the past 24 hours? What was done for them? Was there a head injury, a stiff neck, or a recent headache? Does he have diabetes? Is he on any medication? (p. 641)

STOP, REVIEW, REMEMBER   (PP. 649–651)
MULTIPLE CHOICE

1. d (p. 630)
2. b (p. 634)
3. a (p. 639)

EMERGENCY MEDICAL RESPONDER PRACTICE

1. Any of the following: adult abuser acts in an evasive manner or volunteers little or contradictory information, inconsistent stories from others, caregiver seems inappropriately concerned, child is scared to talk, bruises in various stages of healing, injury not consistent with mechanism of injury, repeat call to same (p. 647)
2. Answers may vary. Confirm environment is safe for you and the patient. Provide necessary emergency care as you would for any patient. Observe the child and caregiver as time permits. Do not be judgmental. Look for signs of neglect. Document thoroughly without being subjective. Provide information to the EMS (p. 648)
3. Any of the following: noisy breathing (wheezing, stridor, crowing, grunting), cyanosis, flaring nostrils, retractions, using accessory muscles, breathing with effort, extreme respiratory rate (either too fast or too slow), altered mental status (p. 629)
4. Altered mental status (p. 629)

IDENTIFICATION

1.

___X___	Altered mental status
_____	Hyperactivity
___X___	Inability to recognize parents
___X___	Rapid weak pulse
_____	Slow strong pulse
___X___	Rapid breathing
_____	Slow breathing
_____	Irregular respirations
___X___	Low blood pressure (late sign)
_____	High blood pressure
___X___	Delayed capillary refill
_____	Rapid capillary refill
___X___	Absence of tears
___X___	Pale, cool, and clammy skin
_____	Warm, dry, and flushed skin (p. 645)

2.
1. When was the child put in the crib?
2. When was the last time the parents looked in on the baby?
3. What were the circumstances concerning the discovery of the infant?
4. What was the position of the baby in the crib?
5. What was the physical appearance of the infant's crib?
6. What else was in the crib?
7. What was the appearance of the room and home?
8. Is there medication present (either for the baby or an adult)?
9. What is the behavior of the people present?
10. What is the general health of the infant—recent illness, medications, or allergies? (p. 647)

CHAPTER REVIEW (PP. 652–655)

MULTIPLE CHOICE

1. c (p. 627)	6. b (p. 640)
2. d (p. 645)	7. c (p. 645)
3. a (p. 641)	8. a (p. 638)
4. b (p. 639)	9. d (p. 648)
5. c (p. 623)	10. b (p. 628)

EMERGENCY MEDICAL RESPONDER PRACTICE

1. Do a general assessment or a "from the doorway" assessment using the pediatric assessment triangle (PAT) to obtain a general impression of the child's condition by observing appearance, breathing, and signs of circulation. (p. 625)
2. Administer oxygen. This is usually done by using the blow-by technique. As the mother is anxious, having her hold the mask near the child's face may help calm the mother. If the mother is too stressed, then you should hold the mask. Be prepared to assist ventilations using a bag-valve mask with supplemental oxygen if the breathing becomes worse. (p. 634)
3. Use the mnemonic SAMPLE to ask the following questions. What are the signs and symptoms? Does the child have any allergies? What medication is the child taking, including medication specifically for this problem? What is the pertinent past medical history? What was the last oral intake and when was it? What were the events that led up to this? (p. 630)
4. Overview of the patient (age and gender), assessment findings including vital signs, care that is being provided (p. 634)
5. Complete a prehospital care report and restock your vehicle so you are prepared for the next call. (p. 634)

MATCHING

1. e (p. 625)	9. h (p. 628)
2. d (p. 647)	10. c (p. 629)
3. k (p. 647)	11. m (p. 634)
4. a (p. 639)	12. f (p. 635)
5. o (p. 639)	13. b (p. 640)
6. j (p. 624)	14. l (p. 645)
7. n (p. 629)	15. g (p. 648)
8. i (p. 638)	

CHAPTER 26

STOP, REVIEW, REMEMBER (PP. 662–663)

MULTIPLE CHOICE

1. a (p. 658)
2. c (p. 659)
3. d (p. 660)

EMERGENCY MEDICAL RESPONDER PRACTICE

1. Any five of the following: fatigue, poor balance, poor coordination—decreased mobility, medication, altered mental status (confusion), high or low blood pressure, decreased night vision, poor peripheral vision (pp. 658–661)
2. scene size-up (Standard Precautions), ensure the airway is open, monitor breathing, control external bleeding, take vital signs, perform a physical exam, get SAMPLE history, update incoming transport unit, comfort, calm, and reassure patient, assist transporting unit with spine stabilization, stabilize pelvis, package for transport. (pp. 667-670)
3. After the call is completed and the patient is transported, attempt to contact someone who can resolve any safety issues such as better lighting, reducing height of curb, or installing safety markings. (p. 665)

MATCHING

1. b (p. 658)
2. e (p. 660)
3. a (p. 658)
4. d (p. 660)
5. c (p. 659)
6. f (p. 661)

STOP, REVIEW, REMEMBER   (PP. 671–672)
MULTIPLE CHOICE

1. b (p. 664)
2. d (p. 665)
3. b (p. 667)

EMERGENCY MEDICAL RESPONDER PRACTICE

1. Any six of the following: depression, substance abuse, abuse, neglect, limited income, unsafe living environment, poor health care, poor nutrition, not taking medication (pp. 663–665)
2. Do a scene size-up and pay attention to "clues" in the environment, patient behavior and hygiene, and where the patient lives. Ask the patient why EMS was called. Evaluate the ABCs. Take a complete set of vital signs. Obtain a SAMPLE history. Do a physical exam. Communicate findings to the responding ambulance. (pp. 667–670)
3. Relay all information to the crew of the transporting ambulance. Let them know that some type of in-home assistance will probably be needed if the patient is discharged to home from the hospital. Make a special point about the heavy drinking and the "poor diet" so they can let the hospital know in order to follow up. (p. 664)
4. Poor hygiene, poor eating habits, disorderly living conditions, (p. 667)
5. Drug interactions, liver may not be as efficient, substance abuse (pp. 662, 664)

MATCHING

1. d (p. 664)
2. a (p. 663)
3. b (p. 664)
4. c (p. 664)
5. e (p. 665)

LIST

1. Any four of the following: fear of hospitals, fear of leaving home, possible hospital admission, losing independence, concern about cost, afraid of leaving spouse behind, concern for pet care (p. 669)
2. The ill or injured elderly patient is likely to show a slow, steady decline, not a sudden change. Don't be lulled into complacency because of little or no change from one set of vital signs to the next. (p. 670)

CHAPTER REVIEW   (PP. 674–676)
MULTIPLE CHOICE

1. b (p. 658)
2. c (p. 658)
3. c (pp. 659–660)
4. a (p. 660)
5. d (p. 660)
6. d (p. 663)
7. a (p. 664)
8. a (p. 666)
9. c (p. 667)
10. b (p. 668)

MATCHING

1. c (p. 659)
2. j (p. 660)
3. k (p. 661)
4. f (p. 661)
5. m (p. 663)
6. b (p. 664)
7. n (p. 667)
8. l (p. 667)
9. e (p. 668)
10. g (p. 668)
11. a (p. 658)
12. o (p. 658)
13. h (p. 657)
14. d (p. 658)
15. i (p. 661)

EMERGENCY MEDICAL RESPONDER PRACTICE

1. The first priority is to establish if the scene is safe. The next concern is your observation using your senses as you approach the patient: the messy room (sight), body odor and urine (smell), and the patient's agitated voice (hearing). You should next take Standard Precautions and move on to the assessment. (p. 667)
2. First evaluate the airway, breathing, and circulation (ABCs). Once this is done and appropriate treatment provided, evaluate the patient to see if he is alert and oriented. Consider evaluating for a stroke using the Cincinnati Stroke Scale. Next obtain a SAMPLE history and a secondary assessment as indicated. (pp. 668–670)
3. Yes. The color, temperature, and condition of the skin show signs of shock that could be caused by internal bleeding. The patient is taking a beta-blocker, which is a medication that will keep the heart rate low even with blood loss. Also, the aspirin can be a contributing factor to the bleeding. (p. 670)

4. The patient seems to live alone in an unhealthy environment and is unable to care for himself properly. This should be checked out if the hospital is considering sending him back home. Also, an evaluation is required to determine what kind of assistance is needed for nutrition, hygiene, and ensuring safety after leaving the hospital. (p. 663)

CHAPTER 27

STOP, REVIEW, REMEMBER   (PP. 680–681)

MULTIPLE CHOICE

1. c (p. 680)
2. a (p. 679)
3. c (p. 679)
4. a (p. 680)
5. b (p. 679)

MATCHING

1. b (p. 680)
2. a (p. 680)
3. c (p. 680)

STOP, REVIEW, REMEMBER   (PP. 686–687)

MULTIPLE CHOICE

1. b (p. 682)
2. a (p. 683)
3. c (p. 685)
4. c (p. 683)
5. a (p. 682)

TRUE/FALSE

1. F (p. 685)
2. T (p. 683)
3. T (p. 683)

CHAPTER REVIEW   (PP. 690–691)

MULTIPLE CHOICE

1. d (p. 682)
2. b (pp. 681–682)
3. d (p. 681)
4. a (p. 680)
5. b (p. 680)
6. c (p. 685)
7. a (p. 680)
8. c (p. 683)
9. c (p. 682)

MATCHING

1. e (p. 682)
2. c (p. 683)
3. a (p. 683)
4. b (p. 685)
5. d (p. 685)
6. f (p. 680)
7. h (p. 685)
8. g (p. 685)

CRITICAL THINKING

1. Various answers will apply based on your local protocol. (pp. 678–679)
2. This question is for discussion and to generate ideas on good communication skills. Answers will vary. (p. 681)

SECTION SIX REVIEW

1. c (p. 591)
   Rationale: The neck of the uterus, which opens to allow childbirth, is called the cervix.
2. c (p. 591)
   Rationale: The placenta attaches to the uterine wall and provides oxygen and nutrients to the fetus through the umbilical cord.
3. a (p. 593)
   Rationale: Uterine contractions during the first stage of labor shorten and dilate the cervix.
4. c (p. 593)
   Rationale: With contractions 5 or more minutes apart there is generally time to transport the patient unless transport will be delayed or prolonged.
5. b (p. 595)
   Rationale: The infant's head entering the birth canal and putting pressure on the rectum causes the sensation of needing to have a bowel movement.
6. d (p. 599)
   Rationale: Placing the hand gently over the baby's head to prevent sudden or "explosive" delivery helps prevent injury to both the baby and the mother.
7. c (p. 600)
   Rationale: Greenish brown amniotic fluid indicates the presence of meconium—the infant's first bowel movement—in the fluid, which may be aspirated into the lungs, causing pneumonia.
8. b (p. 593)
   Rationale: It is normal for amniotic fluid to escape from around the baby during contractions of the uterus.
9. a (p. 601)
   Rationale: This action keeps blood from flowing from the infant's circulation due to gravity until umbilical circulation stops.
10. d (p. 606)
   Rationale: Resumption of contractions and lengthening of the cord indicate separation and impending delivery of the placenta, which will be facilitated by having the mother bear down.
11. a (p. 606)
   Rationale: This amount of blood is normal and expected after delivery.

12. b (p. 610)
    Rationale: Preeclampsia and eclampsia are similar in symptoms, but once seizures occur, the condition is considered eclampsia.

13. d (p. 604)
    Rationale: Chest compressions and ventilations are required in a newborn with a heart rate of less than 60 per minute. All other responses represent normal findings in a newborn.

14. b (p. 623)
    Rationale: The child needs assessment and possibly oxygen. Any respiratory distress will be worsened if being separated from the mother upsets the child. Whenever possible, parents and children are not separated.

15. c (p. 632)
    Rationale: Children have greater body surface for their size and deteriorate quickly once compensatory mechanisms fail. They also require equipment suited to their size and anatomy. The short, flexible trachea of infants and children can be "kinked" like a drinking straw if the neck is overextended.

16. a (p. 626)
    Rationale: A child with a depressed level of responsiveness is very sick and needs immediate intervention, while the other assessments can wait.

17. d (p. 626)
    Rationale: Choice "d" lists the three components of the PAT. The other assessments listed are not part of this initial "from the doorway" assessment.

18. b (p. 626)
    Rationale: Choice "b" lists those things that will tell the most about the child's level of responsiveness.

19. b (p. 628)
    Rationale: The larger head of the infant or small child will cause the neck to flex when the patient is supine unless padding is placed under the shoulders to make them level with the back of the head.

20. a (p. 630)
    Rationale: The most accessible pulse in infants is the brachial pulse in the upper arm.

21. c (p. 631)
    Rationale: Lying and threatening to remove the parent are not appropriate, and restraint is a last resort when assessment and treatment cannot be delayed until the child is calmer. A favorite toy may help calm the patient.

22. c (p. 636)
    Rationale: Proper technique requires caution to avoid overinflating the lungs and causing injury.

23. a (p. 637)
    Rationale: Problems with airway and breathing are the most common cause of cardiac arrest in pediatric patients. Proper airway management is critical, but often overlooked.

24. a (p. 638)
    Rationale: Croup is a viral infection of the larynx, trachea, and bronchi. It characteristically presents with a child who seems well or only mildly ill during the day, only to wake up with the classic "seal bark" cough at night. While not often life threatening, it sometimes is. Children may be quite sick with croup, requiring hospital care.

25. b (p. 640)
    Rationale: Febrile seizures are a common type of seizures in pediatric patients, but there are other causes, many of them life threatening.

26. c (p. 641)
    Rationale: The patient's airway is open and she is breathing adequately. She should be cooled, but not with rubbing alcohol (which can be absorbed through the skin and be toxic) or very cold water (which may cause shivering and increase the body temperature).

27. d (p. 645)
    Rationale: The lack of wet diapers for this period of time in a toddler is an indication of dehydration, which can quickly become quite serious in small children.

28. c (p. 646)
    Rationale: A child's anatomy often results in the lap belt being positioned above, rather than over, the pelvis. Sudden deceleration against the belt can cause abdominal and lower spine injuries.

29. a (p. 646)
    Rationale: A patient who is ventilator-dependent requires immediate, ongoing ventilation. This is the priority, regardless of what the problem with the ventilator is.

30. b (p. 647)
    Rationale: Do not delay resuscitation to gather more information. When additional help arrives, the history and assessment can be performed. Asking when the child was last seen alive implies that the child is being pronounced dead, which is not the EMR's responsibility. Unless rigor mortis is present, CPR is begun.

31. b (p. 658)
    Rationale: The elderly do not sweat as much and may not display diaphoresis, but the other signs of shock listed are still as likely to be present in the elderly as in the young.

32. a (p. 658)
    Rationale: The ability to see close up diminishes with age, as do thickness of the skin, hearing, and appetite.

33. b (p. 664)
    Rationale: Drug and alcohol use are not unusual health concerns in the elderly.

34. d (p. 657)
    Rationale: The patient's primary problem could be something that preceded the fall—something that made her faint or dizzy.

35. c (pp. 667–668)
   Rationale: Although there is an increase in cognitive dysfunction and the senses tend to decline with age, the certainty and degree of these issues is variable.

36. c (pp. 667–668)
   Rationale: It can take elderly patients a bit longer to process information and formulate answers. Don't assume the patient can't hear or can't understand.

37. a (p. 668)
   Rationale: Aspirin is a common drug taken for pain and to prevent strokes and heart attacks. One of aspirin's actions is to interfere with blood clotting.

38. a (p. 670)
   Rationale: The beta-blockers listed in Chapter 26, which are used for some heart problems and high blood pressure, have a similar pattern in their generic names. Metoprolol fits this pattern, making choice "a" an educated follow-up question.

39. d (p. 667)
   Rationale: Elderly patients must be treated with respect by using Mr., Mrs., or Miss. Do not make assumptions that all elderly patients are hearing-impaired.

40. b (p. 664)
   Rationale: While the scene size-up should get your attention regarding possible problems, it is premature to assume the patient is being abused or neglected. It is possible that Alzheimer disease, stroke, or another disorder makes the patient's behavior difficult to manage.

41. d (p. 679)
   Rationale: A congenital problem is one that is present at birth.

42. a (pp. 682–683)
   Rationale: Federal law protects the rights of people with disabilities to keep their service animals with them.

43. b (p. 682)
   Rationale: Choice "b" is the quickest, simplest way to communicate with the least possibility of misunderstanding.

44. c (pp. 682–683)
   Rationale: Many patients with tracheostomies can speak and do not use ventilators. Patients and their families are generally well educated on the care of the tracheostomy.

45. d (p. 683)
   Rationale: An AICD is an automatic implanted cardiac defibrillator, used to detect life-threatening arrhythmias and deliver a shock.

46. a (p. 685)
   Rationale: An indwelling catheter stays in place for an extended period of time so that patients needing frequent doses of drugs do not need to receive multiple IVs. Catheter is a general term for a hollow tube. A urinary catheter drains the bladder, while an IV catheter allows fluid to flow into a vein.

47. a (p. 683)
   Rationale: The tubing that connects the machine to the patient is called a ventilator circuit.

48. d (p. 685)
   Rationale: This is a gastric, or G, tube. A nasogastric, or NG, tube is passed through the nose, throat, and esophagus and into the stomach.

49. b (p. 683)
   Rationale: An AICD is an automatic implanted cardiac defibrillator, used to treat patients with a history of life-threatening heart arrhythmias.

50. c (p. 689)
   Rationale: EMRs are ethically, professionally, and often legally obligated to report any suspected abuse or neglect of a dependent person (child, elderly, mentally or physically disabled), and are protected from civil and criminal penalties when making good-faith reports.

CHAPTER 28

STOP, REVIEW, REMEMBER   (PP. 703–704)

MULTIPLE CHOICE

1. d (p. 702)
2. c (p. 702)
3. c (p. 702)
4. a (p. 702)
5. b (p. 702)

LIST

1. Any six of the following: tire inflation pressure, engine oil, power steering fluid, and transmission fluid, fuel level, headlights, turn signals, backup lights, and scene lights, emergency warning lights, siren, horn, communications equipment, medical equipment, safety equipment (p. 702)

STOP, REVIEW, REMEMBER   (PP. 708–709)

MULTIPLE CHOICE

1. d (p. 704)
2. c (p. 706)
3. c (p. 706)
4. d (p. 706)

TRUE/FALSE

1. F (p. 705)
2. F (p. 706)
3. T (p. 705)
4. T (p. 706)
5. T (p. 707)
6. F (p. 707)
7. F (p. 705)

STOP, REVIEW, REMEMBER   (PP. 711–713)

MULTIPLE CHOICE

1. b (p. 709)
2. d (p. 706)
3. d (p. 711)
4. a (p. 711)
5. c (p. 711)

CASE STUDY

1. This question is for discussion. The student must note why there is agreement or disagreement.
2. Stethoscope, radio or cell phone, blood pressure cuff, oxygen (p. 702)
3. Complete the primary assessment. Check her breathing, respirations, and blood pressure, and take a history. (p. 710)

CHAPTER REVIEW   (PP. 714–715)

MULTIPLE CHOICE

1. b (p. 705)
2. a (p. 702)
3. c (p. 702)
4. d (p. 702)
5. a (p. 706)
6. c (p. 706)
7. b (p. 710)
8. d (p. 707)
9. b (p. 706)
10. b (p. 705)

CHAPTER 29

STOP, REVIEW, REMEMBER   (PP. 719–720)

MULTIPLE CHOICE

1. c (p. 717)
2. a (pp. 717–718)
3. d (p. 717)
4. c (p. 718)
5. a (p. 719)

STOP, REVIEW, REMEMBER   (P. 723)

MULTIPLE CHOICE

1. d (p. 720)
2. b (p. 721)
3. d (p. 721)
4. b (p. 720)
5. a (p. 721)

CHAPTER REVIEW   (PP. 724–725)

MULTIPLE CHOICE

1. c (p. 720)
2. b (p. 719)
3. a (p. 718)
4. a (p. 718)
5. d (p. 719)
6. c (p. 719)
7. d (p. 720)
8. c (p. 721)

MATCHING

1. d (p. 720)
2. a (p. 721)
3. b (p. 721)
4. c (p. 721)
5. e (p. 720)
6. h (p. 718)
7. g (p. 721)
8. f (p. 721)

CRITICAL THINKING

1. The answers to these questions will be based on your local protocol.
2. The answers to these questions will be based on your local protocol.

CHAPTER 30

STOP, REVIEW, REMEMBER   (PP. 733–734)

MULTIPLE CHOICE

1. b (p. 727)
2. b (p. 730)
3. d (p. 731)
4. c (p. 727)
5. b (pp. 727–729)

STOP, REVIEW, REMEMBER   (P. 739)

MULTIPLE CHOICE

1. c (p. 735)
2. b (p. 735)
3. b (p. 735)
4. c (p. 735)
5. d (p. 735)

STOP, REVIEW, REMEMBER   (PP. 742–743)

MULTIPLE CHOICE

1. d (p. 740)
2. a (p. 740)
3. d (p. 740)
4. b (p. 742)
5. d (p. 741)

CHAPTER REVIEW   (PP. 747–748)

MULTIPLE CHOICE

1. d (p. 744)
2. c (p. 744)
3. b (p. 745)
4. a (p. 744)
5. c (p. 743)
6. b (p. 731)
7. b (p. 732)
8. d (p. 737)
9. b (p. 744)
10. a (p. 740)
11. a (p. 732)
12. a (p. 732)
13. c (p. 735)

MATCHING

1. f (p. 740)
2. c (p. 732)
3. d (p. 739)
4. g (p. 742)
5. a (p. 727)
6. j (p. 732)
7. i (p. 732)
8. b (p. 727)
9. h (p. 732)
10. e (p. 740)

CHAPTER 31

STOP, REVIEW, REMEMBER   (PP. 754–755)

MULTIPLE CHOICE

1. d (p. 752)
2. a (p. 753)
3. c (p. 752)
4. c (p. 754)
5. d (p. 757)

TRUE/FALSE

1. T (p. 752)
2. F (p. 752)
3. F (p. 751)
4. T (p. 751)
5. T (p. 755)

MULTIPLE CHOICE

1. d (p. 756)
2. c (p. 757)
3. c (p. 757)
4. d (p. 756)
5. a (p. 759)

TRUE/FALSE

1. T (p. 757)
2. F (p. 757)
3. T (p. 757)
4. T (p. 756)
5. T (p. 757)

CHAPTER REVIEW (PP. 761–762)

MULTIPLE CHOICE

1. c (p. 753)
2. a (p. 755)
3. b (p. 759)
4. d (pp. 755–756)
5. b (p. 757)

FILL IN THE BLANK

1. greater good (p. 753)
2. time, distance, and shielding (p. 752)
3. respirator (N95, P100, or SCBA) (p. 752)
4. Incident Command system (p. 757)
5. 360-degree assessment (p. 756)

CRITICAL THINKING

1. Construction debris of all types, live power lines, water and gas lines, unstable structures (p. 756)
2. Answers will vary. Common feelings include anger, hopelessness, helplessness, and fear.
3. Answers will vary. Common feelings include anger, hopelessness, helplessness, fear, and the need to blame or punish someone.

SECTION SEVEN REVIEW

1. d (p. 702)
   Rationale: Checking and "topping off" fluids are a routine part of daily vehicle inspections.
2. b (p. 702)
   Rationale: A thorough vehicle checklist is completed at least daily. In services with multiple shifts in a 24-hour period, the checklist may be required at the beginning of each shift.
3. b (p. 705)
   Rationale: It is preferable that the driver focuses attention on driving and leaves radio communications to his partner, if possible.
4. a (p. 705)
   Rationale: Lights and sirens permit you to request the right-of-way but do not remove the responsibility of exercising due regard for others. Operating an emergency vehicle unsafely can result in both criminal and civil liability.
5. b (p. 705)
   Rationale: The other three options given are all reasonable actions in exercising due regard. However, text messaging while driving is not a safe practice.
6. a (p. 706)
   Rationale: There is a potential that fumes from leaking gasoline or a running vehicle could ignite other liquids. You should park upwind and uphill whenever possible.
7. c (p. 707)
   Rationale: An N95 respirator is only needed when there is a suspicion that a patient has active tuberculosis.
8. a (p. 707)
   Rationale: Medical calls generally only require Standard Precautions, such as gloves.
9. a (p. 710)
   Rationale: Trust your instinct and wait for help to arrive.
10. c (p. 711)
    Rationale: A complete history is sometimes only obtained by asking the same questions more than once. It is the EMT's responsibility to see if there is any change in the information and is not a reflection on the EMR's abilities. You can often learn by listening to others take a history, but it is not necessary to apologize if you left something out.
11. b (p. 717)
    Rationale: NIMS provides a systematic, yet flexible, system for managing resources and operations at the scene of any large-scale incident and is used by local agencies.
12. a (p. 718)
    Rationale: The command and management component includes a plan for the interaction of multiple agencies.
13. c (p. 721)
    Rationale: In the language of NIMS/ICS, the person ultimately in charge of an incident is the incident commander, regardless of the title or rank assigned by his organization.
14. b (p. 721)
    Rationale: The five common elements of an ICS are incident command, operations, planning, logistics, and finance/administration.
15. d (p. 723)
    Rationale: The EMR still performs within the scope of practice of an EMR, but must know how to work within an ICS.
16. b (p. 718)
    Rationale: Federal funding is not available to systems that do not adopt NIMS/ICS.
17. b (p. 720)
    Rationale: The span of control is from three to seven elements, but ideally not more than five.

18. a (p. 720)
Rationale: Unity of command means that each person has one supervisor. Unified command means that all agencies work together under one command system.

19. d (p. 727)
Rationale: Choice "d" is the definition used by the U.S. Department of Transportation.

20. c (p. 727)
Rationale: The U.S. Department of Transportation developed the placard system used in the transportation of hazardous substances.

21. a (pp. 727–729)
Rationale: The Emergency Response Guidebook is published by the DOT as a reference for the placard system and gives information about important steps in the initial response to hazardous materials incidents.

22. b (p. 730)
Rationale: The NFPA 704 system is used on fixed storage facilities.

23. d (p. 731)
Rationale: The blue area of the placard identifies health risks.

24. c (p. 731)
Rationale: The right side of the placard, which is yellow, gives information about reactivity.

25. d (p. 731)
Rationale: The number system used is from 0 to 4, with 4 representing the highest risk.

26. d (p. 732)
Rationale: Material safety data sheets are required for all hazardous materials in the workplace.

27. c (p. 732)
Rationale: Scene safety is always the highest priority. The EMR must make sure that he is not exposed to the chemical and that the patient is not exposed to additional amounts of the chemical.

28. a (p. 732)
Rationale: The cold zone is the zone in which triage and medical care take place after the patient is decontaminated.

29. b (p. 732)
Rationale: The term used for ridding the patient's body of a toxin or hazardous material is decontamination.

30. d (p. 735)
Rationale: An MCI is defined in relation to the resources available. Any of these events would exceed the routine capabilities of the EMS system.

31. a (p. 735)
Rationale: START is the Simple Triage and Rapid Treatment system of triaging patients, adopted by the Department of Homeland Security in the development of NIMS.

32. b (p. 735)
Rationale: JumpSTART is a modified triage system used for pediatric patients.

33. c (p. 735)
Rationale: In an MCI, resources are not used to treat patients with little likelihood of survival when many more people could be saved. The concept of "greater good" is the basis of triage decisions in MCIs.

34. b (p. 737)
Rationale: Because pediatric patients can often survive if problems with airway and breathing are immediately corrected, JumpSTART includes giving five rescue breaths to the pediatric patient who is not breathing but has a pulse.

35. b (p. 735)
Rationale: In an MCI any adult patient who is not breathing and does not have a pulse is given lowest priority for transport.

36. c (pp. 739–740)
Rationale: During extrication the EMR must wear turnout gear, goggles, helmet, heavy gloves, and protective footwear to prevent injury.

37. a (p. 740)
Rationale: A patient is pinned when a part of his body is entangled with a part of the vehicle.

38. b (p. 740)
Rationale: Stop chocks are used under the wheels to keep the vehicle from moving.

39. c (p. 740)
Rationale: An unstable vehicle presents a hazard to the EMR, as well as the possibility of further injury to the patient. The vehicle must be stabilized before the EMR accesses and assesses the patient.

40. c (p. 742)
Rationale: The laminated glass of the windshield is best removed with a reciprocating saw.

41. a (p. 741)
Rationale: Although it seems like opening the back door might be the best way, most newer cars have doors that automatically lock when the vehicle reaches a certain speed. Chances are, if the driver's door is locked, so are the others. Although the patient may slightly move her neck to unlock the door, she would also likely move her neck at the sound of someone entering the vehicle behind her, prying the door open, or breaking the window.

42. b (p. 744)
Rationale: There are many factors that go into the decision to use air medical resources. Ground transportation is often the best choice.

43. c (p. 745)
Rationale: Always approach the aircraft so that the pilot can see you.

44. b (p. 744)
Rationale: Air medical transportation is typically used for patients in need of immediate surgery, or for interventions for a stroke or heart attack that must be carried out without delay.

45. d (p. 756)

Rationale: Responding to these types of incidents poses many additional challenges and obstacles that are not encountered on routine calls.

46. a (p. 752)

Rationale: The key considerations in protecting yourself from radiation are time (for the radiation to dissipate), distance from the source of the radiation, and shielding to prevent penetration of the radioactive rays or particles.

47. b (p. 752)

Rationale: Although an act of terrorism has not been established, an explosion should always raise the question of this possibility. Keep in mind that many terrorists plan a second explosion to injure or kill those who are responding to the initial explosion.

48. a (p. 757)

Rationale: Avoid the temptation to "jump into" patient care. Accurately sizing up the situation and determining what resources are needed to manage the situation better serve all patients and responders.

49. c (p. 751)

Rationale: As an EMR, your first responsibility is your own safety. Additional resources are needed to assess the situation and decide how to best access and remove the patient from his residence if he is, in fact, there. (The neighbor may be assuming that the patient was home at the time.)

50. d (p. 757)

Rationale: Never enter floodwater (the same goes for the patient). Additional resources are needed to reach this patient. The patient is most likely better off giving birth without your assistance than being swept away by the current, or having would-be rescuers swept away.

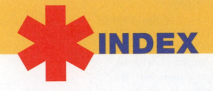

INDEX

Page numbers followed by *f* indicate figures; those followed by *t* indicate tables.

9-1-1, 8
360-degree assessment/survey, 706, 756

A

Abandonment, 62
Abdominal cavity, 75
Abdominal distention, 467
Abdominal pain, 399, 465
  emergency care, 401
  patient assessment, 400, 400*t*, 401*f*
  signs and symptoms, 400*t*
Abdominal quadrants, 78*f*, 399*f*
Abdominal thrusts, 175–176, 175*f*
Abdominal trauma
  closed injuries, 465–466, 466*f*
  emergency care, 466*f*, 468
  gastrointestinal bleeding, 466
  open injuries, 465–466, 465*f*, 466*f*
  patient assessment, 467–468, 468*f*
Abortion, spontaneous, 611
Abrasions, 477, 478*f*. See also Open wounds
Abruptio placentae, 612
Abuse, 647, 688–689, 688*f*
Accessory muscle use, 158, 336, 336*f*
Acute abdomen, 399, 465. See also Abdominal pain
Adolescence/adolescents, 120–121, 121*f*, 121*t*, 622*t*. See also Pediatric patients
Advance directives, 59–61
Advanced EMT (AEMT), 9, 9*f*
AEDs. See Automated external defibrillators
Aeromedical transport, 743, 744*f*
  approach to aircraft, 745, 745*f*
  calling for, 744
  indications, 744
  landing zone, 744, 744*f*
Afterbirth, 593
Agonal breathing, 185, 254
AICD (automated implanted cardiac defibrillator), 683–685, 684*f*
AIDS (acquired immune deficiency syndrome), 27*t*
Air embolism, 487
Air splints, 547, 547*f*
Airborne droplets, 26
Airborne infection, exposure to, 33*f*

Airway. See also Breathing
  anatomy and physiology, 141–146, 141*f*, 142*f*
  assessment, 146–148, 248, 249*f*, 252
  big picture, 140*f*
  burns, 497, 497*f*, 497*t*, 498*f*
  in child versus adult, 143, 144*f*, 637–638, 638*f*
  foreign body obstruction, 175–177, 175*f*, 176*f*, 177*f*
  head-tilt, chin-lift maneuver, 149, 150*f*
  jaw-thrust maneuver, 150, 151*f*
  oropharyngeal, 154–155, 154*f*, 155*f*
  suctioning, 150–154, 152*f*, 153*f*
Allergen, 394
Allergic reaction, 394, 394*f*
Altered mental status, 43, 356, 357*f*
  in behavioral emergency. See Behavioral emergencies
  causes, 356–357
  in diabetic emergency. See Diabetic emergencies
  in drug or alcohol emergency, 378–379, 378*f*, 378*t*
  emergency care, 357–358
  in head injuries, 508
  patient assessment, 357
  in poisoning. See Poisoning
  in seizure. See Seizure
  in stroke. See Stroke
Alveoli, 93, 337
Alzheimer disease, 667
Amniotic sac, 593
Amputation, 477*f*, 487–489, 487*f*, 488*f*, 552
Anaphylactic shock, 394, 435*f*, 449. See also Anaphylaxis; Shock
Anaphylaxis, 394
  causes, 395
  emergency care, 395–398, 397*f*
  signs and symptoms, 395*t*
Anatomical position, 72
Anatomical regions, 76*f*
Anatomical terms, 72, 73*f*
Anatomy, 84
Angina pectoris, 339
Angulated fracture, 539, 539*f*
Animal bites, 489
Antibodies, 394
Anterior/ventral, 73*f*, 74
Antibodies, 394
Apnea, 185
Appendicular skeleton, 537
Arm drift, 366, 366*f*

Arm injuries, 549–550, 549*f*, 550*f*
Arrhythmia(s), 203–204
Arterial bleeding, 439, 440*f*. See also Bleeding
Arteries, 95
Arterioles, 95
Articulation, 506
Assault, 62
Assessment. See Patient assessment
Asthma, 337, 639–640, 639*f*
Asymmetry, 292
Asystole, 203
Atria, 93, 93*f*, 184, 184*f*
Auscultating, 287
Automated external defibrillators (AEDs), 188
  attaching, 205
  continuing quality assurance and call review, 206
  operating, 205–206, 207–208*f*
  in pediatric patients, 206
  public access to, 204
  safety, 204–205
  types, 203–204, 204*f*, 205*f*
Automated implanted cardiac defibrillators (AICD), 683–685, 684*f*
Autonomic nervous system, 96
Avulsion, 477*f*, 478, 489, 489*f*. See also Soft tissue injuries
Axial skeleton, 505, 537
Axillary region, 95*f*

B

Bacteria, 32
Bag-valve-mask (BVM) device, 170*f*, 171*f*, 172–175, 173*f*, 634–637, 636*f*
Bandage(s), 484–486, 485*f*
Bandage compress, 483, 483*f*
Barriers to communication, 307–308, 308*f*, 309*f*
Base station radio, 313
Battery, 62
Battle sign, 509*f*, 510
Behavior, 384
Behavioral emergencies, 384
  calming methods, 385–387
  causes, 384
  emergency care, 386*f*, 387
  patient assessment, 384–385
  signs and symptoms, 384*t*
  suicide risk assessment, 385